GERONTOLOGY

An Interdisciplinary Perspective

Edited by

John C. Cavanaugh
University of Delaware

Susan Krauss Whitbourne
University of Massachusetts

New York   Oxford
OXFORD UNIVERSITY PRESS
1999

Oxford University Press

Oxford   New York
Athens   Auckland   Bangkok   Bogotá   Buenos Aires   Calcutta
Cape Town   Chennai   Dar es Salaam   Delhi   Florence   Hong Kong   Istanbul
Karachi   Kuala Lumpur   Madrid   Melbourne   Mexico City   Mumbai
Nairobi   Paris   São Paulo   Singapore   Taipei   Tokyo   Toronto   Warsaw

and associated companies in
Berlin   Ibadan

Copyright © 1999 by Oxford University Press

Published by Oxford University Press, Inc.
198 Madison Avenue, New York, New York 10016
http://www.oup-usa.org

Oxford is a registered trademark of Oxford University Press

Library of Congress Cataloging-in-Publication Data
Gerontology : an interdisciplinary perspective / edited by John C.
  Cavanaugh and Susan Krauss Whitbourne.
      p.   cm.
    Includes bibliographical references and index.
    ISBN: 978-0-19-511546-8
    1. Gerontology.   2. Aging.   3. Aged.   I. Cavanaugh, John C.
II. Whitbourne, Susan Krauss.
HQ1061.G418   1999
305.26—dc21   98-22404
                                                            CIP

Printed in the United States of America
on acid-free paper

Contents

Preface

The population demographics of the United States and of many other countries is changing dramatically. Most important, the number of older adults in the United States is already higher than at any other point in the country's history. Projections are that this increase will continue into the first third of the twenty-first century as the "baby boom" generation ages.

These demographic trends create an acute need for adequately educated professionals. Career opportunities are expanding rapidly in many fields, such as psychology, social work, health care, education, public administration and policy, and human services. Graduate-level courses have been developed in these fields to meet student and professional demands for appropriate learning opportunities. Separate degree programs and specializations within existing programs have been created at both the master's and doctoral levels.

The growth of courses in gerontology has created a demand for appropriate materials. Although texts in the areas of adult development and aging have been widely available for nearly two decades, parallel texts at the graduate level have not appeared. This has created a serious difficulty for instructors of overview courses on gerontology, especially at the master's level, but also at the beginning of doctoral level. Thus, the need for a comprehensive, single-volume text on gerontology appropriate for graduate students is clearly evident.

The present volume is a comprehensive graduate-level text that will provide a firm foundation in the theory, methodology, and content of gerontology. The text was structured for use in a single semester course. The chapters have been authored by major researchers and practitioners in the field who were selected on the dual criteria of their own substantive contributions and their ability to distill and communicate the extant literature.

The chapters are organized according to a logical sequence that begins with fundamental concepts in gerontological theory and methods of research and then moves into specific areas of specialization within the field. In Chapter 1, Cavanaugh provides an overview of major interdisciplinary views of aging, including life-span theories, and perspectives from the fields of biology, psychology, and sociology. Cavanaugh and Whitbourne then provide a review in Chapter 2 of major research methods in the social sciences as applied to the gerontological enterprise. Traditional and contemporary multivariate methods are described as well as more qualitative analytical approaches. Chapter 3, by Luborsky and McMullen, explores the role of culture and ethnicity among elders in the United States and around the world. In Chapter 4, Whitbourne summarizes the major physical changes that are associated with the normal aging process and discusses the impact of these changes on the individual's psychological functioning and self-concept. The major diseases that occur in the aging population are described in Chapter 5 by Aldwin and Gilmer, who review the connections between these diseases and health-related behaviors and lifestyle. In Chapter 6, Kastenbaum reviews the extensive theoretical and empirical approaches to the study of dying and bereavement, including the experience of dying, working with dying individuals, and grief and bereavement. Stine-Morrow and Soederberg Miller, in Chapter 7, comprehensively describe the changes that occur in cognitive functioning in later life, including attention, working memory, and language. Intelligence and problem solving are covered in Chapter 8 by Dixon and Hultsch. They not only review the traditional psychometric approaches to these areas but also include an analysis of the factors involved in everyday problem solving and creativity. The review of personality theories and research by Labouvie-Vief and Diehl in Chapter 9 covers a wide range of important areas related to changes in midlife personality and self-development. Moving on to a more clinical perspective, Edelstein and Kalish describe issues of assessment in older adulthood in Chapter 10. This comprehensive chapter reviews assessment measures in the areas of cognition, personality, mental health, physical health, and functional assessment. Issues of mental health and intervention are further explored in Chapter 11 by Qualls, who covers major clinical syndromes in older adults, intervention approaches, and prevention strategies. Turning to developmental issues in later life, Stephens and Franks review in Chapter 12 the extensive literature on family relationships and caregiving, including relationships between older adults and their partners, adult children, and siblings and friends. Issues regarding caregiving are also presented in this chapter. Focusing on the workplace and retirement, in Chapter 13 Sterns and Gray examine age discrimination and stereotypes, retirement adjustment, and the use of leisure time by older adults. Institutionalization and the issues involved in providing adequate care for older adults in nursing homes is discussed in Chapter 14 by Smyer and Allen-Burge. Public policy issues are the domain of Binstock in Chapter 15, who discusses current issues in policy relating to older adults, the implications of federal legislation, including the Older Americans Act, and the crucial issues of economic security and health care.

Each chapter was written solely for this volume, and each is written with the intention of providing materials that are of educational value to the student and substantive interest to the professional. The writing style of each chapter is highly readable, avoiding overly technical or abstract discussions that would be lost on the nonspecialist. The authors have also provided section headings that form a descriptive outline for review and study purposes, a list of integrative review questions, and a list of key additional readings that will enable the student to begin building a professional library.

We are hopeful that our text will fill a major gap in the training of future gerontologists. It will enable those who are entering the field at the professional level to have a sophisticated and thorough knowledge of the most current approaches, across disciplines, to understanding the aging process.

January, 1999

J. C. C.
S. K. W.

Contributors

Carolyn M. Aldwin is Professor of Human and Community Development, University of California, Davis.

Rebecca Allen-Burge is Associate Research Psychologist, Applied Gerontology Program, University of Alabama.

Robert H. Binstock, Professor of Aging, Health and Society in the Department of Epidemiology and Biostatistics, School of Medicine, Case Western Reserve University.

John C. Cavanaugh is Professor of Psychology and Individual and Family Studies, and Vice Provost for Academic Programs and Planning, University of Delaware.

Manfred Diehl is Assistant Professor of Psychology, University of Colorado Colorado Springs.

Roger A. Dixon is Professor of Psychology, University of Victoria.

Barry Edelstein is Professor of Psychology, West Virginia University.

Melissa M. Franks is Assistant Professor of Gerontology, Wayne State University.

Diane F. Gilmer is Postgraduate Researcher and Lecturer of Human and Community, Development, University of California Davis.

Jennifer Hurd Gray is Doctoral Candidate in Industrial Gerontological Psychology, University of Akron.

David F. Hultsch is Professor of Psychology, University of Victoria.

Robert Kastenbaum is Professor of Communication, Arizona State University.

Kimberly Kalish is Doctoral Candidate of Psychology, West Virginia University.

Gisela Labouvie-Vief is Professor of Psychology, Wayne State University.

Mark M. Luborsky is Associate Professor and Director of Research of Occupational Therapy, Wayne State University.

Carmit Kurn McMullen is Doctoral Candidate Department of Anthropology, Case Western Reserve University.

Sara Honn Qualls is Professor of Psychology, University of Colorado, Colorado Springs.

ix

Michael A. Smyer, Professor of Psychology and the Dean of the Graduate School of Arts and Science, Boston College.

Lisa M. Soederberg Miller is Postdoctoral Fellow, Department of Psychology, Brandeis University.

Mary Ann Parris Stephens is Professor of Psychology, Kent State University.

Harvey L. Sterns is Professor of Psychology and Director of the Institute for Life-Span Development and Gerontology, The University of Akron.

Elizabeth A. L. Stine-Morrow is Associate Professor of Psychology, University of New Hampshire.

Susan Krauss Whitbourne is Professor of Psychology, University of Massachusetts, Amherst.

GERONTOLOGY

1

Theories of Aging in the Biological, Behavioral, and Social Sciences

John C. Cavanaugh

Why do people grow old? This question has puzzled humanity from the beginning of recorded history, and undoubtedly was pondered for millennia before that. Attempts at answering this question have variously taken religious, philosophical, and scientific turns, with none able to provide a singularly coherent account that is accepted by everyone.

In this chapter, we will consider the range of explanations of aging that enjoys some current support in the biological, behavioral, and social sciences. In anticipation of our review, several things should be noted as guiding principles. First, the sheer diversity of explanations is striking. From molecular biological accounts to those based on the structure of society, virtually every level of analysis has been used to create an account of aging. What this indicates clearly is that aging is a very complex, dynamic process that can be understood only by considering it from multiple perspectives. Second, no single theory has emerged as the primary explanation, even within a particular family of disciplines. This indicates two things. Aging has been a relatively recent focus of biological, behavioral, and social sciences, which creates a rather limited set of data with which to test theories in order to winnow the options. By the same token, the "newness" of aging as a focus of study also creates a fertile arena for speculation, resulting in many competing (and sometimes contradictory) notions of why aging occurs. Overall, this generative period has resulted both in a climate of excitement and discovery unprecedented in science, and of legitimacy in terms of professional and public support for the endeavor. Before we consider the various theories in each of the areas, it is useful first to examine the forces that create development as well as the meaning of age.

Developmental Forces and the Meaning of Age

Irrespective of one's scientific discipline, an understanding of aging requires knowledge of the context in which aging occurs. The process of development, which itself takes a lifetime, is the reflection of a confluence of processes, as we will see. Additionally, the term "age" has several separate meanings, and can be examined in each of these areas.

Forces of Development

As noted earlier, human development is the result of several mutually interactive forces. Developmentalists typically consider four (Cavanaugh, 1997):

- *Biological forces* include all genetic, physiological, and health-related factors affecting development. Examples of biological forces include menopause, facial wrinkling, and changes in the major organ systems.
- *Psychological (behavioral) forces* include all internal perceptual, cognitive, emotional, and personality factors affecting development. Collectively, psychological forces provide the characteristics we notice most obviously about people that make them individuals.
- *Sociocultural factors* include interpersonal, societal, cultural, and ethnic factors that affect development. Sociocultural forces provide diversity and the network of people with whom we interact, and influence how the greater society is structured and operates.
- *Life-cycle forces* reflect differences in how the same event or combination of biological, psychological, and sociocultural forces affects people at different points in their lives. Life-cycle forces provide the context for the developmental differences of interest in adult development and aging. Life-cycle forces are most often incorporated into biological, behavioral, and sociocultural theories of aging.

Each one of us is a product of a unique combination of these forces. Even identical twins growing up in the same family eventually have their own unique friends, partners, occupations, and so on. To see why all of these forces are important, imagine that you want to know how people feel about forgetting. You would need to consider several biological factors, such as whether the forgetting was due, for example, to underlying disease, age-associated neuronal decrements, or genetic factors. You would want to know about behavioral factors such as what the person's memory ability has been throughout his or her life, his or her beliefs about what happens to memory with increasing age, memory capacity, the efficiency of cognitive processing, and sensory functioning. You would need to know about sociocultural factors, such as the influence of social stereotypes about forgetting, the place older adults occupy in society, and social structural factors that place older adults at a relative disadvantage. Finally, within each perspective you would need to know about the age of the person when forgetting experience occurs, as the effects within each arena may vary with age. Focusing on only one (or even two or three) of the forces would provide an incomplete view of how the person feels.

Interrelations among the Forces: Developmental Influences. Each of the forces we have discussed combines to create the developmental experiences people have. One way to consider these combinations is to consider the degree to which they are common or unique. Based on this approach, Baltes (1979) identifies three sets of influences that interact to produce developmental change over the life span: normative age-graded influences, normative history-graded influences, and nonnormative influences.

Normative age-graded influences are those experiences caused by biological, psychological, and sociocultural forces that are highly correlated with chronological age. Some of these—such as menopause—are biological. These normative biological events usually indicate a major change in a person's life; for example, menopause is an indicator that a woman can no longer bear children without medical intervention. Normative psychological events would include focusing on certain concerns at different points in adulthood, such as a concern with socializing the younger generation when a person is middle-aged. Other normative age-graded influences involve sociocultural forces, such as age at which one retires. Normative age-graded influences typically correspond to major time-marker events, which are often ritualized. For example, retirement is often begun with a party celebrating the end of one's employment. These events provide the most convenient way to judge where we are on our social clock.

Normative history-graded influences are events that most people in a specific culture experience at the same point in time. These events may be biological (such as epidemics), psychological (such as particular stereotypes), or sociocultural (such as changing attitudes toward sexuality). Normative history-graded influences often endow a generation with its unique identity, such as the Baby Boom Generation (people born roughly between 1946 and 1960) or Generation X (people born after roughly 1965). These influences can have a profound effect. For example, the emergence of AIDS during the 1980s fundamentally changed the attitudes toward dating and casual sexual relationships that had developed during the preceding decades.

Nonnormative influences are random or rare events that may be important for a specific individual but are not experienced by most people. These may be favorable events, such as winning the lottery or an election, or unfavorable ones, such as an accident or layoff. The unpredictability of these events makes them unique. It is as if one's life is turned upside down overnight.

Life-cycle forces determine the relative importance of the other three influences, as it depends on the specific behaviors examined and the particular point in the life span when they occur (Hultsch & Plemons, 1979). For example, history-graded influences may produce generational differences and conflict; older adults' experiences years ago as middle-aged adults may have little to do with the complex issues faced by today's middle-aged adults. In turn, these interactions have important implications for understanding differences that are apparently age related. That is, differences may be explained in terms of differential life experiences (normative history-graded influences) rather than as an integral part of the aging process itself (normative age-graded influences).

The Meaning of Age and Aging

We have seen that one of the basic forces on development is life-cycle forces, which reflect differences in the effects of events and so forth as a function of age. Consequently, one of the most important aspects of studying adult development and aging is understanding the concept of aging itself. Aging is not a single process. Rather, it consists of at least three distinct processes: primary, secondary, and tertiary aging (Birren & Cunningham, 1985). *Primary aging* refers to the normal, disease-free development during adulthood. Changes in biological, behavioral, sociocultural, or life-cycle processes in primary aging are an inevitable part of the developmental process; examples include menopause, decline in reaction time, and the loss of family and friends. Most of the information in this chapter and throughout this book represents primary aging. *Secondary aging* refers to developmental changes that are related to disease, life style, and other environmentally induced changes that are not inevitable. The progressive loss of intellectual abilities in Alzheimer's disease and related forms of dementia are examples of secondary aging. *Tertiary aging* refers to the rapid losses in most organ and behavioral systems that occur shortly before death. An example of tertiary aging is a phenomenon known as terminal drop, in which intellectual abilities show a marked decline in the last few years preceding death.

Increasingly, researchers and theorists are strongly emphasizing that everyone does not grow old in the same way; that is, individual differences are the rule. Whereas most people tend to show *usual patterns of aging* that reflect the typical, or normative changes with age, other people show *successful aging* in which few signs of change occur. For example, although most people tend to get chronic diseases as they get older, some people never do. What makes people who age successfully different? At this point, we do not really know for sure. It may be a unique combination of genetics, optimal environment, flexibility in dealing with life situations, a strong sense of personal control, and maybe even a bit of luck. For our present discussion, the main point to keep in mind throughout is that everyone's experience of growing old is somewhat different.

Age as an Index.   When most of us think about age, we usually think of how long we have been around since our birth; this way of defining age is known as *chronological age*. Chronological age provides a shorthand method to index time and to organize events and data by using a commonly understood standard, calendar time. Chronological age is not the only shorthand index variable used in gerontology. Gender, ethnicity, and socioeconomic status are others.

No index variable itself actually causes behavior. In the case of gender, for example, it is not whether a person is male or female per se that determines how long he or she will live on average, but rather the underlying forces, such as hormonal effects, that are the true causes. This point is often forgotten when age is the index variable, perhaps because it is so familiar to us and so widely used. However, age (or time) does not directly cause things to happen, either. Iron left out in the rain will rust, but rust is not caused simply by time. Rather, rust is a *time-dependent process* involving oxidation in which time is a measure of the rate by which rust is created. Similarly, human behavior is affected by experiences that occur with the passage of time, not by time itself. What we study in adult development and aging is the result of time- or age-dependent processes, not the result of age itself.

How do we determine whether some behavior is actually time dependent? Birren and Renner (1977) argue that we need to understand the underlying biological, psychological, sociocultural, and life-cycle forces that are all intertwined in an index such as chronological age.

As we will see, index variables are also notoriously poor in providing anything other than the most cursory description of individuals. Although from an index variable one knows the group classification a particular person occupies (e.g., "eighty year olds"), one knows little else. In the end, this is the most problematic aspect of index variables, despite their continued widespread use.

Definitions of Age.   Age can be considered from each of the perspectives of the remaining basic forces on development (Birren & Cunningham, 1985): biological, psychological, and sociocultural. *Biological age* represents where a person is relative to the maximum number of years he or she could possibly live. Biological age is assessed by measuring the functioning of the various vital, or life-limiting, organ systems, such as the cardiovascular system. With increasing age the vital organ systems typically lose their capacity for self-regulation and adaptation, resulting in an increased probability of dying. Through a healthy life style, it is possible to slow some of the age-related change processes and be functionally younger biologically than a much younger (chronologically) person who is inactive. In contrast, someone who has the disease progeria, in which the body ages abnormally rapidly, is biologically much older than his or her chronological peers. In short, biological age accounts for many health-related aspects of functioning in assigning an age to an individual.

Psychological age refers to the functional level of the psychological abilities that people use to adapt to changing environmental demands. These abilities include memory, intelligence, feelings, motivation, and other skills that foster and maintain self-esteem and personal control. For example, Mildred, a 65-year-old English major in college, would be thought of as psychologically young in the intellectual area, because the majority of her classmates are chronologically younger. Many myths about older adults stem from our misconceptions about the abilities that underlie definitions of psychological age. For example, many people believe that all types of memory and other cognitive abilities decline precipitously in later life. Many of these beliefs are wrong, meaning that we need to revise the standards by which we judge psychological aging in these domains.

In every culture there are unwritten expectations of how individuals of a certain chronological age should act. Such unwritten expectations are what is meant by sociocultural age. More formally, *sociocultural age* refers to the specific set of roles individuals adopt in relation to other members of the society and culture to which they belong. Sociocultural age is judged on the basis of many behaviors and habits, such as style of dress, customs, language, and interpersonal style. Most important is the extent to which a person shows the age-graded behavior expected by the society in which one lives; this forms the basis by which a person is judged to be socioculturally younger or older. If one is adopting new roles ahead of one's peers, that person is considered socioculturally older. For example, a woman in her fifties who gives birth to a child through fertility treatments would be considered socioculturally young; most women give birth at earlier ages. Many of the most damaging stereotypes about aging (such as that older people should not be having sex) are based on faulty assumptions about sociocultural age.

As we consider the various theories of aging in the remainder of this chapter, keep in mind that aging is the lifelong product of interactive forces, and that the term aging itself represents a complex set of issues. Putting the theories in this context will help in understanding their relative strengths and weaknesses.

Theories in the Biological Sciences

Among the oldest explanations we have of the aging process are those rooted in biological accounts. These theories vary in terms of level of analysis (e.g., molecular versus systemic) and in whether they are based on purposeful or random events (Hayflick, 1994). In this section, we will organize biological theories along this latter dimension.

Theories Based on Purposeful Events

Theories of biological aging based on purposeful events postulate that there is a "master plan" that governs the aging process. One view of this master plan is that aging is determined by a biological clock based on events that occur within molecules, such as the turning on of "death genes" (e.g., programmed aging theory) or the secretion of certain hormones (e.g., neuroendocrine theory).

Programmed Aging Theory.   Many biogerontologists believe that aging is a highly regulated process based on genetically programmed cell death (e.g., Lock-shin & Zakeri, 1990). In this sense, programmed cell death represents the innate ability of cells to self-destruct, and the ability of dying cells to trigger key processes in other cells. Aging and death are viewed as the logical outcome of this process. The implication is that the DNA in each of our cells provides a master plan of what happens in our bodies from conception through old age and death. The reasoning underlying this theory is that the programming of some cells in the body is a fact universally recognized by biologists (Hayflick, 1994). However, there is considerable disagreement over the issue of when aging begins. To some, aging begins at conception, whereas for other theorists, it begins in the actuarial prime of life, that is, the point in the life span when mortality rates are lowest.

Despite the intuitive appeal of programmed aging theory, it has several major problems (Hayflick, 1994). Most problematic is the need to assume that if a DNA master plan is responsible for aging, then aging must have been selected during the evolutionary process. However, "there never were sufficient numbers of older adults of species, and none of them around long enough, to allow evolution to directly select for aging processes" (Hayflick, 1994, p. 231). For this (and some other) reasons, programmed cell death is less popular among current biogerontologists.

The Neuroendocrine Theory.   Changes in the levels of certain hormones in the bloodstream are considered by some to be linked to why people age. Because hormones help regulate many processes involved in metabolism, reproduction, protein synthesis, immune function, growth, and behavior, they play an enormously important role in normal life processes. Recent research has focused on whether hormonal changes may be possible causes of age-related changes. Decline in reproductive capacity, for example, is as strong a predictor of aging in most species as is increased rates of mortality. Such changes as occur in the reproductive system are controlled by the neuroendocrine system, which in turn is controlled by the hypothalamus (Hayflick, 1994).

To date, the evidence indicates that although hormonal changes occur in many systems, they probably are not the primary cause of aging. One problem is that hormonal changes vary across gender within a species; for example, the hormonal changes associated with aging and reproduction occur precipitously in human women but more gradually in men. Needless to say, though, aging occurs in both, and, in the case of humans, men live roughly seven years less than women. Thus, although hormonal changes are correlated with aging processes, it is unlikely that they are responsible for them (Hayflick, 1994).

Theories Based on Random Events

Many theorists do not believe that aging is the result of some biological master plan. Rather, they believe that aging results from the cumulative effects of random events of various types.

Wear and Tear Theory.   One of the most intuitively appealing theories of biological aging based on random events is based on the notion that death occurs because body systems and organs simply wear out (Whitbourne, 1996).
The analogy here is between humans (or other organisms) and machines; as
we have experienced, all machines eventually wear out. Human aging therefore reflects the cumulative effects of the abuse of everyday life, which can be
viewed as stress. To be sure, there is evidence that some parts of the human
body wear with age; examples include damage to joints, which in severe form
may result in osteoarthritis, and molecular damage caused by certain metabolic processes such as free radicals (discussed later). However, to argue that
such wear and tear *causes* aging is problematic. For example, observable
changes in joints and molecules describe *outcomes* of processes; they do not explain *why* those processes happen in the first place.

Rate of Living Theory.   The rate of living theory is based on the premise that
humans have a certain amount of life energy or physical capacity and that death
occurs once it is depleted (Hayflick, 1994). Various versions of this theory have
been proposed. One of the best known is the relation among metabolic rate,
body size, and longevity (Pearl, 1928), which states that the duration of life is
inversely related to the rate of energy expenditure. Other rate of living theories have proposed heart rate, body temperature, and other such processes. In
general, rate of living theories propose that living in the "fast lane" will result
in death sooner than being "laid back." Although there is some evidence that
these personality characteristics (termed Type A and Type B behavior patterns;
Friedman & Rosenman, 1974) are related to heart attacks, the underlying cause
of this relation is unknown. Moreover, there is considerable evidence among
humans that many centenarians led active lives and many sedentary individuals die young. Thus, rate of living does not explain human aging.

Cross-Linking Theory.   Besides water, protein and proteins combined with
complex carbohydrates or lipids comprise the most common material in cells.
One of the most important and common proteins found in tendons, ligaments,
cartilage, bone, and skin is collagen; in fact, roughly one-third of all the protein in the human body is collagen (Hayflick, 1994). Collagen is what holds
soft tissue together and reinforces bone. Collagen protein consists of parallel
molecules, like rungs of a ladder, that are held together by rungs called cross-
links. In young organisms, the cross-links join only a few nearby ladders,
making the structures flexible and pliant. However, with increasing age more
cross-links are added, resulting in increased rigidity and stiffness. For example, the process of tanning leather involves using chemicals that create
cross-links; aging of skin in humans involves a similar process, which explains why older adults' skin is less soft and pliable. Cross-links may also
happen in other molecules, such as nucleic acids, the molecules that comprise
genes. In this case, the consequence is that faulty genetic blueprints are passed
along as cells divide.

Cross-linking offers a promising approach to understanding biological aging. However, we do not yet fully understand how cross-linking occurs or what causes it. What remains to be seen is whether cross-linking actually interferes with normal biological and physiological processes or causes faulty molecules to be produced. If so, it will emerge as a leading contender. Until then, we must consider cross-linking one of several biochemical changes that occur over time that are correlated with aging.

Free Radical Theory.   Free radical theory is based on a complicated chemical reaction that occurs when certain susceptible molecules in cells encounter oxygen and break apart to form highly reactive components called free radicals (Hayflick, 1994). Free radicals are highly volatile and try to attach themselves to any other molecule that happens to be in the area. When they attach to key molecules, problems may result; the molecule may no longer function properly or may be deactivated.

The free radical theory is supported by several findings, such as that free radicals form age pigments, produce cross-links in some cells, and can damage DNA. They have also been implicated in the formation of neuritic plaques, one of the neuroanatomical symptoms of Alzheimer's disease. Because of the wide range of substances with which free radicals react, they are increasingly being viewed as having an important role in aging.

The best evidence we have about the role of free radicals in aging, though, comes from examining what happens when chemicals known to inhibit free radicals are introduced. These chemicals, called antioxidants, prevent oxygen from combining with susceptible substances and creating free radicals. Some antioxidants, such as vitamin E and vitamin C, occur naturally, and our bodies naturally make others. Enzymes termed superoxide dismutase (SOD), catalase, and glutathione peroxidase destroy free radicals. Antioxidants can be added to food to prevent spoilage; they are often labeled as preservatives on breakfast cereals and baked goods.

Research evidence on the benefits of antioxidants are somewhat mixed, but tend to indicate that animals fed diets containing these substances live as much as 30% longer than control animals (Hayflick, 1994). Additional evidence indicates that free radical production is higher in shorter-lived species. What remains to be discovered is how free radicals operate to affect longevity.

In any case, increasing the levels of antioxidants tends to increase longevity. This effect may not be direct, that is, the mechanism may be to delay the onset of disease rather than to increase longevity itself. For example, the administration of antioxidants delays the appearance of cancer, cardiovascular disease, degenerative diseases of the central nervous system, and declines in the immune system (Hayflick, 1994). Even if the direct effect of antioxidants is to delay disease, increasing the length of healthy life is an important outcome. Because of these positive results, the free radical theory enjoys considerable popularity among biogerontologists.

Immune System Theory.   Because the immune system is the primary defense against any foreign substance that may enter the body, considerable attention is given to age-related changes affecting it. The human immune system is composed of several types of cells that form a network of interacting parts: cell-mediated immunity (consisting of thymus-derived or T lymphocytes), humoral immunity (B lymphocytes), and nonspecific immunity (monocytes and polymorphonuclear neutrophil leukocytes). The primary function of lymphocytes is to defend against malignant cells, viral infection, fungal infection, and some bacteria (Berkow, 1987).

The immune system theory rests on key findings concerning how effectively and efficiently the system works (Lehtonen, Eskola, Vainio, & Lehtonen, 1990). Older adults' immune systems take longer to build up defenses against specific diseases, even after boosts such as immunization injections. This could explain why older adults are more susceptible to bacterial and some viral infections (Abrams & Berkow, 1990). There is some evidence that administering growth hormones may help some specific lymphocyte functioning to return to normal (Weksler, 1990). Natural killer cells, a subpopulation of lymphocytes that provides a broad surveillance system to prevent tumor growth, may also decline with age (Kutza, Kaye, & Murasko, 1995). The general decline in responsiveness in the immune system is believed to be due to the loss of the body's ability to handle multiple invaders at once, the toll of chronic diseases, and a domino effect among lymphocytes (Abrams & Berkow, 1990).

The strength of the immune system theory lies on another key change. In healthy young adults, the immune system is able to recognize organisms that are native to the individual, and the system does not produce antibodies to them. However, with age this self-recognition process breaks down, and the system begins producing autoantibodies that attack the body's naturally occurring proteins (Weksler, 1990). This process can cause autoimmune disorders, such as rheumatoid arthritis.

One of the major unresolved questions about age-related changes in the immune system is whether some other process, such as the neuroendocrine system, or changes in the structure of naturally occurring proteins is actually responsible (Hayflick, 1994). If so, these other changes would be the primary cause of aging. Indeed, if changes occur in proteins, then the immune system would be correctly recognizing them as "foreign" by producing antibodies. Nevertheless, research on immune system changes with age have resulted in significant advances in our understanding of disease processes in older adults.

Theories of Errors and Repairs.   The theory of errors and repairs combines elements of several other theories of aging based on random events. Like wear and tear theory, there is the notion that the human body was not designed to last forever and that aspects of it simply wear out. However, the theory of errors and repairs adds the twist that much like difficulties with our automobile, problems can be and are repaired to the extent possible. However, the repairs are never quite as good as the original, and eventually the repairs themselves fail. Aging and death occur as the result of imperfect repair processes, especially regarding errors in the production of proteins and the reproduction of DNA, which accumulate to a point at which metabolic failure occurs (Hayflick, 1994).

One variation of this theory proposes that normal, healthy people are born with well-behaved genes that operate nearly perfectly in early life but begin to misbehave in later life (Hayflick, 1994). Successful species would be those that were able to suppress the action of misbehaving genes until after reproduction. These genes would not interfere with successful reproduction, but would express themselves later as biological and physiological aging. One example of this is Huntington's disease, an autosomal dominant genetic disorder that occurs most often in middle age in people who showed no signs of the disorder earlier in life. In this sense, error and repair theory relates to the programmed theories of aging we encountered earlier; however, in the present case the genes result from mutations and errors.

Another variation of error and repair theory involves the accumulation of errors in enzyme proteins (Hayflick, 1994). Proteins are extremely complex molecules, consisting of strings of amino acids (of which there are more than 20 kinds) of many lengths and almost limitless shapes. Errors in the twists and turns of proteins are serious, as the function of a protein is determined by its shape. Because proteins must be replaced constantly, there is a reasonable probability that errors in reproduction will result. Such errors may underlie some aspects of aging. In addition, the amino acids that are used to build proteins are either right or left handed. Though chemically identical, right- and left-handed versions of the same amino acid do not work in the same ways. Strangely, virtually all of the amino acids produced in animals are left handed (Hayflick, 1994). After they have joined to form proteins, though, some amino acids slowly and spontaneously convert to the right-handed mirror image of themselves. This process can be measured in tooth enamel because it occurs at a constant rate; if it can be shown to occur at a constant rate in other organs, this conversion rate may provide an accurate measure of biological age. This conversion process may also help explain other age changes as well, although we need considerably more research on the issue.

Finally, several researchers have focused on errors occurring in DNA reproduction (Hayflick, 1994). The exact duplication of DNA in our cells when they divide is essential; indeed, cells have developed ways of repairing the damage if errors occur. However, eventually the ability to repair damaged DNA declines. Research findings to date indicate that longer-lived species maintain the ability to repair DNA longer than do shorter-lived species, providing some evidence that the ability to repair DNA may be central to understanding aging.

Taken together, the various versions of errors and repairs theories indicate that being able to detect and fix errors in molecules may underlie aging, and represent some of the most interesting avenues of contemporary research. It may be that the different aspects of error detection and repair are related, and may provide insights into the processes that are the focus of other theories of aging.

Theories in the Behavioral Sciences

Theories of aging in the behavioral sciences have been driven largely by developments in psychogerontology. For the most part, contemporary theories address the psychology of aging, and integrate approaches that study age differences in behavior as group comparisons and approaches that study the conditions of older adults and later life (Schroots, 1996). For purposes of the present discussion, these theories will be grouped into several general categories: life-span development; basic cognitive processes; modes of thinking; personality, identity, and the self; behavior genetics; and emerging theories.

Life-Span Development

Based on a series of studies, Paul and Margret Baltes and their colleagues (e.g., Baltes, 1987, 1993; Baltes & Baltes, 1990; Baltes, Lindenberger, & Staudinger, in press) proposed that successful aging can be viewed as a process of selective optimization with compensation (SOC). The basic elements of the SOC approach include: antecedent conditions of prior developmental events; processes of selection of goal and behavioral domains, optimization or the goal-related means of achieving success, and compensation or the acquisition of new goals as necessary due to loss or changes in adaptive contexts or domains; and outcomes. In brief, the SOC approach defines successful development as the dual achievement of maximizing gains (desired outcomes or goals) and minimizing losses (avoiding undesirable goals or outcomes). The exact nature of desired goals and outcomes is determined by cultural and personal factors as well as experience, meaning that desired goals or outcomes can (and usually do) change over time. Baltes et al. (in press) use the example of the concert pianist Arthur Rubinstein as an example of the process. At age 80, Rubinstein was asked how he maintained a high level of piano playing expertise; his response was that he played fewer pieces (selection), he practiced these pieces more frequently (optimization), and to counteract his loss of finger speed he used a perceptual device of playing more slowly before fast segments to make the latter appear faster (compensation). Baltes et al. (in press) show that the SOC model can be applied to a wide variety of domains across the life span, demonstrating that the model is flexible.

Schulz and Heckhausen (1996) have extended the basic premises of the life-span model to describe successful aging. In this approach, "successful aging is equated with the development and maintenance of primary control throughout life, which is achieved through control-related processes that optimize the selection and failure compensation functions" (p. 702). The model in based on four principles of human development: (1) there is diversity or variability in the opportunity to sample different performance domains; (2) there is selectivity in resource allocation such that the probability of successful outcomes are maximized; (3) people must compensate and cope with failure and with age-related declines; and (4) people must learn to manage the developmental trade-offs that occur across domains and life stages. Selection and compensation are the key aspects of the model. The selection processes regulate the choice of "action goals" in such a way that a broad range remains and the positive and negative trade-offs between performance domains and life stages are accounted for. Compensation mechanisms maintain, enhance, and remediate competencies and motivational resources after one experiences failure. Selection and compensation processes are motivated primarily by the desire for primary control, and can be described in terms of primary and secondary control processes. Although Schulz and Heckhausen's model has not been directly tested, it provides a reasonable accounting of considerable existing data. They also describe several propositions that flow from the model, which themselves provide specific research directions.

Basic Cognitive Processes

Several explanations of behavioral change have been proposed that point to fundamental declines in various basic cognitive processes, including attention, processing speed, and working memory. All of these perspectives are based on the information-processing model of cognition, which makes three assumptions (Neisser, 1976): (1) people are active participants in cognitive processing; (2) both quantitative (how much information is remembered) and qualitative (what kinds of information are remembered) aspects of performance can be examined; and (3) information is processed through a series of hypothetical stages or stores.

In general, basic cognitive processes theories argue that there is some diminution of processing resources that occurs with age, where processing resources have three properties (Salthouse, 1991): (1) they are limited in quantity, which increases through maturity and declines in later life; (2) they allow or enhance cognitive processing to occur such that performance improves when more resources are available; and (3) they are relevant for a broad range of tasks. In some cases, these theories have emerged as powerful explanatory constructs, although they do not address the question of why processing resources decline in the first place (Birren & Fisher, 1995).

Although attention is a concept that is easy to talk about in general terms, it has proven difficult to define it precisely; about the best theorists do is discuss three interdependent aspects of it: selectivity (how information is chosen for further processing), attentional capacity (how much information can be processed at any given time), and vigilance or sustained attention (how well one is able to maintain attention in performing a task over a long period of time). Most of the focus for our purposes has been on selectivity and capacity. Aging and selective attention theories propose that declines in the abilities to extract information from stimuli and subsequently integrate it underlie aging (Plude & Doussard-Roosevelt, 1989). Feature integration theory (Treisman & Gelade, 1980) is presently the leading approach in this domain, and has been used to explain several different types of attentional difficulties (Plude & Doussard-Roosevelt, 1989). Explanations of age-related decrements in attentional capacity, documented mainly through divided attention tasks on complex tasks, also center on age-related decrements in feature integration. Although originally met with considerable appeal, theories focusing specifically on processing capacity changes have been largely disconfirmed as insufficiently specific (Salthouse, 1991).

One of the most appealing and potentially powerful explanations of age-related decrements in cognitive performance is Salthouse's (1991) processing speed hypothesis. One of the basic facts about aging is that people's cognitive processing slows with increasing age. This general slowing of cognitive processing with age can be linked both with changes in neuronal structures and with higher-order cognitive processes such as reasoning. Thus, processing speed has emerged as a potentially powerful explanatory construct. How processing slows, though, is still a matter of some debate. One view, based on neural networks, argues that as neurons die the new pathways that must be constructed are less efficient (i.e., involve more neuronal connections) than the original pathway (which involved the least number of connections possible); less efficient pathways make processing slower (Cerella, 1990). A contrasting view is the information-loss model, which is based on four assumptions (Myerson, Hale, Wagstaff, Poon, & Smith, 1990): (1) processing occurs in steps; (2) the duration of the step depends on the information available; (3) information is lost during processing; and (4) an age-related increase occurs in the rate of information loss. Both accounts will benefit from more extensive empirical testing.

Working memory refers to processes and structures involved in holding information in mind and simultaneously using that information, sometimes in conjunction with incoming information, to solve a problem, make a decision, or learn new information (Craik & Jennings, 1992). Considerable evidence points to declines in working memory as central to encoding, storing, and retrieving information, as well as undergoing significant declines with age in many circumstances (Craik & Jennings, 1992). Salthouse (1991) argues that declines in working memory probably account for much of the age-related declines in several aspects of memory performance. Whether working memory should be viewed as a separate hypothesis concerning aging, though, is not yet clear; Salthouse (1991), for example, believes that declines in working memory are actually a reflection of declines in processing speed.

One of the most provocative explanations of cognitive aging is the "common cause hypothesis" (Baltes & Lindenberger, 1997; Lindenberger & Baltes, 1994). The common cause hypothesis proposes that the age decrements observed in the sensory and cognitive domains are the result of the integrity of brain structure and function and its age-related changes. This approach is supported by data from a series of studies in which individual differences in cognitive functioning were strongly related to changes in sensory functioning, which in turn may be an index of brain aging. What is especially provocative about these findings is the true representativeness of the samples in these studies. At this point, the exact nature of the common cause (i.e., the link between cognition, sensory function, and brain aging) remains to be discovered, but may indicate a rather global link.

Modes of Thinking

Among the best known theories of development are stage-like descriptions of the progression of modes of thinking (e.g., Piaget, 1970). In gerontology, these descriptions focus on cognitive development beyond formal operations, termed postformal thought. Most of these descriptions focus on young adulthood and middle age (e.g., King & Kitchener, 1994); only a few have discussed implications for older adults. Most notable among these are Kramer's (1989) identification of absolutist, relativistic, and dialectical thinking, and Labouvie-Vief's (1994) view of the integration of thought and emotion. To date, however, these approaches have been largely descriptive of demonstrable age differences; they have not addressed the key question of how and why these differences emerge.

Personality, Identity, and Self

Theories in this domain, perhaps more so than in any other, reflect basic disagreements about terminology. On the one hand, personality, identity, and self can be viewed as underlying dispositional traits; on the other, they reflect dynamic, interactive, constructive processes. Consequently, much of the debate here concerns whether the constructs remain stable or undergo systematic change with age.

The chief proponents of the stability camp are McCrae and Costa (1990), who, based on numerous longitudinal studies of personality traits over long periods of time, concluded that little, if anything, changes across adulthood. They believe that personality can be viewed as a five-factor model: neuroticism, extraversion, openness to experience, agreeableness–antagonism, and conscientiousness–undirectedness. Despite the apparently strong evidence of the stability of dispositional traits, the five-factor model has been criticized as a statistical artifact (Alwin, 1994) and because it does not explain underlying causes of behavior (McAdams, 1992).

Several contrasting theories, based on the dynamic, interactive, constructive view, propose just the opposite. The best known of these is Erikson's (1982) psychosocial theory of development, summarized in Table 1.1. Erikson's the-

TABLE 1.1.
Summary of Erikson's Theory of Psychosocial Development

Approximate age	Psychosocial crisis	Psychosocial strength
Infancy	Basic trust vs. basic mistrust	Hope
Toddler	Autonomy vs. shame and doubt	Will
Preschool	Initiative vs. guilt	Purpose
Middle childhood	Industry vs. inferiority	Competence
Adolescence	Identity vs. identity confusion	Fidelity
Young adulthood	Intimacy vs. isolation	Love
Middle adulthood	Generativity vs. stagnation	Care
Late adulthood	Integrity vs. despair	Wisdom

Adapted from Erikson (1982).

ory proposes that development progresses through eight periods, each characterized by a specific psychosocial crisis. Each crisis is resolved through an interactive process involving both the inner psychological and outer social influences. Resolving each crisis positively sets the stage for future growth by establishing the basic areas of psychosocial competence; failures impair ego development in a particular area and adversely affect the resolution of future crises. The sequence of periods in Erikson's theory is based on the epigenetic principle, which means that each psychosocial strength has its own period of particular importance. The eight periods represent the order of this ascendancy and imply that it takes a lifetime to acquire all of the psychosocial competencies.

From the perspective of aging, the two most important periods in Erikson's theory are generativity–stagnation (the feeling that people must maintain and perpetuate society versus the feeling of self-absorption) and ego integrity–despair (the completion of a life review with a sense of facing old age enthusiastically versus utter despair). Generativity has been the focus of most research (e.g., de St. Aubin & McAdams, 1995) as well as most attention by those providing more detailed descriptions (e.g., Kotre, 1984). Although the universality of the theory has not been adequately demonstrated, it is empirically supported and has given rise to several more focused approaches. Most important, Erikson was the first to construct a truly life-span theory of development.

Among other theories, Whitbourne's (1996) model of identity processes, based on Piaget's ideas of assimilation and accommodation, shows considerable promise for explaining identity development in late life. She believes that people construct a conception of how their lives should proceed, called the life-span construct, which creates a unified sense of past, present, and future.

Loevinger (1976) combined basic concepts from Erikson with a cognitive developmental approach to describe eight stages of ego development more completely. For her, development consists of fundamental changes in the ways in which our thoughts, values, morals, and goals are organized. Kegan (1982) proposed a six-stage model of the development of the self using a similar approach; he focused on how self-concept and cognitive development become integrated. Kegan's ideas emphasize that personality development does not occur in a vacuum; rather, the person must be viewed as an integrated whole. What is common in all of these theories is an explicit recognition that people play an active role in the construction of identity, ego, and self. With the exception of Kegan's theory, each has a substantial body of supportive evidence.

One popular, but problematic, extension of Erikson's theory can be termed life transition theories. Exemplified by Levinson, Darrow, Kline, Levinson, and McKee (1978), these theories proposed that people experience a specified set of life changes in a certain sequence that is highly age related. However, the major premises of these theories have not been replicated, casting serious doubt on their validity.

Behavior Genetics

The application of behavior genetics to aging consists of trying "to apportion the variation found in a population into genetic and environmental components" as a way to answer the question of why people age so differently (Pedersen, 1996, p. 59). Heritability (the genetic component) is a descriptive statistic that refers to the amount of the observed (phenotypic) variation in a population that can be explained by genetic differences across individuals; the rest of the variation is environmental, nongenetic variance.

Plomin and McClearn (1990) and Pedersen (1996) provide substantial evidence that behavior genetics offers powerful analytical approaches that explain many different types of behavioral variations in domains such as personality and cognitive abilities. Pedersen (1996) draws five conclusions from the evidence to date: (1) The relative importance of genetic and environmental influences depends on the domain examined (i.e., is phenotype specific), ranging from low to moderate heritability for personality traits to higher heritability for cognitive abilities. (2) Age differences in heritability exist, but are also phenotype dependent. (3) Across short periods of time (3–6 years), genetic effects are more stable than environmental effects, but both are roughly equally important. (4) Correlations among different aspects of a domain (e.g., different types of cognitive abilities) vary in terms of whether genetic or environmental effects are the key mediator. (5) Heritability of pathological or extreme behaviors may be different than that of the normal range of behaviors. The rapid emergence of behavior genetics since the mid-1980s as a major and influential theoretical framework indicates that it will continue to grow in popularity, with additional domains being examined.

Emerging Theories

Two theories, gerotranscendence (Tornstam, 1989) and gerodynamics/branching theory (Schroots, 1995), represent both a rethinking of older approaches as well as an incorporation of new views. Although neither has been extensively tested empirically, they represent potentially viable approaches to explaining the experience of aging.

Gerotranscendence suggests that aging represents a shift in meta-perspective from a materialistic and rational vision to a more cosmic and transcendent one, which is usually followed by an increase in life satisfaction (Tornstam, 1989). Based on qualitative and quantitative data, Tornstam (1994) described gerotranscendence at three levels of individual development: (1) cosmic—changes in the perception of time, space, and objects, increases of affinity with previous and future generations, changes in the perception of life, loss of a fear of death, acceptance of the mystery dimension in life, and increase in the cosmic communion with the spirit of life; (2) self-discovery of hidden aspects of the self, decrease of self-centeredness, self-transcendence from egoism to altruism, rediscovery of the child within, and achievement of ego-integrity; (3) social and individual relations—less interest in superficial relations, increasing need for solitude, more insight into the differences between self and role, decreasing interest in material things, and increase in reflection. Incorporating aspects of Erikson's notion of integrity and concepts from disengagement theory (discussed later), Tornstam created a view of aging that is both transforming and future oriented. Whether it survives systematic empirical tests remains to be seen.

Schroots' (1995) *gerodynamics* is grounded in general systems theory (especially the second law of thermodynamics) and dynamic systems theory (chaos theory). In brief, this approach proposes that aging is a "nonlinear series of transformations into higher and/or lower order structures or processes, showing a progressive trend toward more disorder than order over the life span, and resulting in the system's death" (Schroots, 1996, p. 747). Gerodynamics is at the basis of a new aspect theory of aging, termed *branching theory*. Branching theory refers to "the bifurcation or branching behavior of the individual at the biological, psychological, or social level of functioning" (Schroots, 1996, p. 747). This means that when a person passes a critical point (the bifurcation point), he or she can branch off into higher or lower structures or processing, which can be translated in terms of mortality (e.g., life expectancy), morbidity (e.g., disease), and quality of life (e.g., well-being).

Although Schroots' ideas have yet to be examined empirically, they nevertheless reflect contemporary thinking in physics and other sciences. Cavanaugh and McGuire (1994) proposed a chaos theory model to account for data on qualitative changes in cognitive development across adulthood. Schroots' approach will require sophisticated methodological and statistical approaches, such as dynamic systems modeling and other mathematical modeling techniques.

Theories in the Social Sciences

In contrast to the other families of theories we have considered thus far, theories of aging in the social sciences focus on the relations people have with each other, as well as how society and culture influence and are influenced by individuals as they age. Most of these theories have their origins in sociology, although more recently the field has seen the influence of economics, cultural anthropology, and feminist theory.

A Classification Scheme

Just as theories of biological and psychological aging vary in their level of analysis, so do theories grounded in the social sciences. As shown in Table 1.2, Marshall (1996) provides a very useful two-dimensional classification scheme that is based on underlying differences in theoretical perspectives: level of analysis (macro, linking, micro) and individual–society assumptions (normative, bridging, and interpretive). Specific theories are listed in the body of Table 1.2.

Although this classification scheme is somewhat idealistic (e.g., not all nuances of feminist theories can be classified as purely bridging), it nevertheless provides a useful heuristic (Marshall, 1996). The micro–macro dimension reflects the traditional range of sociological theories from a social-psychological, individualistic focus to the broader social-structural level of analysis. The normative–interpretive dimension reflects another key aspect of sociological theorizing about aging (e.g., Breytspraak, 1984; Neugarten, 1985). The normative

TABLE 1.2.
Classification of Theories of Aging in the Social Sciences

Level of analysis	Individual-society assumptions		
	Normative	Bridging	Interpretive
Macro	Structuralism	Interest group theory	Political economy
	Modernization theory		
Linking	Activity theory	Life course	Critical theory
	Disengagement theory	Perspective	Symbolic phenomenology
	Age stratification perspective	Feminist theories	
Micro	Role theory	Exchange theory	Continuity theory
	Developmental theory		

Adapted from Marshall (1996).

approach emphasizes the rule-governed nature of social interactions based on societal norms and that explanations are deductive (Wilson, 1970). In contrast, the interpretive approach is based on the notion that people construct and may use norms, but that adherence to them is not automatic. Moreover, explanations do not need to be deductive, and prediction of future outcomes is not necessarily the goal of social science (Marshall, 1996). Another way to conceptualize the normative–interpretive approaches is to consider them as akin to the distinction between consensus (normative) and conflict (interpretive) perspectives (Estes, Linkins, & Binney, 1996).

The remainder of this section consists of a brief overview of the major theories organized along the macrolevel, the microlevel, and the linking levels of analysis. The normative, bridging, and interpretive approaches will be discussed within each.

Macrolevel Theories

Within the normative perspective, macrolevel theories focus on demographic and anthropological views of people as passive agents acted on by society and culture. More recent macrolevel theories view individuals or groups as "actors," especially in the interpretive approach (Marshall, 1996).

Structuralism. In structuralism, individuals and groups are not viewed as conscious or purposive participants; instead, the focus is on universal-historical structural aspects of society (Dowd, 1987). Within the field of aging, this is best represented by approaching aging as a demographic issue. The major issues in structuralism concern whether demographic transitions are universal or specific, relations among population growth, changes in dependency ratios (i.e., the number of older people as compared to younger people), and economic growth (Easterlin, 1991; Marshall, 1996).

Due to its basis in demography, structuralism has had increased attention in two ways: the aging of the Baby Boom generation (those born roughly between 1946 and 1960) has focused considerable attention on social policy issues such as Social Security and Medicare (e.g., Easterlin, 1991), and the rapid increase in older adults in ethnic minority groups has forced researchers and policy makers to reconsider findings based on only one group (e.g., Dannefer, 1996). Additionally, the issue of age norms or the typical age at which individuals achieve certain milestones (e.g., marriage, retirement) is undergoing scrutiny and revision as societal definitions and expectations of older adults continue to evolve (Lawrence, 1996).

Modernization Theory. Modernization theory argues that the status of older adults in society is inversely related to the level of societal industrialization (Cowgill, 1974; Cowgill & Holmes, 1972). Its thesis is that prior to industrialization, older adults were highly valued due to their control of scarce resources and their knowledge of cultural traditions. Cowgill (1974) points to four aspects of modernization that result in the lowered status of older adults: health technology, economic technology, urbanization, and mass education.

Cowgill's ideas are based on the assumption that twentieth-century non-industrialized societies accurately reflect past societies, which, in his view, uniformly held older adults in high esteem. However, ensuing historical analyses conclude that there probably never was a time prior to the Industrial Revolution during which older adults were treated with uniform respect (Achenbaum, 1996; Quadagno, 1982). Although anthropological evidence supports the view that social and cultural contexts shape the status of older adults (Climo, 1992), they do not shape all cohorts equally (Foner, 1984), which is another assumption of modernization theory.

Interest Group Theory.   Interest group theory (e.g., Binstock & Day, 1996), tracing its roots to the beginning of the twentieth century, describes American society as dispersed power at the elite and mass levels, with interest groups competing with each other to get decision makers to respond to them. As applied to aging, this approach views older adults as an interest group whose goal is to shape public policy. Numerous mass membership organizations such as the American Association of Retired Persons (AARP), the Gray Panthers, and the National Committee to Preserve Social Security and Medicare, as well as many organizations with a special emphasis (e.g., Alzheimer's Association, National Hispanic Council on Aging) and professional groups (e.g., Gerontological Society of America, American Geriatrics Society) support the view that interest groups focused on older adults have a major influence on policy and the democratic process as a whole. Because interest group theory has much in common with a demographic view of society (e.g., membership in some organizations, such as AARP, is limited by age), but because members' self-interest, which is open to interpretation, helps set a group's agenda, the theory is considered a bridge between the two extremes.

Political Economy of Aging.   The political economy perspective argues that the treatment of older adults in society and the experience of old age are influenced by economic factors that transcend the United States to include the entire global economy (Estes et al., 1996). This approach adopts a social construction of reality view to explain the role of ideology in systems of domination and social marginalization of older adults, as well as a Marxian emphasis on the relation between age and the means of production (i.e., between aging and exiting from work) (Marshall, 1996). One major contributor to this approach is Myles (1984; Myles & Quadagno, 1991), whose explication of labor's support of pension systems that allow retirement as well as the importance of the socially constructed and politically motivated moral economy has helped explain how older adults are such an important part of the political economy (i.e., through various social programs) yet are largely marginalized in terms of their ability to participate in the process. The major contribution of this approach is that it forces gerontologists to step back and ask whose interests are really be-ing served in efforts to help older adults. However, one drawback is that the approach may overestimate the degree to which older adults are impoverished and, due to its societal focus, overlooks the role of meaning making in older adults' everyday personal experiences (Passuth & Bengtson, 1988).

Microlevel Theories

Microlevel theories attempt to explain aging at the level of the individual. Nor-mative approaches view behavior as predetermined by prior socialization (role theory), biopsychosocial and life-cycle forces (developmental theory), or by in-strumental rational behavior (conventional economic or rational choice theory). Exchange theories focus on the interactions rather than individuals per se. Self, identity, and continuity theories focus on the dynamic meaning making indi-viduals engage in to determine who they are.

Role Theory.   Rosow (1985) uses the terms *status* (the formal position in soci-ety that can be clearly and unambiguously specified and that carries with it certain rights, privileges, prestige, and duties) and *role* (the behaviors appro-priate for any set of rights or duties) to argue that old age in the United States represents a status without a role. This perspective is important in describing the ways in which social structures affect people individually; indeed, Moen (1996) points out that socially constructed gender roles play a major role in people's transitions through various roles in late life. Being on- or off-time in terms of acquiring or losing roles is thought to play a key role in the timing of certain life events (Neugarten, Moore, & Lowe, 1965). Considerable evidence (e.g., Settersten & Hägestad, 1996) supports this view. However, recent cri-tiques of role theory emphasize that roles are partly self-defined, that individ-ual differences are large, and that class, ethnicity, and gender are key consid-erations (e.g., Calasanti, 1996; Moen, 1996).

Developmental Theory.   Developmental theory refers to the class of theories we reviewed in the psychological theories section. In the present context, so-ciologists focus mostly on theories characterized by universal stagelike pro-gressions toward a clear endpoint; as discussed earlier, however, such views are not supported by the preponderance of the data.

Exchange Theory.   Grounded in economic theory, exchange theory is based on a view of social interaction in which people engage in interactions that are rewarding to them and, conversely, withdraw from interactions that are costly (Dowd, 1975). Thus, older adults have less power in social interchange because they have fewer resources to give relative to the number they need; conse-quently, interactions with older adults are differentially costly to younger gen-erations. Such a rational, utilitarian, "profit-motivated" behavioral view, however, cannot account for all social interchange; in other cases, nonrational or other psychological motivations must be identified (Giarrusso, Stallings, & Bengtson, 1995). Applications of exchange theory to aging have been primarily in research on family dynamics (Hogan, Eggebeen, & Clogg, 1993), especially regarding the issues of dependence and caregiving.

Continuity Theory. In an earlier section we considered some specific theories focusing on the active construction of the self in later life. In terms of sociological theory, a similar emphasis is found in continuity theory (Atchley, 1989), which was originally proposed as an alternative to disengagement and activity theory (discussed later). This widely accepted and empirically supported theory argues that the self is a theory about one's interactions with the world, a theory that is tested more frequently with increasing age, in turn producing greater stability or continuity. Continuity of self occurs in two domains: internal and external. Internal continuity occurs when one wants to preserve some aspect of oneself from the past so that the past is sustaining and supporting one's new self. External continuity involves maintaining social relationships, roles, and environments. To the extent that internal and external continuity are maintained, life satisfaction is high.

Linking Theories

To many social scientists, the macro- and microlevel theories fail to provide adequate explanations of aging because they are limited to a societal or individual viewpoint. To many, the social structure must be viewed in interaction with the individual (Marshall, 1994). Whether from a normative or interpretive perspective, each of the theories in this section recognizes the importance of both social structure and the individual.

Activity and Disengagement Theory. One of the earliest theories of aging in the social sciences, activity theory viewed successful aging as the assumption of a large number and variety of "productive" roles, such as volunteering and having hobbies (Cavan, Burgess, Havighurst, & Goldhamer, 1949). Thus, successful aging was a matter of finding one's niche in society, pulling oneself up by one's bootstraps if necessary, to achieve personal adjustment; aging is an individual social problem (Lynott & Lynott, 1996). In reaction to this view, disengagement theory (Cumming & Henry, 1961) puts more emphasis on the social system. The term disengagement refers to the universal, mutual, and inevitable withdrawal of older adults from the roles characterizing middle age; older adults recognize the need to disengage for the good of society. Although disengagement theory was severely criticized on theoretical and empirical grounds (Hochschild, 1975), the activity–disengagement theory debate had an enormous impact on the field. Most important, many subsequent theories can be traced either directly to activity or disengagement theory, or to the issues raised in the debate.

Age Stratification Perspective.   Another highly influential approach is Riley's (1971; Riley, Johnson, & Foner, 1972) age stratification perspective. Riley describes ways in which society makes distinctions in roles on the basis of age, thereby creating age strata that can be viewed much like social class in its effects (Riley, 1971). The approach examines the movement of successive birth cohorts, or groups of people born at the same time who share common experiences, across time as they age (termed "cohort flow"). The age stratification perspective combines aspects of demography and social stratification from mainstream sociology, emphasizes generational (cohort) differences, describes the relations of cohorts within social structure, and emphasizes the importance of historical time in understanding the aging process (Passuth & Bengtson, 1988).

The age stratification perspective has been criticized for its overreliance on chronological age and its overlooking of (sometimes) large individual differences in the experience of aging within cohorts (Passuth & Bengtson, 1988). However, it provided a powerful theoretical framework that forced a rethinking of the meaning of age vs. cohort differences. Moreover, many of its original tenets have been rethought in a more recent emphasis on "age and structural lag" (Riley, Kahn, & Foner, 1994), and it spawned the life course perspective, to which we now turn.

Life Course Perspective.   The life course perspective incorporates explicit acknowledgments that aging occurs from birth through death, involves biological, psychological, and social processes, and is shaped by cohort-historical factors (Passuth & Bengtson, 1988). Hägestad and Neugarten (1985) describe three research emphases: (1) the study of the timing of adult role transitions, (2) the analysis of age norms, and (3) the study of perceptions of age. These emphases and research foci have made the life course perspective the approach of choice in contemporary work on aging within the social sciences (Marshall, 1996), largely because they represent an intellectual openness not found in other theories (George, 1993).

The macro–micro linkages in this approach occur through social institutions such as work or the family. Elder (1995) describes specific modes of interaction, such as the notion that change results in efforts to regain control and adapt, which in turn construct and reconstruct the life course. Social structure is viewed as a structure of roles, and the life course is considered to be a sequence of role transitions, entries, and exits that create a trajectory. However, like the age stratification perspective, the life-course perspective largely ignores within-cohort differences (e.g., Dannefer, 1993).

Feminist Approaches.   In many respects, "gerontological theories are based on the experiences of white, middle-class men" (Calasanti, 1993). Most feminist critiques in aging have drawn from socialist feminism, which argues that women occupy an inferior status in old age as the consequence of living in a patriarchal, capitalist society, a view that also applies to ethnicity (Calasanti, 1996). For example, older women's (especially for women of color) economic hardships are thought to result from a lifetime of disadvantaged employment in a labor market segregated by gender and ethnicity (Lynott & Lynott, 1996). Gender relations, then, are given heavy emphasis in socialist feminist understandings of aging; indeed, Friedan (1993) argues that the negative stereotypes of older adults contribute to an "aging mystique" akin to the "feminine mystique" of the 1950s. Despite the validity of socialist (as well as other) feminist critiques of gerontological theory, they have not as yet coalesced into a true feminist theory applicable to the aging process per se (Lynott & Lynott, 1996).

Critical Theory.   Critical theory takes as a fundamental thesis that prediction and control of behavior are not appropriate goals (Moody, 1988). Rather, gerontological theory must be grounded in the relation between the practical use of facts and their objects of concern; in essence, the key issue is the purpose of knowledge. Drawing mainly on the tradition of the Frankfurt School (Held, 1980) and the work of Habermas (1971), Moody (1993) argues that social gerontological theory must formulate "a positive vision of how things might be different or what a rationally defensible vision of 'a good old age' might be" (p. xvii), which is achieved by applying reflective modes of thought from the humanities. Critical theory has been especially popular in understanding aging as it relates to culture and to the political economy, such as the social construction of dependency (Estes et al., 1996). Although it, too, has not yet developed into a full theory of the aging process, the application of critical theory has expanded traditional views of the field and facilitated self-reflection on the aging experience.

Symbolic Phenomenology.   The social phenomenological approach proposes that social reality is constructed through an ongoing process of negotiations and definitions in which "the meaning of age is presented and negotiated from moment to moment" (Gubrium & Buckholdt, 1977, p. viii). The construction of reality does not occur arbitrarily or capriciously; instead, it is conditioned or constrained "by existing categories for assigning meaning to experience" (Gubrium & Holstein, 1993, p. 67). A clear emphasis in this approach is asking whether research findings fit the everyday social realities of older adults. For example, Gubrium's descriptions of how caregivers of persons with Alzheimer's disease construct meaning from their situation indicates that "objective" research is, at some level, impossible (Gubrium & Lynott, 1992). One criticism of symbolic phenomenology is that its emphasis on microsocial processes underestimates the importance of structural features of society on social life (Passuth & Bengtson, 1988).

Summary and Conclusions

As is clear from our discussion, the range of theories of aging is quite broad. This breadth reflects the wide range of possibilities generated from the four

basic forces on development, as well as the several definitions of age. From this
variety, though, an important question remains: Why do people age?

At the most general level, we must conclude that we still do not have a definitive answer. Nevertheless, we are making substantial progress. Within the
biological sciences, advances in molecular biology have uncovered a wealth of
information concerning genetic and molecular processes. It is likely that within
the next decade enough progress will have been made in the study of both primary and secondary aging from this perspective to conclude something definitive about the role of genetics in the normative aging process. Once this advance has been made, future efforts will likely be focused on either how the
genetic influences operate or, if genetics is eliminated, what other mechanisms
account for aging.

The state of affairs in the behavioral sciences is more muddled, due to the
greater diversity of research than in either the biological or social sciences. In part
this is the result of the fact that the behavioral sciences bridge these other two areas. Consequently, it is essentially impossible to integrate all of the ideas across
all the analytical levels behavioral scientists have examined. Nevertheless, it is
the case that a few conclusions can be drawn. The changes underlying basic cognitive processing, such as speed, are emerging as central to the understanding of
why information processing changes with age. These changes are proving to be
powerful predictors of performance on information-processing tasks. Despite the
growing acceptance of this view, there is little evidence yet linking changes in
basic processes with the changes observed at the more holistic levels examined
by those interested in qualitative changes in thinking and in identity, for example. Whether this lack of connection reflects the need for fundamentally different
types of explanations, or whether it simply reflects a mismatch of methodologies
and a failure to ask the right questions, remains to be seen.

From a social science perspective, the key conclusion is that aging cannot
be understood unless the individual's relationship with the larger society and
culture are taken into account. It is apparent that a unifying theory is needed
that will link the various perspectives currently used to draw distinctions
among the approaches. Unless such a unified view is identified, though, it is
unlikely that any one of the current efforts will emerge as dominant.

In sum, the breadth of the current set of theories of aging is both impressive and challenging. As we continue to improve our methodologies and refine our research questions, it is likely that we will be able to reduce the number of alternatives. Whether we will reach the goal of a theory that transcends
the biological, behavioral, and social sciences is another matter. But it is certainly worth trying.

REVIEW QUESTIONS

1. What are the forces on development? Define each and give examples.

2. What are the various meanings and definitions of age and aging?

3. What biological theories reflect aging as a purposeful event?

4. What biological theories propose that aging is a series of random events?

5. What is life-span development theory? How does it integrate various aspects of development?

6. What theories have been developed to explain cognitive aging?

7. How are change and stability explained in personality development?

8. How does behavior genetics integrate biological and behavioral aspects of aging?

9. What emerging theories have been proposed in the behavioral sciences to explain aging?

10. How can theories of aging in the social sciences be classified?

11. What are the major microlevel theories in the social sciences?

12. What are the major linking theories in the social sciences?

13. What are the major macrolevel theories in the social sciences?

References

Abrams, W. B., & Berkow, R. (Eds.). (1990). *The Merck manual of geriatrics.* Rahwah, NJ: Merck Sharp & Dohme Research Laboratories.

Achenbaum, W. A. (1996). Historical perspectives on aging. In R. H. Binstock & L. K. George (Eds.), *Handbook of aging and the social sciences* (4th ed., pp. 137–152). San Diego: Academic Press.

Alwin, D. F. (1994). Aging, personality, and social change: The stability of individual differences over the adult life span. In D. L. Featherman, R. M. Lerner, & M. Perlmutter (Eds.), *Life-span development and behavior* (Vol. 12, pp. 135–185). Hillsdale, NJ: Erlbaum.

Atchley, R. C. (1989). A continuity theory of normal aging. *The Gerontologist, 29,* 183–190.

Baltes, P. B. (1979). Life-span developmental psychology: Some converging observations on history and theory. In P. B. Baltes & O. G. Brim, Jr. (Eds.), *Life-span development and behavior* (Vol. 2, pp. 255–279). New York: Academic Press.

Baltes, P. B. (1987). Theoretical propositions of life-span developmental psychology: On the dynamics between growth and decline. *Developmental Psychology, 23,* 611–626.

Baltes, P. B. (1993). The aging mind: Potential and limits. *The Gerontologist, 33,* 580–594.

Baltes, P. B., & Baltes, M. M. (1990). Psychological perspectives on successful aging: The model of selective optimization with compensation. In P. B. Baltes & M. M. Baltes (Eds.), *Successful aging: Perspectives from the behavioral sciences* (pp. 1–34). New York: Cambridge University Press.

Baltes, P. B., & Lindenberger, U. (1997). Emergence of a powerful connection between sensory and cognitive functions across the adult life span: A new window to the study of cognitive aging? *Psychology and Aging, 12,* 12–21.

Baltes, P. B., Lindenberger, U., & Staudinger, U. M. (in press). Life-span theory in developmental psychology. In R. M. Lerner (Ed.), *Theoretical models of human develop-*

ment. Volume 1 of W. Damon (Ed. In Chief), *Handbook of Child Psychology* (5th ed.). New York: Wiley.

Berkow, R. (1987). *The Merck manual of diagnosis and therapy* (15th ed.). Rahwah, NJ: Merck Sharp & Dohme Research Laboratories.

Binstock, R. H., & Day, C. L. (1996). Aging and politics. In R. H. Binstock & L. K. George (Eds.), *Handbook of aging and the social sciences* (4th ed., pp. 362–387). San Diego: Academic Press.

Birren, J. E., & Cunningham, W. (1985). Research on the psychology of aging: Principles, concepts, and theory. In J. E. Birren & K. W. Schaie (Eds.), *Handbook of the psychology of aging* (2nd ed., pp. 3–34). New York: Van Nostrand Reinhold.

Birren, J. E., & Fisher, L. M. (1995). Aging and speed of behavior: Possible consequences for psychological functioning. *Annual Review of Psychology, 46,* 329–353.

Birren, J. E., & Renner, V. J. (1977). Research on the psychology of aging. In J. E. Birren & K. W. Schaie (Eds.), *Handbook of the psychology of aging* (pp. 3–38). New York: Van Nostrand Reinhold.

Breytspraak, L. M. (1984). *The development of self in later life*. Boston: Little, Brown.

Calasanti, T. M. (1993). Introduction: A socialist-feminist approach to aging. *Journal of Aging Studies, 7,* 107–109.

Calasanti, T. M. (1996). Incorporating diversity: Meaning, levels of research, and implications of theory. *The Gerontologist, 36,* 147–156.

Cavan, R. S., Burgess, E. W., Havighurst, R. J., & Goldhamer, H. (1949). *Personal adjustment in old age*. Chicago: Science Research Associates.

Cavanaugh, J. C. (1997). *Adult development and aging* (3rd ed.). Pacific Grove, CA: Brooks/Cole.

Cavanaugh, J. C., & McGuire, L. C. (1994). Chaos theory as a framework for understanding adult lifespan learning. In J. D. Sinnott (Ed.), *Interdisciplinary handbook of adult lifespan learning* (pp. 3–21). New York: Greenwood Press.

Cerella, J. (1990). Aging and information-processing rate. In J. E. Birren & K. W. Schaie (Eds.), *Handbook of psychology and aging* (3rd ed., pp. 201–221). San Diego: Academic Press.

Cowgill, D. (1974). Aging and modernization: A revision of the theory. In J. Gubrium (Ed.), *Late life: Communities and environmental policy* (pp. 123–146). Springfield, IL: Charles C. Thomas.

Cowgill, D., & Holmes, L. D. (1972). *Aging and modernization*. New York: Appleton-Century-Crofts.

Craik, F. I. M., & Jennings, J. M. (1992). Human memory. In F. I. M. Craik & S. Trehub (Eds.), *The handbook of aging and cognition* (pp. 51–110). Hillsdale, NJ: Erlbaum.

Cumming, E., & Henry, W. E. (1961). *Growing old: The process of disengagement*. New York: Basic Books.

Dannefer, D. (1993). On the concept of context in developmental discourse: Four meanings of context and their implications. In D. L. Featherman, R. L. Lerner, & M. A. Perlmutter (Eds.), *Life-span development and behavior* (Vol. 11, pp. 83–110). Hillsdale, NJ: Erlbaum.

Dannefer, D. (1996). The social organization of diversity, and the normative organization of age. *The Gerontologist, 36,* 174–177.

de St. Aubin, E., & McAdams, D. (1995). The relations of generative concern and generative action to personality traits, satisfaction/happiness with life, and ego development. *Journal of Adult Development, 2,* 99–112.

Dowd, J. J. (1975). Aging as exchange: A preface to theory. *Journal of Gerontology, 30*, 584–594.

Dowd, J. J. (1987). The reification of age: Age stratification theory and the passing of the autonomous subject. *Journal of Aging Studies, 1*, 317–335.

Easterlin, R. A. (1991). The economic impact of prospective population changes in advanced industrialized countries: An historical perspective. *Journal of Gerontology: Social Sciences, 46*, S299–S309.

Elder, G. H., Jr. (1995). The life course paradigm: Historical, comparative, and developmental perspectives. In P. Moen, G. H. Elder, Jr., & K. Luscher (Eds.), *Examining lives and context: Perspectives on the ecology of human development* (pp. 101–139). Washington, DC: American Psychological Association.

Erikson, E. H. (1982). *The life cycle completed: Review*. New York: Norton.

Estes, C. L., Linkins, K. W., & Binney, E. A. (1996). The political economy of aging. In R. H. Binstock & L. K. George (Eds.), *Handbook of aging and the social sciences* (4th ed., pp. 346–361). San Diego: Academic Press.

Foner, N. (1984). *Ages in conflict: A cross-cultural perspective on inequality between old and young*. New York: Columbia University Press.

Friedan, B. (1993). *The fountain of age*. New York: Simon & Schuster.

Friedman, M., & Rosenman, R. H. (1974). *Type A behavior and your heart*. New York: Random House.

George, L. K. (1993). Sociological perspectives on life transition. *Annual Review of Sociology, 19*, 353–373.

Giarrusso, R., Stallings, M., & Bengtson, V. L. (1995). The "intergenerational stake" hypothesis revisited: Parent-child differences in perceptions of relationships 20 years later. In V. L. Bengtson, K. W. Schaie, & L. M. Burton (Eds.), *Adult intergenerational relations: Effects of societal change* (pp. 227–263). New York: Springer.

Gubrium, J. F., & Buckholdt, D. R. (1977). *Toward maturity: A socio-environmental theory of aging*. San Francisco: Jossey-Bass.

Gubrium, J. F., & Holstein, J. A. (1993). Family discourse, organizational embeddedness, and local enactment. *Journal of Family Issues, 14*, 66–81.

Gubrium, J. F., & Lynott, R. J. (1992). Measurement and the interpretation of burden in the Alzheimer's disease experience. In J. F. Gubrium & K. Charmaz (Eds.), *Aging, self, and community: A collection of readings* (pp. 129–149). Greenwich, CT: JAI Press.

Habermas, J. (1971). *Knowledge and human interests*. (J. J. Shapiro, Trans.). Boston: Beacon.

Hägestad, G. O., & Neugarten, B. L. (1985). Age and the life course. In R. H. Binstock & E. Shanas (Eds.), *Handbook of aging and the social sciences* (2nd ed., pp. 35–61). New York: Van Nostrand Reinhold.

Hayflick, L. (1994). *How and why we age*. New York: Ballantine Books.

Held, D. (1980). *Introduction to critical theory: Horkheimer to Habermas*. London: Hutchinson.

Hochschild, A. R. (1975). Disengagement theory: A critique and proposal. *American Sociological Review, 40*, 553–569.

Hogan, D. P., Eggebeen, D. J., & Clogg, C. C. (1993). The structure of intergenerational exchanges in American families. *American Journal of Sociology, 98*, 1428–1458.

Hultsch, D. F., & Plemons, J. K. (1979). Life events and life-span development. In P. B. Baltes & O. G. Brim, Jr. (Eds.), *Life-span development and behavior* (Vol. 2, pp. 1–36). New York: Academic Press.

Kegan, R. (1982). *The evolving self*. Cambridge, MA: Harvard University Press.

King, P. M., & Kitchener, K. S. (1994). *Developing reflective judgment: Understanding and promoting intellectual growth and critical thinking in adolescents and adults.* San Francisco: Jossey-Bass.

Kotre, J. (1984). *Outliving the self: Generativity and the interpretation of lives.* Baltimore: John Hopkins University Press.

Kramer, D. A. (1989). A developmental framework for understanding conflict resolution processes. In J. D. Sinnott (Ed.), *Everyday problem solving: Theory and applications* (pp. 138–152). New York: Praeger.

Kutza, J., Kaye, D., & Murasko, D. M. (1995). Basal natural killer cell activity of young versus elderly humans. *Journal of Gerontology: Biological Sciences, 50A,* B110–B116.

Labouvie-Vief, G. (1994). *Psyche and Eros.*

Lawrence, B. S. (1996). Organizational age norms: Why is it so hard to know one when you see one? *The Gerontologist, 36,* 209–220.

Lehtonen, L., Esola, J., Vainio, O., & Lehtonen, A. (1990). Changes in lymphocyte subsets and immune competence in very advanced age. *Journal of Gerontology: Medical Sciences, 45,* M108–M112.

Levinson, D. J., Darrow, C., Kline, E., Levinson, M., & McKee, B. (1978). *The seasons of a man's life.* New York: Knopf.

Lindenberger, U., & Baltes, P. B. (1994). Sensory functioning and intelligence in old age: A strong connection. *Psychology and Aging, 9,* 339–355.

Lockshin, R. A., & Zakeri, Z. F. (1990). MINIREVIEW: Programmed cell death: New thoughts and relevance to aging. *Journal of Gerontology: Biological Sciences, 45,* B135–B140.

Loevinger, J. (1976). *Ego development.* San Francisco: Jossey-Bass.

Lynott, R. J., & Lynott, P. P. (1996). Tracing the course of theoretical development in the sociology of aging. *The Gerontologist, 36,* 749–760.

Marshall, V. W. (1996). The state of theory in aging and the social sciences. In R. H. Binstock & L. K. George (Eds.), *Handbook of aging and the social sciences* (4th ed., pp. 12–30). San Diego: Academic Press.

McAdams, D. (1992). The five-factor model in personality: A critical appraisal. *Journal of Personality, 60,* 329–361.

McCrae, R. R., & Costa, P. T., Jr. (1990). *Personality in adulthood.* New York: Guilford.

Moen, P. (1996). Gender, age, and the life course. In R. H. Binstock & L. K. George (Eds.), *Handbook of aging and the social sciences* (4th ed., pp. 171–187). San Diego: Academic Press.

Moody, H. R. (1988). Toward a critical gerontology: The contribution of the humanities to theories of aging. In J. E. Birren & V. L. Bengtson (Eds.), *Emergent theories of aging* (pp. 19–40). New York: Springer.

Moody, H. R. (1993). Overview: What is a critical theory of gerontology and why is it important? In T. R. Cole, W. A. Achenbaum, P. L. Jakobi, & R. Kastenbaum (Eds.), *Voices and visions of aging: Toward a critical gerontology* (pp. xv–xli). New York: Springer.

Myerson, J., Hale, S., Wagstaff, D., Poon, L. W., & Smith, G. A. (1990). The information-loss model: A mathematical theory of age-related cognitive slowing. *Psychological Review, 97,* 475–487.

Myles, J. (1984). *Old age and the welfare state.* Boston: Little, Brown.

Myles, J., & Quadagno, J. (Eds.). (1991). *States, labor markets, and the future of old-age policy.* Philadelphia: Temple University Press.

Neisser, U. (1976). *Cognition and reality.* San Francisco: W. H. Freeman.

Neugarten, B. L. (1985). Interpretive social science and research on aging. In A. Rossi (Ed.), *Gender and the life course* (pp. 291–300). New York: Aldine.

Neugarten, B. L., Moore, J. W., & Lowe, J. C. (1965). Age norms, age constraints, and adult socialization. *American Journal of Sociology, 70*, 710–717.

Passuth, P. M., & Bengtson, V. L. (1988). Sociological theories of aging: Current perspectives and future directions. In J. E. Birren & V. L. Bengtson (Eds.), *Emergent theories of aging* (pp. 333–355). New York: Springer.

Pearl, R. (1928). *The rate of living*. New York: Knopf.

Pedersen, N. L. (1996). Gerontological behavior genetics. In J. E. Birren & K. W. Schaie (Eds.), *Handbook of the psychology of aging* (4th ed., pp. 59–77). San Diego: Academic Press.

Piaget, J. (1970). Piaget's theory. In P. H. Mussen (Ed.), *Carmichael's manual of child psychology: Vol. 1* (3rd ed., pp. 703–732). New York: Wiley.

Plomin, R., & McClearn, G. E. (1990). Human behavioral genetics of aging. In J. E. Birren & K. W. Schaie (Eds.), *Handbook of the psychology of aging* (3rd ed., pp. 67–77). San Diego: Academic Press.

Plude, D. J., & Doussard-Roosevelt, J. A. (1989). Aging, selective attention, and feature integration. *Psychology and Aging, 4*, 98–105.

Quadagno, J. (1982). *Aging in early industrial society: Work, family and social policy in nineteenth century England*. New York: Academic Press.

Riley, M. W. (1971). Social gerontology and the age stratification of society. *The Gerontologist, 11*, 79–87.

Riley, M. W., Johnson, M., & Foner, A. (1972). *Aging and society, Vol. 3: A sociology of age stratification*. New York: Russell Sage Foundation.

Riley, M. W., Kahn, R. L., & Foner, A. (1994). *Age and structural lag: Society's failure to provide meaningful opportunities in work, family, and leisure*. New York: Wiley.

Rosow, I. (1985). Status and role change through the life cycle. In R. H. Binstock & E. Shanas (Eds.), *Handbook of aging and the social sciences* (2nd ed., pp. 62–93). New York: Van Nostrand Reinhold.

Salthouse, T. A. (1991). *Theoretical perspectives on cognitive aging*. Hillsdale, NJ: Erlbaum.

Schroots, J. J. F. (1995). Gerodynamics: Toward a branching theory of aging. *Canadian Journal on Aging, 14*, 74–81.

Schroots, J. J. F. (1996). Theoretical developments in the psychology of aging. *The Gerontologist, 36*, 742–748.

Schulz, R., & Heckhausen, J. (1996). A life span model of successful aging. *American Psychologist, 51*, 702–714.

Settersten, R. A., Jr., & Hägestad, G. O. (1996). What's the latest? Cultural deadlines for family transitions. *The Gerontologist, 36*, 178–188.

Tornstam, L. (1989). Gero-transcendence: A reformulation of the disengagement theory. *Aging, 1*, 55–63.

Tornstam, L. (1994). Gero-transcendence: A theoretical and empirical exploration. In L. E. Thomas & S. A. Eisenhandler (Eds.), *Aging and the religious dimension* (pp. 203–229). Westport, CT: Auburn House.

Treisman, A., & Gelade, G. (1980). A feature-integration theory of attention. *Cognitive Psychology, 12*, 97–136.

Weksler, M. E. (1990). Protecting the aging immune system to prolong quality of life. *Geriatrics, 45(7)*, 72–76.

Whitbourne, S. K. (1996a). *The aging individual*. New York: Springer.

Whitbourne, S. K. (1996b). *Identity and adaptation to the aging process*. Unpublished manuscript, University of Massachusetts.

Wilson, T. P. (1970). Normative and interpretive paradigms in sociology. In J. D. Douglas (Ed.), *Understanding everyday life* (pp. 57–79).

Additional Readings

Birren, J. E., & Bengtson, V. L. (Eds.). (1988). *Emergent theories of aging* (pp. 19–40). New York: Springer.
Hayflick, L. (1994). *How and why we age.* New York: Ballantine Books.
Hayslip, B., Jr., Servaty, H. L., & Ward, A. S. (1995). *Psychology of aging: An annotated bibliography.* Westport, CT: Greenwood Press.
Salthouse, T. A. (1991). *Theoretical perspectives on cognitive aging.* Hillsdale, NJ: Erlbaum.

2

Research Methods

John C. Cavanaugh and Susan Krauss Whitbourne

The study of gerontology adheres to the principles of scientific inquiry. Information concerning aging is gathered in the same ways as in other sciences, such as biology, psychology, sociology, anthropology, and allied health and medical sciences. Gerontologists have the same problems as other scientists: finding appropriate control or comparison groups, limiting generalizations to the types of groups included in the research, and finding adequate means of measurement (Kausler, 1982).

As is evident by the variety of perspectives represented in this text, the study of gerontology involves the additional complexity of being interdisciplinary. The very nature of the topic demands consideration of biological, psychological, sociocultural, and life-cycle forces as they interact over time, requiring the inclusion of a disparate and often very large number of variables. Even relatively straightforward investigations of aging processes require that the researchers consider the many possible influences on the behavior under study. In this chapter, we will identify and describe the many challenges facing gerontologists as they attempt to provide a comprehensive understanding of the aging process.

General Issues in Research Design

Before we consider specific types of research methods, there are several general considerations that should be kept in mind regardless of the technique chosen. The most important of these concern principles of hypothesis testing, issues of validity in research design, and selection and measurement equivalence as specific threats in gerontological research.

33

Principles of Hypothesis Testing

Scientists seek to understand phenomena in such a way as to characterize them accurately and to predict their future behavior (Hertzog & Dixon, 1996). They do so by generalizing from specific events or variables based on carefully designed observations to general principles that govern entire classes of events or variables. Such events or variables reflect constructs that are not directly observed. For example, we may believe that increased anxiety has a deleterious effect on memory. Stated this way, anxiety and memory are hypothetical constructs because we cannot measure them directly. For example, we can measure memory indirectly by observing performance, but that does not reflect the entire essence of memory. The generalizations we form about hypothetical constructs provide the basis for theories, which state substantive hypotheses about the relations among constructs. In turn, these hypotheses inform subsequent observations, which may result in the modification of the theory.

Research design provides a way to translate hypotheses about constructs into a form that is empirically testable (Hertzog & Dixon, 1996). This translation forces us to think about how we will observe or measure the constructs; for example, we must decide how we will observe anxiety or memory. The process also creates an empirical hypothesis, the empirical analog of the substantive hypothesis, about the relation between the observed variables in a specific sample at some specific point in time.

Empirical hypotheses are evaluated through statistical analyses in order to examine the likelihood that the pattern of observations could be found by chance. This evaluation translates the empirical hypothesis into a statistical hypothesis. Common practice differentiates two competing statistical hypotheses: the null hypothesis, which assumes that in the target population of interest two or more variables are statistically independent (i.e., have no relation to each other), and the alternative hypothesis, which indicates that the variables have a nonzero relation in the target population.

The rejection of the null hypothesis for an alternative hypothesis begins a chain of inference from the statistical hypothesis back to the empirical hypothesis and subsequently to the substantive hypothesis. Rejecting the null statistical hypothesis in favor of some alternative hypothesis influences the empirical (and ultimately the substantive) hypotheses. How this influence occurs must be determined in the context of potential rival hypotheses. For example, rejecting the null hypothesis that cardiovascular disease and consumption of dietary fat are unrelated does not necessarily mean that these two variables are related. Only if rival explanations are ruled out can the true existence of a relationship be inferred. We now turn to sources of rival explanations.

Validity and Research Design

The chain of inferences in scientific research rests on the assumption that there are no rival explanations other than the substantive hypothesis for the set of empirical observations one has made. However, there are several threats to the validity of inferences in this chain that raise the possibility that one or more of the rival explanations may not be able to be ruled out. With this in mind, Cook and Campbell (1979) provided a taxonomy of threats to validity: construct validity, internal validity, external validity, and statistical conclusion validity. For a researcher to make valid substantive inferences, the study must be designed in such a way as to guard against these sources of rival explanations. Because it is never possible to design the perfect study, the art of research is to identify the major sources of reasonable validity threats and eliminate them by using appropriate research design techniques.

Construct validity involves the degree to which the measurement method actually assesses the hypothetical constructs of interest and the relation between them (Hertzog & Dixon, 1996). Construct validity is essential for linking substantive and empirical hypotheses (and observations). As Hertzog and Dixon (1996) note, though, behavioral and social science research is often deficient on this count, as the literature is full of examples of inadequately defined concepts and measurement assumptions. The inability to replicate results is typically due to these failures (Hertzog, Hultsch, & Dixon, 1989).

Internal validity refers to the validity of substantive hypotheses within the context of a particular research design about the relation among the variables of interest (Hertzog & Dixon, 1996). In the case of an experiment (discussed in detail later), for example, a threat to internal validity would exist when there is a rival explanation for the relation between the independent variable and the dependent variable other than the manipulation made in the investigation. The issue of internal validity is especially key in quasiexperimental and nonexperimental designs (both of which are described in detail later). Internal validity is particularly an issue in these cases because it is less likely that rival explanations can be eliminated within other than true experimental designs.

External validity represents the degree to which the findings from a particular study can be appropriately generalized beyond the sample and observational context of the investigation to other people, settings, and points in time (Hertzog & Dixon, 1996). Threats to external validity increase as the differences increase between the context of the investigation and the context to which one wishes to generalize. For example, results from research in artificial laboratory environments suffer from low external validity if the desire is to generalize to the "real world." Statistical conclusion validity involves the appropriate use of techniques of statistical inference, such as the correct interpretation of a failure to reject the null hypothesis and the use of statistical tests with adequate statistical power (Hertzog & Dixon, 1996).

It may have occurred to you that these types of validity may be in conflict with each other. For example, a research design with a high degree of internal validity may have low external validity. This is because the need to have high internal validity may lead an experimenter to isolate possible contaminating variables to protect against rival explanations of the relation between the variables of interest. However, such a strategy creates an environment that may be quite unlike the "real world" in which numerous variables are free to exert their influence (and create rival explanations for phenomena). Thus, the art of scientific research is to find the optimal balance of these four types of validity. Finding the balance requires that careful consideration be given to the nature of the substantive hypotheses being examined, the definition of the concepts and their measurement, and clear specification of the statistical techniques that will be used. Unfortunately, too many researchers fail to take the time to complete these essential steps, resulting in ambiguous results. In addition, the nature of the substantive hypothesis may create problems as the researcher attempts to develop just the right measurement instrument. Furthermore, the empirical hypothesis may not lend itself neatly to well-established statistical analytic approaches. The key to conducting good research then is learning to make the proper compromises between competing demands.

Selection and Measurement Equivalence in Gerontological Research

Issues concerning research validity are particularly cogent in gerontological research because several threats to validity cannot be easily addressed (Hertzog & Dixon, 1996). Unfortunately, neither development nor its rival explanations can be manipulated experimentally (e.g., people cannot be assigned randomly to various chronological ages). Thus, few definitive conclusions about causal relations can be drawn in gerontology, especially in the behavioral and social sciences.

Although all threats to validity cannot be eliminated in gerontological research, it is possible to reduce them. In this regard, most attention has been focused on selection and measurement. Selection refers to the process by which units of observation (e.g., people, sections of body tissue) are chosen and assigned within an investigation (e.g., to different groups). Because no two units of observation are exactly identical, concern over selection reflects the possibility that these differences may be systematic and may influence the outcome of the observation process. For example, the people in a particular investigation all come to the situation with unique sets of life experiences that in some cases may give them an advantage (or disadvantage) over others in the study. Unless these differences are taken into account (e.g., by randomization in an experiment), they may create a rival explanation for the outcomes of the research.

Selection factors go beyond choosing who is included in an investigation, though. Selection also refers to the specific exemplars of a phenomenon that are chosen for examination and the times at which observations are taken. Suppose one is interested in studying memory. As you know, there are many different ways of operationalizing memory, such as performance on a rote memory task and study strategies. If the researcher chooses only one way of measuring memory, then the lack of variety introduces threats to validity. Likewise, if measures of memory are taken only once at a specific time of day, there is no way of knowing whether the results are the result of the phenomenon of interest or the time of day. For instance, college students may not perform at optimal levels before noontime, but older adults may be more alert in the early morning compared to the afternoon.

In sum, the issue of selection in gerontological research requires careful decision making about the range of units of observation to be included, exemplars of the phenomenon of interest, and the number of observations made. These decisions frequently reflect a balance of the time and cost of being inclusive and the relative seriousness of the validity threats that result. Research designs that allow multiple variables and exemplars to be examined over multiple occasions are, in general, to be preferred.

The concern with measurement equivalence in gerontological research focuses mainly on the problem of how to make quantitative comparisons mean the same thing across different individuals or across occasions (Labouvie, 1980). Measurement equivalence assumes that the measurement properties of the index used to assess a construct are the same across individuals and time. For example, for a survey in which adults of different ages are asked about whether they are "liberal" or "conservative" to have measurement equivalence, the two labels must mean exactly the same thing to all respondents, and those meanings must be consistent over time. Without measurement equivalence, of course, there would be little idea what the responses meant, and any differences across groups would be impossible to interpret.

Although measurement equivalence is important in all research, more attention has focused on its implications for survey and questionnaire research. As we will see later in this chapter, there are multiple sources of problems in these methods (e.g., the meaning of response categories such as "sometimes" may vary with age; people of different ages may be more or less willing to use extreme categories). Even though measurement equivalence is widely acknowledged as a source of potentially serious threats to validity, few researchers in gerontology, especially in the behavioral and social sciences, establish measurement equivalence in their research. As with selection problems, failure to demonstrate measurement equivalence means that rival hypotheses cannot be ruled out.

Basic Variables: Age, Cohort, and Time of Measurement

The research designs used in gerontology manipulate the variables of age, cohort, and time of measurement. These three factors are thought to influence jointly the individual's performance on any given psychological measure at any point in life. As we shall see, these variables are highly related to each other, making the task of conducting research in gerontology a challenging enterprise.

Age

The study of aging is inherently made difficult by the fact that age cannot be experimentally manipulated. As will be shown later, only when a variable can be manipulated can cause and effect relationships can be inferred. The status of age as a variable is comparable to the status of gender, ethnicity, place of birth, occupation, and other variables that are characteristic of the respondent. At another level, age presents a complication as a variable because it has uncertain meaning in terms of what it represents about the individual. Age is a time-based measure, meaning that the older a person is, the more calendar years that person has experienced. What is the connection between the movement of the calendar and changes going on within the person? The answer is that there is no direct connection. Gerontologists use age as a convenient shorthand, but understand that age is an imperfect index of what we are trying to study.

The fact that age is a function of the passage of time (i.e., the difference between the present time and the date of the individual's birth) relates to another dilemma for gerontologists. As people age, they are exposed to historical events that occur during whatever period of history they happen to be living through. If they are exposed to harsh events such as war, poverty, and political repression they may age differently than people living in different historical time periods, as demonstrated in research on the effects of living through traumatic events or periods (Aldwin, Levenson, & Spiro, 1994; Elder, Shanahan, & Clipp, 1994). There are also less obvious ways in which the historical period influences the individual. Living in highly industrialized areas may lead people to experience a faster rate of physical aging than they would if they lived in rural areas. Historical and social factors make it difficult for researchers to disentangle the so-called "pure" effects of the aging process from the confounding effects of the environment. Fortunately, gerontologists have arrived at some innovative ways to attack this problem, as we shall see shortly.

Cohort

The term "cohort" is used in gerontology to signify the general era in which a person was born. It is determined by the year of an individual's birth. We speak of the "1910" vs. the "1920" cohort, referring to people born in the 10-year period from 1910 to 1919, compared to people born in the 10-year period from 1920 to 1929. Conceptually, the term cohort represents the same sense as the more familiar term "generation," in that it is intended to refer to people who were born in the same period of time and hence lived through some of the same social influences. For example, members of the 1950 cohort were in college during the Vietnam War era and shared certain experiences specific to this period of history. By contrast, the college experiences of people born in the 1960 cohort were far more quiescent.

Time of Measurement

Simply put, "time of measurement" is the year (or period) when testing has taken place. As such, it is a convenient way of representing the social and historical influences on the individual at the point when data are collected. Although it may seem linked to cohort (as in a sense it is), time of measurement is intended to be an index of current environmental conditions. For instance, adults tested in the 1990s were more proficient at using computers than were adults tested in the 1980s, when personal computers were far less available or accessible. A measure of development that depends on computer literacy, then, would be highly influenced by the year in which the study is conducted, apart from any effects due to the aging process. As will be shown later, the inherent connection between time of measurement and cohort creates logical difficulties when investigators attempt to disentangle these indices of social and historical context.

Descriptive Research Designs

Early findings in gerontology were based on two types of research designs: longitudinal and cross-sectional. These two designs still form the basis for the majority of research on psychological gerontology. However, they have been augmented by far more sophisticated designs that attempt to separate the effects of aging from the confounding effects of historical and social influences on performance.

Cross-sectional Designs

The most direct and quickest way to examine the possible effects of aging on a particular variable of interest is to compare people of different ages. The term used to describe this research design is "cross-sectional" because the researcher takes a "cross section" of the population by age. The fact that the cross-sectional design does not take long to complete is its main (and perhaps, only) advantage. An investigator can test a hypothesis regarding possible age differences in as long as it takes to gather the data. There is no need to wait until people actually "age."

Although gerontologists often rely heavily on the cross-sectional design, they realize that to do so involves a high degree of risk. It is never possible to know whether observed differences between people of different age groups reflect the aging process or the fact that the people being compared have lived through different historical periods. The best that the researcher can hope for is that as many confounding factors as possible have been eliminated through careful selection of respondents. One factor in particular is education. When conducting cross-sectional studies most contemporary gerontologists select samples that are equivalent in the amount of education they have received. This strategy sacrifices representativeness, however, as current cohorts of older adults are less likely to have been college educated than are current young adults. This means that the older sample is atypical of the actual over-65 population. Most psychological researchers are willing to sacrifice representativeness, on the grounds that it is better to err on the side of testing a more select older sample than a sample that is clearly handicapped compared to the younger group. Conversely, sociologists look for samples that are more nearly representative of their cohort.

When comparing age groups, researchers must also be sensitive to the age ranges of the groups involved. It would be ideal when comparing, for example, 20 year olds with 70 year olds, to have people as close to 20 and 70 as possible. However, this goal is not always realistically attainable. It is much more difficult to find people who are within a year or two of 70 than people who are within a year or two of 20. As soon as the researcher moves outside the traditional educational setting, it is difficult to capture a group of people similar in age. Unfortunately, not all researchers are sensitive to this problem and it is not unusual to find a study in which samples of "old" people who range over a 20-year span (say, from 60 to 80) are compared with a group of college students ranging from 20 to 22 years old. As a result, it is not clear what the "average" performance within the older group represents.

It is essential for the student to look for these problems when evaluating cross-sectional research. In addition, the final and perhaps most important consideration to keep in mind when evaluating cross-sectional studies is that the design does not permit the researcher to draw inferences about age "changes." Often, a researcher will state that a particular function "increased" or "decreased" across adulthood when in fact all that has been shown is that there are age differences in one direction or another. Even though sophisticated researchers may state that they have found "age changes," the nature of the design prohibits such inferences.

Longitudinal Designs

The longitudinal design is one in which the investigator selects a sample and follows it over a period of years or decades. At the end of that time, or at points along the way, the researcher is then be able to describe changes over the years on the particular set of variables being investigated. This design holds many obvious advantages as a study of the aging process, e.g., the process of development is being observed as it is occurring. Unlike the artificiality of the cross-sectional study, the evidence being accumulated pertains to actual aging processes as they occur within individuals. However, as desirable as the longitudinal design seems to be, it is fraught with many practical and some theoretical difficulties.

Here are some of the practical problems involved in longitudinal research. To embark on a longitudinal study is a major commitment of time and resources on the part of the researcher. It will be many years before the ultimate results are produced, and in the meantime the maintenance of the study files and procedures requires considerable attention. It is also quite likely that a longitudinal study will outlive its originator and arrangements must be made for follow-ups to be conducted by someone else. Most large-scale funded studies are administered by a large staff of investigators so this is less of a problem than was true in the past. Nevertheless, shifts in personnel can have ramifications for the quality of the study. Subjects are also likely to drop out of the study. There is an inevitable "attrition" or loss of participants from the original sample, and so the numbers become smaller and smaller as the years go on. Although measures can be taken to minimize dropouts, there are theoretical difficulties caused by attrition that are even more of a challenge. The "survivors" of a longitudinal investigation are not fully representative of the entire sample that began the study. An extreme form of selective survival is known as "terminal drop," a phenomenon observed in early longitudinal studies of intelligence in which it was noted that those who were dead at Time 2 of the study had performed more poorly on Time 1, even when the times of testing were separated by as much as 5 years.

Of course, the problem of attrition also affects the cross-sectional design. The people who remain alive and are available to be tested in later adulthood are hardier and perhaps smarter than their peers who died at earlier ages from disease or exposure to risk. The cross-sectional finding that older adults are better able to regulate their emotions (Labouvie-Vief, Hakim-Larson, DeVoe, & Schoeberlein, 1989) may reflect the fact that the ones who could not suffered life-shortening stress-related illnesses while in their middle adult years. Even if all the problems noted here were correctable, there remains the problem of separating the effects of social time from the effects of personal aging. The researcher cannot determine whether the changes shown by the sample are due to age per se or to the effects of the environment. Longitudinal studies, then, at best can provide information only on changes over time within a group of people followed up over a particular period of history.

Schaie's General Developmental Model: Sequential Designs

It should be clear by now that the perfect study on aging is virtually impossible to conduct. Age can never be a true independent variable because it cannot be manipulated. Furthermore, age is inherently linked with time and so personal aging can never be separated from social aging. However, researchers have turned to what are called the "sequential" designs in gerontology as a way of separating at least some of the effects of personal aging from the effects of social time.

In a landmark paper, Schaie (1965) outlined the problems involved in traditional cross-sectional and longitudinal designs, as discussed above. His strategy for overcoming these problems was to design "sequential" studies that
would separate the effects of age, cohort, and time of measurement. Each design may be thought of as a 2 × 2 analysis of variance, crossing two of the three
factors (age, cohort, time of measurement) at a time. A complete analysis requires arranging data collections that fit the criteria for all three designs. A layout for such an analysis is shown in Table 2.1. Before describing the sequential designs, it is useful to trace the paths of traditional one-factor designs.
Longitudinal designs are represented by comparisons of cells within each column (e.g., Cells A–E–I). Cross-sectional designs are represented by comparisons of cells within rows (e.g., Cells A–B–C–D).

Cohort-Sequential Design. In the cohort-sequential design, two cohorts are
compared at two different ages (e.g., Cells F + C vs. J + G in Table 2.1). In either case, if the cohort difference is significant, the researcher may conclude
that time of birth has an effect on later adult performance. If both cohorts show
similar scores, or similar patterns of change or stability across the ages they are
studied, the researcher can conclude that the results reflect the influence of intrinsic aging processes. A third possibility is that members of the two cohorts
show different patterns of performance over the two ages tested. Such findings
would lead the researcher to look for differential early life experiences between
the two cohorts that would make their appearance in later life.

Time-Sequential Design. The time-sequential research design involves comparing the effects of age with the effects of time of measurement (e.g., Cells
F + C vs. Cells G + D). Two or more age groups are compared at two or more
times of measurement. The effects of time of measurement would be indicated
if people in the sample, regardless of age, differed in their scores at one testing date compared to another testing date. Age differences across the two times

TABLE 2.1.
Layout of Developmental Research Designs

Years of testing (time of measurement)	Year of birth (cohort)			
	1940	1930	1920	1910
1980	Cell A 40 years old	Cell B 50 years old	Cell C 60 years old	Cell D 70 years old
1990	Cell E 50 years old	Cell F 60 years old	Cell G 70 years old	Cell H 80 years old
2000	Cell I 60 years old	Cell J 70 years old	Cell K 80 years old	Cell L 90 years old

of measurement would lead to the conclusion that age is a significant factor. Finally, the combined effect of age and time of measurement may result in different patterns of age differences for two times of testing.

Cross-Sequential Design. The third sequential design, called "cross-sequential," involves crossing the two factors of cohort and time of measurement (Cells B + F vs. Cells C + G). Two or more birth cohorts are compared at two or more times of measurement in this design, and as a result, age is not even a factor in the analysis. The purpose of this design is to compare these social time effects directly.

The "Sequences" Designs of Baltes

According to Baltes (1968), the separation of cohort from time of measurement effects is not an essential task of the gerontologist. Instead, it is important to attempt to separate ontogenetic (maturational) changes from those that result from exposure to social and historical events taking place during a person's lifetime. The data analytic strategies developed by Baltes directly pit personal aging against social time by repeating either a cross-sectional or longitudinal study at different points of measurement.

Longitudinal Sequences Design. In the longitudinal sequences design, more than one longitudinal study is conducted at different periods of time (Cells F–J vs. C–G). This design overcomes the limitation of a traditional longitudinal study, in which only one cohort is followed over one time period. If the results comparing one age to the other are different, this suggests that social time is interacting with personal aging. Without this check, there would be no way of knowing whether the longitudinal results generalize over time.

Cross-sectional Sequences Design. In the cross-sectional sequences design, the researcher conducts more than one cross-sectional study at two or more different time points (Cells B–C–D vs. E–F–G). The researcher can determine whether cross-sectional findings observed at one time of measurement are comparable to those obtained at another time. If they are not, then the researcher must suspect that social time is influencing the results.

Implications

Schaie proposed that the General Developmental Model could separate personal from social aging. How successful is this model? The answer is, its success is limited. No matter what data collection strategy is used, the fact remains that age, cohort, and time of measurement are inherently related. Once two of these values have been set; the third is automatically determined. There is no way to manipulate all three in a totally independent fashion (i.e., once two of these factors are defined, the value of the third is automatically determined). Consequently, interpretations derived from the sequential studies are always open to alternative explanations. The designs described by Baltes avert this issue as they do not attempt to settle the question of whether time of birth (cohort) is more important than time of measurement. Therefore, there is no third factor that depends on the other two for its definition.

Despite these difficulties, Schaie's exceptionally meticulous strategies as applied to data on intelligence and related variables over the years of adulthood and old age have provided fascinating data with many object lessons for gerontologists regarding the effects of personal vs. social aging. Take, for example, the quality of rigidity–flexibility. A common stereotype of aging is that it leads to greater inflexibility, and that older people are "set in their ways." Research by Schaie and his colleagues using sequential methods (Schaie & Willis, 1991) provided the first real demonstration of how cohort effects have clouded the findings from past studies, both longitudinal and cross-sectional. These analyses showed that over the past 70 years, within Schaie's sample, successive generations have become increasingly more flexible in personality style, behaviors, and attitudes. These generational shifts, concluded Schaie, "have led us to assume erroneously that most individuals become substantially more rigid as they age" (p. P283). Instead, there are modest declines in flexibility beginning in the decade of the 60s, but far more modest than would be predicted on the basis of social views of the elderly or even past cross-sectional studies on the same variable (Chown, 1959). Alternatively, sequential designs may reveal developmental (age-related) similarities across cohorts from different social–historical periods. In research testing the generalizability of Erikson's theory regarding personality changes from college through young adulthood, support was found across two cohorts for the predicted increases in the psychosocial qualities of identity and intimacy (Whitbourne, Zuschlag, Elliot, & Waterman, 1992).

Although the concepts of age, cohort, and time of measurement are easy to translate into numerical values, it is easy to see how quickly they become interwoven and a researcher can lose track of what exactly is being measured. These are the difficulties faced by researchers who try to make sense of developmental data. In reading published findings, it is also important to look for possible threats to the validity of a study's findings. Some of these threats may be based on fairly subtle considerations regarding the comparability of findings across periods of social time. A finding based on research conducted in the 1970s may not hold up to testing in the 1990s. The necessity for researchers to test their findings on various populations is another factor to consider. Many of the results about the "aging process" turn out, on closer inspection, to be descriptive of processes taking place within a culturally narrow group. As the field of gerontology matures, it will be increasingly important for researchers to think "sequentially" with respect not only to social time, but also to socially diverse groups.

Experimental, Quasiexperimental, Nonexperimental, and Correlational Design

When people think of science and how scientific discoveries are made, they tend to think of experiments. Indeed, many would argue that experimentation is the foundation of scientific inquiry. However, conducting experiments in the behavioral and social sciences has been criticized on several grounds, including the ethics involving manipulation and deception, as well as their artificiality. In this section we will consider the necessary elements for experimental design, and consider three common alternatives (quasiexperiments, nonexperiments, and correlation) that are used when at least one key criterion for an experiment is lacking.

Experimental Design

Suppose we are interested in discovering whether having people study a word list in various ways makes a difference in how many items people will remember. We could provide people of different ages with different types of instructions about how to study, and then observe what happens when they are asked to remember the words. For example, we could tell one group each of younger, middle-aged, and older adults to rehearse the words in the list we will show them three times each, and not provide any special hints to a second group.

What we have is a research issue that could be examined through an experiment. In general, an experiment is an investigation "in which at least one variable is manipulated and units are randomly assigned to the different levels or categories of the manipulated variable(s)" (Pedhazur & Schmelkin, 1991). Thus, the two necessary components of an experiment are manipulation (discussed in more detail later) and random assignment. Random assignment means that each of the units of analysis in the experiment (e.g., individuals, families, communities, nursing homes, social service agencies) must have the same odds of being selected for assignment to any of the groups being examined in the study. This strategy is used to control for extraneous factors (i.e., aspects of the units being studied that are not being observed or manipulated) influencing the results of the manipulation. In short, randomization is used to create the situation in which "all other things being equal" any observed differences across groups would be most likely the result of the manipulation.

A lack of either necessary component (manipulation or randomization) results in a nonexperimental design. If no variable is manipulated, thereby creating a situation in which the question of interest is how two or more variables co-vary, then the general approach is one of correlation. If random assignment is lacking but one or more variables is manipulated, then the general approach is one of quasi-experimentation. These latter two designs will be discussed later in this section.

Two aspects of experimental designs need special attention in gerontological research: setting and variable manipulation. The setting of an experiment refers to where the study is conducted. In general, settings include those created specifically for the study (i.e., laboratory experiments) and those that exist naturally (i.e., field experiments). There are well-documented compromises with each setting (Pedhazur & Schmelkin, 1991); for example, laboratory settings may result in limited generalizability of one's results to "real world settings," and field settings may introduce problems in controlling the effects of nonmanipulated variables that may introduce alternative explanations for one's results. In general, the best approach is to select the setting that provides the optimal situation for answering the specific research question being posed.

Key considerations in variable manipulation include ensuring that the variable being manipulated is likely to have the intended outcome (i.e., has sufficient "strength" to create the desired effect), that the manipulation is done as intended, and that the manipulated variable has an effect (Pedhazur & Schmelkin, 1991). Because manipulated variables can have both intended and unintended effects, a good strategy is to conduct a manipulation check (although the check itself could create unintended effects). Paying attention to these issues is especially important in gerontological research. For example, a drug that is effective at a particular dosage level in young or middle-aged adults may prove ineffective (or even toxic) in older adults. Thus, careful planning, including manipulation checks, is essential.

An additional, important distinction is made in experimentation between independent variables, which are the variables manipulated by the experimenter, and dependent variables, which are the behaviors or outcomes that are measured. In our opening example on list learning, the instructions that we give people would be the independent variable and the number of words people remember would be the dependent variable. It is important to note that age cannot be an independent variable because we cannot manipulate it, nor can we randomly assign it to people. Consequently, it is impossible to conduct true experiments to examine the effects of age on a particular person's behavior. At best, we can only find age-related effects of an independent variable on dependent variables.

In general, two types of effects of different levels of the independent variable on the dependent variable are examined: main effects and interaction effects. Main effects occur when the effect of the independent variable does not vary as a function of level; for example, the effectiveness of a particular memory training program may not vary in terms of the number of training sessions. Interaction effects occur when the influence of the independent variable varies with different levels, as when the effectiveness of a memory training program is greater with 10 sessions as opposed to five.

Quasiexperimental and Nonexperimental Designs

The major difference between experimental and quasiexperimental designs is randomization; in quasi-experiments, units are not randomly assigned to groups (Campbell & Stanley, 1963). However, one or more variables is manipulated in both types of designs. Without randomization, researchers have the task of identifying and isolating the effects of the independent variable and all other variables that could potentially affect the dependent variable. Needless to say, this is an extremely difficult task. Approximations of this isolation of effects can be made through various statistical adjustments and techniques, which permit some insight into the causal effects of the independent variable, but none is as good as randomization.

Despite the limitations, quasi-experiments play an important part in gerontological research. For example, it is not possible to ensure random assignment of people to Alzheimer's disease and nondisease groups to examine the effects of a new drug. Quasi-experiments in which predefined groups are given various levels of an independent variable provide a viable alternative, providing that the appropriate caveats are given in terms of the explanation of the outcomes. One common use of quasi-experiments is in program evaluation research. For example, the researcher may need to evaluate the effectiveness of a particular social service program by comparing groups of individuals who have received the program with those who have not. If these individuals were not randomly assigned to the various groups at the outset (which is typically the case), then the evaluation of program outcomes would constitute a quasi-experiment. Nonexperimental designs involve examining group differences between at least two predefined groups such as, for example, people who are employed full time and people who are retired and not employed (Pedhazur & Schmelkin, 1991). In nonexperimental designs, no variable is manipulated; the goal in this case is merely to document differences between the groups in the hopes of accumulating enough evidence to explain the source of such differences. Nonexperimental designs are extremely common in gerontological research, and underlie most of the work using the various descriptive designs described earlier (cross-sectional, longitudinal, and sequential).

As you may have surmised from this discussion, it is very difficult to conduct "true" experiments in gerontology because many of the variables of most interest are not amenable to manipulation or random assignment. For this reason, we have few definitive conclusions about what causes what in the context of aging. Consequently, advances in our knowledge of causal connections in the behavioral and social sciences regarding the aging process occur relatively slowly. To many in the field, though, this is viewed as a challenge to be particularly creative in designing quasi-experiments. It has also fostered the development and acceptance of structural equation modeling, an approach that will be discussed in a later section.

Correlational Design

In correlational studies, the goal is to uncover a relation between two or more observed variables. The design of a correlational study is in contrast to experiments and quasiexperiments, in which the goal is to understand the effects of a manipulated (independent) variable on some behavior, and nonexperiments, in which the goal is to understand group differences on some variable. The strength and direction of a correlation are expressed by a correlation coefficient, abbreviated as r, which can range from -1.0 to 1.0. When $r = 0$, the two variables are unrelated. When r is greater than 0, the variables are positively related; when the value of one variable increases (or decreases), the other variable also increases (or decreases). When r is less than 0, the variables are inversely related; when one variable increases (or decreases), the other variable decreases (or increases).

An example of a correlational study is an investigation by Cavanaugh and Murphy (1986), who were interested in the relationship between anxiety and memory performance. They administered measures of anxiety and memory tests and calculated the correlations between the two. Their results revealed a negative correlation between anxiety and memory performance, meaning that as people's anxiety increases, memory performance decreases.

Correlational studies do not give definitive information concerning cause-and-effect relationships; for example, the correlation between anxiety and memory performance in the Cavanaugh and Murphy (1986) study does not mean that one variable caused the other regardless of how large the relationship was. However, correlational studies do provide important information about the strength of relationship between variables, which is reflected in the absolute value of the correlation coefficient. Moreover, developmental researchers are interested in how variables are related to factors that are very difficult, if not impossible, to manipulate. As a result, correlational techniques are used frequently. In fact, most developmental research is, at some level, correlational because age cannot be manipulated within an individual. What this means is that we can describe a great many developmental phenomena, but we cannot explain very many of them.

Qualitative Methods

In an evolving and interdisciplinary field such as gerontology, there are often instances in which researchers wish to explore a phenomenon of interest in an open-ended fashion. The investigation of contextual factors (see Cavanaugh, Chapter 1) may demand a method that seeks to identify potentially relevant factors within a broad spectrum of possible influences. Qualitative methods allow for the exploration of such complex relationships without the restrictions and assumptions of the scientific model. In other cases, researchers may be working in an area in which conventional methods are neither practical nor

appropriate for the problem under investigation. For example, cultural anthropologists examining the native inhabitants of a rural village cannot use true
experimental procedures and quantitative methods; rather, they gather their
data through observations and conversations with the inhabitants. Typically,
these data are organized on the basis of their content or substance into relevant themes and issues. The product of such an investigation is more likely to
be a written account of what took place instead of a set of numbers. Similarly,
in clinical settings, interviews may provide a more accurate picture of the phenomena under investigation than would questionnaires or other quantifiable
measures. Qualitative methods are also used in the analysis of life history information, which is likely to be highly varied from person to person and not
easily translated into numbers. The main point in using qualitative methods is
that they provide researchers with alternative ways to test their ideas and that
the method can be adapted in a flexible manner to the nature of the problem
at hand.

Interviews

Face-to-face interviews may be regarded by the investigator as the best way to
gather data that are of a highly personal nature, in which self-reports may be
distorted by the individual's desire to appear "good" (a problem known as social desirability). Although the respondent may still attempt to present a favorable impression during an interview, the investigator has more control over
the way that the questions are asked than is the case in a self-report instrument. Follow-up questions (called probes) can be inserted into the interview
as needed to reach greater clarification of a point that the respondent has not
addressed. Interviews are also of great use in clinical settings when the investigator is interested in aspects of personality functioning that lie below the surface and are outside the interviewee's conscious awareness.

    The method of interview administration can range from highly structured,
in which the respondent chooses an answer from a series of preset categories,
to highly unstructured, in which the interviewer and respondent have an extensive conversation about the topic of interest. The data from an unstructured
interview are obviously difficult to analyze, and so many investigators move
after perhaps an initial pilot period into a semistructured interview. There is a
great deal of skill required in using a semistructured interview; the respondent
must be presented with a question and then, on the basis of the answer, presented with a probe question designed to elicit more specific information. To
administer this interview properly, the interviewer should be familiar with how
the responses will ultimately be scored. The semistructured interview also allows the investigator to explore areas of importance in a conditional manner.
Thus, Question #1 might be "Are you married?" If the respondent says "Yes,"
then the interviewer moves to a set of questions about the marriage. If the respondent says "No," then the follow-up questions may pertain to other types

of close relationships in that person's life. Semistructured interviews, then, have a high degree of flexibility, but this flexibility occurs within the parameters of preset categories.

Focus Groups

As a preliminary step in the identification of variables of interest within a certain area, a researcher may arrange for the meeting of a group of respondents to discuss this particular topic. The researcher attempts to identify important themes in the group's discussion and keep the conversation oriented to this theme. For example, the researcher may be interested in the caregiving experiences of elderly minority persons. A group of caregivers would be invited to join the focus group and their conversation would be steered around this issue. Throughout the course of the discussion, issues such as problems they have encountered and the coping methods they have used may arise. At the end of the focus group meeting, the researcher will have identified some concrete questions to pursue in subsequent studies. Themes such as "religion," "finances," and "health problems in the caregiver" that emerge in the discussion can then become the target of a larger and more directed investigation.

Observational Methods

As a qualitative method, the observational study involves the careful examination of the behavior of individuals as noted by individuals trained to watch and record their actions. An observational study may be conducted with the assistance of videotapes or through the live presence of the observer. Videotapes have the advantage of remaining a permanent repository of data, but at the sacrifice of validity if the respondents are reacting in atypical ways to the presence of the camera. In the participant-observation method, employed particularly in sociology and anthropology, the researcher actually takes part in the activities of the individuals being studied. The report of such an investigation includes the subjective experience of the researcher as well as descriptions of the actions of those being observed. For example, a researcher may be interested in the relationships among extended family members living in the same household. The researcher would spend considerable time with these individuals, perhaps even sleeping in their home, to get a sense of what it "feels like" to be a part of this family. It is assumed that the researcher's presence has an effect on the individuals being studied and may distort the data that are being collected. However, as the researcher establishes a longer and more intense relationship with the respondents, this effect of his or her presence may become less pronounced and the data become increasingly valid.

Psychologists working from a behavioral perspective have also developed elaborate procedures for conducting research using observational methods, but these rely on quantitative methods for analysis. A behaviorist using such methods would define precisely the behavior to be observed (such as the number of times a person speaks) and then set up a viewing station to observe the behavior, preferably unobtrusively. The observation would go along for some predetermined period of time (such as 5 minutes every 2 hours for a week). Analysis of the data would involve connecting the individual's responses to "antecedents" or presumable causes in the environment. For example, the individual being observed may speak more frequently if he or she has just been given positive attention by someone else. This finding may be used either to plan an intervention (giving the person more positive attention) or to draw inferences about the relationship between reinforcement and speaking behavior.

Data Analytic Techniques

There are two fundamental approaches to the analysis of qualitative data. In the "pure" use of qualitative methods, the investigator attempts to describe underlying relationships in the data through the use of circular rather than linear methods. In a circular method, the investigator reads through the data (taped or written accounts of interviews or observations) and attempts to discern the presence of themes, issues, or consistencies across respondents. The investigator deliberately attempts to enter the subjective world of the respondents in this procedure rather than adopt the scientific hypothesis-testing mode. For example, in reading through interviews of older divorced women talking about their relationships with their daughters, the researcher may notice that two or three women specifically mention the stress they feel when their daughters talk about their fathers, the ex-husbands of the respondents. The researcher picks up on this theme and then attempts to determine if other respondents may have mentioned this issue, but perhaps less directly. Thus, the researcher initially looks at the data in an open-ended fashion for themes or ideas, and then goes over the data again (and perhaps again) to establish whether these themes are present in the responses of other individuals. Throughout this process, the researcher becomes virtually immersed in the analysis until a clear picture emerges.

The second analytic method, usually derived from semistructured interviews, involves constructing coding categories of open-ended data and then counting the number of responses that fit these categories. This method is actually a quantitative–qualitative approach because it employs elements of both types of strategies. Respondents may be asked, for example, about the quality of various aspects of their retirement such as finances, social relationships, and leisure activities. To analyze the results in the area of leisure activities, the researcher might list all the activities that people mention: golf, tennis, painting, swimming, reading, knitting, playing cards, playing billiards, traveling, going to the movies, and so on. The researcher would then reorganize these responses into groups: athletics (golf, tennis swimming), arts and crafts (knitting, painting), entertainment (movies, reading), and games (billiards, cards). These groupings would then be tested out by other raters, who may not agree with the categories (e.g., "games" vs. "athletics") and then the rating system would be revised accordingly. The final results may be reported as percentages of people who give a particular response, or perhaps as expressed in nonparametric statistics, such as chi-square to determine, for example, if there are sex differences in retirement activities.

Researchers who adopt the second, quantitative version of the qualitative procedure may move to the next step after completing the study of constructing an instrument with preset categories (called closed-ended) based on the responses given by people in the semistructured interview study. Although some areas in gerontology may lend themselves to such a transition, there may be good reasons for the investigator to use qualitative methods throughout the life of the study due to the flexibility of the semistructured interview and its appropriateness for emotionally or personally sensitive areas of investigation.

Structural Equation Modeling

Structural equation modeling (SEM) involves a comprehensive statistical approach to testing hypotheses about relations among observed and latent variables (Hoyle, 1995). The emergence of SEM as a method of choice for testing complex hypotheses in the behavioral and social sciences is a direct result of the development of reasonably user-friendly software in the late 1980s (e.g., Bentler, 1992; Jöreskog & Sörbom, 1993).

Basic Tenets of SEM

SEM begins with the specification of a model, which is a statistical statement about the relations among variables (Hoyle, 1995). These relations involve a set of parameters, which can either be fixed (in which case they are not estimated from the data and their value is fixed by the researcher) or free (in which case the parameters are estimated from the data). Statistical tests of the adequacy of the model involve examining the goodness-of-fit, which indicates the degree to which the pattern of the fixed and free parameters specified in the model is consistent with the pattern of variances and covariances from the observed data (Hoyle, 1995).

Structural equation models are most easily communicated in a path diagram (see Figure 2.1 for an example). Path diagrams have three principal components: rectangles, ellipses, and arrows. Rectangles typically represent observed or measured variables. Ellipses most often represent latent or unobserved variables, as well as errors of prediction and of measurement. Arrows indicate associations between variables: straight arrows point in one direction and represent the direction of prediction (from predictor to outcome);

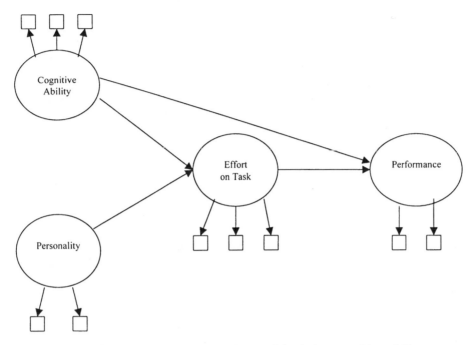

Figure 2.1. Hypothetical structural equation model relating cognitive ability, personality, effort on task, and performance. Circles represent latent variables and squares represent measures of the latent variables (see text).

curved arrows point in two directions and represent nondirectional associations (i.e., correlations). Path diagrams are typically oriented so that the overall flow of the model is from left to right. Although errors of measurement and prediction are always present, they are often omitted from the depiction for clarity.

The structural equation model itself has two components defined by the pattern of fixed and free parameters: the measurement model and the structural model (Hoyle, 1995). The measurement model consists of the specification of relations between the observed indicators (such as scores on tests) and unobserved latent variables (such as intelligence or personality characteristics). The structural model describes the relations among the latent variables and any observed variables that are not indicators of latent variables. When combined, the measurement and structural models provide a comprehensive statistical model that can be used to evaluate relations among variables that are free of measurement error (Hoyle, 1995).

The relations among variables in a structural equation model can be of three types: association, direct effect, and indirect effect. An association represents a nondirectional relation analogous to the correlation between variables. The building block of structural equation models is the direct effect, which is a directional relation between two variables (an independent variable and a dependent variable) usually evaluated by analysis of variance or multiple regression. The dependent variable in one direct effect may be the independent variable in another direct effect, and one independent variable may be related to multiple dependent variables (or vice versa). An indirect effect is the effect of an independent variable on a dependent variable through one or more mediating variables. The combination of all direct and indirect effects of an independent variable on a dependent variable is called the total effect of the independent variable.

A key consideration when creating models in SEM is identification, which depends on whether a single, unique value for each free parameter can be obtained from the observed data (Hoyle, 1995). If a value for each free parameter can be obtained through one and only one manipulation of the observed data, then the model is said to be just identified and has zero degrees of freedom. If a value for a free parameter can be obtained in more than one way from the observed data, then the model is overidentified and has degrees of freedom greater than zero. If values for one or more free parameters cannot be obtained, the model is underidentified. Only those models that are just identified or overidentified can be estimated through SEM. Unfortunately, determining the identification status of a complex model is often difficult, and the statistical programs do not always provide information on the exact location of a specification problem (Chou & Bentler, 1995; MacCallum, 1995).

Once the model has been specified, the next step is to compute estimates of the free parameters from a set of observed data. The preferential approach to achieve these estimates is to use iterative methods such as maximum likelihood or generalized least squares (Hoyle, 1995). Each iteration creates an implied (estimated) covariance matrix that is compared to the actual covariance matrix observed in the data set. Because the estimation process produces only rarely an exact duplicate of the observed covariance matrix, the goal of the analysis is to minimize the difference between the estimated and observed matrices, termed the residual matrix. Iterations (i.e., repetitions of the analysis) continue until the residual matrix cannot be reduced any further, at which point the estimation procedure is said to have converged on a solution, which becomes the final model.

How good a given estimation is defines the fit of the model to the observed data. This determination is a statistical one that takes into account features of the data, the model, and aspects of the estimation method (Hoyle, 1995). The latter point is important; for example, sampling error becomes increasingly problematic as sample size decreases, and the likelihood of reasonable fit increases with the number of free parameters estimated because these are derived from the data. Common statistical fit indexes include the c^2 goodness-of-fit test, as well as several adjunct fit tests (e.g., incremental fit indexes, absolute fit indexes) (Hu & Bentler, 1995). Each of these statistical indexes has limitations, resulting in the relatively common practice of reporting multiple indicators of fit. An extension of tests of fit involves comparing two or more models of the same data. Such comparisons can be the key in testing competing theories, for example, and are similar conceptually to comparing different models in hierarchical regression. The computation of estimated parameters and tests of fit is achieved most often through the use of specialized computer programs such as LISREL and EQS. It is important to realize that although both programs provide parameter estimates and tests of fit, they do so based on different mathematical approaches, especially when the data are not normally distributed (Byrne, 1995). These different approaches can, under certain conditions, result in dramatically different solutions. Thus, researchers should be familiar with these differences to more adequately evaluate the results of SEM.

One controversial aspect of SEM involves modification of models based on the results of an estimation that resulted in poor fit. If a theory-based rationale for freeing parameters that were initially fixed (or vice versa) can be articulated, then model modification can be justified more easily (MacCallum, 1995). The controversy involves model modification that occurs solely on the basis of inspection of the statistical output of the analysis; for example, the modification index or the Wald test (provided by EQS) provides a statistical estimate of the change in the c^2 goodness-of-fit test that would result if parameters were freed (if initially fixed) or fixed (if initially free), respectively. As MacCallum (1995) points out, model modification increases the chances of Type I error, and opens the possibility that indiosyncracies in data may be interpreted as reliable results.

Interpreting Structural Equation Models

Making sense of the statistical results of SEM is rarely simple and unambiguous. Assuming that the overall fit indexes are acceptable, individual estimates are evaluated in terms of their difference from some specific null value, usually zero (Hoyle, 1995). Fortunately, the ratio of each estimate to its standard error is distributed as a z statistic, establishing its significance from the null value (e.g., >1.96 if the null value is zero) is straightforward. Perhaps the most useful basis for interpretation is with standardized parameter estimates, which remove scaling information and are based on the number of standard deviations change in the dependent variable per standard deviation change in the independent variable when all other independent variables are at zero. These estimates correspond to effect size estimates derived from ANOVA analyses, for example, and provide a level playing field of sorts for informal comparisons of estimated parameters throughout the model.

The most difficult aspect of interpreting the results of SEM, though, involves making sense of the relations among the variables. Despite the predilection of researchers to infer causality from statistically significant relations in structural equation models, SEM tests the relations among the variables only as they were measured in a nonexperimental context (Hoyle, 1995). For a causal relation to be demonstrated, three necessary conditions must be demonstrated

(Bollen, 1989): association, isolation, and directionality. It is the case that SEM establishes association, and offers considerably more flexibility in isolating potential "causal" variables from other variables than is true of partial correlation or ANOVA. The latter is the case because SEM allows the specification of complex models that include as many key (and potential causal) variables as is practical, as well as (ideally) multiple measures of each variable. However, SEM usually cannot test the hypothesis of directionality, that is, whether variable A causes variable B, or whether the reverse is the case. In particular, the primary shortcoming of a single application of SEM is its inability to eliminate competing theories of directionality; achieving this takes an experiment. Nevertheless, if additional research is conducted with SEM that cumulatively and systematically eliminates alternative theories, then the evidence amassed across these investigations may indicate causal connections.

In sum, SEM is both similar and different from the related approaches of correlation, multiple regression, and ANOVA (Hoyle, 1995). It is similar in that all of these approaches are based on linear models, the statistical tests are true only if certain assumptions about the observed data are met (e.g., for SEM they are independence of observations and multivariate normality), causality is not tested in one model, and modifications to the model increase the likelihood that the results will be sample specific.

However, SEM differs from these other approaches in three key ways. First, SEM requires a formal specification of the model to be estimated and tested. Thus, the researcher must state explicitly all the hypothesized relations among the variables of interest, requiring considerable thought. Second, SEM provides the capacity to test relations among latent variables isolated from the effects of unreliability and uniqueness. Third, the statistical indicators obtained in SEM are ambiguous compared to those obtained in other approaches.

Overall, SEM is a more comprehensive and flexible approach to research design and data analysis than any other single approach in common use (Hoyle, 1995). Indeed, ANOVA, multiple regression, and factor analysis are all special instances of SEM. Clearly, SEM provides a way to test more complex and specific hypotheses, thereby providing an extremely powerful research tool.

Survey and Questionnaire Methods

Without doubt, the most common research tools in the social and behavioral sciences are surveys and questionnaires. They are truly an ubiquitous part of life, from the checklists one completes at a physician's office about prior illnesses to the national polls about attitudes toward government leaders. Much of the popularity of surveys and questionnaires can be attributed to the ease with which they can be constructed. For use in scientific research, however, great care needs to be taken to meet the necessary criteria of measurement equivalence discussed earlier. In this section we will briefly consider the primary elements of good surveys and questionnaires, including the issues of reliability, validity, and scale development.

Reliability and Validity

The reliability of a survey or questionnaire formally refers to the proportion of variance attributable to the true score of a latent variable (Ghiselli, Campbell, & Zedeck, 1981); less formally, reliability refers to the consistency with which the instrument measures the phenomenon of interest. Reliability underlies all measurement; indeed, a scale is worthless if it is unreliable. Several methods for computing reliability have been developed. The most common, internal consistency, concerns the homogeneity of items in a scale. A scale is said to be internally consistent to the extent that all of the items are highly intercorrelated, which implies that all of the items are measuring the same latent variable (DeVellis, 1991). Such a scale is also said to be unidimensional; multidimensional scales are families of related, unidimensional scales. Other types of reliability include test–retest (in which scores from one administration are correlated with scores from a second administration separated over some period of time), alternate forms reliability (in which scores from two versions of the same scale are correlated), and split-half reliability (in which scores from half of the items on a scale are correlated with items from the other half). Test–retest reliability is often problematic, in that the lack of correlation over time may indicate either that the measure is unstable or that the phenomenon of interest changes over time; for this reason, it is not recommended unless it is already well established that the phenomenon of interest is stable (Nunnally, 1978). Such measures tend to be found among personality trait indicators.

The validity of a survey or questionnaire refers to the degree to which the scale measures what it purports to measure; that is, the latent variable that the scale measures is the latent variable of interest (DeVellis, 1991). Simply because a scale is reliable does not guarantee that the scale is valid; indeed, validity is demonstrated separately from reliability. Validity is inferred from the manner in which the scale was constructed (content validity), its ability to relate to other similar measures and predict specific events (concurrent and predictive validity), or its relation to measures of other constructs (convergent and discriminant validity). Content validity involves demonstrating that the items in a particular scale reflect and are representative of the content domain in question (e.g., a vocabulary test would include a representative sample of words). Content validity could be established by having a panel of experts judge the items for relevancy and representativeness. Concurrent validity is demonstrated through correlations with another measure that is widely agreed to be the "gold standard" for measuring a particular construct; for example, a new scale could be shown to correlate with an established scale. Predictive validity refers to the ability to predict some future score or behavior on the basis of a present score or behavior. Convergent validity exists to the extent that the scale correlates with measures of related constructs (e.g., mathematical test scores correlating with problem-solving test scores) and not correlating with unrelated constructs (e.g., mathematical test scores not correlating with scores on a test of artistic ability) as predicted by a theory (e.g., that mathematical ability is related to problem solving but not to artistic ability). Discriminant validity refers to the appropriate lack of correlation with measures of unrelated concepts.

Scale Development

Creating a scale from scratch is a difficult endeavor that entails eight discrete steps (DeVellis, 1991). Step 1 entails determining what one wants to measure, a deceptively simple operation that is actually much more difficult than it seems. Three key elements to maximize success at this step involve using theory to clarify the central constructs to be measured, being very specific in defining the constructs, and being clear about what to include (and what to leave out) in the measure.

Step 2, generating the item pool, involves generating a large pool of possible items for eventual inclusion in the scale. Several good principles should be followed in this regard. Each of the items chosen should reflect the latent variable, keeping in mind that each item can be viewed as a separate "test" of the underlying construct. Redundancy of item content should be included, especially at the beginning stages of scale construction. The number of items in the pool should be considerably greater than the number required in the final scale. Great care should be exercised in writing items, with special attention paid to clarity of wording, grammatical construction, length, and reading difficulty level. Items that are positively worded (e.g., "I am a good person") should be combined with negatively worded items (e.g., "I sometimes feel that I am not a worthwhile person") to provide items with both high and low levels of the latent variable and to avoid response bias (e.g., agreeing with all items). However, caution should be taken when both types of items are included in the same scale, as they may be confusing to respondents.

Step 3 in scale development entails selecting a response format. Several popular options exist. The most popular, the Likert scale, involves presenting items as declarative statements followed by a response format with varying levels of agreement and disagreement. A Guttman response format involves presenting progressively higher levels of an attribute and noting the point at which the respondent shifts endorsements (e.g., from agree to disagree). Response category scales reflect a continuum along which respondents make discriminations (e.g., "always," "sometimes," "never"). In all of these cases, the decision of how many options to include is often a difficult one. More options may increase the variance of scores across respondents, but may prove difficult to use because they force people to make finer-grained discriminations than is reasonable. Thus, the art of constructing a response format is to balance the opportunity for variance with the need to provide a format that is easy to use and understand.

Step 4 involves having the initial item pool and response format reviewed by experts. The goal here is to make a determination about the relevance of each item to the construct being measured, as well as its clarity and conciseness. In the process, the experts may also note aspects of the construct that are not reflected in the pool.

Step 5 concerns considering whether to include items to detect flaws in the scale. One possible approach would be to include items designed to detect responding that reflects respondents' attempts to answer in the manner they think they are supposed to or in a way that will make them appear "good" (social desirability). Such items would serve to designate such respondents, and to question the validity of their responses.

Step 6 entails administering the items to a large and diverse sample of individuals so that the scale can be tested. The more representative the sample is of the types of individuals ultimately targeted for study, the more useful this developmental stage will be.

Step 7 involves evaluating the items for inclusion in the next or final version of the scale. This step includes examining reliability estimates, as well as scale means and individual item variances.

Finally, Step 8 entails optimizing scale length to maximize reliability and validity. This typically involves dropping "bad" items based on a preestablished criterion, such as a certain level of item reliability.

Together, these steps, if followed carefully, will create a sound scale. One of the difficulties in behavioral and social science research in gerontology, however, is that many researchers fail to take even the most elementary precautions in developing scales prior to using them in research. As a result, the measures may even lack reliability, making it extremely difficult to learn much of value from their use. Moreover, such poor research methods are a major contributing factor to the failure to replicate findings from one study to another, and a major reason why there is often a failure to establish equivalence of measurement across age groups, a concept discussed earlier.

Ethics in Research

The individuals who participate in research are asked to give of their time and, on some occasions, to provide information about themselves that is very private or potentially embarrassing. In some types of experimental studies, the researchers may need to use deception to study the variables of interest. For instance, in a study of attitudes toward the elderly, the subject may be told that the experiment is about "social interactions" and that he or she is about to meet a new person. The characteristics of the person are described as either old or young (manipulating the variable of age) and the respondent is then asked some questions about what he or she thinks the person is like. There actually is no person that the respondent will be meeting, however, because the researcher was interested only in what the respondent's expectations were. The deception was needed to set up the experimental manipulation. In research on intervention, respondents are randomly placed into a treatment group vs. no treatment group. Depending on the nature of the design, respondents will not be told everything about the study until it is over. In both of these cases, it is important for the researcher to protect the rights of the respondent because there is information that he or she does not have about the study prior to agreeing to participate in it.

Institutional Review Boards

The need to protect the rights of participants became increasingly evident in the 1960s and 1970s with the publicity attached to several notorious studies in social psychology, particularly the series of experiments on obedience to authority carried out by Stanley Milgram at Yale. In the mid-1970s, all institutions receiving federal funding for research being carried out on human subjects were required to establish Institutional Review Boards (IRBs) that would review all proposed studies to be carried out at that institution or by anyone employed by that institution. The purpose of such reviews was to ensure that the rights of the subjects were adequately protected. The American Psychological Association also developed a set of ethical guidelines to ensure that studies specifically in psychology meet predetermined criteria for protection of human (and animal) subjects.

Informed Consent

The most important ethical guideline to be followed in conducting research is to ensure that participants have as much information as possible prior to being in the study about what they are being asked to do. Although this information might be limited by the nature of the study (i.e., if deception is involved), the respondent should at least be "informed." Furthermore, the prior review of the study by the IRB would ensure that the benefits of being in the study outweigh the risks to the individual.

Informed consent is usually accomplished by giving the respondent a consent form that describes the study in as much detail as possible. Clear information must be given about risks and benefits of participation. Furthermore, respondents should be given the right to refuse to participate, so that they do not feel that they are being coerced into participation. For example, it would be unethical to make an elderly medical patient's treatment contingent on agreement to be in a study being carried out by hospital researchers. Similarly, the informed consent form must include a statement regarding a subject's right to withdraw without penalty. At any time, the individual may decide that the experiment has become too long, stressful, or in some other ways problematic and no negative outcome will ensue when this happens. Thus, the provision of a service will not be discontinued nor will there be any sort of financial or other penalty if the respondent chooses to leave the study. The consent form also specifies that the names of participants in the study will remain either anonymous or confidential (to be known only by the researchers). In the case of anonymity, the respondent is told that the responses are going to be summed in the form of group data and there will be no reason to examine the respondent's data specifically. In cases where confidentiality but not anonymity is guaranteed (as in a longitudinal study where it is necessary to know people's names), the investigator makes it clear that the data will be coded or in other ways made inaccessible to other parties.

In cases where the older person is cognitively impaired, consent for participation in research must be obtained from a family member (or other individual, such as a lawyer) who has the power of attorney. The protection of the rights of individuals who are not competent to make decisions about their welfare is particularly important so that they are not victims of abuse. Following the conclusion of the study, ethical guidelines dictate that respondents should be fully informed about the study's purpose. This debriefing should include the variables of interest and the expected relationships. If deception was involved, the debriefing form should state clearly what that deception was and why it was needed. Respondents should also be given the opportunity to find out where to read the study's results when it is published. Generally, both debriefing and information about the results are accomplished by giving the respondent a written sheet of paper that fully describes the study's purpose and gives the address and telephone number of the principal investigator (or in the case of a graduate student, the professor advising the student). In the case of a longitudinal investigation, the debriefing process becomes more complicated because the investigator may not want to reveal completely what the study was about or provide information on possible results. Such feedback could bias the findings during the next round of the study. Researchers involved in follow-up studies must still provide a debriefing form, but it may not divulge such specific facts about the study.

Finally, researchers may choose to or be advised by the IRB that they should have some type of back-up or referral agency to send respondents to should the study lead to emotional or medical problems. For example, if the study is on the effect of aerobic exercise on cardiac output, the researchers must be prepared to provide emergency medical care (or transport the respondent to an emergency room) if a respondent suffers adverse physical reactions. In research dealing with more emotional topics, where respondents might become distressed over questions regarding relationships with others, losses in their lives, or psychiatric history, it is necessary for the researchers to have the number of a mental health clinic that provides walk-in treatment. In other cases, the researchers may be encouraged to provide respondents automatically with the names of educational or other referral services at the time of debriefing.

Concluding Comments

The issues raised in this chapter form the very foundation for all of the data on substantive issues presented in the remainder of this book. Asking good, clear, and insightful research questions is only the beginning. Unless the investigator uses sound methodologies, the data that are gathered will not further understanding of the issues being studied. As you continue through this book, reflect on the techniques used to provide the data being discussed, and keep a healthy skepticism about the results.

REVIEW QUESTIONS

1. How does the chain of inferences relate to the validity of research designs?

2. What are the basic variables in developmental research, and how are they related in descriptive designs?

3. What are the primary characteristics of experimental, quasiexperimental, nonexperimental, and corrleational designs?

4. What are the major components of qualitative methods? How are they different from quantitative methods?

5. What are the major elements of structural equation modeling?

6. How are good scales and questionnaires constructed and evaluated?

7. What are the major concerns regarding ethics in research?

References

Aldwin, C. M., Levenson, M. R., & Spiro, A. (1994). Vulnerability and resilience to combat exposure: Can stress have lifelong effects? *Psychology and Aging, 9,* 34–44.
Baltes, P. B. (1968). Longitudinal and cross-sectional sequences in the study of age and generation effects. *Human Development, 11,* 145–171.
Bentler, P. M. (1992). *EQS structural equation program manual.* Los Angeles: BMDP Statistical Software.
Bollen, K. A. (1989). *Structural equations with latent variables.* New York: Wiley.
Byrne, B. M. (1995). One application of structural equation modeling from two perspectives: Exploring the EQS and LISREL strategies. In R. H. Hoyle (Ed.), *Structural equation modeling: Concepts, issues, and applications* (pp. 138–157). Thousand Oaks, CA: Sage Publications.
Campbell, D. T., & Stanley, J. C. (1963). Experimental and quasi-experimental designs for research on teaching. In N. L. Gage (Ed.), *Handbook of research on teaching* (pp. 171–246). Chicago: Rand McNally.

Cavanaugh, J. C., & Murphy, N. Z. (1986). Personality and metamemory correlates of memory performance in younger and older adults. *Educational Gerontology, 12,* 387–396.

Chou, C.-P., & Bentler, P. M. (1995). Estimates and tests in structural equation modeling. In R. H. Hoyle (Ed.), *Structural equation modeling: Concepts, issues, and applications* (pp. 37–55). Thousand Oaks, CA: Sage Publications.

Chown, S. M. (1959). Rigidity—A flexible concept. *Psychological Bulletin, 56,* 353–362.

Cook, T. D., & Campbell, D. T. (1979). *Quasi-experimentation: Design and analysis issues for field settings.* Chicago: Rand McNally.

DeVellis, R. F. (1991). *Scale development: Theory and applications.* Newbury Park, CA: Sage Publications.

Elder, G. H., Jr., Shanahan, M. J., & Clipp, E. C. (1994). When war comes to men's lives: Life-course patterns in family, war and health. *Psychology and Aging, 9,* 5–16.

Ghiselli, E. E., Campbell, J. P., & Zedeck, S. (1981). *Measurement theory for the behavioral sciences.* New York: Freeman.

Hertzog, C., & Dixon, R. A. (1996). Methodological issues in research on cognition and aging. In F. Blanchard-Fields & T. M. Hess (Eds.), *Perspectives on cognitive change in adulthood and aging* (pp. 66–121). New York: McGraw-Hill.

Hertzog, C., Hultsch, D. F., & Dixon, R. A. (1989). Evidence for the convergent validity of two self-report metamemory questionnaires. *Development Psychology, 25,* 687–700.

Hoyle, R. H. (1995). The structural equation modeling approach: Basic concepts and fundamental issues. In R. H. Hoyle (Ed.), *Structural equation modeling: Concepts, issues, and applications* (pp. 1–15). Thousand Oaks, CA: Sage Publications.

Hu, L., & Bentler, P. M. (1995). Evaluating model fit. In R. H. Hoyle (Ed.), *Structural equation modeling: Concepts, issues, and applications* (pp. 76–99). Thousand Oaks, CA: Sage Publications.

Jöreskog, K. G., & Sörbom, D. (1993). *LISREL 8: User's reference guide.* Chicago: Scientific Software.

Kausler, D. H. (1982). *Experimental psychology and human aging.* New York: Wiley.

Labouvie, E. W. (1980). Identity versus equivalence of psychological measures and constructs. In L. W. Poon (Ed.), *Aging in the 1980's: Psychological issues* (pp. 493–502). Washington, DC: American Psychological Association.

Labouvie-Vief, G., Hakim-Larson, J., DeVoe, M., & Schoeberlein, S. (1989). Emotions and self-regulation: A life-span view. *Human Development, 32,* 279–299.

MacCallum, R. C. (1995). Model specification: Procedures, strategies, and related issues. In R. H. Hoyle (Ed.), *Structural equation modeling: Concepts, issues, and applications* (pp. 16–36). Thousand Oaks, CA: Sage Publications.

Nunnally, J. C. (1978). *Psychometric theory* (2nd ed.). New York: McGraw-Hill.

Pedhazur, E. J., & Schmelkin, L. P. (1991). *Measurement, design, and analysis: An integrated approach.* Hillsdale, NJ: Erlbaum.

Schaie, K. W. (1965). A general model for the study of developmental change. *Psychological Bulletin, 64,* 92–107.

Schaie, K. W., & Willis, S. L. (1991). Adult personality and psychomotor performance: Cross-sectional and longitudinal analyses. *Journal of Gerontology: Psychological Sciences, 46,* P275–284.

Whitbourne, S.K., Zuschlag, M.K., Elliot, L.B. & Waterman, A.S. (1992). Psychosocial development in adulthood: A 22-year sequential study. *Journal of Personality and Social Psychology, 63,* 260–271.

Additional Readings

Berg, B. L. (1998). *Qualitative research methods for the social sciences* (3rd ed.). Boston: Allyn & Bacon.
DeVellis, R. F. (1991). *Scale development*. Newbury Park, CA: Sage Publications.
Hoyle, R. H. (Ed.). (1995). *Structural equation modeling: Concepts, issues, and applications*. Thousand Oaks, CA: Sage Publications.
Rossi, P. H., Wright, J. D., & Anderson, A. B. (1983). *Handbook of survey research*. San Diego, CA: Academic Press.
Schaie, K. W., Campbell, R. T., Meredith, W., & Rawlings, S. C. (Eds.). (1988). *Methodological issues in aging research*. New York: Springer.

3

Culture and Aging

Mark R. Luborsky and Carmit Kurn McMullen

What Is Culture and Why Is It Important to Gerontology?

Culture shapes the status, social settings, living conditions, and personal experiences of the elderly and contributes to many of the psychosocial and physical processes of aging. Culture is also at work guiding the historical development of the discipline of gerontology. It directs our attention to particular questions and problems for study and instills notions of proper and improper ways to conduct research (Cavanaugh & Whitbourne, 1998; Achenbaum, 1978; Luborsky & Sankar, 1993).

Our goal in this chapter is to provide the reader with the skills needed to identify and understand the cultural dimensions of aging. We will provide definitions of key terms and concepts, show how culture links communities and individual lives, and provide a brief overview of aging in a cross-cultural and historical perspective. Illustrations and examples in each section provide a lively perspective on these concepts and facts.

Culture Defined

Culture is a distinctive feature of humanity, a vital and pervasive force that patterns our basic social and political institutions, ideals, and norms for a "good life." Major transformations in our history have occurred with the rise of new visions of cultural ideals and practices embodied in innovative social systems. Perhaps because culture is so interwoven in human life, it is hard to provide a definition that encompasses all aspects of culture. However, culture is generally defined as shared basic value orientations, norms, and beliefs, as well as customary habits and ways of living. Culture defines the basic cosmology, or *worldview* of a society in that it provides the fundamental explanations about the meanings and goals of life, the makeup and forces in the universe, and proper relationships among them. An ethnographer discovers culture by interviewing and observing people to discover the beliefs, values, and ideals they share and that they believe distinguishes them as members of an identifiable culture. At the same time, researchers pay particular attention to discovering the evaluative standards used to judge the meaning of events and actions— what is "right" and "wrong" in that society.

Although a culture is often identified with a particular social group or nation, it is typical to find a plurality of cultural traditions existing within such groups. Multiple cultural traditions may result from contact with other groups through trade, immigration, and conquest, as well as through innovations originating within the social group. A plurality of cultural traditions within social groups has been a fact of human existence throughout history and is found in technologically simple societies (e.g., foraging or nomadic peoples) as well as industrialized nations. Cultural *syncretism* occurs when multiple traditions are combined into a new whole. In other situations, cultural traditions may coexist without much interaction. This is called cultural *pluralism*.

Conceptualizing Culture in Gerontological Research

We argue that at least three important aspects of culture must be recognized to conduct rigorous research and program development related to culture and aging. The first aspect is that culture provides core values during childhood that instill deeply motivating beliefs and emotions. In this regard, cultural values, norms, and beliefs are a framework that guides individuals' interpretation of their sense of well-being and direction in life. The second and interrelated aspect is that culture exerts a continuing force during ongoing adult socialization over the lifetime (Rosow, 1974). It may serve as both a stabilizing force through the provision of traditions and norms, or as an agent of potential change as cultures evolve and thus pose new challenges to individuals socialized in earlier eras. We will focus on these first two aspects of culture in our discussion of personhood, the life course, and biography.

Third, culture should not be idealized. We must examine its potential for both positive and negative influences on individuals and communities. Culture can be a positive force by providing individuals and groups with an orienting sense of meaningful values and ideals. These may become particularly important with the onset of adversities such as health problems, financial woes, family, and relationship hassles. Here culture helps to provide explanations for the occurrence of problems and guidelines for their resolution. Yet culture can also be the source of deep distress and hardship. It may set ideals, goals, and expectations that cannot be met in a given community or historic era. Culture also provides negative stereotypes, stigma, and devaluation of some people or traits. For example, a person who survives paralysis from childhood polio or stroke in later life may, after strenuous rehabilitation, regain the ability to walk with crutches or a walker. This person may feel enormous pride in the attainment of "successful" rehabilitation and in the personal triumph over adversity.

North American culture values that foster a "mind over matter" attitude, when internalized as personal goals, may have a beneficial impact on the individual's health. On the other hand, our cultural values also emphasize the need for autonomy and independence, and lead that individual to be viewed negatively in wider society because his or her residual disability requires use of an adaptive device. Similarly, despite economic success, which is the criteria for the "American dream," members of minority ethnic groups in the United States may remain devalued due to historic factors and the cultural biases of majority groups. Thus, it is always important to explore culture both as a positive resource and as a source of distress.

Within a community, culture often poses value dilemmas and value conflicts to individuals. Between groups, many calamitous wars and conflicts have been rooted in intolerance about differing core ideologies and traditions. Similarly, failure to ascribe equal recognition of other people's cultural traditions has led to the mistreatment of individuals and whole societies, as evidenced in slavery or brutality toward prisoners of war. *Ethnocentrism*, the tendency to see one's own culture as superior to others, seems to be a universal aspect of human culture. Part of taking an anthropological perspective involves thinking reflexively about one's own ethnocentric judgments in order to minimize them. Instead of ethnocentrism, anthropologists aim for a perspective on other cultures called *cultural relativism*, whereby each culture is understood on its own terms, without judgment. Cultural relativism is a perspective that is hard to learn and perhaps impossible to uphold in all situations. Nonetheless, it is absolutely essential for cross-cultural research. In our discussion of elder neglect, we will discuss cultural relativism in more detail.

Culture as Cognitive Blinders

Although the basic anthropological perspective we have outlined was developed as a tool for understanding vastly different cultural worlds, it can also help us understand the cultural basis of aging in our own culture, exemplified in the case of disability mentioned above. The quiet hand of culture is also manifest in gerontology's continuing debate about how to define and label the ultimate goal of the discipline. Energetic arguments continue to rage about the "proper" modern vision for aging—whether research and policy should be framed in terms of "normal aging," "aging well," "successful aging," or "productive aging" (e.g., Rowe & Kahn, 1998). Each viewpoint poses a different benchmark for judging individuals' success and failure in the aging endeavor and provides different evaluation criteria for programs designed to improve the status and care of the elderly.

Culture can foster a kind of intellectual blindfold. By this we mean culture provides underlying assumptions about how things work that we take for granted. What seems natural or common sense in one culture may seem absurd in another. Basing research, policy, and practice on common-sense assumptions can lead to misinterpretations of the aging process across cultures. Failing to reflect on our own cultural biases makes it easy to pass ethnocentric judgment on values and practices that are beneficial when they do not seem right according to our own cultural sensibilities. Improved awareness of the specific cultural viewpoint that we habitually utilize can also open up new insights for programs and treatment in our own culture. For example, there are many unquestioned assumptions about the value of life story telling in gerontological research. "Life story telling is beneficial, according to current wisdom, because it 'empowers' the narrator to represent, in public, *personal* experiences and meaning . . . it promotes our cherished modern ideal of freeing people to voice their own experiences (Gilligan, 1982; Tannen, 1989) without control by others. An appeal of the life story derives from our view of them as self-directed and self-reflexive expressions" (Luborsky, 1993, p. 445). These assumptions have remained largely unquestioned because they "make sense" in our culture. However, critical empirical studies of life story telling have suggested that our assumptions may be misguided (Luborsky, 1993).

Another example of culture as cognitive blinders comes from the field of rehabilitation. Common sense, cultural assumptions that loss of physical functioning was a "normal" part of aging, combined with the historical development of rehabilitation as an intervention for young adults, delayed recognition of the life-enhancing benefits of rehabilitation for elderly individuals (Becker & Kaufman, 1988).

An important part of conducting research involves developing models and identifying constructs and variables for data collection. Sometimes these models, constructs, and variables are *predetermined* by researchers without considering the perspective of the individuals or populations being studied. The cognitive blinders of researchers may lead them to overlook issues that are fundamental to their research endeavor. The need to understand cultural dimensions of aging becomes very salient when identifying, for example, issues in adjustment and coping. An anthropological perspective asks, *what is it that individuals are adjusting to?* That is, how do individuals perceive social and personal expectations, as well as the range of desirable options and appropriate styles of adjusting. These kinds of questions contrast with others that ask only how and how well people cope, without investigating the meanings and rationales that people use in actively defining their situation and choosing a particular course of action. Without learning what people perceive as the important challenges and appropriate coping styles in their own lives, we can glimpse only a part of the picture related to predetermined notions of coping and adjustment.

What Is Ethnicity?

Ethnicity is a concept that exists within complex societies and often at the boundaries between societies. Ethnic identity is a topic that has been examined with growing interest in our century. It refers to both an individual and collective sense of identity derived from historical and cultural group membership and related behaviors and beliefs. Obeyesekere (1982) makes a compelling argument for the situational nature of ethnic identity, in that it emerges most prominently under conditions of contact between groups and not as a within-group phenomena. A shared ethnic identity, with its explicit and implicit values, beliefs, and behaviors, may be considered a subculture within the larger shared culture.

It is important to recognize ethnic identity as something with both "solid" and "fluid" properties (Luborsky & Rubinstein, 1987, 1997). By this we mean that, on the one hand, there is something ideally unchanging or irreducible about ethnic identity, and yet, on the other hand, ethnic identity is situationally malleable. Thus, while ethnic identity exists as a trait that people have to differing degrees, it is not a fixed trait. Instead, it is sensitive to a variety of historic, social, cultural, personal, and life-span developmental events. At the individual and group levels, ethnic identity changes in different contexts and over time.

There is often confusion about the relationship between ethnic identity, religion, and family life. In one view, the family is the focal point of ethnic identity, because it is within the family that ethnic values and behaviors are transmitted. Ethnicity may serve as a language particular to psychological events and processes within families (Luborsky & Rubinstein, 1987; Friedman, 1982). Ethnic background and religion do not always coincide. Some religions and ethnic identities—for example Judaism—correspond, while others—for example Catholicism—may not. Our view, however, is that both family life and religion are themselves important manifestations of ethnic identity. While Catholicism may be equally important to Poles, Italians, and Irish, each of these ethnic groups manifests distinctive religious traditions and for members of each group, participation in religious activities may be an important expression of its own ethnic identity.

Social gerontologists and others who study old age and the elderly are increasingly aware of the relationship of ethnic identity to aging. Questions these scholars raise are crucial to understanding the aging process: Does membership in specific ethnic groups make the experience of old age different? How do age and ethnic identity intertwine in people's lives? How do older people use ethnic identity as a resource to cope with the stresses and strains of later life? Are there differences between ethnic groups in patterns of care for older people?

These are intriguing questions, but they are difficult to answer. One reason for the difficulty is that ethnic identity is built up from the interweaving of conscious and unconscious behaviors and beliefs. Thus, for example, a person may willfully behave in an ethnic way, as when choosing to attend an ethnic festival or when deliberately selecting ethnically appropriate food. But a person may also be unconscious of ethnic behavior, as in ethnically-distinctive reactions to the experience of pain (Zborowski, 1969). Likewise, an individual may consciously reject his or her ethnic group, but may retain ethnically-derived beliefs. Regardless of these conceptual difficulties, however, there is little doubt that ethnicity accounts for significant differences between people in a wide variety of life experiences including how they face physical pain (Zborowski, 1969), their concepts of illness (Suchman, 1964), variability in family configurations (Cohler & Grunebaum, 1981), the context of life crises and ritual (Myerhoff, 1978), beliefs about death (Kalish & Reynolds, 1976), and the patterning and meanings of alcohol consumption (Greeley, 1980), institutionalization (Markson, 1979), and mental illness (Jenkins, Kleinman, & Good, 1991; Kleinman, 1988). Students who are interested in learning more about ethnicity and aging in the United States should consult a recent publication on minority elderly as a starting point for further research (Gerontological Society of America, 1994). Several excellent examples of ethnographic studies of aging and ethnicity in the United States include Johnson's (1985) study of Italian-Americans, Ikels' (1983) study of Chinese in Hong Kong and Boston, and Myerhoff's (1978) study of a Jewish senior center.

Linking Culture and Individual Lives: Personhood, the Life Course, and Biography

Anthropologists have identified several "cultural units" that influence the experience of aging. These cultural units are recognizable elements in nearly every culture, yet there is a high degree of variability in the ways they are defined and evaluated cross-culturally. They are part of the shared, collective cultural repertoire and thus transcend the individual (Fry, 1990). In this section, we will discuss three cultural units with particular importance for understanding the linkages between culture as a collective and personal force that shapes the process of aging.

Personhood

The notion of a "person" is a cultural construct. It does not exist as a tangible entity in nature. The category of the "person" is found in all societies, but the identities and capacities that make it up are culture specific (Geertz, 1984; Hallowell, 1954; Shweder & Bourne, 1984). Personhood is bestowed by society and is earned by achieving and maintaining expected social roles and ideals. It is not an intrinsic property of the individual nor can it be seized merely by individual fiat (Fortes, 1984). By *person* we refer to the cultural category of adulthood or personhood. The term *individual* is used to refer to the concrete biological organism. Personhood is not an automatic or intrinsic property of the individual nor can it be gained by personal claim. It must be socially legitimated, that is, validated by other members of the community.

For example, in America when a baby leaves its mother's body at birth it is recognized as a person. We grant official places for babies as persons in society by assigning family and personal names, federal social security numbers, and legal rights (although these are exercised in proxy by the parents until legally defined adulthood is achieved). But we watch eagerly for babies to become more of "real" persons as they come to master the movement of their arms and legs, demonstrate awareness of people, and begin to speak. In American society full personhood is earned during the adult phase of the life course by being a responsible and (re)productive worker, spouse, family member, and community member. It is necessary to both achieve entry to and remain competent in these areas to have socially recognized full personhood. Individuals who are unemployed, disabled, or childless may be stigmatized and share a sense of not being a complete person.

Researchers are split as to whether, in theory, the category of full person is fixed once achieved or if it can be retracted. In the case of people with disabilities or the elderly, there appears to be evidence that it is diminished. Certain categories of persons are held in lower esteem and their legal and moral autonomy and recognition as self-determining individuals are bridged. These categories include, for example, people with dementia, physical disabilities that prevent communication, or people whose failure to uphold social norms and expectations results in moral and legal sanctions. In the later instances, citizens convicted of capital crimes and treasons are deprived of their liberty of free movement and free association by imprisonment or even death. Even though there is some distinction between those who willfully break social norms (thus the recent emergence of the "temporary insanity defense") and those whose physical condition stymies their ability to meet expected social behaviors, both are deprived of recognition as culturally competent and complete persons. It seems that in many cultures, elderly individuals who become frail and decrepit are no longer classified as full persons (cf. Barker, 1997). Understanding the dynamics and meanings underlying the loss of full personhood for frail elderly is an important step toward understanding the status and treatment of elderly cross-culturally (Luborsky, 1994).

The Life Course

The life course is another cultural unit that powerfully shapes the aging experience. Sociological studies of the life course have focused on the effects of social change on the life patterns of cohorts in historical context (Elder, 1985). In other words, the aggregate experiences of individuals in cohorts over time constitute the life course as conceptualized in sociology. In anthropology, the term life course has been used to refer to a shared, normative and cognitive model of life stages (Fry, 1990; Keith et al., 1994). This cultural life course is shaped by the aggregate of individual life patterns, but only loosely corresponds to them. In fact, it is not only a reflection of, but a model for individual life patterns. All cultures recognize the life course as a cultural unit, although there is a great deal of variability in the following: the salience of the life course as a meaningful construct for members of the culture, the uniformity or diversity in possible life course trajectories, the parameters of the life course (defined by age, achievements, capacities, etc), the number of stages in the life course, the ways individuals make transitions between life course stages, and the evaluation of various life course stages as better or worse times of life (Fry, 1990). Keith et al. (1994) used a research tool called the "Age Game" to systematically compare the life course in various settings. They found that a chronologically staged life course was not always meaningful, and that the interactions of demography, political economy, cohort experiences, patterns of social interaction, and subsistence activities had a great influence on concepts of the life course in different societies.

How do cultural definitions of the life course affect individual choices? Levine (1978) studied the relationships between individual and cultural life pathways among the present-day Gusii (a society in Africa) and eighteenth-century residents of Essex county, Massachusetts. His conceptual framework is a concise and insightful statement of the relationship between the collective and individual aspects of the life course: "the life course [consists of] pathways through the age-differentiated life span and subjective representations of it. These pathways embody both continuities and discontinuities for the individual, and their subjective representations can be collective or individual. The collective representations of the life course in cultural beliefs and values is a set of ideals that may not be realized but serve as standards against which individuals evaluate themselves" (Levine, 1978, pp. 289–290).

Bernice Neugarten's work on social age also explores how cultural values become norms for individual behavior. Fry claims that the life course is structured by social age. "[Age-salient] roles and the attributes they entail (e.g. such things as responsibilities) are markers punctuating the life course and rendering a social clock" (Fry, 1990, p. 139). These social clocks work only if individuals feel pressure to conform to the expectations of the cultural life course. As such, they are open to change. Finally, the notion of multiple "careers" suggests that social age may be assessed somewhat differently across various arenas of an individual's life, such as work, childrearing, or health. Thus, social age captures many of the complexities of the individual aging process that chronological age cannot.

The "expected life history" (ELH) is another interesting heuristic for understanding the links between the cultural life course and actual life patterns. The ELH is an "affectively weighted individual model of the generalized future," which is created through a dialectical, reflexive process that reshapes future expectations in light of the past and present (Seltzer & Troll, 1986, p. 758). The cultural life course, social age, and ELH all provide a shared timetable for evaluating how "on-time" or "off-time" an individual is with respect to age-appropriate life course stages from birth to death. For an individual, threats to a desirable ELH, or the sense of being "off-time" with respect to the normative life course, may result in psychological distress. In some cases, being "off-time" poses a threat to personhood, as in the example of a middle-aged adult who experiences the onset of disability in our culture.

Biography and Self-Representation

The previous discussion has illustrated that the process of aging involves individuals negotiating their lives with respect to cultural norms. This negotiation is perhaps most profoundly reflected in a person's ongoing construction of a life story of personal biography. This story is not only an individual creation, but also a culturally patterned template (Luborsky, 1993). Life stories, because they are stories, reflect and are evaluated according to cultural norms of what constitutes a good story. "The form of narrative is based on a socially shared expectation that stories should have a beginning, middle, and an end, in which the meaning of expective and eruptive life events is understood in terms of socially shared definitions" (Cohler, 1982, p. 205). Thus, the life story, like the life course, can be treated as a cultural unit. Individual variations in life stories certainly exist, but there is also a patterning in the ways in which stories are told (Luborsky, 1993).

The life story is highly flexible and often contradictory. Individuals generally have complex and somewhat conflicting self-representations, and the situations in which self-representations are evoked will have a significant impact on the stories people tell about themselves (Ewing, 1990). People do not usually experience these inconsistencies; rather they experience wholeness and continuity in their biography and self-representation. Such continuity in meaning is assumed to be a major goal of the self-representations of one's life, and a mechanism for preserving a sense of self in the face of life events and changing circumstances. Memories and the meaning of experiences are continually recognized to give meaning to the present and to frame the future (Luborsky & Rubinstein, 1987; Myerhoff, 1984; Cohler, 1982, 1991; Seltzer & Troll, 1986). In some situations, such as bereavement, disablement, or retirement, people can no longer maintain a sense of wholeness across different settings and are unable to ignore normally unproblematic inconsistencies in their self-representations. In response, people try to reorient and integrate their self-representations to create a renewed, more coherent sense of self. This process of narrative reorganization is both an individual and cultural act, in that an individual creatively draws on goals, symbols, and meanings, all of which are cultural phenomena, to recreate his or her life story.

The Case Study of a Kwakiutl Healer

A compelling example of the complex relationship between the normative and creative (Adams-Price, 1998) dimensions of culture over the life span is illustrated by the life of Quesalid, a male Native American of the Pacific Northwest Coast culture area (Levi-Strauss, 1968). His case illustrates how culture, community, and individual values and norms do not exist in isolation, but are deeply intertwined. It is difficult if not fruitless to attempt to understand them separately. Quesalid's life story also exemplifies how biographical meaning-making processes shape both the individual who makes meanings and the consequences of those meanings as they unfold over time in the community.

Quesalid lived in the early 1900s. His early childhood and adolescence followed the traditional pattern of statuses and life cycle transitions. But in early adulthood his life was redefined as he became skeptical of the implicit cultural suppositions that were used to rationalize the careers of socially important and renowned medical practitioners in the region. The outcome of his struggle to reshape the traditional life course into an individualized one was unpredictable. Rather than changing basic healing practices as he originally intended, he eventually came to reaffirm them.

As a young man he grew deeply critical of the healers who practiced the traditional "bloody cotton" form of healing. The family of a sick person would bring the patient to a healer who would diagnose the cause of the affliction. The central procedure in the curing ceremony occurred when the healer appeared to draw a wad of bloodied cotton from the person's body and held it aloft, revealing it as the embodied source of the disease. Quesalid sought to debunk this curing ceremony by revealing that is was merely a deft sleight of hand by the healers who produced a cotton wad they had previously hidden away. He dedicated himself to learning to be a healer to be able to discredit the teachers and practitioners. After completing his apprenticeship, Quesalid's practice grew and he was able to discredit other prominent healers. In the process he too became a renowned and powerful healer because his patients declared themselves healthy. Soon, using the traditional techniques, he cured cases that eluded the elderly experts. In the end he established a great reputation despite his disbelief in the healing techniques he practiced.

Quesalid's career illustrates how challenges to creativity emerge differently according to the situations in which an individual's intentions are negotiated. At its start he led a traditional life, but after questioning the basic assumptions underlying a fundamental healing practice in his society, he devoted himself to revealing it as a hoax. In the process he became a leading practitioner. He set out with a remarkably clear and simple agenda. Over time the course of the activities and meanings to his life biography yielded unforeseeable paths and outcomes.

To summarize, one important and little studied question is, what challenges are posed by the ways people work to construct a personally meaningful life narrative within the context of or in opposition to the parameters defined by a normative life course? The case of Quesalid can serve as a heuristic to help explore how the normative life course serves as an implicit category that structures the life story meaning-making process. The form and content of one's life story emerge from factors beyond those dictated by the objective events and specific circumstances of the lifetime. In studying the processes of biography and the life course, we must also consider a person's stance toward life events and intent in living and telling his or her biography. We can observe that the socially given normative life course can be either revitalized to reaffirm the person's sense of living a traditional life, or reorganized and transformed to express a sense of rebellion or nonconformity to the normative sequences and statuses in life.

Comparative Perspectives on Culture and Aging

A fundamental part of the anthropological perspective involves using a comparative approach to the study of human beings and their cultures. Comparisons across cultures and over time highlight commonalities and differences that are otherwise easily overlooked. Part of the reason that anthropologists shy away from making broad generalizations about human nature is because the comparative perspective prevents them from doing so. In this next section we will provide a broad, comparative introduction to some of the commonalities and differences in the aging experience that we hope will encourage you to further investigate the fascinating literature on aging in different cultures.

Historical and Cross-Cultural Variation in the Demography of Aging

In considering the demographic aspects of aging, one must remember that "old age" is a cultural construct that is defined by factors beyond the abstract numbers of chronological age. Who is considered old varies enormously both across cultures and within cultures over time. The definition of old age depends in part on how long people in a society tend to live. It may also be defined in social terms that are tied only loosely to chronological age, such as having grandchildren or achieving a certain position in the community. Nonetheless, demographic models are based on chronological age.

As a rule (and China is an important exception), developed and developing countries vary in the proportion of elderly in their populations. The demography of aging roughly corresponds to economic development (Albert & Cattell, 1994). In Table 3.1 three demographic measures related to aging—life expectancy, the proportion of the population under 15, and the proportion over 60—are presented for countries at different levels of economic development. European and other industrialized societies have undergone a demographic transition in which their population structure was transformed from having a high proportion of the population under the age of 15 to having relatively similar proportions of young, middle-aged, and elderly. This transition was caused by reductions in the rates of mortality and fertility, and was accompanied by population aging—an increase in the absolute number and proportion of elderly in society.

76 Luborsky and McMullen

National Life Expectancy and Percentage of the Population Under 15 Years and 60+
Years by Gender

Country and income level	Life expectancy at birth (years)		Total population age < 15 (%)	Total population age 60+ (%)	
	Male	Female		Male	Female
Low income					
China	68.2	71.7	26	9	10
Ethiopia	48.4	51.6	47	4	5
Nepal	57.6	57.1	43	5	5
Pakistan	62.9	69.0	42	5	5
Middle income					
Mexico	69.5	75.5	35	6	7
Papua New Guinea	57.2	58.7	39	5	5
High income					
Germany	73.4	79.9	16	17	25
Japan	76.9	82.9	16	19	23
Singapore	75.1	79.5	23	9	10
Sweden	76.2	80.8	19	19	24
United States	73.4	80.1	22	14	18

Sources: Sex & Age Annual 1950–2050 (1996 revision). New York: United Nations Statistical Division of the UN Secretariat; The World Bank (1993). *World Tables.* Baltimore, MD: The Johns Hopkins University Press.

   United Nations data from 1996 show that life expectancy at birth (the average number of years remaining in life) worldwide was 64 years. But the worldwide picture is more complex. Higher than average life expectancies are found in more developed countries, and lower than average life expectancies are found in less developed ones. It is important to keep in mind that life expectancy at birth is strongly influenced by infant mortality rates (Handwerker, 1990). In a country with high infant mortality rates, life expectancy at birth may be very low, but life expectancy at the age of 10 may compare more favorably with the global average. In other words, if life expectancy at birth is 35, as it is among the Ju/'hoansi of Botswana, this does not mean that few adults survive beyond the age of 35. Rather, it usually indicates high rates of infant mortality (Albert & Cattell, 1994).

Although population aging has largely been concentrated within the world's wealthiest countries, dramatic increases in the absolute number of elderly will occur in developing countries. In fact, this process is already underway. As Kinsella and Taeber (1992) note, "sixty percent of the increase in the world's elderly population occurs in developing countries." The global dynamics of population aging point to the importance of cross-cultural and anthropological research on aging for the international field of gerontology.

Ethnic or cultural diversity is also becoming increasingly important for gerontologists conducting research in the United States. Within the United States the proportion of elderly in immigrant and minority groups has and will continue to rise relative to nonimmigrant white elderly (Godziak, 1988; Angel & Hogan 1994). Most notably, these rates are expected to be the greatest among Hispanics (Markides, 1996).

In the next section we will sketch an overview of cross-cultural and historical variation in the status of the elderly. Examples are intended to be an introduction to the variety of aging experiences in other cultures. As mentioned earlier, one of the most valuable benefits of anthropology is that in learning how other people do things, you become equipped with the tools to ask new questions about and to find new solutions to the problems in your own society. Hopefully, thinking carefully about aging in other cultures will also provide you with new perspectives for understanding aging in our own society.

Studying Cross-Cultural Variation

One way of describing patterns of cross-cultural variation in anthropology is to examine a specific issue, such as the social status of the aged, by using archives designed for comparing data from a large number of societies. These archives are created when ethnographers deposit copies of their raw data and results from field expeditions around the world. Research that uses these archives as data is called *holocultural* research. This technique is best suited for research on worldwide and historical patterns of cultural variation. Holocultural studies of aging have suggested several key issues surrounding the status of the elderly cross-culturally. They have documented significant cross-cultural variations in elders' contribution to and control over cultural resources (religious, ritual, artistic, and subsistence skills), elders' political power, intergenerational relationships and exchanges of wealth, caregiving, and the treatment of infirm elderly (Simmons, 1945, 1960; Cowgill & Holmes, 1972; Palmore & Manton, 1974; Maxwell, Silverman, & Maxwell, 1982; McArdle & Yeracaris, 1981; Maxwell, 1980; Sheehan, 1976; Glascock & Fineman, 1980, 1981; Glascock, 1997). These major research topics, generated through holocultural research, have formed the basis of the field of anthropology and aging. For example, Simmons (1945) used a holocultural study to examine variations in the status of the elderly in so-called primitive societies. Drawing a sample of 71 societies, he systematically examined several dimensions across each culture. He proposed several cross-cultural universals in the aging experience, such as the desire to continue actively participating in social life, and pointed to productivity, political control, and integration in family life as determinants of well-being among the elderly.

While holocultural studies are extremely useful for hypothesis and theory building, they also have several important drawbacks. Since holocultural studies rely on existing research reports, they are limited by problems of data quality and the thoroughness of existing descriptions on the topic of study. Furthermore, holocultural studies compare traits, such as residence in extended households, without carefully examining the *cultural meaning, prevalence, and intragroup variation* in the practice of these traits. Consider for a moment the importance of intra-group variation. We can easily recognize that American elders live in a variety of different situations, have different emotional and financial support systems, and are neither uniformly happy nor dissatisfied in old age. Similarly, it is important to consider the diversity of aging experiences among elders in different cultures. We have to be careful not to present other cultures as uniform, cohesive societies. Other cultures are as complex as our own, and are equally subject to conflict, deviance, activism, and other forces of intracultural diversity.

Cross-Cultural Variability in the Aging Experience

We will briefly present several case studies to illustrate how culture affects the status and well-being of the elderly. This list illustrates key ideas. It is not a comprehensive account of cultural variability with respect to the aging experience, but is intended to give you a sense of just how different aging can be in different cultures.

Value Systems and the Experience of Aging: Independence and Dependency in the United States and China.   Cultural values about morality and the fundamental nature of social interactions have a significant impact on the experience of aging. As mentioned earlier, cultural values can present individuals with moral dilemmas as well as solutions as they go about life. The United States and China present striking contrasts in terms of cultural values surrounding independence, dependency, reciprocity and obligation. Margaret Clark (1972) vividly portrays the crisis of dependency experienced by many American elders who live in a culture that places extraordinarily high importance on individualism, independence, and self-sufficiency. Many elderly Americans prefer to live independently and resist dependency on their children for as long as possible (Albert & Cattell, 1994). As mentioned in our recurrent example of adult-onset disability, the reluctance to use adaptive devices to minimize the impact of physical impairments among many Americans may also be linked to the fundamental importance of independence as a criteria for full adult personhood in our culture (Luborsky, 1994).

Dependency, one of Americans' greatest fears, is not perceived as such a threat in other cultures. In China, positive values associated with reciprocity and dependency in old age present a stark contrast to American culture. Davis-Freedman (1991) writes that Chinese elderly are generally portrayed as "dependents in need of help and support." Both Americans and Chinese hope to delay the onset of health decline and dependency in old age, but Chinese culture provides for an easier transition into a dependent role. Old age is seen as a period of physical decline, yet elders seem to greet old age with acceptance and high self-esteem. Frailty is taken as an "unpleasant but inevitable" fact of life (Davis-Freedman, 1991, p. 13), and elders readily accept help without embarrassment. Several fundamental values help to buffer the negative aspects of aging for Chinese. First, all social interactions, and especially those among relatives, are grounded in an ethic of reciprocity and mutual obligation. Second, Confucianism places paramount importance on filial piety, the obligation of children to honor and obey their parents, to give priority to parents' needs while they are alive, and to honor them through elaborate funerals. Filial piety is closely related to the notion of reciprocity: parents provide all they can for their children, and, in return, children must do their best to repay their parents. Third, Daoism and Buddhism elevate the status of the elderly by emphasizing their veneration after death. Government ideology and programs have generally reinforced these traditional supports for the elderly (Davis-Freedman, 1991).

Kinship Systems and Elders' Living Arrangements. Living arrangements are of obvious importance to elders. Many of the most important issues in gerontology—caregiving, dependency, frailty, and social integration—are closely related to elders' living arrangements. To understand the cultural dynamics behind living arrangements, we also need to consider broader patterns of kinship as they affect family and household structure.

There is enormous cross-cultural variation in the ways that cultures define kinship. Kinship refers to the definition and classification of the relationships between individuals linked through biological descent and marital ties. One difference between kinship systems is whether the family unit is centered around the relationship between parents, children, and siblings, *or* between a husband and wife. Generally, these two types of kinship system result in different household composition. When the emphasis is placed on parent-to-child relationships, the preferred living arrangement tends to be extended households in which members of several generations, including siblings and their wives and children, live together. When the emphasis is placed on the relationship between husband and wife, each couple will prefer to set up their own household, resulting in nuclear households. For elders, as Ikels (1983, 1991) documents for elderly Chinese living in the United States and in China, living in an extended household may lead to several outcomes for elderly. It may

buffer the effects of disablement or dementia; it may also correspond to a position of seniority and control over household affairs and supportive intergenerational relationships. Alternatively, it may increase intergenerational conflict or result in an unwanted sense of dependency on one's children.

There is a trend worldwide for elders in developing countries to live in extended households, whereas elders in developed countries live on their own
or with a spouse (Albert & Cattell, 1994). From a cross-cultural perspective, a
remarkably low percentage of U.S. elderly co-reside with their children. Crimmins and Ingeneri (1990) report that only 18% of elders who have living children share households with a child. In fact, 31% of American elders live alone.
The proportion of elderly living alone in developed countries ranges enormously worldwide from under 9% in Japan to 40% in Sweden. In the developing nations of Southeast Asia, Latin America, and Africa the proportion of
elderly living alone is generally below 10% (Albert & Cattell, 1994).

Cross-cultural studies of kinship and living arrangements suggest two important qualifications to these global trends. First, household structure does
not have a consistent relationship with elders' position within families (Martin, 1990; Goldstein, Schuler, & Ross, 1983). A second qualification to industri-
alized/nonindustrialized residence patterns is that elders' living arrangements
are determined by a complex interaction of economic, emotional, and ideo-
logical forces that differs between and within cultures (Palmore & Maeda, 1985).
Interviews with elder Hindus in an urban area of Nepal did not find that living in an extended household was a guarantee of economic security. Elders
were very anxious about handing over control of household affairs to the
younger generation, and complained that they were given no money of their
own out of the household income. These concerns were highly evident despite
religious and cultural ideals that encourage younger household members to
support their elder parents. Researchers noted that "Several elderly respondents actually commented that they were like strangers in their own family;
no one talked to them or paid them any attention. They were taken care of, but
only in a manner they perceived as both demeaning and alienating" (Goldstein
et al., 1983, p. 720).

Those examples illustrate the problems of assuming a direct link between
household structure and elders' status. Careful, qualitative studies of household relations should be used in conjunction with quantitative census data on
living arrangements. Doing so provides a richer understanding of the impact
that living arrangements have on the elderly.

Succession to Seniority: Power and Resource Control.   An important aspect
of aging and intergenerational relationships surrounds issues of power and resource control. Anthropologists have pointed to two important and interrelated
questions regarding what happens when people reach the stage in life that is
defined as "old age" (and this is defined differently cross-culturally). First,
when people reach old age, how much control do they have over economic
and cultural resources (religious, ritual, artistic, and subsistence skills)? Sec-

ond, what political power and authority is reserved for elders in family and public roles?

In many agricultural and pastoral societies, positions of power and authority are specifically designated for elders (Halperin, 1984). Lowell and Eleanor Holmes present the case of Samoan elders, who are highly esteemed community members and are expected to hold important political and religious positions in their society (Holmes & Holmes, 1995). Before World War II, Samoans were relatively isolated from American and other Western influences. They lived in small villages and farmed a variety of food plants, raised chickens and pigs, and supplemented their diet with deep-sea and reef fishing. Old age in Samoa was not defined by chronological age, but by the inability to perform strenuous agricultural or domestic work. Old age was seen as a positive stage of life, with time for relaxation and socializing. Elders lived within extended households numbering between 8 and 12 people. Many elderly men, and occasionally elderly women, were elected by their extended families to positions of political authority called *matai*, or other religious positions. *Matai* served on village-level councils and were widely respected in their community. While *matai* were predominantly male, many elderly women were members of a parallel, women's village council. Women also filled significant religious positions. The association between the position of *matai* and old age was so strong that when a middle-aged man was elected to the position, he was expected to behave like an old man. Old age, in this case, was defined by status and roles, not by chronology. Consider the following statement from a *matai* who was not chronologically old:

> Always I must act as if I were old. I must walk gravely and with measured step . . . Old men of sixty are my companions and watch my every word, lest I make a mistake. Thirty-one people live in my household. For them I must plan. I must find food and clothing, settle their disputes, arrange their marriages. There is no one in my whole family who dares to scold me or even to address me familiarly by my first name. It is hard to be so young and yet to be a chief. (Mead 1928, p. 36, as cited in Holmes & Holmes, 1995, p. 162)

Gender Differences in Succession to Seniority.   Gender, along with age, is one of the most important axes along which power and prestige are culturally patterned. In traditional Hindu culture, gender analysis is critical for understanding elders' control over resources. As a rule, upper-caste Hindu men are highly esteemed in old age. They have several sources of power, whereas elderly women, who are often widows, are considered dangerous and impure, and have few sources of power or influence. As heads of households in a strongly patriarchal society, elderly men have power over their wives and descendants. Male elders in influential families also exercise considerable political power on a local level. Elders who no longer manage their households have other avenues of prestige, since old age is also widely recognized and respected as a time for religious devotion (Vatuk, 1980). Elderly women, on the other hand, are in a more precarious situation as they age. As long as their husbands are heads of households, older women in Indian society actively manage the domestic affairs of the household. Widows, on the other hand, face a precarious situation in old age.

Traditionally upper-caste Hindu women could achieve power only through their connections with male relatives—their husbands, brothers, or sons. In old age, many of these connections are severed through death or the division of extended households. The Indian example points to the significance of gender in shaping the experience of old age cross-culturally. In contrast to Hindu society, the status of the elderly men and women is relatively undifferentiated in many groups. Among the Samoans and the Hausa of Nigeria (Coles, 1990), men and women each have separate avenues for power and prestige in old age.

Death-Hastening Practices and Elder Neglect.   When we learn that in some places, the elderly have regularly been buried alive, stabbed to death by their eldest son, or left in a cave to die, these acts seem almost incomprehensible. In fact, they may represent our deepest fears. However, such death-hastening behaviors are embedded within specific cultural contexts that lend them meaning and justification (Glascock, 1997). Anthropological research on death-hastening behaviors has pointed to several generalizations about the practice. The presence of death-hastening behaviors in a given culture does not mean that its elderly have low status or are generally neglected. In fact, death hastening occurs when elders pass from a life-course stage that corresponds to healthy, intact old age into a final stage of life variously understood as decrepitude. This transition is marked by changes in the elder's family and social relationships, and in some cases by changes in the relationship of the elder to the supernatural world (Barker, 1997; Glascock, 1997).

Second, death hastening tends to occur as an option of last resort among technologically simple societies in harsh environments, societies that are mobile, and societies that face periodic food shortages (Halperin, 1984). In most foraging and nomadic societies, an abundant food supply, egalitarianism, and a strong ethic of sharing generally ensure that elders' needs are provided for even when they are no longer able to collect their own food. Elders are also respected and valuable members of society because they possess a lifetime of knowledge about religion, ritual, and many skills necessary for survival. However, Halperin (1984) suggests that in resource-scarce environments such as the Arctic, or during periods of drought or famine, elders and young children can place a serious burden on the rest of their group. These situations have led to neglect or abandonment among foraging groups including the Arctic Eskimos and the Tiwi of Australia (Guemple, 1987; Hart & Pilling, 1961).

However, not all foraging societies abandon their elderly, as the following example will show. The Ju/'hoansi of Botswana and Namibia (who are also known as the San or !Kung) are a well-studied foraging group whose elders frequently complain about abuse and neglect by caregivers. Without understanding the cultural context of such complaints, it would be easy as an outsider to accept that the harsh environment of the Kalahari Desert can lead to death-hastening or neglectful behaviors toward elders. However, Ju/'hoansi culture strongly emphasizes egalitarianism and reciprocity. Elders feel a strong sense of entitlement to be cared for, and caregiving is organized in such a way to provide an ample supply of caregivers to elders (Rosenberg, 1997). Decades of fieldwork among the Ju/'hoansi have failed to corroborate reports by elders that they are often neglected and mistreated.

How can we understand elders frequent complaints of neglect, then? Rosenberg (1997) found that complaining is a standard form of discourse among the Ju/'hoansi. Complaining about being neglected is a way for Ju/'hoansi elders to exert pressure on their caregivers and to ensure that they will not be neglected. It is a culturally patterned way of talking that resembles a performance. We should not take this example to generalize that in other cultures complaints about elder neglect are unfounded. Rather, Rosenberg's work (1997) is a wonderful illustration of the need to consider the specific context of a given aspect of a culture in order to understand its meaning.

Modernization Theory and Culture Change over Time

Earlier we mentioned that the demographics of global aging are closely linked with economic development. It is no surprise, then, that modernization theory, which attempts to explain patterns of economic and social development, has been one of the most important frameworks for explaining the patterning of cross-cultural variation in the status of the elderly. Modernization theories have been used to explain changes in many areas of society, including individual psychology, social institutions, economic production, and family structure. In fact, the concept of modernization as a force of change can be traced back to the very beginnings of social science (Cowgill, 1986).

In an attempt to explain the relationship between modernization and the status of the elderly, Cowgill and Holmes (1972) selected 15 societies, each corresponding to what they defined as different levels of modernization (from preliterate, to peasant, to industrial societies). Their hypothesis that the status of elders would decline with the degree of modernization was generally confirmed, and their study marked the beginning of a heated debate among anthropologists over the definition of modernization and its impact on the status of the elderly. Cowgill (1974) proposed four central aspects of modernization that threaten the position of the elderly: modern health technology, modern economic technology, urbanization, and education. Building on Cowgill and Holmes' original study, Holmes and Holmes (1995) summarized 10 key propositions regarding the relationship between modernization and aging. These are listed in Table 3.2.

It is impossible to summarize the vast writing in support and in critique of modernization theory in this chapter, but we will present three crucial short-

TABLE 3.2.
Proposed Relationships between Modernization and Aging

---

1. "The concept of old age itself appears to be relative to the degree of modernization."

2. "Longevity is directly and significantly related to the degree of modernization."

3. "Modernized societies have a relatively high proportion of old people in their populations."

4. "The aged are the recipients of greater respect in societies where they constitute a low proportion of the total population."

5. "Societies that are in the process of modernizing tend to favor the young, while the aged are at an advantage in more stable, sedentary societies."

6. "Respect for the aged tends to be greater in societies in which the extended family is prevalent, particularly if it functions as the household unit." [The implication here is that modernization breaks down the extended family.]

7. "In nonindustrial societies the family is the basis social group providing economic security for dependent aged, but in industrial ones the responsibility tends to be partially or totally that of the state."

8. "The proportion of aged who retain leadership roles in modern societies is lower than in industrial ones."

9. "Religious leadership is more likely to be a continuing role of the aged in preindustrial than in modern societies."

10. "Retirement is a modern invention found only in modernized, high-productivity societies."

Adapted from Holmes and Holmes (1995, pp. 257–270).

comings of this model. Students are referred to several excellent and accessible review of this literature for more detail (Cowgill, 1986; Foner, 1984; Holmes & Holmes, 1995).

One of the most important critiques of modernization has come from a historical perspective. Fischer (1978), Laslett (1976), Nydegger (1983), and Quadango (1982) have all argued that modernization theory presents a nostalgic view of the past as a "golden age" for the elderly, a view that is out of touch with the facts. Recent work in historical demography has made important strides toward a more accurate and nuanced account of intergenerational relationships in the past (Hareven, 1996; Kertzer & Laslet, 1995). For example, careful studies of family composition and household structure in India have refuted claims that Indian society is moving from "traditional" extended households to "modern" nuclear ones (Biswas, 1985; Martin, 1990). Changes in Indian family structure are much more complex and heterogeneous to be accounted for in a linear model such as modernization theory. In fact, long-term community-based research in a North Indian village has documented that an increase in extended households has corresponded to improvements in health and expanding economic opportunities—the very factors that modernization theory predicts would bring the demise of extended households (Wadley & Derr, 1993).

A second critique of modernization theory points to the problems of classifying societies according to a scale of modernization. There are serious conceptual flaws in a theory that ranks present-day societies according to their degree of modernization, because doing so implies an evolutionary trajectory of social development. The modernization framework explicitly assumes an evolutionary trajectory from "traditional" to "modern" society, categories that are extremely problematic considering the legacy of social Darwinism, colonialism, and imperialism. We have to be very cautious not to use the experience of present-day foragers, horticultural, or peasant societies to make inferences about our past. Current anthropology does not view societies with simple economic subsistence strategies as any less "modern" or "developed" than our own. Rather, the variations in social and economic systems found cross-culturally have more to do with particular differences in historical, political, and ecological transformations over time than with any sweeping evolutionary force. There are obvious methodological difficulties in using cross-sectional data to generalize about long-term historical processes.

A third critique emphasizes the fact that modernization does not replace historically situated and deeply entrenched cultural institutions with a new, generic "modern" culture. The process of culture change often involves the incorporation of new cultural practices, values, and institutions, but these are always articulated against existing cultural forms. "Modernity" in Hong Kong, for example, may be constructed very differently then "modernity" in Great Britain. Studies on the impact of early industrialization on intergenerational family dynamics from these two settings reveal that despite similarities in the process of industrialization, family in Great Britain and Hong Kong experienced economic change very differently. Whereas in Hong Kong industrialization reinforced notions of filial piety by enabling unmarried daughters to provide support for their parents (Ikels, 1983), the situation in Great Britain produced the opposite effect (Tilly & Scott, 1978). These differences result from antecedent cultural traditions, global and local political–economic forces, as well as responses to and interpretations of change.

Conclusion

In this chapter we have provided you with some of the basic tools and concepts that are used to study the cultural context of aging. We have presented examples that hopefully will challenge you as novice anthropologists to adopt an anthropological perspective on the social problems and moral dilemmas that you will study and encounter throughout your careers. Some of these examples, such as death hastening, can raise deeply felt emotional and moral reactions—for the actors involved, the ethnographers who observe and interpret their actions, and the readers of ethnographers' reports. These layers of interpretation, and even confusion, are what culture is all about. The challenge as an anthropologist is to take a stance of cultural relativism, to stubbornly critique your own assumptions about the way things work, and to try to understand other cultures from the perspectives of their members. In doing so, you often learn new ways of seeing your own culture as well.

REVIEW QUESTIONS

1. How is culture defined and conceptualized in the chapter?

2. What are some of the challenges that culture can place on individuals in the process of aging?

3. Define the terms ethnocentrism and cultural relativism. Provide examples of each from throughout the chapter.

4. What do we mean by taking an *anthropological perspective* on aging? Identify several aspects of an anthropological perspective on aging.

5. Try to outline the normative life course in your own culture, specifying the various stages, criteria for each stage, and transitions between stages. Has the normative life course been a force shaping your own personal biography and decision making?

References

Achenbaum, A. (1978). *Old age in the new land: The American experience since 1970.* Baltimore: Johns Hopkins Press.

Adams-Price, C. (1998). *Aging and creativity: Theoretical and empirical approaches.* New York: Springer.

Albert, S. M., & Cattell, M. G. (1994). *Old age in global perspective: Cross-cultural and cross-national views.* New York: G. K. Hall.

Angel, J., & Hogan, D. (1994). The demography of minority aging populations. In *Minority elders: Five goals toward building a public policy base* (2nd ed.). Washington, DC: Gerontological Society of America.

Barker, J. (1997). Between humans and ghosts: The decrepit elderly in a Polynesian society In J. Sokolovsky (Ed.), *The cultural context of aging* (pp. 407–424). New York: Bergin and Garvey.

Becker, G., & Kaufman, S. (1988). Old age, rehabilitation, and research: A review of the issues. *Gerontologist, 28(4),* 459–468.

Biswas, S. K. (1985). Dependency and family care of the aged in village India: A case study. *Journal of the Indian Anthropological Society, 20,* 238–257.

Cavanaugh, J., & Whitbourne, S. (1998). *Gerontology: Interdisciplinary perspectives,* New York: Oxford University Press.

Clark, M. (1972). An anthropological view of retirement. In F. Carp (Ed.), *Retirement* (pp. 117–156). New York: Human Sciences Press.

Cohler, B. (1982). Personal narratives and life course. In P. B. Baltes & O. G. Brim (Eds.), *Life-span development and behavior* (vol. 4, pp. 205–234). New York: Academic Press.

Cohler, B. (1991). The life story and the study of resilience and response to adversity. *Journal of Life History avid Narrative, 1(2 & 3),* 169–200.

Cohler, B., & Grunebaum, H. (1981). *Mothers, grandmothers and daughters: Personality and child care in three generation families.* New York: Wiley.

Coles, C. (1990). The older woman in Hausa society: Power and authority in urban Nigeria. In J. Sokolovsky (Ed.), *The cultural context of aging: Worldwide perspectives* (pp. 57–82). Westport, CT: Bergen & Garvey.

Cowgill, D. O. (1974). Aging and modernization: A revision of the theory. In J. F. Gubrium (Ed.), *Late life: Communities and environmental policy* (pp. 123–146). Springfield, IL: Charles C Thomas.

Cowgill, D. O. (1986). *Aging around the world.* Belmont, CA: Wadsworth.

Cowgill, D. O., & Holmes L. D. (1972). *Aging and modernization.* New York: Appleton-Century-Crofts.

Crimmins, E. M., & Ingeneri, D. G. (1990). Interaction and living arrangements of older parents and their children. *Research on Aging, 12,* 3–35.

Davis-Freedman, D. (1991). *Long lives: Chinese elderly and the Communist revolution.* Stanford: Stanford University Press.

Elder, G. (1985). *Life course dynamics: Trajectories and transitions, 1968–1980.* Ithaca, NY: Cornell University Press.

Ewing, K. (1990). The illusion of wholeness: Culture, self and the experience of inconsistency. *Ethos, 18(3),* 251–278.

Fischer, D. H. (1978). *Growing old in America.* New York: Oxford University Press.

Foner, N. (1984). *Ages in conflict: A cross-cultural perspective on inequality between old and young.* New York: Columbia University Press.

Fortes, M. (1984). Age, generation, and social structure. In D. Kertzer & J. Keith (Eds.), *Age and anthropological theory* (pp. 99–122). Ithaca, NY: Cornell University Press.

Friedman, E. (1982). The myth of the shiksa. In M. McGoldrick, J. Pearce, & J. Giordano (Eds.), *Ethnicity and family therapy.* New York: Guilford.

Fry, C. (1990). The life course in context: Implications for comparative research. In R. Rubinstein (Ed.), *Anthropology and aging: Comprehensive reviews.* Boston: Kluwer Academic Publishers.

Geertz, C. (1984). Anti-anti relativism. *American Anthropologist, 86(2),* 263–277.

Gerontological Society of America. (1994). *Minority elders: Five goals toward building a Public Policy Base* (2nd ed.). Washington, DC: Gerontological Society of America.

Gilligan, C. (1982). *In a different voice: Psychological theory and women's development.* Cambridge, MA: Harvard University Press.

Glascock, A., & Fineman, S. (1981). Social asset or social burden: Treatment of the aged in non-industrial societies. In C. L. Fry (Ed.), *Dimensions: Aging, culture, and health.* New York: J. F. Bergin.

Glascock, A. (1997). When is killing acceptable: The moral dilemma surrounding assisted suicide in America and other societies. In J. Sokolovsky (Ed.), *The cultural context of aging: Worldwide perspectives* (pp. 56–70). New York: Bergin & Garvey.

Glascock, A., Fineman, S. (1980). A holocultural analysis of old age. *Comparative Social Research, 3,* 311–333.

Godziak, E. (1988). *Older refugees in the United States: From dignity to despair.* Washington, DC: Refugee Policy Group.

Goldstein, M. C., Schuler, S., & Ross, J. L. (1983). Social and economic forces affecting intergenerational relations in extended families in a third world country: A cautionary tale from South Asia. *Journal of Gerontology, 38(6)*, 716–724.

Greeley, H. (1980). *Ethnic drinking subcultures*. Brooklyn: J. F. Bergin.

Guemple, L. (1987). Growing old in Inuit society. In J. Sokolovsky (Ed.), *Growing old in different societies; Cross cultural perspectives*. Acton, MA: Copley.

Hallowell, I. (1954). *Culture and experience*. Philadelphia: University of Pennsylvania.

Halperin, R. (1984). Age in cultural economics: An evolutionary approach. In D. Kertzer & J. Keith (Eds.), *Age and anthropological theory* (pp. 159–194). Ithaca, NY: Cornell University Press.

Handwerker, W. P., (1990). Demography. In T. M. Johnson & F. Sargent (Eds.), *Medical anthropology: Contemporary method and theory* (pp. 319–348). Westport, CT: Praeger.

Hareven, T. (1996). *Aging and generational relations over the life course: A historical and cross cultural perspective*. Berlin: Walter de Gruyter.

Hart, C., & Pilling, A. (1961). *The Tiwi of North Australia*. New York: Holt, Reinhart & Winston.

Holmes, E. R., & Holmes, L. (1995). *Other cultures, elder years*. Thousand Oaks, CA: Sage.

Ikels, C. (1983). *Aging and adaptation: Chinese in Hong-Kong and the United States*. Hamden, CT: Archon.

Ikels, C. (1991). Aging and disability in China: Cultural issues in measurement and interpretation. *Social Science and Medicine, 32(6)*, 649–655.

Jenkins, J. H., Kleinman, A., & Good, B. (1991). Cross-cultural aspects of depression: Introduction. In A. Kleinman & J. Becker (Eds.), *Psychosocial aspects of depression* (pp. 67–97). Hillsdale, NJ: Lawrence Erlbaum.

Johnson, C. (1985). *Growing up and growing old in Italian-American families*. New Brunswick, NJ: Rutgers University Press.

Kalish, R. & Reynolds. (1976). *Death and ethnicity: A psychocultural study*. Los Angeles: Ethel Percy Andrus Gerontology Center, University of Southern California.

Keith, J., Fry, C., Glascock, A. P., Ikels, C., Dickerson-Putman, J., Harpending, H. C., & Draper, P. (1994). *The aging experience: Diversity and commonality across cultures*. Thousand Oaks, CA: Sage.

Kertzer, D., & Laslet, P. (1995). *Aging in the past: Demography, society, and old age*. Berkeley, CA: University of California Press.

Kinsella, K., & Taeber, C. (1992). *An aging world II*. Washington, DC: U. S. Bureau of the Census, International Population Reports.

Kleinman, A. (1988). *Rethinking psychiatry*. New York: Free Press.

Laslett, P. (1976). Social development and aging. In R. Binstock & E. Shanas (Eds.), *Handbook of aging and the social sciences*. New York: Van Nostrand Reinhold.

Levi-Strauss, C. (1968). *Structural anthropology*. Paris: Ecole Etude.

Levine, R. (1987). Comparative notes on the life course. In T. Haraven (Ed.), *Transitions: The family and the life course in historical perspective*. New York: Academic Press.

Luborsky, M. R. (1993). The romance with personal meaning in gerontology: Cultural aspects of life themes. *The Gerontologist, 33(4)*, 445–452.

Luborsky, M. (1994). The cultural adversity of physical disability: Erosion of full adult personhood. *Journal of Aging Studies, 8(3)*, 239–253.

Luborsky, M., & Rubinstein, R. (1987). Ethnicity and lifetimes: Self-concepts and situational contexts of ethnic identity in late life. In D. Gelfand & C. Barresi (Eds.), *Ethnic dimensions of aging* pp. 35–50. New York: Springer.

Luborsky, M., & Rubinstein, R. (1997). The dynamics of ethnic identity in elderly widowers' reactions to bereavement. In J. Sokolovsky (Ed.), *The cultural context of aging: Worldwide perspectives* (pp. 304–315). New York: Bergin & Garvey.

Luborsky, M., & Sankar, A. (1993). Extending the critical gerontology perspective: Cultural dimensions. *The Gerontologist, 33(4),* 440–444.

Markides, K. (1996). Race, ethnicity, and aging: Impact of inequality. In R. Binstock & L. George (Eds.), *Handbook of aging and social sciences* (4th ed.). New York: Academic Press.

Markson, E. (1979). Ethnicity as a factor in the institutionalization of the elderly. In D. Gelfand & A. Kutzik (Eds.), *Ethnicity and aging: Theory, research, and policy* (pp. 341–356). New York: Springer.

Martin, L. G. (1990). The status of South Asia's growing elderly population. *Journal of Cross Cultural Gerontology, 5,* 93–117.

Maxwell, R. (1980). Contempt for the elderly: A cross-cultural analysis. *Current Anthropology, 24,* 569–570.

Maxwell, R., Silverman, P., & Maxwell, E. (1982). The motive for gerontocide. *Studies in Third World Societies, 22,* 67–84.

McArdle, J., & Yeracaris, C. (1981). Respect for elderly in preindustrial societies as related to their activity. *Behavior Science Research, 16(3/4),* 307–339.

Mead, M. (1928). *Coming of age in Samoa.* New York: William Morrow.

Myerhoff, B. G. (1978). *Number our days.* New York: Dutton.

Myerhoff, B. G. (1984). Rites and signs of ripening: The intertwinig of ritual, time and growing older. In D. Kertzer & J. Keith (Eds.), *Age and anthropological theory* (pp. 305–330). Ithaca, NY: Cornell University Press.

Nydegger, C. (1983). Family ties of the aged in cross-cultural perspective. *The Gerontologist, 23,* 26–32.

Obeyesekere, G. (1982). Sinhalese-Budhist identity in Ceylon. In G. DeVos & L. Romanucci-Ross (Eds.), *Ethnic identity: Cultural continuities and change.* Chicago: University of Chicago Press.

Palmore, E. B., & Maeda, D. (1985). *The honorable elders: A cross-cultural study of aging in Japan.* Durham, NC: Duke University Press.

Palmore, E. B., & Manton, K. M. (1974). Modernization and status of the aged: International correlations. *Journal of Gerontology, 29(2),* 205–210.

Quadango, J. (1982). *Aging in early industrial society.* New York: Academic Press.

Rosenberg, H. G. (1997). Complaint discourse, aging, and caregiving among the Ju/'hoansi of Botswana. In J. Sokolovksy (Ed.), *The cultural context of aging: Worldwide perspectives* (pp. 33–55). New York: Bergin & Garvey.

Rosow, I. (1974). *Socialization to old age.* Berkeley, CA: University of California Press.

Rowe, J., & Kahn, J. (1989). *Successful aging.* New York: Pantheon Books.

Seltzer, M., & Troll, L. (1986). Expected life history, a model in nonlinear time. *American Behavioral Scientist,* 746–764.

Sheehan, T. (1976). Senior esteem as a factor of socioeconomic complexity. *The Gerontologist, 16,* 433–440.

Shweder, R., & Bourne, E. (1984). Does the concept of person vary cross-culturally? In R. Shweder & R. LeVine (Eds.), *Culture theory: Essays on mind, self, and emotion* New York: Cambridge University Press.

Simmons, L. (1945). *The role of the aged in primitive society.* New Haven, CT: Yale University Press.

Simmons, L. (1960). Aging in pre-industrial societies. In C. Tibbits (Ed.), *Handbook of so-cial gerontology* (pp. 62–91). Chicago: University of Chicago Press.

Suchman, E. (1964). Sociomedical variations among ethnic groups. *American Journal of Sociology 70*, 328–329.

Tannen, D. (1989). *Talking voices. Repetition, dialogue, and imagery in conversational dia-logue.* Cambridge: Cambridge University Press.

Tilly, L., & Scott, J. (1978). *Women, work and family.* New York: Holt, Reinhart & Win-ston.

Vatuk, S. (1980). Withdrawal and disengagement as a cultural response to aging in In-dia. In C. L. Fry (Ed.), *Aging in culture and society: Comparative viewpoints and strate-gies* (pp. 126–148). New York: Praeger.

Wadley, S., & Derr, B. (1993). Karimpur families over sixty years. In P. Uberoi (Ed.), *Family, kinship and marriage in India.* New York: Oxford University Press.

Zborowski, M. (1969). *People in pain.* San Francisco: Jossey-Bass.

4

Physical Changes

Susan Krauss Whitbourne

Physical Aging

The physical aging process occurs against a backdrop of a lifetime of accumulated experiences in which the individual has come to know and understand the functioning and appearance of his or her unique body. In this chapter, the most significant age-related changes in physical functioning will be summarized and analyzed in terms of their impact on the individual's sense of self. The concept of "physical identity" as used here refers to the individual's self-perception of the body's appearance, competence, and limitations. A model of the aging of physical identity will be presented that will form the backdrop for a discussion of age-related changes in specific areas of functioning. Implications for health professionals will also be discussed in the context of these changes.

After reading this chapter, it should be clear that the physical changes associated with the aging process are complex, multifaceted, and multidirectional. Individuals age in their own unique ways, due to their genetic inheritance and life-style choices. Of particular importance is the necessity of distinguishing between the processes of normal aging and alterations in functioning that are the result of specific diseases. Although it is true that older individuals are at heightened risk of developing chronic health problems such as arthritis, cardiovascular disease, cancer, and diabetes, these are diseases rather than normal age-related changes. Clinicians should be aware that they need to persist in the treatment of an elderly client rather than assume that the symptoms of chronic disease represent inevitable losses due to aging.

The Multiple Threshold Model of Physical Aging and Identity

The aging process is a constant challenge to the maintenance of a stable sense of identity over time. The multiple threshold model of aging (Whitbourne,

1996b) relates age changes to identity, coping processes, adaptational outcomes, and age-related control behaviors. The term "threshold" in this model refers to the point at which an age-related change is recognized by the individual. Before this threshold is reached, the individual does not think of the self as "aging" or "old," or even perhaps as having the real potential to be "aging" or "old." After crossing the threshold, the individual recognizes the possibility that functions may be lost through aging (or disease) and begins to adapt to this possibility by changing identity accordingly (see Figure 4.1).

The term "multiple" in this model refers to the fact that the aging process involves potentially every system in the body, so that there is in actuality no single threshold leading into the view of the self as aging. The individual may feel "old" in one domain of functioning, such as in the area of mobility, but feel "not old," "middle-aged," or possibly "young" in other domains, such as in the area of sensory acuity or intellectual functioning. Whether a threshold is crossed depends in part on the actual nature of the aging process and whether it has affected a particular area of functioning. However, it is also the case that individuals vary widely in the areas of functioning that they value. Mobility may not be as important to an individual whose major source of pleasure is derived from sedentary reading activities. Changes in the area of mobility will not have as much relevance to the individual's direct adaptation to the environment or to identity as would be the case for losses in vision or memory. In the multiple threshold model, it is assumed that changes in areas important to adaptation and competence have the greatest potential for affecting identity. It is further assumed that individuals vary in their ability to integrate the crossing of a threshold into their physical identities and that some individuals respond by overreacting and others by minimization or denial of the particular

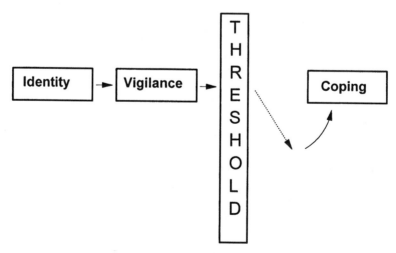

Figure 4.1. A multiple threshold model of identity and physical aging.

age change. Ideally, the individual is able to reach a point of having incorporated knowledge of the aging change into identity in a flexible and adaptive manner.

Effects of Age on Appearance and Mobility

Skin

Age Changes. A variety of changes contribute to the phenomena of wrinkling and sagging, the most apparent age-related effects on the skin. The epidermis, the outer layer of the skin, becomes flattened, and cells in the epidermis form less organized patterns. These changes at the microscopic level are reflected in geometric furrows on the skin's surface. Many changes in the skin's appearance and structure can be explained by photoaging—exposure to the ultraviolet rays of the sun (Takema, Yorimoto, Kawai, & Imokawa, 1994; Yang, Lee, & Wei, 1995). Throughout the body, wrinkling and sagging occur due to decreases in collagen (Kligman, Grove, & Balin, 1985) and the increasing brittleness of elastin. The subcutaneous fat on the limbs decreases, and there is a decrease in muscle mass, further adding to the loss of firmness in the skin's appearance.

There are also significant changes in the sweat and oil-producing glands that maintain body temperature and lubricate the skin surface (Kurban & Bhawan, 1990). The skin becomes rougher, dryer, and more vulnerable to surface damage. These changes lead to medical problems such as dermatitis, pruritis (excessive itching), and general discomfort (Kligman, 1989). Age-related alterations also occur in the coloring of the skin. There are fewer melanocytes, and those that remain develop irregular areas of dark pigmentation. Under the skin surface, capillaries and small arteries become dilated, creating small irregular colored lines.

Psychological Implications. For many individuals, particularly in middle age (Whitbourne, 1996b), age changes in the skin that lead to wrinkling are very noticeable and can have an impact on the individual's identity. In particular, comparisons of present appearance with pictures or memories of early adulthood can cause unhappiness in older people who valued their youthful image (Kleinsmith & Perricone, 1989). Age-related changes in the skin and supporting tissues alter the skin's protective functions as well as its appearance. Even if the individual is not particularly concerned about the effects of age on appearance, these changes in comfort level can trigger the crossing of an aging threshold.

There are many steps that older individuals can take to slow or compensate for aging of the skin. First and foremost, fair-skinned people should avoid direct exposure to the sun and use sunblocks when they cannot avoid exposure (Gilchrest, 1989). To counteract the fragility, sensitivity, and dryness of the skin, the individual can use sunscreens, emollients, and fragrance-free cosmetics (Ditre et al., 1996). Although there is considerable skepticism in the academic community toward the bold claims of facial care advertisers, there is some supportive evidence emerging for these treatments, including facial massage and vitamin E (Iida & Noro, 1995; Nachbar & Korting, 1995).

Hair

Age Changes. With increasing age, the hair on the head and body loses pigmentation and takes on a white appearance due to a decrease in melanin production in the hair follicles. The rate at which hair color changes varies from person to person due to variations in the timing of onset and rate of melanin production decrease across the surface of the scalp.

Gradual and general thinning of scalp hair occurs in both sexes over adulthood. Hair loss results from destruction or regression of the germ centers that produce the hair follicles underneath the skin surface. Men may also experience thinning of the hairs in their whiskers and a growth of coarse hair on the eyebrows and inside the ear. Patches of coarse terminal hair may develop on the face in women, particularly around the chin.

Psychological Implications. As is true for wrinkles, the threshold for age-related changes in the hair, at least for graying, appears to be crossed at some point in the 30s or 40s (Whitbourne, 1996b). Unlike wrinkles, gray hairs can be returned to virtually their original state through the use of hair dye. Changes in hair thickness, however, are not so easily reversed. The desire to disguise or stop the apparent signs of aging through surgery or the wearing of hairpieces is widespread, as is evident in the many advertisements for hair loss replacement.

Body Build

Age Changes. Over the course of adulthood standing height is reduced, occurring at a greater rate after the 50s; this is particularly pronounced in women (de Groot, Perdigao, & Deurenberg, 1996). The major cause is loss of bone mineral content in the vertebrae, which leads to collapse and compression in the length of the spine; changes in the joints and flattening of the arches of the feet can further contribute to height loss (Kenney, 1989).

Total body weight increases from the 20s until the mid-50s, after which it declines. Most of the weight gain in middle adulthood is due to an accumulation of body fat, particularly around the waist and hips. The weight loss that occurs in the later years of adulthood is not due to a slimming of the torso but to a loss of lean body mass consisting of muscle and bone (Baumgartner, Heymsfield, & Roche, 1995). Consequently, very old adults may have very thin extremities but fatty areas in the chin, waist, and hips. There are secular trends, however, in these patterns. For example, cohorts of older women are showing a decrease rather than an increase in body fat (Rico, Revilla, Hernandez, Gonzalez-Riola, & Villa, 1993), possibly related to changes in life-style and dietary habits. Conversely, more recent cohorts of older men are more likely to be heavier than earlier cohorts of men at comparable ages (Grinker, Tucker, Vokonas, & Rush, 1995).

Psychological Implications. Changes in body fat that lead to the appearance of a sagging or heavier body shape can result in increased identification of the self as moving away from the figure of youth. These developments may occur well before the first gray hairs have sprouted. Indeed, awareness of changes in body composition can occur surprisingly early in adulthood, perhaps by the 30s (Whitbourne, 1996b).

Fortunately, the crossing of the body fat threshold may be readily compensated. Participation in active sports and exercise can offset the deleterious effects of aging on body fat accumulation. Endurance athletes do not gain weight and they maintain their muscular physiques throughout adulthood for as long as they continue to train (Suominen, Heikkinen, Parkatti, Forsberg, & Kiiskinen, 1980). Participation in exercise training programs can even be of value for middle-aged and elderly adults who were sedentary throughout their lives. By engaging in vigorous walking, jogging, or cycling for 30–60 minutes a day for 3–4 days a week, the sedentary adult can expect to achieve positive results in a period as short as 10–20 weeks (Whitbourne, 1996a). Resistance training can also promote loss of body fat in middle aged and older adults (Campbell, Crim, Young, & Evans, 1994; Fielding, 1995). The same activities that middle-aged people might engage in to combat body fat changes can also have very positive cardiovascular and general health benefits. Thus, vanity might actually serve a protective function in this area.

Mobility

Age Changes. The individual's ability to move around in the physical environment is a function of the integrity of the muscles, bones, joints between the bones, tendons and ligaments that connect muscle to bone, and contractility of flexor and extensor muscles. Mobility changes in important ways over the course of the adult years such that movement becomes more difficult, more painful, and less effective.

Between 40 and 70, there is a loss of muscle strength (Booth, Weeden, & Tseng, 1994), amounting to approximately 10–20% (Skelton, Greig, Davies, & Young, 1994) with more severe losses of 30–40% after ages 70 to 80; these losses are referred to as sarcopenia. However, there are individual variations that can lead to important deviations from such a general pattern of decline. The extent to which aging affects loss of muscle strength depends in part on which gender is being tested, the general level of activity in which the individual has typically engaged, the particular muscle group being tested, and whether the type of muscle strength being assessed is static (isometric) or dynamic.

Similarly, the overall course of bone development in adulthood is toward loss of bone strength (Currey, Brear, & Zioupos, 1996), resulting in diminished ability of the bones to withstand mechanical pressure and to show greater vulnerability to fracture. The decrease in various measures of bone strength ranges from 5 to 12% per decade from the 20s through the 90s (McCalden, McGeough, Barker, & Court-Brown, 1993). Microcracks that develop in response to stress placed upon the bones further exacerbate the likelihood of fracture (Courtney, Hayes, & Gibson, 1996; Schaffler, Choi, & Milgrom, 1995).

The period of maximum bone loss is between the 50s and the 70s. The explanation of the underlying process that causes loss of bone mineral content is that the rate of resorption exceeds that of new bone growth in later adulthood, giving a net result of a reduction in bone mass (Sherman et al., 1992). Body weight is positively related to bone mineral content, meaning that heavier individuals lose less bone mineral content and that less bone loss occurs in weight-bearing limbs (Edelstein & Barrett-Connor, 1993). Genetic factors also play a role (Dargent & Breart, 1993; Kelly et al., 1993) as does life-style, including factors such as physical activity, smoking, alcohol use, and diet, which can account for 50–60% of the variation in bone density (Krall & Dawson-Hughes, 1993) and can also influence the rate of fractures (Seeley, Kelsey, Jergas, & Nevitt, 1996). African-American women have higher bone mineral density than do white women, although women in both races are at risk of bone fracture due to reduced density (Perry et al., 1996). There are also hormonal influences on bone mass. Bone mineral loss in women proceeds at a higher rate in postmenopausal women who are no longer producing estrogen in monthly cycles (Garnero, Sornay Rendu, Chapuy, & Delmas, 1996). In men, testosterone levels are positively related to several measures of bone mineral formation (Clarke et al., 1996).

Declines in joint functioning throughout adulthood can be accounted for by age losses in virtually every structural component of the joint. Starting in the 20s and 30s, the arterial cartilage begins to thin, fray, shred, and crack so that the underlying bone eventually begins to wear away. At the same time, outgrowths of cartilage develop and these interfere with the smooth movement of the joint (Ralphs & Benjamin, 1994). Age-related weakening of the muscles further contributes to restrictions in range of movement due to changes in the joints themselves (Vandervoort et al., 1992). Furthermore, the joints are subjected to an extreme amount of trauma throughout life, including the strains and sprains encountered during everyday activities and strenuous exercise, activities that further contribute to their deterioration.

Psychological Implications.   For many individuals, thresholds of aging become painfully crossed with each newly discovered joint ache or mobility restriction, sometimes beginning in the 40s (Whitbourne, 1996b). Changes in the structures that support movement have many pervasive effects on the individual's life, resulting in restrictions in activity and pain, which can interfere with the individual's psychological adaptation and sense of well-being (Hughes, Edelman, Singer, & Chang, 1993).

One of the most serious outcomes of reduced muscle strength, bone strength, and joint mobility is the heightened susceptibility of older individuals, particularly women, to falls (Dargent & Breart, 1993; Roberto, 1992). After a fall, individuals may develop a maladaptive "fear of falling" (Downton & Andrews, 1990) or lowered sense of self-efficacy regarding the ability to avoid a fall (Tinetti & Powell, 1993). As a result, they become less stable on their feet and avoid physical activities that might benefit their strength and stability. Other adults may react to falls by repressing their occurrence (Wright et al., 1990), which might maintain their sense of self-efficacy but place them at risk for further serious injury.

There are many interventions individuals can take in response to changes in mobility, primarily involving exercise. A regular program of exercise can help compensate for the loss of muscle fibers (Morganti et al., 1995) even in persons as old as 90 years (Fiatarone et al., 1990). Older individuals can also benefit from resistance training exercises that, within limits, increase the stress placed upon the bone (Sinaki, 1996). Supplement of the diets of older women with vitamin D can retard bone loss (Dawson Hughes, 1996). Balance and flexibility training can be an effective intervention to minimize the risk of falls in older women (Province et al., 1995), as can Tai Chi (Wolf et al., 1996).

Much attention has been focused on growth hormone as a "treatment" for various age-related changes in muscle and bone. Unfortunately, consumers are misled by the exaggerated claims of advertisers into believing that growth hormones will reverse or retard the aging process. The research on which the original claims for the effectiveness of hormone therapy are based was conducted on individuals (not necessarily elderly) with growth hormone deficiency. Some positive effects of growth hormone therapy on muscle and bone have been demonstrated in studies on normal aging (Welle, Thornton, Statt, & McHenry, 1996). However, the majority of findings fail to support the advertised benefits of this form of intervention (Taaffe, Jin, Vu, Hoffman, & Marcus, 1996) and in fact there are indications that such treatments may have harmful side effects (Riedel, Brabant, Rieger, & von zur Muhlen, 1994).

Effects of Age on Vital Functions

Cardiovascular System

Age Changes. The aging process results in serious limitations of the heart's ability to pump blood through the circulatory system at a rate that adequately perfuses the body's cells. The reduction in the heart's pumping capacity is due to a variety of changes affecting the structure and function of the heart muscle walls, particularly the left ventricle, which becomes progressively thicker with each decade in adulthood and less elastic (Kitzman & Edwards, 1990) as the number of myocardial cells decreases and the remaining cells become hypertrophied (Olivetti, Melissari, Capasso, & Anversa, 1991). The decreased capacity of the ventricle walls to expand results in a reduced and delayed filling of the left ventricle and the ejection of less blood into the aorta (Arrighi et al., 1994). The cardiac muscle also becomes less responsive to the neural stimulation of the "pacemaker" cells in the heart that initiate each contraction (Montamat & Davies, 1989). Effects of aging on the arteries further compromise the system's ability to distribute blood to the body's cells (Shimojo, Tsuda, Iwasaka, & Inada, 1991).

Under normal conditions these changes in the heart and arteries are not particularly pronounced or noticable. The effects of aging of the circulatory system are most apparent while the individual is engaging in aerobic exercise, when there is a reduction both in maximum oxygen consumption (aerobic capacity) and the maximum attainable heart rate (Lakatta, 1987). Aerobic capacity decreases in a linear fashion throughout the adult years, so that the average 65-year-old individual has 30–40% of the aerobic capacity of the young adult (McArdle, Katch, & Katch, 1991). This decrease is significantly lower, however, in very active individuals, amounting to 5–7% per decade (Trappe, Costill, Vukovich, Jones, & Melham, 1996). Other functional variables decrease to a commensurate degree, such as the amount of blood pumped at each beat of the heart and the cardiac output per minute. These decreases in the functional capacity of the heart mean that less oxygen reaches the muscles during exercise.

Psychological Implications. The functioning of the cardiovascular system is an important influence on the individual's feelings of well-being and identity. The efficiency of the cardiovascular system is essential to life so that threats to the integrity of this system are perceived as highly dangerous. Awareness of reduced cardiovascular efficiency can therefore serve as reminders of one's own personal mortality.

On the positive, side, there is a wealth of research pointing to the effectiveness of exercise in slowing or reversing the effects of the aging process. The results of this research consistently reveal improved functioning in long-term endurance athletes, master athletes, exercisers, and previously sedentary adults (Whitbourne, 1996a). Even moderate or low intensity exercise can have beneficial effects on healthy sedentary elderly (Hamdorf, Withers, Penhall, & Haslam, 1992). Further, aerobic exercise training has the positive effect of lowering the heart rate and improving work load intensity and duration in submaximal exercise (Morey et al., 1991), ultimately placing less stress upon the heart during exertion. Other benefits of exercise training are improvements in the peripheral vasculature (Blumenthal et al., 1989), lipid metabolism (Tamai et al., 1988), and blood pressure during or immediately after exertion (Webb, Poehlman, & Tonino, 1993). A word of caution, however; as noted above, even highly trained individuals lose aerobic capacity by the time they reach their 60s (Trappe et al., 1996). In addition to the advantages of exercise training for the cardiovascular system, adults who become involved in aerobic activities experience a variety of positive effects on mood, anxiety levels, and particularly feelings of mastery and control, leading to enhanced feelings of self-esteem (McAuley, Lox, & Duncan, 1993; Strawbridge, Cohen, Shema, & Kaplan, 1996).

Respiratory System

Age Changes. The airways in the respiratory system permit gas exchange between the blood and air, making it possible for the body's cells to receive support for their metabolic activities. Aging reduces the quality of gas exchange in the lungs, vital capacity, the amount of air that is moved into and out of the lungs at maximal levels of exertion (Reddan, 1981), and forced expiratory volume, the amount of air that can be breathed out during a short amount of time (Smith, Cunningham, Patterson, Rechnitzer, & Koval, 1992). These reductions result from changes in pulmonary structures such that the airways, and particularly lung tissue, lose the elastic ability to resist expansion as they fill with air. These changes mean that less than the maximal amount of air can be brought into and out of the lungs, particularly under conditions of exertion (Teramoto, Fukuchi, Nagase, Matsuse, & Orimo, 1995).

Psychological Implications. Age changes in respiration can lead to the unpleasant feelings of dyspnea and fatigue, which in turn may lead the individual to avoid strenuous activities, a consequence that further impairs the individual's cardiovascular and respiratory efficiency. Because both of these functions are so crucial to life, and because shortness of breath is so frightening, the individual might prematurely conclude that death is around the corner.

The effects of exercise training on respiratory functioning are encouraging (Blumenthal et al., 1989), but the specific effects of exercise on respiratory functioning are not as dramatic as are the effects on the cardiovascular system. Equally, if not more, beneficial to the respiratory function is the avoidance of cigarette smoking (Hermanson et al., 1988).

The Effects of Age on Regulatory Systems

Excretory System

Age Changes. There are significant and widespread changes in the structure of the kidneys that are reflected in cross-sectional studies in impaired efficiency across adulthood on every measure of renal functioning studied (Rowe, Shock,

& DeFronzo, 1976; Saltzman, Kowdley, Perrone, & Russell, 1995). There are also independent losses in the kidney mechanisms responsible for concentrating urine (Rowe, 1982). Particularly challenging to the aging kidney is aerobic exercise, because it diverts blood to the working skeletal muscles and thereby causes a further reduction in the blood flow through the kidneys. Equally important, the urine-concentrating mechanism begins to fail during exercise or under extreme conditions of heat when the individual begins to perspire. Fatigue, changes in body chemistry, and potentially harmful changes in bodily fluid levels occur more rapidly in the older adult who cannot adequately conserve sodium and water under these conditions.

The effects of aging on the bladder are of great importance to the individual's conscious experience of aging. Adults past the age of 65 years experience a reduction in the total amount of urine they can store before feeling a need to void, and more urine is retained in the bladder after the individual has attempted to empty it. These alterations are due to changes in the connective tissue of the bladder causing the organ to lose its expandability and contractility. Furthermore, recognition of the need to void may not occur until the individual's bladder is almost or even completely filled. This means that the individual has less or perhaps no time to reach a lavatory before leakage or spillage occurs.

The most significant effect of changes with age in the bladder is on patterns of urinary incontinence. The prevalence of incontinence among the population 60 years and older is estimated to be 19% for women and 8% for men (Herzog, Diokno, Brown, Normolle, & Brock, 1990) but can reach as high as 36% among community-dwelling elderly with dementia (Ouslander & Abelson, 1990). Women are more likely to suffer from stress incontinence—loss of urine at times of exertion. Urge incontinence, which is more prevalent in men, involves urine loss following an urge to void or lack of control over voiding with little or no warning (Diokno, Brock, Brown, & Herzog, 1986); it is related to prostatic disease or incomplete emptying of the bladder. Among the community-dwelling elderly, each of these conditions is reversible and may disappear within a year or two of its initial development (Herzog et al., 1990).

Psychological Implications.   Age effects on renal functioning significantly reduce the older person's ability to excrete medications, a fact that can be of great importance in a therapeutic context. Unless the dosage is adjusted to take into account this lower rate of tubular transport, drugs may have an adverse impact instead of their intended benefits (Lamy, 1988; Montgomery, 1990).

Age-related changes in the bladder can be important threshold phenomena (Whitbourne, 1996a). Incontinence is highly disruptive to the older individual's everyday life, causing distress and embarrassment (Hunskaar & Vinsnes, 1991). Such occasions involve shame, and also they feed into the association in many people's minds between "senility" and urinary incontinence. Given the many associations to urinary continence, it would not be unreasonable to suppose that even a single episode of stress incontinence could create a painful if not traumatic threshold experience. On the positive side, incontinence cases often be managed through behavioral strategies, sometimes involving only very simple exercises (Burns et al., 1993).

Digestive System

Age Changes. The documented effects of aging on digestion in the empirical literature are relatively minor. There is a reduction in the metabolism of certain nutrients in the stomach and small intestine, and changes in gastric juice secretion, but structures such as the esophagous, liver, pancreas, and large intestine appear to be spared by the aging process (Whitbourne, 1996a). More important are the beliefs that people hold as communicated through the media, the social context in which food is eaten, other physical and cognitive deficiencies, and the individual's lifelong patterns of nutrition (Costello & Moser-Veillon, 1992; Ryan, Craig, & Finn, 1992).

Psychological Implications. Although age changes in digestion are relatively minor, there are important ramifications of age changes in patterns of nutrition that may lead to symptoms mimicking those of psychological or cognitive impairment disorders. Unchecked, a vicious cycle may be created, as depression can lead to loss of interest in food and food preparation (Rosenbloom & Whittington, 1993). Conversely, the establishment of healthy dietary patterns can serve to compensate for declines in other areas of physiological functioning (Sone, 1995).

Another issue related to digestion concerns fecal incontinence. Although, at least for women, there are changes in the anal sphincters that can eventually lead to incontinence (Haadem, Dahlstrom, & Ling, 1991), this condition does not affect the majority of the aged population. However, older adults may associate irregularities in defecation with feared diseases and the prospects of institutionalization in later life (Holt, 1991; Wald, 1990). The anxiety created by this concern may contribute further to gastrointestinal problems, so that what originates as a temporary problem comes to have a more prolonged course. Interventions by professionals that involve sensitive discussion of this very personal and potentially frightening area of daily life can be extremely beneficial.

Immune System

Age Changes. There is substantial evidence of reduced immune system functioning across age groups of adults. T cells, which destroy antigens (foreign substances that enter the body), lose effectiveness over the adult years (Bloom, 1994; Trebilcock & Ponnappan, 1996) in part due to changes in the thymus gland. Autopsy studies have revealed that the deterioration of the thymus gland begins shortly after sexual maturity is reached, so that by the time the individual is 45–50 years old, the thymus retains only 5–10% of its peak mass. Consequently, there are fewer effective T cells present both within the thymus gland and in the bloodstream. Other immune system cells, including NK cells, K cells, and macrophages, appear to retain their functioning into old age (Kutza, Kaye, & Murasko, 1995), and there is some evidence that the remaining T cells are able to produce an enhanced response despite their smaller numbers (Born et al., 1995).

Psychological Implications. Recent investigations are providing important data in the field of psychoneuroimmunology, in which the intricate connections are examined between affective states such as stress and depression, nervous system functioning, and the immune system (Kiecolt Glaser & Glaser, 1995). For example, elderly individuals with high levels of life stress experience lower T-cell functioning (McNaughton, Smith, Patterson, & Grant, 1990). Conversely, social support, at least among women, was found to be positively related to immune system competence measured in terms of lymphocyte numbers and response to mitogens (Thomas, Goodwin, & Goodwin, 1985).

There are many ways professionals can take advantage of the potential interactions between psychological variables and immune system functioning. The crossing of an aging threshold in any salient area of functioning, to the extent that it triggers a stressful reaction, can lead to deleterious effects on immune functioning. Various methods of stress reduction can help older individuals who have become overly preoccupied with changes in their body's functioning so that more harmful effects on overall health status can be avoided.

Effects of Age on the Reproductive System and Sexuality

Female Reproductive System

Throughout her 40s, a woman's reproductive capacity becomes gradually reduced until, by the age of 50–55, it ceases altogether. Associated with the ending of the monthly phases of ovulation and menstruation is a diminution of the hormones estrogen and progesterone. Other changes in sexual functioning are related to aging of the tissues in other bodily systems. For example, sagging of the breasts and torso results from decreased skin elasticity. Subcutaneous fat accumulates around the waist, leading to uneven bulges. The appearance and functioning of the genital organs also change after the menopause. The pubic hair on the mons veneris and around the vulva becomes thin and coarser. The labia majora and minora become thinner and wrinkled, the skin in the vulva atrophies, and the surface cells of the vaginal wall become thin, dry, pale, and smooth. The vagina also becomes narrower and shorter. These changes are significant not only for their effects on sexual functioning but for their effects on the woman's enjoyment of sexual intercourse.

The older woman may experience discomfort during intercourse due to changes in the vagina and vulva, and the rhythmic contractions of the uterus may become painful.

Male Reproductive System

Men experience a climacteric of sorts in which there is a reduction in the number of viable sperm they produce due to degenerative changes in the seminiferous tubules of the testes (Harman, 1978). With increasing age, men may experience changes in the prostate gland that lead to a reduction of the volume and pressure of semen expelled during ejaculation. Age-related changes also include overgrowth or hypertrophy of the glandular and connective tissue in the parts of the prostate that surround the prostatic urethra. This condition, called benign prostatic hypertrophy, is increasingly prevalent in men past 50 years, rising to an estimated 50% of men 80 years and older. The adjacent penile urethra may become constricted due to this overgrowth, and urinary retention may ensue. Discomfort and embarrassment may result from difficulties in urination and from the occurrence of involuntary penile erections (Masters & Johnson, 1966). If urinary retention becomes a chronic condition, kidney problems may develop, leading to more serious health threats.

Penile erectility is a physiological index of reproductive function that has a decidedly noticable effect on the older man's sense of his sexuality. Older men experience fewer nightly episodes of penile erections compared to younger males (Karacan, Williams, Thornby, & Salis, 1975). By contrast, there are inconsistencies in the findings regarding increase in penile circumference during erection; in some research decreases are noted across age groups (Solnick & Birren, 1977), and in other research no age differences are observed (Schiavi & Schreiner-Engel, 1988).

As is true for women, there is a general slowing down in men of the progression through the human sexual response cycle. Compared to young adults, orgasm is shorter, involving fewer contractions of the prostate and ejection of a smaller amount of seminal fluid (Masters & Johnson, 1970). These findings may carry some negative implications for the aging male's sexual relations. However, the gains for the older man's ability to enjoy sexuality are also compelling. He may feel less driven toward the pressure to ejaculate, be able to prolong the period of sensual enjoyment prior to orgasm, and have the control to coordinate his pleasure cycle to correspond more to his female partner.

A man's pattern of sexuality in the earlier years of adulthood is a strong predictor of his sexuality in old age (George & Weiler, 1985), second only to health and the presence of physical disease or use of medications (Segraves & Segraves, 1995). The sexually active middle-aged man, given good health, has the potential to remain sexually active well into his later years.

Psychological Implications

Difficulties in adjusting to age changes in the sexual response cycle may present a problem if the partners are unfamiliar with the fact that sexual responsivity naturally becomes altered in later adulthood. The woman may worry that she has lost her orgasmic capacity because it takes her longer to become aroused, excited, and stimulated. The aging male may be at high risk for developing symptoms of secondary (nonphysiological) impotence.

The professional's responsibility in these areas is to explore in a patient and careful manner the level of concern the individual or couple may have about their functioning. Given cohort differences in attitudes toward sexuality, it is likely that the average older person finds it difficult to discuss specific details about problems in sexual functioning. The general level of anxiety associated with sexual matters can lead to heightened potential reactions to actual age changes in physiological functioning. Furthermore, in this area perhaps more so than in any other, it might be necessary for the professional's own attitudes toward sexuality in the aged to become an area of personal focus and reflection before proceeding to the level of intervention.

Effects of Age on the Nervous System

Central Nervous System (CNS)

Age Changes.   In the CNS, as in the other major organ systems, changes that are due to aging alone are difficult to separate from changes that are the result of disease (Morris & McManus, 1991). Neurofibrillary tangles and amyloid plaques are deleterious changes that occur in Alzheimer's disease, but are also found to a lesser extent in normal aging brains (Price, Davis, Morris & White, 1991). Decreases are reported in acetylcholine in the hippocampus of normal individuals (Court et al., 1993; Perry, Piggott, Court, Johnson, & Perry, 1993), changes that are also associated with Alzheimer's disease. Although there have been earlier reports of a decline in the number of neurons in the hippocampus, more recent evidence on "normal" aging calls these findings into question (Davies, Horwood, Isaacs, & Mann, 1992). Similarly, decreased amounts of dopamine in the substantia nigra-basal ganglia pathway are reported in conjunction with the normal aging process (Cruz Sanchez, Cardozo, & Tolosa, 1995), but these changes are hallmarks of Parkinson's disease.

Conflicting results abound in this rapidly emerging field, such as contradictory data on age-related changes in the nucleus basalis of Meynert, a subcortical area of the brain thought to be a major contributor to age-related cortically based memory losses (Baloyannis, Costa, Psaroulis, Arzoglou, & Papasotiriou, 1994; Szenborn, 1993). New findings on larger samples (Leuba & Kraftsik, 1994) are also challenging established conclusions regarding the effect of aging on cortical structures (Devaney & Johnson, 1980), such as the primary visual cortex. As knowledge of the brain and the quality of measurement techniques continue to become refined, these contradictory findings may become resolved. For example, regional variations in neurotransmitter levels and neuron numbers may be found that account for apparent discrepancies between investigations (Mozley et al., 1996).

The most significant new contributions to the literature on aging emerge from investigations employing brain measures in living individuals. A key conclusion emerging from these studies is that there is considerable interindividual variability in patterns of brain changes. Whereas previous studies on neuron counts throughout brain regions tended to focus on overall changes, more recent investigators using brain scans document variation as well. Thus, in one large study using magnetic resonance imaging (MRI) techniques, percentages of atrophy ranging from 6 to 8% per year were reported, but there was wide individual variation in patterns of cortical atrophy and in ventricular enlargement (Coffey et al., 1992). Some of this variability may be accounted for by health status, as indicated by contrasting findings from two MRI studies of temporal lobe volume in which the declines found in one study (Convit et al., 1995) were not observed in a second investigation of individuals selected on the basis of their excellent health (DeCarli et al., 1994). There also may be significant gender variations, with greater reductions in both the frontal and temporal lobes in men (Cowell et al., 1994) but more in the hippocampus and parietal lobes of women (Murphy et al., 1996).

In studies of the frontal lobes using both MRI and positron-emission tomography (PET) scans, age reductions appear to be more conclusively demonstrated than in studies of other cortical areas amounting, perhaps, to 1% per decade (De Santi et al., 1995; DeCarli et al., 1994). Such findings, in conjunction with alterations in the limbic system with age, are interpreted as providing a neurological basis for the behavioral observations of memory changes in older adults (Nielsen Bohlman & Knight, 1995).

Psychological Implications.   Aging of the central nervous system has direct effects on a variety of sensory, motor, and cognitive capacities. However, the view of the aging brain as a degenerating system does not take into account what is known about the compensatory processes of redundancy and plasticity (Diamond, 1990). The impact of these processes is most likely to occur in the association areas of the cerebral cortex that mediate abstract thinking. In fact, these abilities may improve in the later years of adulthood as the individual stores more experiences into the long-term memory association areas on which decisions and judgment are based.

Autonomic Nervous System (ANS)

Age Changes.   Although in many aspects the ANS operates without significant age-related alterations throughout adulthood, there are important effects of aging on two functions served by the ANS that have a considerable impact on the individual's daily life: bodily temperature control and sleep patterns.

It is well established both through population health statistics and experimental studies that individuals over age 65 are impaired in their responses to extremely hot and cold temperatures. Older adults have a diminished perception that the core body temperature is low (Taylor, Allsopp, & Parkes, 1995) and impaired vasoconstrictor response, the ability to raise core temperature when the body's peripheral temperature becomes lowered (Budd, Brotherhood, Hendrie, & Jeffery, 1991). However, there is considerable variability within the older adult population in responses to cold (Inoue, Nakao, Araki, & Ueda, 1992).

Responses to extremes of heat are impaired due to decreased secretion by the sweat glands in the skin (Inoue, Nakao, Araki, & Murakami, 1991). However, well-trained older men with greater aerobic power seem to be less susceptible to hyperthermia (Tankersley, Smolander, Kenney, & Fortney, 1991). Older adults also appear to be less likely to drink water under conditions of heat stress due mainly to reduced thirst sensitivity (Phillips, Bretherton, Johnston, & Gray, 1991), a phenomenon that could contribute to less efficient behavioral responses to overheating.

There are also well-established age differences in sleep patterns. Older adults take more time to fall asleep, are awake more at night, and spend more time lying awake in the morning (Bliwise, 1992). The primary causes of sleep disturbance include sleep apnea (Ancoli-Israel & Kripke, 1991), periodic leg movements, heartburn, and frequent needs to urinate (Friedman et al., 1992). Electroencephalographic sleep patterns show some corresponding age alterations, including a rise in Stage 1 sleep (drowsiness without actual sleep) and a large decrease in Stage 4 sleep (slow wave or heavy sleep). By the 60s and 70s, rapid eye movement (REM) sleep starts to diminish as well, as do the observable behaviors associated with REM sleep. Perhaps related to changes in sleep patterns is the preference for (Atkinson & Reilly, 1995) and actual superiority of work performed in the morning by older adults (Harma, 1996).

Psychological Implications. The knowledge gained from personal experience and media exposure that one's aging body is less adaptable to outside temperatures may cause older adults living in areas with cold winters to restrict their outdoor activities. They may also limit their outdoor exposure during the summer. An overreaction to this information can reduce the well-being of the older adult who may unnecessarily feel forced to remain indoors even on days when the temperature would not pose a threat. Conversely, for the older adult to ignore completely actual age changes in temperature control can also have dangerous consequences. Fortunately, changes in the autonomic nervous system occur gradually over a period of years. Consequently, there are many opportunities for the individual to learn to adjust to the effects of aging and find new behavioral accommodations as these become necessary.

Similarly, the function of sleep in everyday life is crucial to the individual's sense of well-being, and there is a strong relationship between quality of sleep and psychological symptoms (Hays, Blazer, & Foley, 1996). Older adults who overreact to slight sleep change patterns are perhaps the ones fated to experience the most significant changes in their ability to get a good night's sleep. They need to be given the information that a night's sleep need not consist of more than 7 hours and that the longer the time spent in bed awake, the harder it will be for the individual to develop a normal nightly rhythm based on this more realistic sleep requirement. It is also important for the older individual to develop healthy sleep habits (Riedel, Lichstein, & Dwyer, 1995), and especially to avoid daytime naps, because these interfere with nighttime sleep (Hays et al., 1996).

Effects of Age on Sensory Functioning

Vision

Age Changes.   Many of the age effects on visual functions can be explained in terms of the effects of normal aging on the eye's structures (Scheie & Albert, 1977). The image reaching the retina is clouded by increased density and opacity of the lens and by the formation of opacities in the vitreous. Adding to these structural changes are changes in the retina itself, including declines in the number of photoreceptors, the accumulation of debris in the outermost layer of the retina, and the detachment of the vitreous from the surface of the retina. The amount of light reaching the retina is diminished by the condition known as senile meiosis, the reduction in the size of the pupil due to atrophy of the iris dilator (Carter, 1982).

In addition to these changes that reduce the quality of the visual image on the retina are changes in the lens that decrease its capacity to accommodate to changes in focus as objects move closer or further away. In addition to becoming denser, the lens fibers become harder and less elastic and the nucleus of the lens moves forward in the capsule (Cook, Koretz, Pfahnl, Hyun, & Kaufman, 1994). The loss of accommodative power of the lens, called presbyopia, is a condition that typically requires correction by age 40 to 50. By 60 years, the lens is completely incapable of accommodating to focus on objects at close distance (Moses, 1981). The lens also becomes yellowed due to an accumulation of yellow pigment, leading to poorer color discrimination in the green–blue–violet end of the spectrum (Mancil & Owsley, 1988).

There is a reduction in visual acuity that is especially severe at low levels of illumination, such as driving at night and when tracking moving objects (Kline, 1994). Dark adaptation is reduced so that older adults have greater difficulty adjusting to movement from bright to dim lighting and lower absolute levels of ability to see in the dark. There is also a reduction in the individual's ability to react to scotomatic glare, or sudden exposure to bright light, such as a flashbulb or the headlights of an oncoming car at night. Stereopsis, the perception of three-dimensional space resulting from the varying input that reaches the two eyes, appears to be stable, at least up to age 65 years (Yekta, Pickwell, & Jenkins, 1988).

Psychological Implications.   Given the centrality of vision to many activities, changes with age in the eye's basic functions can have profound psychological effects. One set of problems relates to discomfort and frustration caused by poorer acuity and reduced focusing power. Even if visual problems can be corrected, there are residual symptoms that may remain in special circumstances such as after overwork or when reading small print. Older adults report experiencing sensitivity to glare, difficulty seeing in dim light, and problems focusing on near objects (Kosnik, Winslow, Kline, Rasinski, & Sekuler, 1988).

Presbyopia, although reached after a gradual process of changes in the lens, is often perceived with relative suddenness by the individual. The immediacy of this apparent change, given the association that many people have between presbyopia and the infirmities of age, makes it more likely that the change will be negatively interpreted. The necessity of wearing bifocals adds the complication of requiring the individual to adjust to a new and awkward way of using corrective lenses.

Visual problems have many effects on everyday life, including heightened vulnerability to falls (McMurdo & Gaskell, 1991), increased dependence on others (Hakkinen, 1984), and interference with the ability to complete basic tasks of living such as driving, housekeeping, grocery shopping, and food preparation (Owsley, Ball, Sloane, Roenker, & Bruni, 1991; Rudberg, Furner, Dunn, & Cassel, 1993; Salive et al., 1994). Apart from the practical implications, these changes can further erode the individual's physical identity.

Many changes in visual functioning can be compensated by corrective lenses, increases in the ambient lighting, and efforts to reduce glare and heighten contrast between light and dark. Cataract surgery can have widespread positive effects on daily life (Brenner, Curbow, Javitt, Legro, & Sommer, 1993). The success of these efforts depends on the individual's willingness to persist in trying new ideas when the old methods no longer work. Nevertheless, a point may be reached within each sphere of functioning in which the individual's range of movement becomes compromised. Furthermore, the situation may not permit compensation, as is true for night driving. Sensitivity by family and professionals plays an important role in helping the older person adapt to this age-related change in a valued function.

Hearing

Age Changes.   Presbycusis, the general term used to refer to age-related hearing loss, includes several specific subtypes reflecting different changes in the auditory structures. The most common form of hearing loss reduces sensitivity to high-frequency tones earlier and more severely than sensitivity to low-frequency tones (Van-Rooij & Plomp, 1990). The loss of high-frequency pitch perception is particularly pronounced in men. Speech perception is affected both by the various forms of presbycusis operating at the sensory level and by changes in the central processing of auditory information at the level of the brain stem and above (Van-Rooij & Plomp, 1992).

In addition to the effects of aging on speech discrimination due to the loss of high-pitched tone sensitivity are the effects of aging on the ability to hear when there is interference or distraction. Age effects begin to appear even as early as 40 years in the understanding of sentences under a variety of distorting conditions, particularly when the speech signal is interrupted (Bergman et al., 1976). Other conditions known to impair speech perception include higher rate of presentation, deletion of parts of the message, competition from background noise or competing messages, and reverberation (Heller & Wilber, 1990; Neils, Newman, Hill, & Weiler, 1991).

Psychological Implications. Hearing deficits greatly interfere with interpersonal communication, leading to strained relationships and greater caution by the elder in an attempt to avoid making inappropriate responses to uncertain auditory signals. They also reduce the older person's ability to hear noises such as a siren or a door knock (Gatehouse, 1990). Furthermore, hearing deficits can indirectly affect cognitive processes. Listening is more effortful for the older adult with hearing loss and, consequently, is more draining of cognitive resources (Pichora-Fuller, Schneider, & Daneman, 1995). These changes are almost impossible to avoid noticing and it is perhaps for this reason that hearing loss forms a threshold for a large percentage of individuals over the age of 70 and particularly those in their 80s (Whitbourne, 1996b). There is evidence linking hearing loss to impaired physical functioning (Ives, Bonino, Traven, & Kuller, 1995) and psychological difficulties including loneliness (Christian, Dluhy, & O'Neill, 1989) and depression (Kalayam, Alexopoulos, Merrell, & Young, 1991).

Those who interact with hearing-impaired elders can benefit from learning ways to communicate that lessen the impact of age-related changes (Slawinski, Hartel, & Kline, 1993). Modulating one's tone of voice, particularly for women, so that it is not too high, and avoiding distractions or interference can be important aids to communicating clearly with older adults (Souza & Hoyer, 1996).

Balance

Age Changes. The effects of age on the vestibular organs involve the losses occurring in the sensory structures as well as in the pathways to the higher levels of the nervous system (Rosenhall & Rubin, 1975). The results of these changes in the vestibular system are increased dizziness and vertigo in older adults (Toglia, 1975).

However, structural changes in the vestibular system do not account entirely for the phenomena of dizziness and vertigo. The loss of information from another sensory system, such as vision, can make it more difficult for the older person to compensate successfully (Alexander, 1994; Salive et al., 1994; Tanaka, Hashimoto, Noriyasu, & Ino, 1995). Slowing of central integrative processes responsible for maintaining postural stability can also contribute to increased likelihood of falls. It may take longer for the older adult to integrate information from the vestibular, visual, and somesthetic systems, resulting in less efficient control of posture under changing body positions (Teasdale, Stelmach, & Breunig, 1991). Dizziness, a contributor to falling, may also be exacerbated or caused by psychological disorders, use of certain medications, and physical illnesses including cardiac and vascular problems (Anderson et al., 1995).

Psychological Implications.   Balance is an essential element of moving about effectively in the environment. Aging of the vestibular system brings with it the potential for the individual to feel insecure in moving, particularly under conditions that are less than ideal, such as sloping, steep, or uneven surfaces. Fear of falling due to other changes in mobility can increase the individual's anxiety and perhaps exacerbate any true deficits in vestibular functioning (Maki, Holliday, & Topper, 1991; Myers et al., 1996). Conversely, individuals who ignore dizziness and vertigo may place themselves in danger as they may not be able to avoid a fall when and if they do lose their balance.

Professionals can encourage the older individual to benefit from the coping strategies that involve seeking other cues, such as those provided by the somesthetic system. During episodes of dizziness or vertigo, the individual can learn to pay attention to stance and bodily orientation, learning to judge the position of the lower body limbs to make better use of feedback in adjusting posture (Hu & Woollacott, 1994a; Hu & Woollacott, 1994b; Meeuwsen, Sawicki, & Stelmach, 1993). Balance training and Tai Chi, mentioned earlier in the context of changes in mobility, can also be of great value in fall prevention (Province et al., 1995b; Wolfson et al., 1996).

Taste and Smell

Age Changes.   Although there are general decreases in taste sensitivity across age groups of older adults, there is nevertheless wide variability across individuals and within the same individual among the four primary tastes (Cowart, Yokomukai, & Beauchamp, 1994; Stevens, Cruz, Hoffman, & Patterson, 1995). Similarly, although there are general cross-sectional decreases in the ability to recognize and detect odors, there are wide individual variations in part due to differences within the older population in health status (Weiffenbach & Bartoshuk, 1992). Different odors also show differential sensitivity to age effects (Wysocki & Gilbert, 1989).

Contributing to the observed age differences in sensitivity to taste and smell are apparent cognitive differences in the ability to identity odors and food tastes (Corwin, 1992; Russell et al., 1993; Stevens, Cain, Demarque, & Ruthruff, 1991). Age effects in these higher order cognitive and perceptual processes may lead to a distorted picture of the effects of aging on the sensory processes involved in taste and smell.

Psychological Implications.   The ability to enjoy food is vitally important not only to the individual's health, but also to the ability to enjoy the sensory pleasures associated with the experience of eating. Thus, if the individual suffers age-related changes in taste and smell, a potentially satisfying aspect of daily life is lost. The real or perceived effects of aging on digestive functioning can further exacerbate any sensory losses. On the other hand, age changes in taste and smell are neither inevitable nor universal, and there is tremendous variation among older adults based on their health habits and past eating patterns. Furthermore, laboratory studies of functioning in the areas of taste and smell, involving threshold levels of detection, may present an exaggerated picture of age losses as they are experienced in everyday life.

Age-related changes in smell, in particular, may have another set of implications for the individual's daily functioning. Older adults who have lost olfactory sensitivity may not be able to detect the presence of dangerous odors such as leakage of natural gas from a faulty heating system or stove. Similarly, they may fail to be sensitive to the foul taste of spoiled food (Whitbourne, 1996a). Again, most older individuals are able to detect smells that are above threshold levels; precipitous losses that occur in this area of functioning may signal a more serious underlying medical condition in need of treatment.

Concluding Observations

In this chapter, a number of age-related changes have been described that occur throughout the body's organ systems and sensory processes. The multiple threshold model postulates that an individual's reactions to these changes varies according to how central the area of functioning is to identity as well as how the individual approaches the age change. Older adults who overreact to physical changes may experience an unnecessary and potentially harmful sense of discouragement or despair. Conversely, those who deny or minimize the presence of age-related limitations in physical functioning may place themselves at risk due to overexertion or failure to take preventative actions.

Authors in the field of gerontology have, for years, advised professionals to examine their own age biases and attitudes toward elderly people. This admonition definitely applies with regard to the aging of the body, as professionals who are a product of Western culture have undoubtedly acquired a number of negative attitudes toward the loss of functioning that is so generally associated with old age. Less well recognized, though, is the need for the gerontologist to examine his or her own personal aging thresholds and take these into account when dealing with older individuals.

Finally, it is crucial for gerontologists to recognize the independence, autonomy, and vitality of spirit seen in many elders, even those with severe losses or age-related limitations. They are coping daily with physical changes that would daunt the younger professional or specialist. Gerontologists who condescend to the elderly or patronize them (perhaps as a result of their own fears of aging) are missing important treatment opportunities as well as important opportunities to learn from the wisdom of their elders.

REVIEW QUESTIONS

1. What are the major normal age-related changes that occur in each of the body's major organ systems? Summarize these in chart form.

2. How does the multiple-threshold model relate changes in physical functioning to identity processes? What are some of the specific coping strategies that individuals can use to adapt to changes in valued physical functions?

3. Describe the three most important positive interventions that individuals can take advantage of to slow down the rate of the physical aging process.

4. What are the most important interactions between psychological functioning and physical functioning in later adulthood?

5. How do social attitudes toward aging influence the way that individuals adapt to the aging of their bodies? Be sure to distinguish between changes in outward appearance and changes in the functioning of vital organ systems.

6. What are the most important educational goals that gerontologists can implement in working with elderly clients to help them adapt to changes in normal physical functioning?

References

Alexander, N. B. (1994). Postural control in older adults. *Journal of the American Geriatrics Society, 42*, 93–108.

Ancoli-Israel, S., & Kripke, D. F. (1991). Prevalent sleep problems in the aged. *Biofeedback and Self Regulation, 16*, 349–359.

Anderson, D. C., Yolton, R. L., Reinke, A. R., Kohl, P., & Lundy-Ekman, L. (1995). The dizzy patient: A review of etiology, differential diagnosis, and management. *Journal of the American Optometric Association, 66*, 545–558.

Arrighi, J. A., Dilsizian, V., Perrone Filardi, P., Diodati, J. G., Bacharach, S. L., & Bonow, R. O. (1994). Improvement of the age-related impairment in left ventricular diastolic filling with verapamil in the normal human heart [see comments]. *Circulation, 90*, 213–219.

Atkinson, G., & Reilly, T. (1995). Effects of age and time of day on preferred work rates during prolonged exercise. *Chronobiology International, 12*, 121–134.

Baloyannis, S. J., Costa, V., Psaroulis, D., Arzoglou, L., & Papasotiriou, M. (1994). The nucleus basalis of Meynert of the human brain: A Golgi and electron microscope study. *International Journal of Neuroscience, 78*, 33–41.

Baumgartner, R. N., Heymsfield, S. B., & Roche, A. F. (1995). Human body composition and the epidemiology of chronic disease. *Obesity Research, 3*, 73–95.

Bergman, M., Blumenfeld, V. G., Cascardo, D., Dash, B., Levitt, H., & Margulies, M. K. (1976). Age-related decrement in hearing for speech: Sampling and longitudinal studies. *Journal of Gerontology, 31*, 533–538.

Bliwise, N. G. (1992). Factors related to sleep quality in healthy elderly women. *Psychology and Aging, 7*, 83–88.

Bloom, E. T. (1994). Natural killer cells, lymphokine-activated killer cells, and cytolytic T lymphocytes: Compartmentalization of age-related changes in cytolytic lymphocytes? *Journal of Gerontology: Biological Sciences, 49*, B85–92.

Blumenthal, J. A., Emery, G. F., Madden, D. J., George, L. K., Coleman, R. E., Riddle, M. W., McKee, D. C., Reasoner, J., & Williams, R. S. (1989). Cardiovascular and behavioral effects of aerobic exercise training in healthy older men and women. *Journal of Gerontology: Medical Sciences, 44*, M147–157.

Booth, F. W., Weeden, S. H., & Tseng, B. S. (1994). Effect of aging on human skeletal muscle and motor function. *Medicine and Science in Sports and Exercise, 26*, 556–560.

Born, J., Uthgenannt, D., Dodt, C., Nunninghoff, D., Ringvolt, E., Wagner, T., & Fehm, H. L. (1995). Cytokine production and lymphocyte subpopulations in aged humans. An assessment during nocturnal sleep. *Mechanisms of Ageing and Development, 84*, 113–126.

Brenner, M. H., Curbow, B., Javitt, J. C., Legro, M. W., & Sommer, A. (1993). Vision change and quality of life in the elderly: Response to cataract surgery and treatment of other chronic ocular conditions. *Archives of Ophthalmology, 3*, 680–685.

Budd, G. M., Brotherhood, J. R., Hendrie, A. L., & Jeffery, S. E. (1991). Effects of fitness, fatness, and age on men's responses to whole body cooling in air. *Journal of Applied Physiology, 71*, 2387–2393.

Burns, P. A., Pranikoff, K., Nochajski, T. H., Hadley, E. C., Levy, K. J., & Ory, M. G. (1993). A comparison of effectiveness of biofeedback and pelvic muscle exercise treatment of stress incontinence in older community-dwelling women. *Journal of Gerontology: Medical Sciences, 38*, M167–174.

Campbell, W. W., Crim, M. C., Young, V. R., & Evans, W. J. (1994). Increased energy requirements and changes in body composition with resistance training in older adults. *American Journal of Clinical Nutrition, 60*, 167–175.

Carter, J. H. (1982). Predicting visual responses to increasing age. *Journal of the American Optometric Association, 53*, 31–36.

Christian, E., Dluhy, N., & O'Neill, R. (1989). Sounds of silence: Coping with hearing loss and loneliness. *Journal of Gerontological Nursing, 15*, 4–9.

Clarke, B. L., Ebeling, P. R., Jones, J. D., Wahner, H. W., O'Fallon, W. M., Riggs, B. L., & Fitzpatrick, L. A. (1996). Changes in quantitative bone histomorphometry in aging healthy men. *Journal of Clinical Endocrinology and Metabolism, 81*, 2264–2270.

Coffey, C. E., Wilkinson, W. E., Parashos, I. A., Soady, S. A., Sullivan, R. J., Patterson, L. J., Figiel, G. S., Webb, M. C., Spritzer, C. E., & Djang, W. T. (1992). Quantitative cerebral anatomy of the aging human brain: A cross-sectional study using magnetic resonance imaging. *Neurology, 42,* 527–536.

Convit, A., de Leon, M. J., Hoptman, M. J., Tarshish, C., De Santis, S., & Rusinek, H. (1995). Age-related changes in brain: I. Magnetic resonance imaging measures of temporal lobe volumes in normal subjects. *Psychiatric Quarterly, 66,* 343–355.

Cook, C. A., Koretz, J. F., Pfahnl, A., Hyun, J., & Kaufman, P. L. (1994). Aging of the human crystalline lens and anterior segment. *Vision Research, 34,* 2945–2954.

Corwin, J. (1992). Assessing olfaction: Cognitive and measurement issues. In M. J. Serby & K. L. Chobor (Eds.), *Science of olfaction* (pp. 335–354). Berlin: Springer-Verlag.

Costello, R. B., & Moser-Veillon, P. B. (1992). A review of magnesium intake in the elderly. A cause for concern? *Magnesium Research, 5,* 61–7.

Court, J. A., Perry, E. K., Johnson, M., Piggott, M. A., Kerwin, J. A., Perry, R. H., & Ince, P. G. (1993). Regional patterns of cholinergic and glutamate activity in the developing and aging human brain. *Brain Research and Developments in Brain Research, 74,* 73–82.

Courtney, A. C., Hayes, W. C., & Gibson, L. J. (1996). Age-related differences in post-yield damage in human cortical bone. Experiment and model. *Journal of Biomechanics, 29,* 1463–1471.

Cowart, B. J., Yokomukai, Y., & Beauchamp, G. K. (1994). Bitter taste in aging: Compound-specific decline in sensitivity. Kirin International Symposium: On bitter taste (1993, Tokyo, Japan). *Physiology and Behavior, 56,* 1237–1241.

Cowell, P. E., Turetsky, B. I., Gur, R. C., Grossman, R. I., Shtasel, D. L., & Gur, R. E. (1994). Sex differences in aging of the human frontal and temporal lobes. *Journal of Neuroscience, 14,* 4748–4755.

Cruz Sanchez, F. F., Cardozo, A., & Tolosa, E. (1995). Neuronal changes in the substantia nigra with aging: A Golgi study. *Journal of Neuropathology and Experimental Neurology, 54,* 74–81.

Currey, J. D., Brear, K., & Zioupos, P. (1996). The effects of ageing and changes in mineral content in degrading the toughness of human femora. *Journal of Biomechanics, 29,* 257–260.

Dargent, P., & Breart, G. (1993). Epidemiology and risk factors of osteoporosis. *Current Opinions in Rheumatology, 5,* 339–345.

Davies, D. C., Horwood, N., Isaacs, S. L., & Mann, D. M. (1992). The effect of age and Alzheimer's disease on pyramidal neuron density in the individual fields of the hippocampal formation. *Acta Neuropathologica Berlin, 83,* 510–517.

Dawson Hughes, B. (1996). Calcium and vitamin D nutritional needs of elderly women. *Journal of Nutrition, 126,* 1165s-1167s.

DeCarli, C., Murphy, D. G., Gillette, J. A., Haxby, J. V., Teichberg, D., Schapiro, M. B., & Horwitz, B. (1994). Lack of age-related differences in temporal lobe volume of very healthy adults. *American Journal of Neuroradiology, 15,* 689–696.

de Groot, C. P., Perdigao, A. L., & Deurenberg, P. (1996). Longitudinal changes in anthropometric characteristics of elderly Europeans. SENECA Investigators. *European Journal of Clinical Nutrition, 50,* 2954–3007.

De Santi, S., de Leon, M. J., Convit, A., Tarshish, C., Rusinek, H., Tsui, W. H., Sinaiko, E., Wang, G. J., Bartlet, E., & Volkow, N. (1995). Age-related changes in brain: II. Positron emission tomography of frontal and temporal lobe glucose metabolism in normal subjects. *Psychiatric Quarterly, 66,* 357–370.

Devaney, K. O., & Johnson, H. A. (1980). Neuron loss in the aging visual cortex in man. *Journal of Gerontology, 35,* 836–841.

Diamond, M. C. (1990). An optimistic view of the aging brain. In A. L. Goldstein (Ed.), *Biomedical advances in aging* (pp. 441–449). New York: Plenum.

Diokno, A. C., Brock, B. M., Brown, M. B., & Herzog, A. R. (1986). Prevalence of urinary incontinence and other urological syptoms in the noninstitutionalized elderly. *Journal of Urology, 136,* 1022–1025.

Ditre, C. M., Griffin, T. D., Murphy, G. F., Sueki, H., Telegan, B., Johnson, W. C., Yu, R. J., & Van Scott, E. J. (1996). Effects of alpha-hydroxy acids on photoaged skin: A pilot clinical, histologic, and ultrastructural study. *Journal of the American Academy of Dermatology, 34,* 187–195.

Downton, J. H., & Andrews, K. (1990). Postural disturbance and psychological symptoms amongst elderly people living at home. *International Journal of Geriatric Psychiatry, 5,* 93–98.

Edelstein, S. L., & Barrett-Connor, E. (1993). Relation between body size and bone mineral density in elderly men and women. *American Journal of Epidemiology, 138,* 160–169.

Fiatarone, M. A., Marks, E. C., Ryan, N. D., Meredith, C. N., Lipsitz, L. A., & Evans, W. J. (1990). High-intensity strength training in nonagenarians. Effects on skeletal muscle. *Journal of the American Medical Association, 263,* 3029–34.

Fielding, R. A. (1995). The role of progressive resistance training and nutrition in the preservation of lean body mass in the elderly. *Journal of the American College of Nutrition, 14,* 587–594.

Friedman, L. F., Bliwise, D. L., Tanke, E. D., Salom, S. R., et al. (1992). A survey of self-reported poor sleep and associated factors in older individuals. *Behavior, Health, and Aging, 2,* 13–20.

Garnero, P., Sornay Rendu, E., Chapuy, M. C., & Delmas, P. D. (1996). Increased bone turnover in late postmenopausal women is a major determinant of osteoporosis. *Journal of Bone and Mineral Research, 11,* 337–349.

Gatehouse, S. (1990). Determinants of self-reported disability in older subjects. *Ear and Hearing, 11 (Suppl.).*

George, L. K., & Weiler, S. J. (1985). Sexuality in middle and late life. In E. Palmore, J. Nowlin, E. Busse, I. Siegler, & G. Maddox (Eds.), *Normal aging III .* Durham, NC: Duke University Press.

Gilchrest, B. A. (1989). Skin aging and photoaging: An overview. *Journal of the American Academy of Dermatology, 21,* 610–613.

Grinker, J. A., Tucker, K., Vokonas, P. S., & Rush, D. (1995). Body habitus changes among adult males from the normative aging study: Relations to aging, smoking history and alcohol intake. *Obesity Research, 3,* 435–446.

Haadem, K., Dahlstrom, J. A., & Ling, L. (1991). Anal sphincter competence in healthy women: clinical implications of age and other factors. *Obstetrics and Gynecology, 78,* 823–827.

Hakkinen, L. (1984). Vision in the elderly and its use in the social environment. *Scandanavian Journal of Social Medicine, 35,* 5–60.

Hamdorf, P. A., Withers, R. T., Penhall, R. K., & Haslam, M. V. (1992). Physical training effects on the fitness and habitual activity patterns of elderly women. *Archives of Physical Medicine and Rehabilitation, 73,* 603–608.

Harma, M. (1996). Ageing, physical fitness and shiftwork tolerance. *Applied Ergonomics, 27,* 25–29.

Harman, S. M. (1978). Clinical aspects of the male reproductive system. In E. L. Schneider (Ed.), *Aging: Vol. 4. The aging reproductive system* . New York: Raven Press.

Hays, J. C., Blazer, D. G., & Foley, D. J. (1996). Risk of napping: excessive daytime sleepiness and mortality in an older community population. *Journal of the American Geriatrics Society, 44,* 693–698.

Heller, K. S., & Wilber, L. A. (1990). Hearing loss, aging, and speech perception in reverberation and noise. *Journal of Speech and Hearing Research, 33,* 149–155.

Hermanson, B., Omenn, G. S., Kronmal, R. A., & Gersh, B. J. (1988). Beneficial six-year outcome of smoking cessation in older men and women with coronary artery disease. *New England Journal of Medicine, 24,* 1365–1392.

Herzog, A. R., Diokno, A. C., Brown, M. B., Normolle, D. P., & Brock, B. M. (1990). Two-year incidence, remission, and change patterns of urinary incontinence in noninstitutionalized older adults. *Journal of Gerontology: Medical Sciences, 45,* M67–74.

Holt, P. R. (1991). General perspectives on the aged gut. *Clinics in Geriatric Medicine, 7,* 185–189.

Hu, M.-H., & Woollacott, M. H. (1994a). Multisensory training of standing balance in older adults: I. Postural stability and one-leg stance balance. *Journal of Gerontology: Medical Sciences, 49,* M52–61.

Hu, M.-H., & Woollacott, M. H. (1994b). Multisensory training of standing balance in older adutls. II. Kinetic and electromyographic postural responses. *Journal of Gerontology: Medical Sciences, 49,* M62–71.

Hughes, S. L., Edelman, P. L., Singer, R. H., & Chang, R. W. (1993). Joint impairment and self-reported disability in elderly persons. *Journal of Gerontology: Social Sciences, 48,* S84–92.

Hunskaar, S., & Vinsnes, A. (1991). The quality of life in women with urinary incontinence as measured by the Sickness Impact Profile. *Journal of the American Geriatrics Society, 39,* 378–382.

Iida, I., & Noro, K. (1995). An analysis of the reduction of elasticity on the ageing of human skin and the recovering effect of a facial massage. *Ergonomics, 38,* 1921–1931.

Inoue, Y., Nakao, M., Araki, T., & Murakami, H. (1991). Regional differences in the sweating responses of older and younger men. *Journal of Applied Physiology, 71,* 2453–2459.

Inoue, Y., Nakao, M., Araki, T., & Ueda, H. (1992). Thermoregulatory responses of young and older men to cold exposure. *European Journal of Applied Physiology, 65,* 492–498.

Ives, D. G., Bonino, P., Traven, N. D., & Kuller, L. H. (1995). Characteristics and co-morbidities of rural older adults with hearing impairment. *Journal of the American Geriatrics Society, 43,* 803–806.

Kalayam, B., Alexopoulos, G. S., Merrell, H. B., & Young, R. C. (1991). Patterns of hearing loss and psychiatric morbidity in elderly patients attending a hearing clinic. *International Journal of Geriatric Psychiatry, 6,* 131–136.

Karacan, I., Williams, R. L., Thornby, J. I., & Salis, P. J. (1975). Sleep-related penile tumescence as a function of age. *American Journal of Psychiatry, 132,* 932–937.

Kelly, P. J., Nguyen, T., Hopper, J., Pocock, N., Sambrook, P., & Eisman, J. (1993). Changes in axial bone density with age: A twin study. *Journal of Bone Mineral Research, 8,* 11–17.

Kenney, A. R. (1989). *Physiology of aging* (2nd ed.). Chicago: Year Book Medical.

Kiecolt Glaser, J. K., & Glaser, R. (1995). Psychoneuroimmunology and health consequences: Data and shared mechanisms. *Psychosomatic Medicine, 57,* 269–274.

Kitzman, D. W., & Edwards, W. D. (1990). Age-related changes in the anatomy of the normal human heart. *Journal of Gerontology: Medical Sciences, 45*, M33–39.

Kleinsmith, D. M., & Perricone, N. V. (1989). Common skin problems in the elderly. *Clinics in Geriatric Medicine, 5*, 189–211.

Kligman, A. M. (1989). Psychological aspects of skin disorders in the elderly. *Cutis, 43*, 498–501.

Kligman, A. M., Grove, G. L., & Balin, A. K. (1985). Aging of human skin. In C. E. Finch & E. L. Schneider (Eds.), *Handbook of the biology of aging* (2nd ed.). New York: Van Nostrand Reinhold.

Kline, D. W. (1994). Optimizing the visibility of displays for older observers. Special Issue: Human factors and the aging driver. *Experimental Aging Research, 20*, 11–23.

Kosnik, W., Winslow, L., Kline, D., Rasinski, K., & Sekuler, R. (1988). Visual changes in daily life throughout adulthood. *Journal of Gerontology: Psychological Sciences, 43*, P63–70.

Krall, E. A., & Dawson-Hughes, B. (1993). Heritable and life-style determinants of bone mineral density. *Journal of Bone Mineral Research, 8*, 1–9.

Kurban, R. S., & Bhawan, J. (1990). Histologic changes in skin associated with aging. *Journal of Dermatology and Surgical Oncology, 16*, 908–914.

Kutza, J., Kaye, D., & Murasko, D. M. (1995). Basal natural killer cell activity of young versus elderly humans. *Journal of Gerontology: Biological Sciences, 50A*, B110–116.

Lakatta, E. G. (1987). Why cardiovascular function may decline with age. *Geriatrics, 42*, 84–94.

Lamy, P. P. (1988). Actions of alcohol and drugs in older people. *Generations, 12*, 9–13.

Leuba, G., & Kraftsik, R. (1994). Changes in volume, surface estimate, three-dimensional shape and total number of neurons of the human primary visual cortex from midgestation until old age. *Anatomy and Embryology Berlin, 190*, 351–366.

Maki, B. E., Holliday, P. J., & Topper, A. K. (1991). Fear of falling and postural performance in the elderly. *Journals of Gerontology, 46*, M123–M131.

Mancil, G. L., & Owsley, C. (1988). `Vision through my aging eyes' revisited. *Journal of the American Optometric Association, 59*, 288–294.

Masters, W. H., & Johnson, V. E. (1966). *Human sexual response.* Boston: Little, Brown.

Masters, W. H., & Johnson, V. E. (1970). *Human sexual inadequacy.* Boston: Little, Brown.

McArdle, W. D., Katch, F. I., & Katch, V. L. (1991). *Exercise physiology: Energy, nutrition, and human performance* (3 ed.). Philadelphia: Lea & Ferbiger.

McAuley, E., Lox, C., & Duncan, T. E. (1993). Long-term maintenance of exercise, self-efficacy, and physiological change in older adults. *Journal of Gerontology: Psychological Sciences, 48*, P218–224.

McCalden, R. W., McGeough, J. A., Barker, M. B., & Court-Brown, C. M. (1993). Age-related changes in the tensile properties of cortical bone. The relative importance of changes in porosity, mineralization, and microstructure. *Journal of Bone and Joint Surgery, 75*, 1193–1205.

McMurdo, M. E., & Gaskell, A. (1991). Dark adaptation and falls in the elderly. *Gerontology, 37*, 221–224.

McNaughton, M. E., Smith, L. W., Patterson, T. L., & Grant, I. (1990). Stress, social support, coping resources, and immune status in elderly women. *Journal of Nervous and Mental Disease, 178*, 460–461.

Meeuwsen, H. J., Sawicki, T. M., & Stelmach, G. E. (1993). Improved foot position sense as a result of repetitions in older adults. *Journal of Gerontology: Psychological Sciences, 48*, P137–141.

Montamat, S. C., & Davies, A. O. (1989). Physiological response to isoproterenol and coupling of beta-adrenergic receptors in young and elderly human subjects. *Journal of Gerontology: Medical Sciences, 44,* M100–105.

Montgomery, S. A. (1990). Depression in the elderly: Pharmacokinetics of antidepressants and death from overdose. *International Clinical Psychopharmacology, 5,* 67–76.

Morey, M. C., Cowper, P. A., Feussner, J. R., DiPasquale, R. C., Crowley, G. M., Kitzman, D. W., & Sullivan, R. J., Jr. (1991). Two-year trends in physical performance following supervised exercise among community-dwelling older veterans. *Journal of the American Geriatrics Society, 39,* 549–554.

Morganti, C. M., Nelson, M. E., Fiatarone, M. A., Dallal, G. E., Economos, C. D., Crawford, B. M., & Evans, W. J. (1995). Strength improvements with 1 yr of progressive resistance training in older women. *Medicine and Science in Sports and Exercise, 27,* 906–912.

Morris, J. C., & McManus, D. Q. (1991). The neurology of aging: normal versus pathologic change. *Geriatrics, 46,* 47–48.

Moses, R. A. (1981). Accommodation. In R. A. Moses (Ed.), *Adler's physiology of the eye.* St. Louis: C.V. Mosby.

Mozley, P. D., Kim, H. J., Gur, R. C., Tatsch, K., Muenz, L. R., McElgin, W. T., Kung, M. P., Mu, M., Myers, A. M., & Kung, H. F. (1996). Iodine-123–IPT SPECT imaging of CNS dopamine transporters: nonlinear effects of normal aging on striatal uptake values. *Journal of Nuclear Medicine, 37,* 1965–1970.

Murphy, D. G. M., DeCarli, C., McIntosh, A. R., Daly, E., Mentis, M. J., Pietrini, P., Szczepanik, J., Schapiro, M. B., Grady, C. L., Horwitz, B., & Rapoport, S. I. (1996). Sex differences in human brain morphometry and metabolism: An in vivo quantitative magnetic resonance imaging and positron emission tomography study on the effect of aging. *Archives of General Psychiatry, 53,* 585–594.

Myers, A. M., Powell, L. E., Maki, B. E., Holliday, P. J., Brawley, L. R., & Sherk, W. (1996). Psychological indicators of balance confidence: Relationship to actual and perceived abilities. *Journal of Gerontology: Medical Sciences, 51,* M37–43.

Nachbar, F., & Korting, H. C. (1995). The role of vitamin E in normal and damaged skin. *Journal of Molecular Medicine, 73,* 7–17.

Neils, J., Newman, C. W., Hill, M., & Weiler, E. (1991). The effects of rate, sequencing, and memory on auditory processing in the elderly. *Journal of Gerontology: Psychological Sciences, 46,* P71–75.

Nielsen Bohlman, L., & Knight, R. T. (1995). Prefrontal alterations during memory processing in aging. *Cerebral Cortex, 5,* 541–549.

Olivetti, G., Melissari, M., Capasso, J. M., & Anversa, P. (1991). Cardiomyopathy of the aging human heart. Myocyte loss and reactive cellular hypertrophy. *Circulation Research, 68,* 1560–1568.

Ouslander, J. G., & Abelson, S. (1990). Perceptions of urinary incontinence among elderly outpatients. *Gerontologist, 30,* 369–372.

Owsley, C., Ball, K., Sloane, M. E., Roenker, D. L., & Bruni, J. R. (1991). Visual/cognitive correlates of vehicle accidents in older drivers. *Psychology and Aging, 6,* 403–415.

Perry, E. K., Piggott, M. A., Court, J. A., Johnson, M., & Perry, R. H. (1993). Transmitters in the developing and senescent human brain. *Annals of the New York Academy of Science, 695,* 69–72.

Perry, H. M., 3rd, Horowitz, M., Morley, J. E., Fleming, S., Jensen, J., Caccione, P., Miller, D. K., Kaiser, F. E., & Sundarum, M. (1996). Aging and bone metabolism in African American and Caucasian women. *Journal of Clinical Endocrinology and Metabolism, 81,* 1108–1117.

Phillips, P. A., Bretherton, M., Johnston, C. I., & Gray, L. (1991). Reduced osmotic thirst in healthy elderly men. *American Journal of Physiology, 261*, R166–171.

Pichora-Fuller, M. K., Schneider, B. A., & Daneman, M. (1995). How young and old adults listen to and remember speech in noise. *Journal of the Acoustical Society of America, 97*, 593–608.

Price, J. L., Davis, P. B., Morris, J. C., & White, D. L. (1991). The distribution of tangles, plaques and related immunohistochemical markers in healthy aging and Alzheimer's disease. *Neurobiology of Aging, 12*, 295–312.

Province, M. A., Hadley, E. C., Hornbrook, M. C., Lipsitz, L. A., Miller, J. P., Mulrow, C. D., Ory, M. G., Sattin, R. W., Tinetti, M. E., & Wolf, S. L. (1995). The effects of exercise on falls in elderly patients. A preplanned meta-analysis of the FICSIT Trials. Frailty and Injuries: Cooperative Studies of Intervention Techniques. *Journal of the American Medical Association, 273*, 1341–1347.

Ralphs, J. R., & Benjamin, M. (1994). The joint capsule: Structure, composition, ageing and disease. *Journal of Anatomy, 184*, 503–509.

Reddan, W. G. (1981). Respiratory system and aging. In E. L. Smith & R. C. Serfass (Eds.), *Exercise and aging: The scientific basis* (pp. 89–107). Hillside, NJ: Enslow.

Rico, H., Revilla, M., Hernandez, E. R., Gonzalez-Riola, J. M., & Villa, L. F. (1993). Four-compartment model of body composition of normal elderly women. *Age and Ageing, 22*, 265–268.

Riedel, B. W., Lichstein, K. L., & Dwyer, W. O. (1995). Sleep compression and sleep education for older insomniacs: Self-help versus therapist guidance. *Psychology and Aging, 10*, 54–63.

Riedel, M., Brabant, G., Rieger, K., & von zur Muhlen, A. (1994). Growth hormone therapy in adults: Rationales, results, and perspectives. *Experimental and Clinical Endocrinology, 102*, 273–283.

Roberto, K. (1992). Coping strategies of older women with hip fractures: Resources and outcomes. *Journal of Gerontology: Psychological Sciences, 47*, P21–26.

Rosenbloom, C. A., & Whittington, F. J. (1993). The effects of bereavement on eating behaviors and nutrient intakes in elderly widowed persons. *Journal of Gerontology: Social Sciences, 48*, S223–229.

Rosenhall, U., & Rubin, W. (1975). Degenerative patterns in the aging human vestibular neuroepithelia. *Acta Otolaryngolica, 76*, 208–220.

Rowe, J. W. (1982). Renal function and aging. In M. E. Reff & E. L. Schneider (Eds.), *Biological markers of aging* . Bethesda MD: National Institutes of Health, Publication Number 82–2221.

Rowe, J. W., Shock, N. W., & DeFronzo, R. A. (1976). The influence of age on the renal response to water deprivation in man. *Nephron, 17*.

Rudberg, M. A., Furner, S. E., Dunn, J. E., & Cassel, C. K. (1993). The relationship of visual and hearing impairments to disability: An analysis using the longitudinal study of aging. *Journal of Gerontology: Medical Sciences, 48*, M261–265.

Russell, M. J., Cummings, B. J., Profitt, B. F., Wysocki, C. J., Gilbert, A. N., & Cotman, C. W. (1993). Life span changes in the verbal categorization of odors. *Journal of Gerontology: Psychological Sciences, 48*, P49–53.

Ryan, A. S., Craig, L. D., & Finn, S. C. (1992). Nutrient intakes and dietary patterns of older Americans: A national study. *Journal of Gerontology: Medical Sciences, 47*, M145–150.

Salive, M. E., Guralnik, J., Glynn, R. J., Christen, W., Wallace, R. B., Ostfeld, A. M. (1994). Association of visual impairment with mobility and physical function. *Journal of the American Geriatrics Society, 42*, 287–292.

Saltzman, J. R., Kowdley, K. V., Perrone, G., & Russell, R. M. (1995). Changes in small-intestine permeability with aging. *Journal of the American Geriatric Society, 43,* 160–164.

Schaffler, M. B., Choi, K., & Milgrom, C. (1995). Aging and matrix microdamage accumulation in human compact bone. *Bone, 17,* 521–525.

Scheie, H. G., & Albert, D. M. (1977). *Textbook of ophthalmology* (9 ed.). Philadelphia: Saunders.

Schiavi, R. C., & Schreiner-Engel, P. (1988). Nocturnal penile tumescence in healthy aging men. *Journal of Gerontology, 43,* M146–150.

Seeley, D. G., Kelsey, J., Jergas, M., & Nevitt, M. C. (1996). Predictors of ankle and foot fractures in older women. The Study of Osteoporotic Fractures Research Group. *Journal of Bone Mineral Research, 11,* 1347–1355.

Segraves, R. T., & Segraves, K. B. (1995). Human sexuality and aging. *Journal of Sex Education and Therapy, 21,* 88–102.

Sherman, S. S., Tobin, J. D., Hollis, B. W., Gundberg, C. M., Roy, T. A., & Plato, C. C. (1992). Biochemical parameters associated with low bone density in healthy men and women. *Journal of Bone and Mineral Research, 7,* 1123–1130.

Shimojo, M., Tsuda, N., Iwasaka, T., & Inada, M. (1991). Age-related changes in aortic elasticity determined by gated radionuclide angiography in patients with systemic hypertension or healed myocardial infarcts and in normal subjects. *American Journal of Cardiology, 68,* 950–953.

Sinaki, M. (1996). Effect of physical activity on bone mass. *Current Opinions in Rheumatology, 8,* 376–383.

Skelton, D. A., Greig, C. A., Davies, J. M., & Young, A. (1994). Strength, power and related functional ability of healthy people aged 65–89 years. *Age and Ageing, 23,* 371–377.

Slawinski, E. B., Hartel, D. M., & Kline, D. W. (1993). Self-reported hearing problems in daily life throughout adulthood. *Psychology and Aging, 8,* 552–562.

Smith, W. D. F., Cunningham, D. A., Patterson, D. H., Rechnitzer, P. A., & Koval, J. J. (1992). Forced expiratory volume, height, and demispan in Canadian men and women aged 55–86. *Journal of Gerontology: Medical Sciences, 47,* M40–44.

Solnick, R. L., & Birren, J. E. (1977). Age and male erectile responsiveness. *Archives of Sexual Behavior, 6,* 1–9.

Sone, Y. (1995). Age-associated problems in nutrition. *Applied Human Science, 14,* 201–210.

Souza, P. E., & Hoyer, W. J. (1996). Age-related hearing loss: Implications for counseling. *Journal of Counseling and Development, 74,* 652–655.

Stevens, J. C., Cain, W. S., Demarque, A., & Ruthruff, A. M. (1991). On the discrimination of missing ingredients: Aging and salt flavor. *Appetite, 16,* 129–140.

Stevens, J. C., Cruz, L. A., Hoffman, J. M., & Patterson, M. Q. (1995). Taste sensitivity and aging: High incidence of decline revealed by repeated threshold measures. *Chemical Senses, 20,* 451–459.

Strawbridge, W. J., Cohen, R. D., Shema, S. J., & Kaplan, G. A. (1996). Successful aging: predictors and associated activities. *American Journal of Epidemiology, 144,* 135–141.

Suominen, H., Heikkinen, E., Parkatti, T., Forsberg, S., & Kiiskinen, A. (1980). Effect of lifelong physical training on functional aging in men. *Scandanavian Journal of the Society of Medicine, 14 (Suppl.),* 225–240.

Szenborn, M. (1993). Neuropathological study on the nucleus basalis of Meynert in mature and old age. *Patologia Polska, 44,* 211–216.

Taaffe, D. R., Jin, I. H., Vu, T. H., Hoffman, A. R., & Marcus, R. (1996). Lack of effect of recombinant human growth hormone (GH) on muscle morphology and GH-insulin-like growth factor expression in resistance-trained elderly men. *Journal of Clinical Endocrinology and Metabolism, 81,* 421–425.

Takema, Y., Yorimoto, Y., Kawai, M., & Imokawa, G. (1994). Age-related changes in the elastic properties and thickness of human facial skin. *British Journal of Dermatology, 131,* 641–648.

Tamai, T., Nakai, T., Takai, H., Fujiwara, R., Miyabo, S., Higuchi, M., & Kobayashi, S. (1988). The effects of physical exercise on plasma lipoprotein and apolipoprotein metabolism in elderly men. *Journal of Gerontology: Medical Sciences, 43,* M75–79.

Tanaka, T., Hashimoto, N., Noriyasu, S., & Ino, S. (1995). Aging and postural stability: Change in sensorimotor function. *Physical and Occupational Therapy in Geriatrics, 13,* 1–16.

Tankersley, C. G., Smolander, J., Kenney, W. L., & Fortney, S. M. (1991). Sweating and skin blood flow during exercise: Effects of age and maximal oxygen uptake. *Journal of Applied Physiology, 71,* 236–242.

Taylor, N. A., Allsopp, N. K., & Parkes, D. G. (1995). Preferred room temperature of young vs aged males: The influence of thermal sensation, thermal comfort, and affect. *Journal of Gerontology: Medical Sciences, 50,* M216–M221.

Teasdale, N., Stelmach, G. E., & Breunig, A. (1991). Postural sway characteristics of the elderly under normal and altered visual and support surface conditions. *Journal of Gerontology: Biological Sciences, 46,* B238–244.

Teramoto, S., Fukuchi, Y., Nagase, T., Matsuse, T., & Orimo, H. (1995). A comparison of ventilation components in young and elderly men during exercise. *Journal of Gerontology: Biological Sciences, 50A,* B34–39.

Thomas, P. D., Goodwin, J. M., & Goodwin, J. W. (1985). Effect of social support on stress-related changes in cholesterol, uric acid level, and immune function in an elderly sample. *American Journal of Psychiatry, 142,* 735–737.

Tinetti, M. E., & Powell, L. (1993). Fear of falling and low self-efficacy: A cause of dependence in elderly persons. *Journals of Gerontology, 48,* 35–58.

Toglia, J. U. (1975). Dizziness in the elderly. In W. Fields (Ed.), *Neurological and sensory disorders in the elderly*. New York: Grune & Stratton.

Trappe, S. W., Costill, D. L., Vukovich, M. D., Jones, J., & Melham, T. (1996). Aging among elite distance runners: A 22-yr longitudinal study. *Journal of Applied Physiology, 80,* 285–290.

Trebilcock, G. U., & Ponnappan, U. (1996). Evidence for lowered induction of nuclear factor kappa B in activated human T lymphocytes during aging. *Gerontology, 42,* 137–146.

Vandervoort, A. A., Chesworth, B. M., Cunningham, D. A., Paterson, D. H., Rechnitzer, P. A., & Koval, J. J. (1992). Age and sex effects on mobility of the human ankle. *Journal of Gerontology: Medical Sciences, 47,* M17–21.

Van-Rooij, J. C., & Plomp, R. (1990). Auditive and cognitive factors in speech perception by elderly listeners: II. Multivariate analyses. *Journal of the Acoustical Society of America, 88,* 2611–2624.

Van-Rooij, J. C., & Plomp, R. (1992). How much do working memory deficits contribute to age differences in discourse memory? Special Issue: Cognitive gerontology. *Journal of the Acoustical Society of America, 91,* 1028–1033.

Wald, A. (1990). Constipation and fecal incontinence in the elderly. *Gastroenterology Clinics of North America, 19,* 405–418.

Webb, G. D., Poehlman, E. T., & Tonino, R. P. (1993). Dissociation of changes in metabolic rate and blood pressure with erthrocyte Na-K pump activity in older men after endurance training. *Journal of Gerontology: Medical Sciences, 48*, M47–52.

Weiffenbach, J. M., & Bartoshuk, L. M. (1992). Taste and smell. *Clinics in Geriatric Medicine, 8*, 543–555.

Welle, S., Thornton, C., Statt, M., & McHenry, B. (1996). Growth hormone increases muscle mass and strength but does not rejuvenate myofibrillar protein synthesis in
healthy subjects over 60 years old. *Journal of Clinical Endocrinology and Metabolism,
81*, 3239–3243.

Whitbourne, S. K. (1996a). *The aging individual: Physical and psychological perspectives.* New
York: Springer.

Whitbourne, S. K. (1996b). *Identity processes and perceptions of physical functioning in adults:
A test of the multiple threshold model.* Paper presented at the American Psychological Association 104th Annual Meeting, Toronto, Ontario, Canada.

Wolf, S. L., Barnhart, H. X., Kutner, N. G., McNeely, E., Coogler, C., Xu, T., & the At-
lanta FICSIT Group. (1996). Reducing frailty and falls in older persons: An investigation of Tai Chi and computerized balance training. *Journal of the American Geriatrics Society, 44*, 489–497.

Wolfson, L., Whipple, R., Derby, C., Judge, J., King, M., Amerman, P., Schmidt, J., &
Smyers, D. (1996). Balance and strength training in older adults: Intervention gains
and Tai Chi maintenance. *Journal of the American Geriatrics Society, 44*, 498–506.

Wright, B. A., Aizenstein, S., Vogler, G., Rowe, M., & Miller, C. (1990). Frequent fallers:
Leading groups to identify psychological factors. *Journal of Gerontological Nursing,
16*, 15–19.

Wysocki, C. J., & Gilbert, A. N. (1989). The National Geographic smell survey: Effects
of age are heterogenous. *Annals of the New York Academy of Sciences, 561*, 12–28.

Yang, J. H., Lee, H. C., & Wei, Y. H. (1995). Photoageing-associated mitochondrial DNA
length mutations in human skin. *Archives of Dermatological Research, 287*, 641–648.

Yekta, A. A., Pickwell, L. D., & Jenkins, T. C. (1988). Binocular vision, age and symptoms. *Ophthalmic Physiological Optics, 9*, 115–120.

Additional Readings

Cohen, G. (1988). *The brain in human aging.* New York: Springer.

Hayflick, L. (1994). *How and why we age.* New York: Ballantine Books.

Lee, I., Hsieh, C., & Paffenbarger, R. S., (1996). Exercise intensity and longevity in men:
The Harvard Alumni Health Study. *Journal of the American Medical Association, 273*,
1179–1184.

Shephard, R.J. (1982). *Physiology and biochemistry of exercise.* New York: Praeger.

Selkoe, D.J. (1997). Alzheimer's disease: Genotypes, phenotypes, and treatments. *Science, 275*, 630–631.

Sone, Y. (1995). Age-associated problems in nutrition. *Applied Human Science, 14*,
201–210.

Strawbridge, W. J., Cohen, R. D., Shema, S. J., & Kaplan, G. A. (1996). Successful aging:
Predictors and associated activities. *American Journal of Epidemiology, 144*, 135–141.

Whitbourne, S.K. (1996). *The aging individual: Physical and psychological perspectives.* New
York: Springer.

5

Immunity, Disease Processes, and Optimal Aging

Carolyn M. Aldwin and Diane F. Gilmer

"What are old women made of? . . . Moans and groans
and aches in their old bones. . . What are old men made
of? . . . Whisky, brandy, anything you've handy."

—*Leadbelly*

Well-being in late life is a tightly knit amalgam of physical, psychological, and social health. Disruptions in any one system may have negative implications for the others. For example, a simple broken ankle, in the absence of adequate social support, can rapidly turn an otherwise healthy, well-functioning elder into a frail, institutionalized one. Urinary incontinence can lead to social isolation, which in turn can create a whole host of problems. Conversely, a perturbation in the social domain, such as bereavement, can lead to depression, which in turn impairs appetite. Poor eating habits can result in inadequate nutrition, which can impair cognitive functioning, as can depression itself.

Complicating this effort to understand the interrelationships among physical, mental, and social health is the fact that physical health problems can manifest in the older adults in ways that are different than in younger adults. A simple bladder infection, for example, causes some discomfort in urination in the young; in older adults, the same infection may be more likely to disrupt other systems in the body, which in turn can impair cognitive functioning and result in pseudodementia. Many illnesses have rather similar symptoms, rendering differential diagnosis difficult. For example, both hypo- and hyperthyroidism can manifest as simple fatigue in older adults, as do a number of leukemias and cardiovascular disorders such as congestive heart failure, while bone cancers such as multiple myeloma may be confused with simple arthritis. Thus, it is very important to understand both the types of physical problems common to older adults and the ways in which they can affect psychological and social health.

123

That physical problems can have such dramatic effects on multiple domains in older adults is probably due to two factors. The first is lack of adaptive reserves. While the vast majority of elders have enough physical capacity
to cope with every day demands, extraordinary demands may be more likely
to overtax the system. For example, a slight balance problem may not impair
ordinary walking, but if an elder breaks an ankle, it may make learning to use
crutches very difficult, if not impossible. Second, the ability to meet adaptive
challenges adequately depends upon a highly complex coordination across a
variety of systems. In older adults, regulation among systems is often impaired,
and an adaptive challenge may end up affecting multiple systems in a cascade
effect.

This chapter will first discuss impairment in the regulatory systems (immune, nervous, and endocrine), as well as the diseases thereof. It will then describe common illnesses in different organ systems, as well as their effect on
functioning in other domains. However, in acknowledgment of the fact that
psychosocial factors also affect physical health, we also describe how optimal
aging in those systems may be promoted for each organ system.

Regulatory Systems

The nervous, endocrine, and immune systems are complex systems whose primary purpose is to coordinate and regulate body functions. As such, they communicate both with each other and with every cell in the body, providing feedback to regulatory centers in the brain. Immune cells have receptor cites for
neurotransmitters, and the distinction between neurotransmitters, peptides,
and endocrine hormones is becoming blurred. Deregulation or impairment in
these systems underlies many of the diseases common late in life, such as cancer, heart disease, and diabetes. Thus, this chapter will describe the immune
system in some detail, as its workings tend to be less familiar to psychologists,
before turning to disorders in the other systems.

Immune System

The immune system is the primary defense against bacterial, viral, and parasitic infections, as well as their toxic byproducts, and abnormal cells such as
precancerous and tumor cells. Although we have known for decades that white
blood cells, or leukocytes, increase dramatically during infections, it is only
very recently that we have begun to comprehend the enormous complexity,
flexibility, and specificity of immune functioning. New components and cell
subtypes continue to be discovered, and there is much that is still unknown
about exactly how the immune system works.

One of the great mysteries of the immune system is that it learns to differentiate between self and other, in part by recognizing identifying antigens

on the surfaces of invading bacteria and cells that have been taken over by viral DNA or RNA. Once the immune system has learned to recognize an external invader, it generates a defense against that specific antigen. This happens by maturing naive or immature lymphocytes, stored in the bone marrow. In the thymus, T cells develop receptor cites for both specific antigens and for human leukocyte-associated (HLA) proteins, which can be considered patterns of proteins that are specific to each individual and form the basis for self-recognition in the immune system. Sometimes errors can arise, leading the immune system to generate autoantibodies that can attack normal cells, which can result in autoimmune diseases such as rheumatoid arthritis. Furthermore, the immune system has a memory component called memory T cells that store patterns for each antigen for future use. Recognition of an antigen can stimulate proliferation of the specific cells that can attack that invader. How exactly learning, memory, and proliferation occur is still a mystery, but immunologists are slowly beginning to understand at least some of these processes.

There are three basic types of immune responses, humoral, cellular, and delayed hypersensitivity (Miller, 1996a). In humoral immunity, B lymphocytes generate antibodies or immunoglobulins, complex protein chains that either agglutinate cells to help clear them from the body or that simply identify antigens to the cellular components. The cellular components then destroy the invaders by lysing or splitting open their cells. There are five major types of antibodies (IgA, IgD, IgE, IgG, and IgM), each of which has multiple subtypes. Antibodies have different functions. For example, IgE mediates allergies and asthma, and also fights parasitic infections, while IgG, also known as gamma globulin, helps combat hepatitis. While antibodies are usually specific to particular antigens, if the molecular shapes of antigens are similar enough, some cross-reactivity may occur. Multispecificity occurs when an antibody can react to more than one antigen.

Cellular immunity is mediated primarily by T cells, of which there are many different subtypes. Effector cells recognize and lyse abnormal cells. CD4 cells, also known as helper T cells, assist B cells in identifying and destroying antigens. They generate cytokines that stimulate other parts of the immune system. Cytokines such as interleukin-4 (IL-4) stimulate B cells to produce antigens, while IL-2 can assist in cell maturation. CD8 cells, also known as suppressor T cells, serve to dampen immune reactions. The ratio of CD4 to CD8 cells may be a better indicator of the healthiness of the immune system rather than the absolute level of either component.

In delayed hypersensitivity reaction, antigen-specific T cells can attract other immune cells such as macrophages or neutrophils to the site of an infection (Miller, 1996a). This type of immune reaction typically takes longer to occur, but grows in strength with repeated exposure. Allergic reactions to bee stings are an example of delayed hypersensitivity. This type of immune response mediates anaphylaxis, which is an extreme allergic response that can result in death.

Natural killer (NK) cells are another important component of the immune system. These cells have a surveillance function to fight against viral infection and parasites, but, more importantly, they are our primary protection against cancer. NK cells constantly circulate in the blood system and are able to identify precancerous cells and lyse them before they can proliferate (Adler & Nagel, 1994).

It is tempting to believe that many of the diseases in late life are due to immunosenescence, or aging of the immune system. However, at this point in time, research on the immune system is relatively new, and there is little consensus as to what exactly are age-related changes. Immune system functioning can be affected by a wide variety of factors, including nutrition, stress levels, exercise, and disease, thus making it difficult to differentiate between normative changes and those secondary to other problems. Further, there are marked inconsistencies in findings across species, for different strains within species, in similar cells taken from different parts of the body, and even in the same individuals across time (Miller, 1996b).

Nonetheless, it is widely believed that immunodeficiencies occur with age. We know that older adults are more prone to certain types of infectious agents, such as *Escherichia coli* and pneumococcus (responsible for some types of pneumonia), and have a much higher incidence of cancer. The number of autoantibodies also increases slightly, although this does not appear to result in an increase in autoimmune diseases with age (Miller, 1996a).

Miller (1996a, 1996b) has provided exhaustive reviews of the often contradictory results, and believes that a few age changes do occur consistently in humans. Although there do not appear to be consistent findings vis-à-vis changes in the number of B and T cells in humans, there do appear to be age-related differences in the types of T cells. In particular, there appears to be a decrease in the number of immature T cells and relatively greater proportions of mature, antigen-specific T cells. This is consistent with thymic involution, and suggests that the immune system in late life may be less effective when exposed to new strains of bacteria or viruses. Delayed hypersensitivity weakens with age, and T cells may also decrease in their ability both to produce and respond to cytokines. B cells also produce fewer antigens, but this may be due to a decrease in cytokines rather than any intrinsic age-related changes in the B cells themselves. Interestingly, the older immune systems may respond less well to vaccines, and there is some indication that vaccinations may temporarily impair immune responses to other pathogens. Surprisingly, though, there is no evidence for a decrease in NK cells with age.

There are several immune system diseases that increase with age, including multiple myeloma, chronic lymphatic leukemia, and chronic myelocytic leukemia, which are cancers of different types of immune cells (Rothstein, 1994). Diagnosing leukemias such as these may be problematic in older adults, as the symptoms at onset are often vague and easily confused with more common problems, which can delay early recognition. For example, multiple myeloma often causes bone pain, which can be confused with arthritis. Not only are they serious health problems in and of themselves, but they may create anemias that can aggravate other chronic conditions, such as cardiovascular disease. Thus, early detection of leukemia is very important in late life.

Besides disease, there are a number of factors that can affect immune functioning, including nutrition, exercise, and stress. The immune system is very sensitive to nutritional deficiencies, especially to micronutrients, and one study in older adults showed that a daily vitamin supplement did enhance immune functioning (Chandra, 1992). Sone's (1996) review suggests that vitamins E and B_6 and trace mineral zinc may be helpful in boosting immune systems in older adults.

The relationship between exercise and immune function is complex. Moderate exercise apparently increases immune function, although very heavy exercise may impair it (Nieman, 1997). Cross-sectional studies have found that older adults who had participated in endurance training on a long-term basis had better immune functioning and fewer upper respiratory tract infections than sedentary elders (Nieman et al., 1993; Venjatraman & Fernandes, 1997). However, cross-sectional comparisons cannot prove causality, and short-term training programs in sedentary elders have showed either no effect on, or sometimes resulted in, impaired immune function (Nieman et al., 1993; Rall et al., 1996). This may be due to the tendency for vigorous exercise to result in subclinical muscle injury and an associated inflammatory response, and establishing the appropriate exercise levels may be particularly important for older individuals (Shepard & Shek, 1996). One study showed that rats subjected to both dietary restriction and long-term physical exercise did show delayed immunosenescence (Utsuyama, Ichikawa, Konno-Shirakawa, Fujita, & Hirokawa, 1996), suggesting a possible causal relationship, but this has not yet been firmly established in humans.

Finally, there is growing evidence that stress affects immunocompetence (Cohen & Herbert, 1996). Although studies in psychoneuroimmunology (PNI) have shown direct links between stress, immunosuppression, and the development of illness in animal models, connecting all of these links in humans is more difficult. This is due to a number of factors, including our longer life spans, in which cancers, for example, can take 20 years or more to develop and the robustness of human immune response, which fortunately ensures that the relationship between stress and illness in humans is relatively weak. There are also ethical conerns about subjecting individuals to stress levels sufficient to create major illness, and most of the studies are correlational in design, creating difficulties in causal interpretation. However, carefully controlled studies by Cohen and his colleagues (Cohen, Tyrrell, & Smith, 1993) have shown that stress can impact immune function, which results in more respiratory illness among individuals exposed to a cold virus.

There is also some evidence that how individuals cope with stress can bolster immune functioning. Studies by Fawzy and his colleagues (Fawzy et al., 1990, 1993) showed that individuals who had received coping interventions did use more effective means of coping with malignant melanoma. This coping resulted in less emotional distress, better immune function, and, most impressively, better survival after 6 years. Nearly a third of the control subjects had died, but less than 10% of the intervention subjects had died.

PNI studies in older adults, however, are fairly rare, in part because elders often have illnesses or on medications that can affect immune response, making them unsuitable subjects (for reviews see Aldwin, Spiro, Clark, & Hall, 1991). PNI studies are also sometimes difficult to interpret, because stress can result in either immunosuppression or activation, depending on its temporal and contextual characteristics (cf. Aldwin, 1994). Thus, McIntosh, Kaplan, Kubena, and Landmann (1993) showed that life events were associated with both increased and decreased lymphocyte counts in their aged sample, whereas marital conflict impaired immune responsiveness among long-term married couples (Kiecolt-Glaser et al., 1997). Reacting to stress with depressive symptoms may be particularly problematic for immune function in older adults (Aldwin et al., 1991).

Nervous System

Aging of the nervous system can also contribute to age-related changes in other systems. For example, slowing of neural transmission may affect the ability to regulate homeostasis as well as decrease response times. There may also be age-related changes in the levels of neurotransmitters. For example, blood levels of norepinephrine increase with age (DiGiovanna, 1994). Stress-related increases in norepinephrine appear heightened, and return to baseline levels less quickly.

Problems in ANS maintenance of homeostasis may be most noticeable in cardiovascular function. Many older adults suffer from orthostatic hypotension, which is a dramatic decrease in blood pressure when changing from a supine to a standing position, which can result in dizziness and falls. Normally, the sympathetic nervous system (SNS) maintains adequate levels of blood pressure by stimulating cardiac activity and constricting blood vessels. However, the norepinephrine receptors may be less responsive to SNS stimulation (which perhaps accounts for the higher levels of blood norepinephrine), and thus the heart and the blood vessels do not respond rapidly enough to maintain blood pressure.

One of the more intriguing hypotheses concerns the effect of stress on neurological aging. The hippocampus is particularly susceptible to neuronal loss with age, which Sapolsky (1992) suggests may be partially stress related. Glucocorticoids released by the adrenal cortex as part of the stress response do appear to have detrimental effects on neuronal loss in the hippocampus in animals (which in turn results in increasing levels of glucocorticoid, resulting in a cascade effect).

The three most common nervous system disorders in late life are strokes, dementia, and Parkinson's disease. Strokes, or cerebral vascular accidents (CVAs), are caused when a blockage in an artery prevents blood from flowing to part of the brain, probably due to atherosclerosis, or when a break in an artery results in a hemorrhage in the brain. Both can result in neuronal death. Neurons are postmitotic cells and may not replicate, and neuronal loss can have serious implications. The type of symptoms that result depends in large part on the location of the stroke and the pathways that it interrupts. For example, CVAs in the occipital region may result in blindness, in the sensory motor cortex may result in paralysis, in Broca's area in the frontal cortex may result in impaired language production, and damage in Wernicke's area in the temporal lobe may present with problems in language comprehension. However, if the loss is relatively minor, recovery of function can be achieved. Axons are capable of self-repair and increased dendritic branching may occur to restore neuronal pathways. Nerve growth factor (NGF) may assist in recovery of function processes in part by stimulating dendritic branching.

Dementia also increases with age, and there are many different types. Some are related to a series of transient ischemic attacks (TIAs), small strokes that result in cumulative damage. Pseudodementias may be due to inadequate nutrition, drug side effects, alcohol consumption, bladder infections, and so on, and may be reversible if adequately diagnosed. Brain tumors in older adults may clinically present as dementia and also appear to be increasing. However, by far the most common of the dementias is senile dementia of the Alzheimer's type (SDAT).

SDAT is characterized by an increase in neurofibrillary tangles and senile plaques, and a massive loss of neurons, especially cholinergic neurons. The brain atrophies and the ventricles become enlarged, as do the sulci. The exact symptoms of SDAT vary from individual to individual, in part as a function of which structures the neurofibrillary tangles and plaques infiltrate. They are found primarily in the hippocampus and the frontal and temporal lobes of the cortex, and eventually infiltrate subcortical structures, including the brain stem (Scheibel, 1996). SDAT is always characterized by impairment in both short- and long-term memory. Memory losses eventually become so severe that the individual may fail to recognize even very close loved ones. SDAT may also be associated with impairment in abstract thinking and judgment, difficulty in finding and defining words, copying three-dimensional figures, visuospatial disturbances resulting in an inability to find one's way around the neighborhood and house, and rapid personality change, often increases in aggression and inappropriate social behavior. Eventually, SDAT results in loss of the self, an inability to perform such basic tasks as feeding and toileting, and infiltration of the brain stem results in death. Currently, there is no good treatment for SDAT. The drugs currently approved for treatment have shown at best modest results, but there are several promising clinical trials for new treatments (Marx, 1996).

Parkinson's disease is the third most common neurological disorder in late life, and is characterized by a loss of cells in the substantia nigra, resulting in lower dopamine levels (McDowell, 1994). There are several different kinds of Parkinson's, but they are all characterized by motor tremors of the hands, arms, and legs, which decrease when performing voluntary tasks and during sleep. Increased muscle stiffness and decreased control of muscle contracts result in balance and gait problems as well as difficulty in completing voluntary movements. Eventually Parkinson's is also associated with dementia. Treatment with L-Dopa, a dopamine precursor, can mitigate the effects of Parkinson's.

Given that strokes are the leading cause of brain injury in late life, care of the cardiovascular system, through exercise, diet, and perhaps a daily aspirin, is also important for cognitive health. There is also evidence in animals that exercise directly benefits neurological functioning through an increase in the production of neurotrophic factors such as nerve growth factor, which can decrease neuronal death (Cotman & Neeper, 1996). However, whether exercise directly affects cognitive function in older humans is still a matter of debate. Exercise does improve cognitive function for the extremely sedentary, and long-term exercisers exhibit better cognitive function, but short-term interventions in older adults have generally shown little effect (Stones & Kozma, 1996).

There is also the intriguing suggestion that cognitive stimulation may help maintain cognitive function in late life. Enriched environments, in which animals receive extra stimulation, have been shown to increase the size of the cortex, even in elderly rats (Diamond, 1993). Education appears to be a protective factor for SDAT (Butler, Ashford, & Snowdon, 1996), although Pedersen, Reynolds, and Gatz (1996) caution that higher education may reflect better initial neurological functioning rather than function as a protective factor per se. Interestingly, Shimamura and his colleagues (1995) have shown that emeritus professors at Berkeley who do not have serious chronic disease show few cognitive decrements with age.

Interestingly, recent studies have suggested that estrogen replacement therapy may reduce the risk of Alzheimer's (Kawas et al., 1997), either through the protective effect of estrogen on vascular disease (Birge, 1997) or because estrogen may block the neurotoxic consequences of the stress response (Henderson, 1997). Nonetheless, given that the exact etiology of SDAT and Parkinson's disease are as yet poorly understood, it is difficult to specify behaviors that might avoid or defer onset of these disorders.

Endocrine System

Aging of the endocrine system may also underlie disease processes in a variety of organ systems. For example, the drop in estrogen with menopause enhances the risk of cardiovascular disease and osteoporosis, and may be associated with memory problems (Paganini-Hill & Henderson, 1996a, 1996b). Although most women do not experience menopausal depression, a dramatic decrease in estrogen, due, for example, to surgical menopause or a late life child, can result in clinical depression, as can a particularly long perimenopausal transition (Avis, Brambilla, McKinlay, & Vass, 1994).

In women, menopause signals a dramatic shift in sex hormones. The perimenopausal stage typically starts around age 45. The menstrual cycle shortens, perhaps due to age-related decrease in the responsiveness of the ovaries to luteinizing hormone (LH) and follicle-stimulating hormone (FSH), resulting in decreasing estrogen and progesterone levels. Eventually, the estrogen levels become low enough that ovulation ceases. On average, progesterone levels have decreased sufficiently by age 51 so that menstruation ceases, resulting in menopause. By the fourth year after menopause, the ovaries stop secreting estrogen, although there is some circulating estrogen because the adrenal cortex produces small amounts, and because the testosterone and androstenedione can be converted to estrogen, albeit in a less potent form.

There is currently a debate as to the origin and regulating mechanisms of menopause. Some argue that it is a function of decreasing numbers of follicles in the ovaries; others argue that it is centrally regulated via the hypothalamus. Wise, Krajnak, and Kashon (1996) argue that both the ovary and the brain are key pacemakers in menopause, and research is needed to study the interaction of these multiple regulators.

As mentioned earlier, the drop in estrogen levels has serious consequences. We now recognize that estrogen and other sex hormones affect a variety of other functions, including urinary incontinence, nutrient absorption and metabolism, cardiovascular function, memory and cognition, and bone and mineral metabolism. Estrogen declines also lead to characteristic age-related changes in appearance, including changes in body fat distribution and skin wrinkling. Interestingly, women who have more fat reserves may have less decline in estrogen, because fat cells convert androstenedione to estrogen. However, higher estrogen levels and delayed menses have also been associated with increase risk of breast and cervical cancers.

It is also important to recognize many hormones do not appear to show normal age-related changes, including thyroid hormones and insulin. However, there may be disease-related changes in their functioning.

Older adults seem particularly susceptible to both hypo- and hyperthyroidism (Gregerman & Katz, 1994). Both may result in fatigue and apathy. Older individuals with hyperthyroidism may lose weight and report nervousness, tremors, and heart palpitations, but their thyroid glands are not enlarged, unlike younger adults. Hypothyroidism in late life is probably an autoimmune disorder resulting in atrophy of the thyroid gland. About one-third of cases in older adults show classical signs of slowness of speech, thought, and movement, cold intolerance, and a coarsening of the skin and hair, but about two-thirds manifest only fatigue and can be difficult to diagnose. Arthritis-like conditions are also common in hypothyroidism, as are depression and ataxia (poor balance and gait problems), which are often dismissed as "simply aging." Elders presenting with these symptoms should be screened for hypothyroidism, as treatment is often effective in reversing these symptoms.

There is a dramatic increase in non-insulin-dependent diabetes mellitus (NIDDM) with age. Estimates for the prevalence of NIDDM in older adults range from 12 to 18%, with perhaps an additional 20% showing glucose intolerance (Stolk et al., 1997). Diabetes is especially problematic in African-Americans, who show 60% higher rates of diabetes compared to whites with comparable weights (Cowie, Harris, Silverman, Johnson, & Rust, 1993). Insulin and glucagon are released by the islets of Langerhans in the pancreas. Insulin removes glucose from the blood in several ways, promoting its entry into cells and storing it by either converting it to glycogen for storage in the muscle cells or by storing glucose in fat cells. In contrast, glucagon stimulates liver cells to release glucose into the blood. Although levels of circulating insulin do increase with age, this appears to be primarily related to a high carbohydrate diet, an increase in body fat, especially in the abdomen, and a reduction in physical fitness. The increase in insulin is probably due to the lower target cell responsiveness, which removes relatively little blood glucose even when insulin levels are high.

The consequences of diabetes are very severe. High blood glucose levels lead to the manufacture of sorbitol, which results in damage to blood vessels. This can cause cataracts and diabetic retinopathy, the leading cause of blindness in the aged. Sorbitol also causes degeneration of nerves, which can lead to fecal and urinary incontinence, impaired recovery from injury and gangrene of the feet, and perhaps cognitive impairment (Strachan, Deary, Ewing, & Frier, 1997). High blood glucose levels can also lead to glycosylation, which creates cross-linkages in proteins such as collagen fibers. This results in damage to the circulatory system, leading to heart attacks, strokes, gangrene of the lower extremities, and kidney failure. Finally, high blood glucose levels create high osmotic pressure, resulting in dehydration in cells, increased urination, and mineral loss, which can result in brain malfunction, circulatory failure, coma, and death. Classic signs of diabetes include weight loss, an increase in appetite and thirst, an increase in urination, greater susceptibility to infections, and the presence of glucose in the urine.

Exercise and diet are clearly important for the health of some portions of the endocrine system, including insulin and growth hormone levels and their effectiveness. For example, vigorous exercise and weight loss in older adults improve insulin sensitivity literally within days, but must be continued to be maintained (DiGiovanna, 1994).

Hormone replacement therapies (HRT) have generated much interest. Administration of both growth hormones and testosterone in older adults can improve body weight and lean muscle mass, but do not necessarily improve functional ability and may result in harmful side effects (Papadakis et al., 1996). In contrast, synthetic calcitonin, especially when administered in nasal sprays, may be effective in preventing or delaying the onset of osteoporosis and may even increase bone density slightly. Although it does not appear to affect bone density once osteoporosis is established, it may decrease pain and reduce the risk of fracture (Plosker & McTavish, 1996). Dehydroepiandrosterone (DHEA) is an androgen secreted by the adrenal gland that increases growth factors, lean muscle mass, and perhaps immune and cognitive function; some have recommended it as a way to enhance quality of life in older adults (Yen, Morales, & Khorram, 1995). Others, however, caution that DHEA may increase the risk of breast cancer (Dorgan et al., 1997) and argue that many of these effects have not been found in humans (Miller, 1996a).

The most common form of HRT is the administration of estrogen or estrogen–progesterone combinations in postmenopausal women. Estrogen treatment delays the onset of osteoporosis and decreases the risk of heart disease and perhaps Alzheimer's disease (Kawas et al., 1997). Although it can increase the risk of breast cancer, this is likely to be due to the effect of delaying menopause rather than an additional risk (Collaborative Group on Hormonal Factors in Breast Cancer, 1997).

Specific Organ Systems

This section has two purposes. The first is to describe diseases that are common in late life, and what effects they may have on psychosocial function. The second is to discuss ways of preventing or delaying the onset of these diseases.

Cardiovascular System

Cardiovascular diseases include not only problems with the heart but also the vascular system. The incidence of all cardiovascular diseases increases with age and includes hypertension, heart disease, congestive heart failure, stroke (cerebral vascular disease), and peripheral vascular disease. Arteriosclerosis refers to narrowing of the arteries, due to changes in the collagen fibers in the arterial walls. This causes them to harden and become less elastic. Atherosclerosis refers to the buildup of plaque on the walls, which causes arteries to narrow. Plaque is an amalgam of cholesterol, dead blood cells, and fibrotic fibers resulting from a complex interaction of heredity, diet, health behavior habits such as exercise and smoking, and immune system functioning. Atherosclerosis starts in childhood in Western countries and is slowly progressive throughout most of life. The most recent research suggests that arteriosclerosis is the more general condition, of which atherosclerosis is the most common subtype.

Hypertension, the persistent elevation of the systolic and/or diastolic arterial blood pressure, increases steadily with age and is the most common medical diagnosis in people over the age of 60 (Menscer, 1992). Generally, blood pressure that is maintained below 140 mm Hg (systolic) and 90 mm Hg (diastolic) is considered healthy, although there is great variation in these numbers. In the majority of cases, the cause of hypertension is unknown, and probably reflects both genetic and environmental factors. Secondary causes of hypertension in older adults include an increase in renal and hormonal diseases, as well as use of certain medications (sinus and cold preparations, as well as steroids). Hypertension is a major risk factor for cardiovascular disease, including atherosclerotic heart disease, congestive heart failure, and cerebrovascular accidents.

Coronary artery disease (CAD) is the leading cause of morbidity and mortality in late life (Hall, 1992). Men are affected by coronary artery disease at much younger ages than women and it is only by age of 75, 10 to 15 years after menopause, that the prevalence of CAD becomes equal for men and women (Wei, 1994). A heart attack, or myocardial infarction (MI), occurs when blood flow to cells in the heart muscle is interrupted, usually due to atherosclerosis. The arteries that feed the heart muscle become blocked and fail to deliver blood to the heart muscle. The seriousness of the MI reflects the amount of muscle tissue that is damaged. The heart can recover fairly well from minor attacks, but if too much muscle tissue is lost, disability or even death can result. Diagnosis of an MI is more difficult in the older person because symptoms of the problem are usually different from those found in a younger person. In a younger person chest pain, pallor, and perspiration are the classic indicators of an MI. However, in an older person, an MI may be signaled by confusion, weakness, vertigo, or abdominal pain. Furthermore, the older person has a higher frequency of complications following an MI, including life-threatening arrhythmias and heart failure (Wei, 1994).

Congestive heart failure occurs when the left side of the heart is weakened and is no longer able to pump blood effectively through the body. As well as a decreased perfusion of blood to the body, there is a resultant buildup of pressure in the left ventricle, raising venous and capillary pressure, which creates congestion in the lungs, and making it difficult to breathe. There are several causes of this disorder, including diseases of the cardiac valves and CAD. Congestive heart failure is a relatively common condition in the older population, and symptoms can range from mild to very severe. Congestive heart failure limits the ability to carry out normal activities due to shortness of breath. Treatment centers around the use of diuretics during acute episodes to eliminate excessive water and salt and the use of digitalis to increase the efficiency of the heart.

Strokes (cerebral vascular accidents or CVAs) are also a major problem in the older population. Most CVAs are secondary to atherosclerosis or hypertension. There are two causes of CVAs, a blockage of an artery in the brain or a hemorrhage from a ruptured artery. In both cases there is a lessened perfusion of oxygen and nutrients to the brain. As noted earlier, after a CVA the prognosis for the patient, both in mortality and in functional recovery, is dependent on coexisting medical problems of the person, the area of the brain where the damage occurs, and the extent of the damage. If damage occurs to a large enough area, recovery of function is much more difficult and often very limited. Transient ischemic attacks (TIAs), temporary blockage of blood to the arteries, are often warning signs of strokes. Both CVAs and TIAs can result in cognitive loss, which may be confused with Alzheimer's disease.

Prevention of cardiovascular disease starts early in life, although changes in life-style practices as an older person have also proven to be beneficial.

Weight control, smoking cessation, stress reduction, exercise, and a low-fat diet are primary factors in maintaining a healthy cardiovascular system. Epidemiologic studies closely link saturated fat and cholesterol levels to the development of atherosclerosis and coronary artery disease. Other preventive therapies include the use of aspirin to prevent blood clots from forming. Estrogen replacement therapy is also effective in reducing the incidence of heart attacks in women, although when used with progesterone its protective effect may be somewhat attenuated (Grodstein & Stampfer, 1995).

The protective effect of exercise on the cardiovascular system has been studied extensively. Various studies have shown that individuals who have followed a lifelong program of exercise and who avoid disease show less decline in cardiovascular function with age and may even live longer (Paffenbarger et al., 1993).

Gastrointestinal System

Older adults complain of a variety of digestive disorders. One of the most common problems in late life is periodontal disease, as nearly half of those over 65 have lost all of their teeth. Further, older people who are poor have a higher incidence of tooth loss than do adults from other socioeconomic groups (Henry, 1996). Hopefully, this will decrease in future generations with improved dental practices and preventive care, as oral health is essential to adequate nutritional intake.

Constipation, colitis, and hemorrhoids are also common complaints in later years. Most of these conditions likely stem from poor eating habits, lack of exercise, and medication use rather than aging per se. There is a danger, however, that these common complaints can obscure more serious disease processes. For example, an elder may assume that blood in the stool is due to a long-standing hemorrhoid problem rather than colon cancer. Due to lack of exercise, inadequate nutrition, and restriction of fluid intake, gastrointestinal problems are nearly universal in bed-bound elders. Sorting out the complaints in older persons requires extensive time, attention, and knowledge on the part of the health care provider.

Diverticular disease is one of the most frequently occurring gastrointestinal disorders of aging, found in at least one-third of people over the age of 60 (Nelson & Castell, 1990). Diverticula, sacs or pouches in the wall of the colon, develop as a result of changes in the elasticity of the colon, while diverticulitis is the inflammation that occurs when there is a perforation in one or more of the diverticula. The lack of dietary fiber is the most probable cause of the disease, since vegetarians and others with a lifelong high intake of fiber have a much lower incidence of the disease. However, why a high fiber diet is protective against diverticular disease is not clear at this time (Cheskin & Schuster, 1994a).

As with a number of other diseases, symptoms of diverticulitis are often different for young and older adults. Younger adults typically report fever, pain, constipation, diarrhea, and nausea, while the elders may not have a fever and complain less of pain. Diverticulitis is a very serious disease for both the young and old, and major problems can occur, including an abdominal abscess from leakage of intestinal contents into the abdominal cavity. Diverticulitis is usually treated conservatively in older adults, and includes rest, antibiotics, and hydration, but surgery may be necessary (Cheskin & Schuster, 1994a).

Cancers of the colon and rectum are fairly prevalent in the elderly and the incidence almost doubles with each decade over the age of 50. Risk factors include diet low in fiber and high in fat, as well as a family history of the disease and long-standing colitis or polyps. Early detection of the disease is crucial for survival; when colon cancer is confined to the mucosal layer of the bowel, there is an 80–90% 5-year survival rate (Cheskin & Schuster, 1994a). Independent of the age of the person, this type of cancer is invariably treated surgically, with the addition of chemotherapy and radiation, if necessary. Although some practitioners may hesitate to subject elders to surgery, their long-term survival rate is no different than younger cancer victims, although they have more postoperative complications (Mulcahy, Patchett, Daly, & O'Donoghue, 1994).

Gallbladder disease also occurs throughout adulthood but is far more common in older people. Risk factors include a diet high in cholesterol and fat, inactivity, high blood pressure, diabetes, and smoking. Women, especially those using estrogen replacement, are also at higher risk of the disease. The most common symptoms of gallbladder disease are indigestion, pain when fat is eaten, nausea, and vomiting. The treatment of choice is to remove the gallbladder, because blockage in the common bile duct may be a dangerous complication. Even in the most frail patient, aggressive treatment is recommended over more conservative methods, e.g., weight loss and avoidance of fatty foods (Gilliam, 1994). Recent advances in treatment include laparoscopic removal of the gallbladder, which is less invasive than regular surgery, and the use of ultrasound to break down the stones.

Finally, undernutrition can be a problem for older people. About 16% of elderly people in the United States consume less than 1000 calories a day, placing them in danger of undernourishment. This increases dramatically among the ill or institutionalized (Nelson & Franzi, 1992). Risk factors for undernutrition are chronic disease and functional losses, low income, social isolation, depression or cognitive impairment, and use of drugs or alcohol.

To have a healthy gastrointestinal system, it is important to develop lifelong habits of good nutrition and exercise. This includes eating a diet high in fiber, that is, whole grains and fresh fruits and vegetables, as well as drinking fluids, especially water. The nutritional needs of older adults are somewhat different from those who are younger, in particular their need for adequate levels of protein, vitamins, and minerals to decrease vulnerability to disease and enhance recovery from illness and injury (Rosenberg, 1994). Almost all essential nutrients are required for adequate brain function, including glucose. Interestingly, adequate nutrition in the current cohort of elders may largely reflect their oral health. For example, missing teeth, poor fitting dentures, and periodontal disease may limit the types of food that they are able to eat and the pleasure of eating, which may result in inadequate nutrition.

Respiratory System

The respiratory system is particularly vulnerable to disease in late life. Although many respiratory diseases occur throughout the life span, they are both more prevalent and more virulent in late life. For example, pneumonia is the fifth leading cause of death in people over the age of 65 (Bartlett, 1994). It is one of the few acute infectious diseases to which the older adults are more susceptible than the young and it is much more likely to result in death. Pneumonia was termed "the friend of the aged" in early days of medicine, as it hastened the death of an aged person suffering multiple illnesses. It is still a prevalent disease of the aged and a difficult one to diagnosis and to treat. Symptoms of pneumonia often present differently in older versus younger individuals, making accurate diagnosis difficult. Younger individuals typically complain of fever or chills, whereas the older person may suffer from poor appetite, weakness, or forgetfulness. Pneumonia is one of the leading causes of hospitalization in the aged. However, it is preferable that the illness be treated in the home, if possible, as older adults are especially vulnerable to nosocomial infections, that is, those acquired in a hospital or institution.

Frail elders are also susceptible to tuberculosis, a disease that is being seen more often in the United States, in part due to the growing population of homeless and the lack of health prevention programs for new immigrants. Tuberculosis is difficult to diagnosis because its symptoms resemble those of other respiratory illnesses (cough, low-grade fever, weakness, and loss of weight) and often goes unrecognized. Older adults who live in close quarters, such as institutions, are at particular high risk as the bacteria is airborne. There are medications available to cure the illness, but the regimen is long (9–18 months), making compliance difficult for many frail elders (Stead & Dutt, 1994).

Chronic obstructive pulmonary disease (COPD) is an umbrella term for several respiratory illnesses, including chronic bronchitis, emphysema, and asthma. The hallmark of all COPD illnesses is reduced expiratory airflow or inability to rid the lungs of trapped air. Symptoms of COPD are often insidious, usually disabling, and very uncomfortable, frequently leading to extreme distress as the person is not able to eliminate old air or take in fresh oxygen. Individuals with COPD often use the sternocleidomastoid muscles in the upper chest to aid in expanding the lungs, failing to use the diaphragm muscles properly. Over time, diaphragm and intercostal muscle strength declines, challenging physical endurance and further inhibiting adequate respiration (Adair, 1994). Risk factors for COPD include cigarette smoking, age, and occupational exposure to asbestos, coal dust, smoke, and other environmental pollutants.

Two of the most common COPD diseases are chronic bronchitis and emphysema. Chronic bronchitis is the fifth leading cause of death in the United States, and most deaths occur in people over the age of 55 (Adair, 1994). In this condition, the cells of the respiratory tract produce thickened mucous, in a process called hypersecretion, which makes it difficult to clear the respiratory tract. On the other hand, emphysema is characterized by damage to the alveoli, which limits their ability to take in or get rid of air. Long-term insult results in scarring on the surface of the alveoli, as well as hypersecretion of mucous. Air becomes trapped behind mucous plugs, further causing prolonged inflation of the alveoli. The thickening of the alveoli cell walls, their hyperinflation, and the trapped air render gas exchange problematic. In truth, it is often difficult to differentiate between the two conditions, bronchitis and emphysema, as they may co-occur and result in similar damage and symptoms.

Lung cancer is the leading cause of cancer death in men and women (Perry, 1994). Cigarette smoking accounts for 85–90% of lung cancers, and the risk of death from lung cancer is directly related to cigarette smoking, often calculated in pack years (number of packs smoked per year times the number of years smoked). As is well known at this time, even passive exposure to cigarette smoke increases the risk of the disease. Diagnosis of lung cancer is difficult because warning signs, chronic cough, blood in sputum, or shortness of breath, are similar to symptoms of other respiratory illnesses. Although early diagnosis is beneficial, general prognosis for the disease is poor, with only a 5–10% survival rate over 5 years (Perry, 1994). In general, surgery and radiation are treatment modes for lung cancer. Even with the recent trends for more aggressive treatment of the disease, survival rate has changed very little over the years (Kaesberg, 1996). There are some age differences in the disease course of lung cancer: at diagnosis, it is more likely to have metastasized in middle-aged patients than in older ones. Thus, the older person may have a greater likelihood of being cured (Perry, 1994). Further, aggressive treatment may be appropriate for all ages as there are reports that patients in their seventh decade of life benefit as much from surgical treatment as those at younger ages (Santambrogio, Nosotti, Bellaviti, & Mezzetti, 1996).

There are enormous individual variations in respiratory change with age, usually dependent on exercise history and health of the older person. Further, regular aerobic exercise, even at older ages, enhances the ability to maintain pulmonary capacity and recover from illness, and adds to longevity (Lee, Hsieh, & Paffenbarger, 1995). In addition, older people are encouraged to get vaccines to protect themselves against influenza and pneumonia, although there is some question as to the ability of the immune system of the very frail older person to respond to these vaccines (Pomidor, 1992).

One of the most important ways of maintaining respiratory health is to avoid smoking. Pulmonary function declines are accelerated in smokers, and cessation of smoking decreases the rate of decline, although not to the extent of nonsmokers (Lavizzo-Mourey, 1994). Even for individuals with COPD, cessation of smoking is a high priority in their treatment. Although it is difficult to reverse the damage that has been done by these diseases (especially emphysema), management can reduce symptoms and improve functional status. In fact, new advances in pulmonary rehabilitation programs have proven to be beneficial in both old and young people, measured by an increase in walking distance and improved self-assessment scores (Couser, Guthmann, Hamadeh, & Kane, 1995).

It is impossible to underestimate the importance of lifelong respiratory care. Pulmonary fitness as a young person is predictive of respiratory health in later years, but exercise that challenges the respiratory system is beneficial even into very old years.

Urinary/Renal System

Urinary incontinence in not a normal consequence of aging, but a physiological disorder that can be highly embarrassing and socially isolating. Consequently, urinary incontinence frequently results in a poorer quality of life. The prevalence of urinary incontinence increases with age, is slightly higher in women, and is more common in older persons in institutions (70%) than those who live in the community (20%) (Ham, 1992). Further, incontinence has been shown to be a primary risk factor for permanent institutionalization (Baker & Brice, 1995). This overlooked and undertreated ailment of older people can usually be comfortably managed and even cured.

There are four basic types of urinary incontinence: stress, urgency, overflow, and functional (Ouslander, 1994). Stress-related incontinence is due to weakness of the pelvic floor muscles, which in turn reflects previous vaginal deliveries or sphincter weakness, often due to low levels of estrogen. With this type of incontinence, laughing or sneezing may result in dribbling. In urge incontinence, there is an irritation that stimulates the bladder to empty frequently. This can be due to local infection, obstruction due to a tumor, or a CNS disorder, e.g., stroke. In overflow incontinence, there is anatomic obstruction that prevents the bladder from emptying completely, resulting in constant dribbling of urine. This is usually due to an enlarged prostate. However, overflow incontinence may also be due to poor regulation of the sphincter muscles because of a neurogenic disorder, e.g., spinal cord lesion. Finally, functional incontinence refers to inappropriate micturition due to a variety of causes, including dementia, medication use, or depression.

With age, almost all men have a gradual enlargement of the prostate gland. The growth of the gland causes it to compress the urethra, leading to nocturia (nighttime urination), urinary hesitancy, decreased urinary stream, and, occasionally, incontinence. These symptoms of benign prostatic hyperplasia (BPH) begin around the age of 50 in most men. The probable causes of this disorder are aging and age-associated changes in hormones, primarily androgens. Men are often hesitant to seek help for this disorder, although symptoms can become very bothersome. Surgery involving partial prostatectomy is the treatment of choice at this time, although alternatives to surgery, such as hormone therapy and indwelling metal shunts, are being tested (Brendler, 1994).

Prostate cancer seldom occurs in men under the age of 50. The cause of this illness is unknown, although there may be a familial connection. It does not appear to be related to BPH. African-American men are most at risk of prostate cancer, although they are also the least aware of symptoms and/or methods that are available for screening (Price, Colvin, & Smith, 1993). Although there are no early symptoms of prostate cancer, in later stages the disease resembles symptoms of BPH as the growth pushes on the urethra and hampers urination (Brendler, 1994).

Prostate cancer tumors vary in their rate of growth and it is difficult at biopsy to determine the aggressiveness of the tumor, which makes it difficult to determine prognosis of the disease. However, mortality rates due to prostate cancer are higher for men under the age of 65, and thus the disease is generally treated very aggressively in that age group, using surgery, radiation, or some combination thereof. In older men, however, aggressive treatment is questionable as they are more likely to die of an illness other than prostate cancer. Further, surgery and radiation can result in incontinence and impotence. Nevertheless, Mazur and Merz (1995) found that older men with prostate cancer chose treatment and the risks of side effects (impotence but not incontinence) over a shorter life expectancy.

The most common screening test for prostate cancer is a rectal examination to feel for irregularities or hardening of prostatic tissue. Another screening tool, prostatic-specific antigen (PSA), is a blood test that is currently being used to test for cancer in prostatic tissue, although there are limitations to this test as it is also elevated in men with BPH. Of further consideration is that screening for prostate cancer has been questioned because, as mentioned above, treatment in older age groups is controversial and medical outcomes can be detrimental to the quality of life of the man. However, at this time, recommendations are for men over the age of 50 to have PSA and a rectal exam yearly (Brendler, 1994). Again, there are heated discussions among health professionals about the advisability of screening for prostate cancer (Collins & Barry, 1996), except for those men at particular risk of prostate cancer.

Diseases that affect the kidneys of younger people also are found in those over the age of 65, including glomerulonephritis, nephritis, and renal failure, both acute and chronic. However, because of the existence of concurrent illnesses in older persons, e.g., diabetes and hypertension, the course and management of these diseases are more complicated. Renal disorders can result in problems with water metabolism, hyponatremia (low sodium), and hypokalemia (low potassium), which can exacerbate other health problems. For example, an older person with congestive heart failure needs to be able to maintain fluid and electrolyte homeostasis, but this is compromised in the aging or diseased kidney. Less well known is the fact that fluid and electrolyte imbalances can cause confusional states, and make elders more susceptible to environmental stressors such as heat and cold. In a recent heat wave in Chicago, for example, hundreds of elders died from hyperthermia and the inability to maintain homeostasis, which stressed the heart and other organs.

Contrary to popular opinion, appropriate management can alleviate many of the symptoms of incontinence (Ouslander, 1994). Both men and women can use Kegel exercises, repetitive contractions of the pelvic floor muscles, to prevent stress incontinence, and estrogen replacement can be helpful for women. A recent development has been the use of a collagen implant into the tissues surrounding the urethra, which adds bulk to the tissues and prevents leakage of urine. Antibiotics, bladder relaxant medications, behavioral procedures, or surgery (dependent on the cause) are used in the treatment of urge incontinence. Surgery and catheterization have been used successfully in overflow incontinence and behavioral therapy and/or incontinence undergarments are commonly helpful for people who have functional incontinence (Ouslander, 1994).

Further, elders and their caregivers should be alerted to the dangers of dehydration. Due to worries about incontinence, many elders fail to consume adequate fluid levels, which is especially problematic during heat waves. Interestingly, dementia may be one of the presenting symptoms for bladder and kidney infections (Tunkel & Kaye, 1994). Thus, health practitioners should check for infections, as well as dehydration and electrolytic imbalance, when assessing for possible dementias.

Musculoskeletal System

Musculoskeletal pathology is nearly universal in late life, and is a leading cause of morbidity and functional loss for old people. The two most common skeletal disorders in late life are osteoporosis and osteoarthritis. (These two disorders should not be confused with rheumatoid arthritis, associated with severe deformity of the joints, which is actually an autoimmune system disorder that can strike at any age.)

Osteoporosis reflects bone loss that has progressed to the point where bones break under little or no stress. Fractures occur primarily in the vertebrae, wrist (distal radius), and "hip" (actually, usually the top of the femur) (Chestnut, 1994). Groups that are at risk of developing this illness are Caucasians and Asian women, and those with low body weight and/or with a family history of osteoporosis. African-Americans are less likely to develop the disease, in part due to larger frame sizes and higher levels of body fat. Estrogen deficiency is the major determinant of postmenopausal osteoporosis, although the lifestyle factors of inactivity and low calcium intake are also implicated.

The consequences of osteoporosis are very severe, affecting not only body structure but other systems of the body. The loss of bone mass in the vertebrae, the round, disk-like bones that make up the spinal column, can result in compression of the spine, with a possible decrease in height. Multiple vertebral fractures will often result in a severe skeletal deformity, called skeletal kyphosis, or dowager's hump. In this condition, many of the vertebra are fused together and the spinal column is bowed, sometimes to the extent that the lowest rib is actually resting on the iliac crest of the pelvis, which results in abdominal distention and diminished respiratory function. Colles' fracture of the wrist are another common complication of osteoporosis, in fact the most frequent type of fracture in Caucasian women under age 75 (Meier, 1990). Although this type of fracture often heals rapidly, even this temporary functional loss results in decreased independence and need for outside assistance.

Contrary to popular belief, hip fractures do not reflect breaks in the pelvic bone, but rather the top of the femur or thigh bone. Consequences of this type of fracture are very severe and include hospitalization, surgery, morbidity, nursing home placement, and even death. In fact, more than 25% of all patients with hip fractures are discharged to nursing homes and, of those, almost 35% never resume walking again (Meier, 1990). Mutran, Reitzes, Mossey, and Fernandez (1995) found that poor social support, as well as depression, resulted in less improvement in walking among women 59 years of age and older.

Prevention of osteoporosis is problematic, as there are few symptoms of the disease until a fracture occurs. Early diagnosis and therapy can reduce the risk of a fracture, but currently there is no precise and accurate screening mechanism that is also reasonably priced (Chestnut, 1994). Treatment for osteoporosis centers around the use of calcium and vitamin D supplementation for both men and women, bone metabolism regulators, including hormones such as estrogen and calcitonin, as well as antiresorptive agents (Bone et al., 1997).

The incidence of osteoarthritis, a chronic inflammatory disease of the joints, is another condition that increases with age. This disease affects about 80% of people over the age of 65, women more so than men, and is the most common form of arthritis in the aged (Spirduso, 1995). It is characterized by a slowly progressive deterioration of joint cartilage, particularly in the fingers, hips, and knees. Obesity, persistent wear and tear, and prior injury are precursors to osteoarthritis. There may also be a familial relationship, in at least some forms of the disease.

When osteoarthritis occurs in the hip, knee joints, or feet, pain and discomfort can seriously impair mobility, creating a change in normal walking gait. The short, shuffling steps seen in many elders are a direct consequence of arthritis in the hips. Treatment for osteoarthritis consists of maintaining an active life-style (including physical therapy), heat, and the use of analgesics (Fife, 1994). Older people who have severe disability from this disease often will have very successful surgical replacement of the injured joint (Studenski, Rigler, & Robbins, 1996).

Finally, falling in the senior population is seen as a major public health problem. There are a number of reasons as to why the older person is at risk of falling: loss of muscle mass interfering with balance, changes in gait and sensory deficits, and neuromotor slowing. Further, fractures in later life take longer to heal, require longer recovery times, and are more likely to result in the person becoming confined to a wheelchair or bed bound (Grisso & Kaplan,

1994). Immobility further exacerbates bone and muscle loss, leading to a cascade effect. Finally, Brummel-Smith (1992) found that older adults were less likely to receive adequate rehabilitation, although active rehabilitation is one of the keys to recovery at all ages.

Adequate calcium and vitamin D intake as well as physical activity are the keys to maintaining bone density in later years. Taking both calcium and vitamin D may be well advised in later years, both for men and women, as the the manufacture of vitamin D decreases with age, a problem that is made worse because older people spend less time outdoors and are exposed less to the sun. A study in New York City of aged adults residing in nursing homes in the winter and spring showed that they had insufficient vitamin D levels, suggesting the need for supplementation (O'Dowd, Clemens, Kelsey, & Lindsay, 1993). In addition, exercise has beneficial effects on bone maintenance, muscle mass, and balance, even in very late life (see Whitbourne, Chapter 4, this volume).

Integumentary System

Skin disorders can affect both the health and physical appearance of the older person. Some are simply bothersome and/or unsightly, but others can be life threatening. One of most common skin problem that occurs with age is xerosis, or dry skin. The cause of this condition is unknown, but it results in scaling of the skin, itching, and inflammation. Xerosis is worse for older people in winter months when people stay inside in a warm, dry environment. Hot or frequent baths and irritating detergents can also exacerbate the condition. People with this condition are usually advised to avoid frequent hot baths, to use mild soaps, and to use topical ointments after bathing, although the use of oils in bathing is dangerous as they can leave the bathtub slippery.

There are a number of benign lesions that are common in late life. One of the most common is seborrheic keratosis, brown to black colored irregular lesions that appear to be stuck to the skin. They are usually removed for cosmetic reasons as well as to differentiate the lesion from a malignant one (Kaminer & Gilchrest, 1994).

Prevalence of skin cancers increases with age and with exposure to the sun. Basal cell carcinoma, a small, fleshy bump or nodule, is the most common type of skin cancer in late life, and, although these types of cancer are not considered deadly, if they are not removed extensive injury to the skin can occur. Squamous cell carcinoma, usually appearing as red, scaly patches, is the second most common form of skin cancer. This type of cancer generally occurs in areas where there has been chronic ulceration or extreme exposure to the sun. Because squamous cell carcinomas can metastasize, they are removed surgically. Further, many older people find them bothersome or unattractive, and thus wish to have them taken off.

Of particular importance is a malignant melanoma, a type of skin cancer that can be fatal. People who are most at risk are those who have pale skin, have had a history of blistering sunburns, and/or have a family history of a malignant melanoma (Kaminer & Gilchrest, 1994). There is a decreased risk in dark brown or black-skinned people. The classic description of a malignant melanoma is a red, white, blue, or black growth that has an irregular border. Successful treatment depends on its early detection and removal. Any mole that changes in shape or other characteristics is suspect and needs to be checked by a health care professional.

The decubitus ulcer or bed sore is a serious noncancerous skin disorder that is not only very painful but also difficult to treat. Spending long hours in bed or sitting in a wheel chair without frequent changes of position creates pressure points in the body, eventually creating a sore or tear in the skin and surrounding tissue. The resulting ulcers are not only unsightly and painful, but are extremely difficult to heal, especially given the decrease in vascularization and immunocompetence of the skin. The existence of decubitus ulcers may be one indicator of the elder neglect in institutionalized settings, but, for the very frail elder, is almost unavoidable (Allman, 1994).

Care of the skin can include both preventive and ameliorative actions. While moisturizers cannot decrease wrinkles, they can mitigate their appearance. Special creams, or even Vaseline or Crisco, can alleviate some of the discomfort due to xerosis, or dry skin. Further, a new topical medication, Retin-A, has been shown to improve sun-damaged skin and help to increase skin smoothness (Goldfarb, Ellis, & Voorhees, 1990). Sun block should be used to prevent damage from ultraviolet rays and decrease wrinkling, maldistribution of melatonin, and the probability of skin cancers. Finally, estrogen replacement therapy has been used with good results to increase skin thickness in post-menopausal women (Cortes-Gallego, Villanueva, Sojo-Aranda, & Santa Cruz, 1996).

Sensory System

Although diseases of the sensory system are usually not directly life-threatening, they can have a devastating effect on an older adult's quality of life. Problems in either vision or hearing can decrease an elder's ability to move about effectively in the environment, interfere with social interaction, and increase his or her susceptibility to accidental injury.

Cataracts, cloudiness or opacity of the lens of the eye, can occur at any age, but are found much more frequently in later years. Although painless, with time they can interfere with vision, particularly at nighttime or in bright sunlight. Surgery is usually done when the person complains that the cataract interferes with their daily life. In the meantime, patients are advised to use sunglasses to protect their eyes against the sun's rays.

Glaucoma is a leading cause of blindness in late life. It is caused by an increasing buildup of fluid in the eyeball, which results in pressure and damage to the optic nerve. This disease can be present for many years without any symptoms, quietly doing its damage. People most of risk of glaucoma include those of African-American descent or with a family history of glaucoma. High blood pressure and diabetes are also risk factors. There are several ways to control the damage of glaucoma, including medications and laser therapy, but early detection is the key to prevention of retinal damage (Reuben, 1991).

One of the most deleterious retinal diseases is macular degeneration, a relatively newly diagnosed disorder. In this condition the macula of the eye, or the part of the retina where central vision occurs, is damaged. The cause of the disease is unknown, although a precursor may be age-related thinning of the retina. Laser treatment is being used with some success to stop the disease process, but there is no cure at this time (Michaels, 1994). Again, sunglasses to screen out ultraviolet rays is believed to help prevent the condition.

Although there can be many causes of poor hearing, including excess cerumen or wax in the ear, the major reason is damage to the minuscule hair cells that line the inner ear. It is believed that this damage, in part, is due to loud noises or what is termed "environmental pollution." Other causes of hearing loss include familial tendency to deafness and being male. Interestingly, African-American men have less hearing loss, suggesting that genetics does play a role in hearing loss (Mhoon, 1990).

Hearing loss with age, or presbycusis, profoundly affects the life of the older person. There is the issue of safety when the ability to hear car horns, smoke alarms, or barking dogs is gone. There can be loss of connectiveness to the environment as the ability to determine the presence of others, or to hear birds singing or water running, declines or disappears. Further, willingness to communicate with others, or to mingle in social settings, is often diminished. Thus, loss of hearing can lead to depression and sometimes paranoia. Use of hearing aids has long been considered a sign of aging, and not a very popular one. On the other hand, with President Clinton (age 50) wearing a newly acquired hearing devise, this stigma may decrease.

Functional Health

As we have seen, normative age-related changes tend to have little impact on day-to-day functioning, although they may impair our ability to respond to environmental challenges. There is also a shift in the nature of illness with age, from acute to chronic illnesses such as hypertension, arthritis, and cardiovascular disease—indeed, the majority of older Americans have one or more of these illnesses. However, the existence of chronic disease does not necessarily result in disability, and the stereotype of the frail elder is simply not applicable to most of the young-old (individuals in their 60s and 70s). Thus, gerontologists and geriatricians are becoming more interested in functional health, that is, the degree of impairment of the individual, regardless of type of disease, or, usually, combination of diseases.

There are two basic ways of assessing functional health (Kovar & Lawton, 1994). Activities of daily living (ADLs) consist of those basic activities required of an adult to be independent, such bathing, dressing, toileting, eating, transferring from bed to chair, and walking. Individuals with deficiencies in these areas are at risk of institutionalization. ADLs are typically used to determine treatment requirements, eligibility for health care services, and adequacy of institutional care (Stone & Murtaugh, 1990).

Instrumental activities of daily living (IADLs) tap higher order skills that are also necessary for independent living. Although the content of IADL scales varies, most include questions about the ability to use the telephone, manage money, prepare meals, do light or heavy housework, and shop. Indications of IADL difficulties in an older person may warn of impending problems and an intervention at this stage may help prevent further deterioration of the environment, reduce the danger of institutionalization, and allow the person to remain self-sufficient.

Prevalence of disability increases substantially with age, both in ADLs and IADLs. According to the 1989 National Long Term Care Survey only about 10% of older persons have limited ability with the ADL bathing, and the percentage reporting losses in indoor activities such as walking, transferring, using the toilet, or eating is even smaller (Jette, 1996). On the other hand, older people have more difficulty with IADLs. Nearly 24% of community-dwelling elders in one study had difficulty doing heavy housework and 11% had difficulty shopping (Kovar & Lawton, 1994).

ADL and IADL impairments are predictive of both morbidity and mortality. Older people who have functional losses are more likely to be institutionalized, to recover more slowly after institutionalization, and to be at greater risk of mortality (Guralnik & Simonsick, 1993; Manton, Corder, & Stallard, 1993). ADL scores indicating low functional status are associated with less likelihood of patients returning home after institutionalization and are indicative of new and worsened impairment during hospitalization and a delayed functional recovery after discharge (Hirsch, Sommers, Olsen, Mullen, & Winograd, 1990). Thus, knowing the functional abilities of an elder is often more useful than simply having an illness diagnosis.

Summary

Normal age-related changes are generally mild and do not seem to impair normal functioning, but they do make individuals more susceptible to disease, which can severely impact individuals' quality of life. Diagnosis is often difficult in the aged adults because many diseases present differently in young and old individuals, and vague symptoms can be indicative of many different kinds of problems. Cognitive impairment in particular may have many different etiologies, such as infections, cardiovascular disease, electrolyte imbalances, poor nutrition, depression, and hormonal deficiencies, as well as neuronal disorders, and adequate diagnosis is essential for proper treatment. Further, illnesses tend to have cascade effects, with perturbations in one system leading to problems in others.

It is encouraging that the rate of decline in health can be modified in late life. Most important is adequate exercise and nutrition, and an avoidance of toxins such as cigarette smoking and excessive alcohol intake. Even in late life, improvements in exercise and diet can have salutary effects. Although severe caloric restriction as an antiaging mechanism is still controversial in humans, obesity can lead to many problems in metabolism, skeletal integrity, and perhaps cancer, and thus should be avoided. Hormone replacement therapies in particular hold great promise for delaying or mitigating the aging process. Although death is inevitable, decreases in functional impairment due to diseases can greatly improve the quality of life in older adults.

Acknowledgments

Preparation of this chapter was supported by a grant from the National Institute on Aging (AG13006). We would like to thank Drs. Lois Aldwin and Michael R. Levenson for their helpful comments on earlier drafts of this paper.

REVIEW QUESTIONS

1. What are the three types of immunity?

2. What are the effects of the decrease in estrogen at menopause?

3. What are the different types of urinary incontinence, and how would you treat them?

4. What are the causes and consequences of osteoporosis?

5. Why is it harder for older adults to maintain homeostasis?

6. How does the immune system change with age?

7. What are the different types of cardiovascular disease in the elderly?

8. What are the major causes of malnutrition in the elderly?

9. What are the consequences of diabetes?

10. What types of disorders can result in confusional states in the elderly?

11. What are the effects of exercise on the aging processes?

12. What is the effect of stress on the aging processes?

References

Adair, N. (1994). Chronic airflow obstruction and respiratory failure. In W. R. Hazzard, E. L. Bierman, J. P. Blass, W. H. Ettinger, & J. B. Halter (Eds.), *Principles of geriatric medicine and gerontology* (3rd ed., pp. 583–595). New York: McGraw-Hill.

Adler, W. H., & Nagel, J. E. (1994). Clinical immunology and aging. In W. R. Hazzard, E. L. Bierman, J. P. Blass, W. H. Ettinger, & J. B. Halter (Eds.), *Principles of geriatric medicine and gerontology* (3rd ed., pp. 67–75). New York: McGraw-Hill.

Aldwin, C. (1994). *Stress, coping, and development: An integrative approach.* New York: Guilford.

Aldwin, C., Spiro, A. III, Clark, G., & Hall, N. (1991). Thymic hormones, stress and psychological symptoms in older men: A comparison of different statistical techniques for small samples. *Brain, Behavior and Immunity, 5,* 206–218.

Allman, R. M. (1994). Pressure ulcers. In W. R. Hazzard, E. L. Bierman, J. P. Blass, W. H. Ettinger, & J. B. Halter (Eds.), *Principles of geriatric medicine and gerontology* (3rd ed., pp. 1329–1336). New York: McGraw-Hill.

Avis, N. E., Brambilla, D., McKinlay, S. M., & Vass, K. (1994). A longitudinal analysis of the association between menopause and depression. Results from the Massachusetts Women's Health Study. *Annals of Epidemiology, 4,* 214–220.

Baker D. I., & Brice T. W. (1995). The influence of urinary incontinence on publicly financed home care services to low-income elderly people. *Gerontologist, 35,* 360–369.

Bartlett, J. G. (1994). Pneumonia. In W. R. Hazzard, E. L. Bierman, J. P. Blass, W. E. ttinger, & J. B. Halter (Eds.), *Principles of geriatric medicine and gerontology* (3rd ed., pp. 565–573). New York: McGraw-Hill.

Birge, S. J. (1997). The role of estrogen in the treatment of Alzheimer's disease. *Neurology, 48* (Suppl. 7), S36–41.

Bone, H. G., Downs, R. W., Tucci, J. R., Harris, S. T., Weinstein, R. S., Licata, A. A., McClung, M. R., Kimmel, D. B., Gertz, B. J., Hale, E., & Polvino, W. J. (1997). Dose-response relationships for alendronate treatment in osteoporotic elderly women. *Journal of Clinical Endocrinology and Metabolism, 82,* 265–274.

Brendler, C. B. (1994). Disorders of the prostate. In W. R. Hazzard, E. L. Bierman, J. P. Blass, W. H. Ettinger, & J. B. Halter (Eds.), *Principles of geriatric medicine and gerontology* (3rd ed., pp. 657–664). New York: McGraw-Hill.

Brummel-Smith, K. (1992). Rehabilitation. In R. J. Ham & P. D. Sloane (Eds.), *Primary care geriatrics: A case-based approach* (2nd ed., pp. 137–161). St. Louis: Mosby Year Book.

Butler, S. M., Ashford, J. W., & Snowdon, D. A. (1996). Age, education, and changes in the Mini-Mental State Exam scores of older women: Findings from the nun study. *Journal of the American Geriatrics Society, 44,* 675–681.

Chandra, R. K. (1992). Effect of vitamin and trace-element supplementation on immune responses and infection in elderly subjects. *Lancet, 340,* 1124–1127.

Cheskin, L. J., & Schuster, M. M. (1994a). Colonic disorders. In W. R. Hazzard, E. L. Bierman, J. P. Blass, W. H. Ettinger, & J. B. Halter (Eds.), *Principles of geriatric medicine and gerontology* (3rd ed., pp. 723–732). New York: McGraw-Hill.

Chestnut, C. H. (1994). Osteoporosis. In W. R. Hazzard, E. L. Bierman, J. P. Blass, W. H. Ettinger, & J. B. Halter (Eds.), *Principles of geriatric medicine and gerontology* (3rd ed., pp. 897–907). New York: McGraw-Hill.

Cohen, S., & Herbert, T. B. (1996). Health psychology: Psychological factors and physical disease from the perspective of human psychoneuroimmunology. *Annual Review of Psychology, 47,* 113–142.

Cohen, S., Tyrrell, D. A., & Smith, A. P. (1993). Negative life events, perceived stress, negative affect, and susceptibility to the common cold. *Journal of Personality & Social Psychology, 64,* 131–140.

Collaborative Group on Hormonal Factors in Breast Cancer (1997). Breast cancer and hormone replacement therapy: Collaborative reanalysis of data from 51 epidemiological studies of 52,705 women with breast cancer and 108,411 women without breast cancer. *The Lancet, 350,* 1047–1059.

Collins, M. N., & Barry, M. (1996). Controversies in prostate cancer screening: Analogies to the early lung cancer screening debate. *Journal of the American Medical Association, 276,* 1976–1979.

Cortes-Gallego, V., Villanueva, G. L., Sojo-Arnada, I., & Santa Cruz, F. J. (1996). Inverted skin changes induced by estrogen and estrogen/glucocorticoid on aging dermis. *Gynecological Endocrinology, 10,* 125–128.

Cotman, C., & Neeper, S. (1996). Activity-dependent plasticity and the aging brain. In E. L. Schneider & J. W. Rowe (Eds.), *Handbook of the biology of aging* (4th ed., pp. 284–299). San Diego: Academic Press.

Couser, J. I., Guthmann, R., Hamadeh, M. A., & Kane, C. S. (1995). Pulmonary rehabilitation improves exercise capacity in older elderly patients with COPD. *Chest, 107,* 730–734.

Cowie, C. C., Harris, M. I., Silverman, R. E., Johnson, E. W., & Rust K. F. (1993). Effect of multiple risk factors on differences between blacks and whites in the prevalence of non-insulin-dependent diabetes mellitus in the United States. *American Journal of Epidemiology, 137,* 719–732.

Diamond, M. C. (1993). An optimistic view of the aging brain. *Generations, 17,* 31–33.

DiGiovanna, A. G. (1994). *Human aging: Biological perspectives.* New York: McGraw Hill.

Dorgan, J. F., Stanczyk F. Z., Longcope C., Stephenson H. E., Jr., Chang L., Miller R., Franz C., Falk, R. T., & Kahle, L. (1997). Relationship of serum dehydroepiandrosterone (DHEA), DHEA sulfate, and 5–androstene-3 beta, 17 beta-diol to risk of breast cancer in postmenopausal women. *Cancer Epidemiology, Biomarkers and Prevention, 6,* 177–181.

Fawzy, F. I., Cousins, N., Fawzy, N. W., Kemeny, M. E., Elashoff, R., & Morton, D. (1990). A structured psychiatric intervention for cancer patients: I. Changes over time in methods of coping and affective disturbance. *Archives of General Psychiatry, 47,* 720–725.

Fawzy, F. I., Fawzy, N. W., Hyun, C. S., Elashoff, R., Guthrie, D., & Fahey, J. L., & Morton, D. L. (1993). Malignant melanoma: Effects of an early structured psychiatric intervention, coping, and affective state on recurrence and survival 6 years later. *Archives of General Psychiatry, 50,* 681–689.

Fife, R. S. (1994). Osteoarthritis. In W. R. Hazzard, E. L. Bierman, J. P. Blass, W. H. Ettinger, & J. B. Halter (Eds.), *Principles of geriatric medicine and gerontology* (3rd ed., pp. 981–986). New York: McGraw-Hill.

Gilliam, J. H. (1994). Hepatobiliary disorders. In W. R. Hazzard, E. L. Bierman, J. P. Blass, W. H. Ettinger, & J. B. Halter (Eds.), *Principles of geriatric medicine and gerontology* (3rd ed., pp. 707–715). New York: McGraw-Hill.

Goldfarb, M. T., Ellis, C. N., & Voorhees, J. J. (1990). Dermatology. In C. K. Cassel, D. E. Riesenberg, L. B. Sorensen, & J. R. Walsh (Eds.), *Geriatric medicine* (2nd ed., pp. 383–393). New York: Springer-Verlag.

Gregerman, R. I., & Katz, M. S. (1994). Thyroid diseases. In W. R. Hazzard, E. L. Bierman, J. P. Blass, W. H Ettinger, & J. B. Halter (Eds.), *Geriatric medicine and gerontology* (pp. 807–824). New York: McGraw-Hill.

Grisso, J. A., & Kaplan, F. (1994). Hip fractures. In W. R. Hazzard, E. L. Bierman, J. P. Blass, W. H. Ettinger, & J. B. Halter (Eds.), *Principles of geriatric medicine and gerontology* (3rd ed., pp. 1321–1327). New York: McGraw-Hill.

Grodstein, F., & Stampfer, M. (1995). The epidemiology of coronary heart disease and estrogen replacement in postmenopausal women. *Progress in Cardiovascular Diseases, 38,* 199–210.

Guralnik, J. M., & Simonsick, E. M. (1993). Physical disability in older Americans. *Journals of Gerontolog: Social Sciences, 48* (Special Issue), S3–S10.

Hall, N. K. (1992). Health maintenance and promotion. In R. J. Ham & P. D. Sloane (Eds.), *Primary care geriatrics: A case-based approach* (2nd ed., pp. 95–118). St. Louis: Mosby Year Book.

Ham, R. J. (1992). Incontinence. In R. J. Ham & P. D. Sloane (Eds.), *Primary care geriatrics: A case-based approach* (2nd ed., pp. 381–405). St. Louis: Mosby Year Book.

Henderson, V. W. (1997). The epidemiology of estrogen replacement therapy and Alzheimer's disease. *Neurology, 48* (Suppl. 7), S27–35.

Henry, R. G. (1996). Oral diseases and disorders. In D. B. Reuben, T. T. Yoshikawa, & R. W. Besdine (Eds.), *Geriatrics review syllabus* (3rd ed., pp. 280–284). Dubuque, IA: Kendall/Hunt.

Hirsch, C. H., Sommers, L., Olsen, A., Mullen, L., & Winograd, C. (1990). The natural history of functional morbidity in hospitalized older patients. *Journal of the American Geriatrics Society, 38,* 1296–1303.

Jette, A. M. (1996). Disability trends and transitions. In R. H. Binstock & L. K. George (Eds.), *Handbook of aging and the social sciences* (4th ed., pp. 94–116). San Diego: Academic Press.

Kaesberg, P. R. (1996). Oncology. In D. B. Reuben, T. T. Yoshikawa, & R. W. Besdine (Eds.), *Geriatrics review syllabus* (3rd ed., pp. 321–328). Dubuque, IA: Kendall/Hunt.

Kaminer, M. S., & Gilchrest, B. A. (1994). Aging of the skin. In W. R. Hazzard, E. L. Bierman, J. P. Blass, W. H. Ettinger, & J. B. Halter (Eds.), *Principles of geriatric medicine and gerontology* (3rd ed., pp. 411–429). New York: McGraw-Hill.

Kawas, C., Resnick, S., Morrison, A., Brookmeyer, R., Corrada, M. Zonderman, A., Bacal, C., Lingle, D. C., & Metter E. (1997). A prospective study of estrogen replacement therapy and the risk of developing Alzheimer's disease: The Baltimore Longitudinal Study of Aging. *Neurology, 48,* 1517–1521.

Kiecolt-Glaser, J. K., Glaser, R., Cacioppo, J. T., MacCallum, R. C., Snydersmith, M., Kim, C., & Malarkey, W. B. (1997). Marital conflict in older adults: Endocrinological and immunological correlates. *Psychosomatic Medicine, 59,* 339–349.

Kovar, M. G., & Lawton, M. P. (1994). Functional disability: Activities and instrumental activities of daily living. In M. P. Lawton & J. A. Teresi (Eds.), *Annual review of gerontology and geriatrics* (Vol. 14, pp. 57–75). New York: Springer Publishing Co.

Lavizzo-Mourey, R. (1994). Promoting health and function among older adults. In W. R. Hazzard, E. L. Bierman, J. P. Blass, W. H. Ettinger, & J. B. Halter (Eds.), *Principles of geriatric medicine and gerontology* (3rd ed., pp. 213–220). New York: McGraw-Hill.

Lee, I. M., Hsieh, C. C., & Paffenbarger, R. S. (1995). Exercise intensity and longevity in men: The Harvard Alumni Health Study. *Journal of the American Medical Association, 273,* 1179–1184.

Manton, K. G., Corder, L. S., & Stallard, E. (1993). Estimates of change in chronic disability and institutional incidence and prevalence rates in the U. S. elderly population from the 1982, 1984, and 1989 National Long Term Care Survey. *Journals of Gerontology: Social Sciences, 48*, S153–S166.

Marx, J. (1996). Searching for drugs that combat Alzheimer's. *Science, 273*, 50–53.

Mazur, D. J., & Merz, J. F. (1995). Older patients' willingness to trade off urologic adverse outcomes for a better chance at five-year survival in the clinical setting of prostate cancer. *Journal of the American Geriatrics Society, 43*, 979–984.

McDowell, F. H. (1994). Parkinson's disease and related disorders. In W. R. Hazzard, E. L. Bierman, J. P. Blass, W. H. Ettinger, & J. B. Halter (Eds.), *Geriatric medicine and gerontology* (3rd ed., pp. 1051–1062). New York: McGraw-Hill.

McIntosh, W. A., Kaplan, H. B., Kubena, K. S., & Landmann, W. A. (1993). Life events, social support, and immune response in elderly individuals. *International Journal of Aging and Human Development, 37*, 23–36.

Meier, D. (1990). Disorders of skeletal aging. In C. K. Cassel, D. E. Riesenberg, L. B. Sorensen, & J. R. Walsh (Eds.), *Geriatric medicine* (2nd ed., pp. 164–183). New York: Springer-Verlag.

Menscer, D. (1992). Hypertension. In R. J. Ham & P. D. Sloan (Eds.), *Primary care geriatrics: A case-based approach* (2nd ed., pp. 561–575). St. Louis: Mosby Year Book.

Mhoon, E. (1990). Otology. In C. K. Cassel, D. E. Riesenberg, L. B. Sorensen, & J. R. Walsh, (Eds.), *Geriatric medicine* (2nd ed., pp. 405–419). New York: Springer-Verlag.

Michaels, D. D. (1994). The eye. In W. R. Hazzard, E. L. Bierman, J. P. Blass, W. H. Ettinger, & J. B. Halter (Eds.), *Principles of geriatric medicine and gerontology* (3rd ed., pp. 441–456). New York: McGraw-Hill.

Miller, R. A. (1996a). Aging and the immune response. In E. L. Schneider & J. W. Rowe (Eds.), *Handbook of the biology of aging* (4th ed., pp. 355–392). San Diego: Academic Press.

Miller, R. A. (1996b). The aging immune system: Primer and prospectus. *Science, 273*, 70–74.

Mulcahy, H. E., Patchett, S. E., Daly, L., & O'Donoghue, D. P. (1994). Prognosis of elderly patients with large bowel cancer. *British Journal of Surgery, 81*, 736–738.

Mutran, E. J., Reitzes, D. C., Mossey, J., & Fernandez, M. E. (1995). Social support, depression, and recovery of walking ability following hip fracture surgery. *Journals of Gerontology: Social Sciences, 50B*, S354–S361.

Nelson, J. B., & Castell, D. O. (1990). Gastroenterology. In C. K. Cassel, D. E. Riesenberg, L. B. Sorensen, & J. R. Walsh (Eds.), *Geriatric medicine* (2nd ed., pp. 347–361). New York: Springer-Verlag.

Nelson, R. C., & Franzi, L. R. (1992). Nutrition. In R. J. Ham & P. D. Sloane (Eds.), *Primary care geriatrics: A case-based approach* (2nd ed., pp. 162–193). St. Louis: Mosby Year Book.

Nieman, D. C. (1997). Exercise immunology: Practical applications. *International Journal of Sports Medicine, 18* Suppl 1:S91–100.

Nieman, D. C., Henson, D. A., Gusewitch, G., Warren, B. J., Dotson, R. C., Butterworth, D. E., & Nehlsen-Cannarella, S. L. (1993). Physical activity and immune function in elderly women. *Medicine and Science in Sports and Exercise, 25*, 823–831.

O'Dowd, K. J., Clemens, T. L., Kelsey, J. L., & Lindsay, R. (1993). Exogenous calciferol (vitamin D) and vitamin D endocrine status among elderly nursing home residents in the New York City area. *Journal of the American Geriatrics Society, 41*, 414–421.

Ouslander, J. G. (1994). Incontinence. In W. R. Hazzard, E. L. Bierman, J. P. Blass, W.

H. Ettinger, & J. B. Halter (Eds.), *Principles of geriatric medicine and gerontology* (3rd ed., pp. 1229–1249). New York: McGraw-Hill.

Paffenbarger, R. S., Hyde, R. T., Wing, A. L., Lee, I. M., Jung, D. L., & Kampert, J. B. (1993). The association of changes in physical-activity level and other lifestyle characteristics with mortality among men. *New England Journal of Medicine, 328,* 538–545.

Paganini-Hill, A., & Henderson, V. W. (1996a). Estrogen replacement therapy and risk of Alzheimer disease. *Archives of Internal Medicine, 156,* 2213–2217.

Paganini-Hill, A., & Henderson, V. W. (1996b). The effects of hormone replacement therapy, lipoprotein cholesterol levers, and other factors on a clock drawing task in older women. *Journal of the American Geriatrics Society, 44,* 818–822.

Papadakis, M. A., Grady, D., Black, D., Tierney, M. J., Gooding, G. A., Schambelan, M., & Grunfeld C. (1996). Growth hormone replacement in healthy older men improves body composition but not functional ability. *Annals of Internal Medicine, 124,* 708–716.

Pedersen, N. L., Reynolds, C. A., & Gatz, M. (1996). Sources of covariation among mini-mental state examination scores, education, and cognitive abilities. *Journal of Gerontology: Psychological Sciences, 51B,* P55–P63.

Perry, M. C. (1994). Lung cancer. In W. R. Hazzard, E. L. Bierman, J. P. Blass, W. H. Ettinger, & J. B. Halter (Eds.), *Geriatric medicine and gerontology* (3rd. ed., pp. 607–613). New York: McGraw-Hill.

Plosker, G. L., & McTavish, D. (1996). Intranasal salcatonin (salmon calcitonin). A review of its pharmacological properties and role in the management of postmenopausal osteoporosis. *Drugs and Aging, 8,* 378–400.

Pomidor, A. (1992). Pneumonia. In R. J. Ham & P. D. Sloan, (Eds.), *Primary care geriatrics: A case-based approach* (2nd ed., pp. 603–611). St. Louis: Mosby Year Book.

Price, J. H., Colvin, T. L., & Smith, D. (1993). Prostate cancer: Perceptions of African-American males. *Journal of the National Medical Association, 85,* 941–947.

Rall, L. C., Roubenoff, R., Cannon, J. G., Abad, L. W., Dinarello, C. A., & Meydani, S. N. (1996). Effects of progressive resistance training on immune response in aging and chronic inflammation. *Medicine and Science in Sports and Exercise, 28,* 1356–1365.

Reuben, D. B. (1991). Hearing and visual impairment. In J. C. Beck (Ed.), *Geriatrics review syllabus* (pp. 160–172). New York: American Geriatrics Society.

Rosenberg, I. H. (1994). Nutrition and aging. In W. R. Hazzard, E. L. Bierman, J. P. Blass, W. H. Ettinger, & J. B. Halter (Eds.), *Principles of geriatric medicine and gerontology* (3rd ed., pp. 49–59). New York: McGraw-Hill.

Rothstein, G. (1994). White cell disorders. In W. R. Hazzard, E. L. Bierman, J. P. Blass, W. H. Ettinger, & J. B. Halter (Eds.), *Principles of geriatric medicine and gerontology* (3rd ed., pp. 749–761). New York: McGraw-Hill.

Santambrogio, L., Nosotti, M., Bellaviti, N., & Mezzetti, M. (1996). Prospective study of surgical treatment of lung cancer in the elderly patient. *Journals of Gerontology: Biological and Medical Sciences, 51,* M267–M269.

Sapolsky, R. M. (1992). *Stress, the aging brain, and the mechanism of death.* Cambridge, MA: MIT Press.

Scheibel, A. B. (1996). Structural and functional changes in the aging brain. In J. E. Birren & K.Warner Schaie (Eds.), *Handbook of the psychology of aging* (pp. 105–128). San Diego: Academic Press.

Shepard, R. J., & Shek, P .N. (1996). Impact of physical activity and sport on the immune system. *Reviews on Environmental Health, 11,* 133–147.

Shimamura, A. P., Berry, J. M., Mangels, J. A., & Rusting, C. L. (1995). Memory and cognitive abilities in university professors: Evidence for successful aging. *Psychological Science, 6,* 271–277.

Sone, Y. (1996). Age-associated problems in nutrition. *Applied Human Science, 14,* 201–210.

Spirduso, W. W. (1995). *Physical dimensions of aging.* Champaign, IL: Human Kinetics.

Stead, W. W., & Dutt, A. K. (1994). Tuberculosis: A special problem in the elderly. In W. R. Hazzard, E. L. Bierman, J. P. Blass, W. H. Ettinger, & J. B. Halter (Eds.), *Principles of geriatric medicine and gerontology* (3rd ed., pp. 575–582). New York: McGraw-Hill.

Stolk, R. P., Pols, H. A., Lamberts, S. W., de Jong, P. T., Hofman, A., & Grobbee, D. E. (1997). Diabetes mellitus, impaired glucose tolerance, and hyperinsulinemia in an elderly popuation. The Rotterdam Study. *American Journal of Epidemiology, 145,* 24–32.

Stone, R. I., & Murtaugh, C. M. (1990). The elderly population with chronic functional disability: Implications for home care eligibility. *Gerontologist, 30,* 491–496.

Stones, M. J., & Kozma, A. (1996). Activity, exercise, and behavior. In J. E. Birren & K. W. Schaie (Eds.), *Handbook of the psychology of aging* (4th ed., pp. 338–352). San Diego: Academic Press.

Strachan, M. W., Deary, I. J., Ewing, F. M., & Frier, B. M. (1997). Is type II diabetes associated with an increased risk of cognitive dysfunction? A critical review of published studies. *Diabetes Care, 20,* 438–445.

Studenski, S. A., Rigler, S. K., & Robbins, J. M. (1996). Musculoskeletal diseases and disorders. In D. B. Reuben, T. T. Yoshikawa, & R. W. Besdine (Eds.), *Geriatrics Review Syllabus* (3rd ed., pp. 234–251). Dubuque, IA: Kendall/Hunt.

Tunkel, A. R., & Kaye, D. (1994). Urinary tract infections. In W. R. Hazzard, E. L. Bierman, J. P. Blass, W. H. Ettinger, & J. B. Halter (Eds.), *Principles of geriatric medicine and gerontology* (3rd ed., pp. 625–635). New York: McGraw-Hill.

Utsuyama, M., Ichikawa, M., Konno-Shirakawa, A., Fujita, Y., & Hirokawa, K. (1996). Retardation of the age-associated decline of immune functions in aging rats under dietary restriction and daily physical exercise. *Mechanisms of Ageing and Development, 91,* 219–228.

Venjatraman, J. T., & Fernandes, G. (1997). Exercise, immunity and aging. *Aging, 9,* 42–56.

Wei, J. Y. (1994). Disorders of the heart. In W. R. Hazzard, E. L. Bierman, J. P. Blass, W. H. Ettinger, & J. B. Halter (Eds.), *Principles of geriatric medicine and gerontology* (3rd ed., pp. 517–532). New York: McGraw-Hill.

Wise, P. M., Krajnak, K. M., & Kashon, M. L. (1996). Menopause: The aging of multiple pacemakers. *Science, 273,* 67–70.

Yen, S. S., Morales, A. J., & Khorram, O. (1995). Replacement of DHEA in aging men and women. Potential remedial effects. *Annals of the New York Academy of Sciences, 774,* 128–142.

Additional Readings

Cohen, S., & Herbert, T. B. (1996). Health psychology: Psychological factors and physical disease from the perspective of human psychoneuroimmunology. *Annual Review of Psychology, 47,* 113–142.

Collaborative Group on Hormonal Factors in Breast Cancer (1997). Breast cancer and hormone replacement therapy: Collaborative reanalysis of data from 51 epidemiological studies of 52,705 women with breast cancer and 108,411 women without breast cancer. *The Lancet, 350,* 1047–1059.

Cotman, C., & Neeper, S. (1996). Activity-dependent plasticity and the aging brain. In E. L. Schneider & J. W. Rowe (Eds.), *Handbook of the biology of aging* (4th ed., pp. 284–299). San Diego: Academic Press.

Jette, A. M. (1996). Disability trends and transitions. In R. H. Binstock & L. K. George (Eds.), *Handbook of aging and the social sciences* (4th ed., pp. 94–116). San Diego: Academic Press.

Kovar, M. G., & Lawton, M. P. (1994). Functional disability: Activities and instrumental activities of daily living. In M. P. Lawton & J. A. Teresi (Eds.), *Annual review of gerontology and geriatrics* (Vol. 14, pp. 57–75). New York: Springer Publishing Co.

Miller, R. A. (1996b). The aging immune system: Primer and prospectus. *Science, 273,* 70–74.

Paffenbarger, R. S., Hyde, R. T., Wing, A. L., Lee, I. M., Jung, D. L., & Kampert, J. B. (1993). The association of changes in physical-activity level and other lifestyle characteristics with mortality among men. *New England Journal of Medicine, 328*(8), 538–545.

Sapolsky, R. M. (1992). *Stress, the aging brain, and the mechanism of death.* Cambridge, MA: MIT Press.

Shimamura, A. P., Berry, J. M., Mangels, J. A., & Rusting, C. L. (1995). Memory and cognitive abilities in university professors: Evidence for successful aging. *Psychological Science, 6,* 271–277.

Stones, M. J., & Kozma, A. (1996). Activity, exercise, and behavior. In J. E. Birren & K. W. Schaie (Eds.), *Handbook of the psychology of aging* (4th ed., pp. 338–352). San Diego: Academic Press.

6

Dying and Bereavement

Robert Kastenbaum

What we call aging flows from what we call developing.
What we call dying flows from what we call living.
What we call grieving flows from what we call loving.
Social and behavioral scientists have tended to regard both aging and death as special topics. In human development courses these "peripheral" topics frequently are placed at semester's end where, with any luck, they can be dispatched quickly if not completely evaded. One thinks of Jean Baudrillard's (1993, p. 126) Foucault inspired contention that all ghettos had their origin in society's displacement of the dead:

> At the very core of the 'rationality' of our culture . . . is an exclusion that precedes every other, more radical than the exclusion of madmen, children, or inferior races, an exclusion preceding all these and serving as their model: the exclusion of the dead and of death.

It is no longer tenable to restrict the topics of dying, death, and bereavement to the academic equivalent of a ghetto that is of interest only to specialists with a morbid turn of mind. Understanding human development and experience without attention to death is as possible as understanding the physical universe without attention to gravity. Neither mortality nor gravity cease operation where ignored. This chapter is based on the premise that we stand to improve the quality of our lives as individuals and the quality of our work as gerontologists by serious consideration of what it is that brings us down and how we live with this prospect. We will be looking at the aging individual's encounters with mortality within the frame of the total life-course and the interpersonal relationships and symbolic interactions that link each person with the community. Dying and grieving are not appendages *to* living; rather, these terms designate critical episodes and dimensions *within* the experience of living.

We begin with the overall picture of age and mortality: what are the major causes of death for elderly men and women and what trends are in evidence? This exploration will help to provide a context for understanding individual and societal responses to death in the later adult years. We then follow a topic sequence that parallels the events and experiences occurring prior to and during the last phase of life: (1) attitudes and behavior patterns before death is imminent; (2) major causes of death; (3) end-of-life issues, including management of the dying process and other decision points, including the options of suicide and euthanasia; and (4) bereavement, grief, and recovery. We conclude with a brief consideration of implications for life-course theory and interventions.

How Do Elderly Men and Women Meet Their Deaths?

Dying and grieving occur within the ever-changing sociocultural flow. The principal risks to life and the odds of surviving to one's next birthday are conditioned by each society's *death system* (Kastenbaum, 1997), i.e., the ways in which mortality is interpreted and the pattern of actions that either increase or decrease vulnerability to death and the ability to recover from grief. Medical advances have reduced the risk of death from some causes and lenghened the duration of the preterminal and terminal phases of life for many people. At the same time, our ability to care for the terminally ill and to support the grieving has been affected by changes in family size, mobility and stability (Stephens & Franks, Chapter 12, this volume), the movement toward a consumer society, and many other factors.

Death Becomes More Patient

At the turn of the century infants, children, and youth were at particularly high risk for death, as were women going through the child-bearing process. The general mortality rate was 17.2 per 1000 people. The mortality rate has since declined significantly. The most recent statistics available show a mortality rate of 8.9 per 1000 people in 1995. To put it another way: longevity has increased remarkably. More than 25 years have been added to life expectation at birth since the turn of the century. Furthermore, life expectation has increased for elderly adults as well. Women who have reached age 75 now have an average expectancy of 12 more years if white and 11 if African-American. Men at 75 have nearly a decade of life awaiting them on the average (African-American: 8.7; white: 9.5). The reduction in mortality rate, increase in longevity, and graying of America are three facets of the same trend toward a longer-lived population. The rapid development of gerontology and geriatrics itself is part of the broad spectrum of societal responses to a longer-lived population.

Much of this improvement is attributable to the sharp reduction in contagious diseases that had for centuries decimated the ranks of infants and youth (Aldwin & Gilmer, Chapter 5, this volume). The hazards faced by child-bearing women have been sharply reduced and a newborn's chances of surviving into adulthood have markedly increased. Society has found ways to protect its young more effectively, and so we have had larger and larger survivor cohorts venturing into the later adult years.

Societal Images of Life and Death

There has been a subtle alternation in the sociocultural image of death as the force of mortality has increasingly found its expression among long-lived people. At present in the United States about 80% of all deaths occur after age 60. The same general trend is apparent throughout much of the world. *Paradoxically, there is both more life (increased expectancy) and more death (higher percentage of total population mortality) in the later adult years.* Death had long been portrayed in poetry, song, and the visual arts as a personified force that tore a child from the arms of its mother or one young lover from another. Today there is a tendency to soften the image of death by personifying him (usually male) as a "gentle comforter" (Kastenbaum & Herman, 1997) who comes for the old and weary. There is also a tendency to enhance this image with the supposition that elders have completed their lives and therefore are ready to accept death's invitation—a supposition that speaks more about society's needs and wishes than about an elderly person's actual state of mind.

Unlike the situation at the turn of the century, we now expect children to grow up, grow old, and then die when life supposedly does not matter so much to them, or their lives matter so much to others. As a society we are devastated by the "untimely" (i.e., nonnormative) death of the young, but consider death to be "natural" for the aged. This attitude cluster was not unknown in the past, but has become more salient today. Of particular concern for gerontologists is the cultural assumption that the death of elderly men and women is an anti-climactic event that fulfills Nature's plan, a dry branch snapping off in the breeze. We are therefore relieved of responsibility as researchers, educators, caregivers, and advocates. But are we?

Major Causes of Death

Each pathway to death has distinctive characteristics, as illustrated by Glaser and Strauss's (1968) useful concept of *trajectories of dying.* Family and friends have no chance to prepare themselves for the loss or engage in leave-taking interactions with a person whose life ends through the *unexpected quick trajectory.* By contrast, a person who is moving toward death on the *lingering trajectory* will be available for continued contact over a protracted period of time, but

will require both physical care and emotional support month after month. Pathways to death also differ in the type of symptomatology that is likely to be experienced, each configuration of stress and loss having distinctive effects on
the individual and those providing care.

We would not want to lose sight of the fact that people do not just die—
people die with specific patterns of physical change that affect their functional
abilities, relationships, mood, and self-concept in distinctive ways. The brief
summary that follows represents but an invitation to attend carefully to the total sociophysical context within which elderly people end their lives.

Heart Disease and Cancer

Heart disease became the most common cause of death in the United States in
1940, and cancer moved up to the second position. These causes have remained
in their dominant positions up to the present day, having displaced pneumonia, influenza, and tuberculosis after these conditions were brought under improved control by public health measures and medical advances (Aldwin &
Gilmer, Chapter 5, this volume). The 10 major causes of death for the general
population today are presented in Table 6.1. It can be seen that heart disease
and cancer take by far the heaviest toll, accounting for more deaths each year
than the other leading causes combined.

TABLE 6.1.
10 Leading Causes of Death in the United States: All Ages

Rank	Cause of death	Number	Rate
1	Heart disease	2,322,421	875.4
2.	Malignant neoplasms	733,834	276.6
3.	Cerebrovascular diseases	160,431	60.5
4.	Chronic obstructive pulmonary disease & allied conditions	106,146	40.0
5.	Accidents & adverse effects	93,874	35.4
6.	Pneumonia & Influenza	82,579	31.1
7.	Diabetes mellitus	61,559	23.2
8.	Human immunodeficiency virus infection	32,655	12.3
9.	Suicide	30,862	11.6
10.	Chronic liver disease & cirrhosis	25,325	9.5

Rates per 100,000. Preliminary 1996 data.
Source: National Center for Health Statistics

Heart disease continues to be the leading cause of death in the later adult years despite a notable and sustained decline in rate. In 1970, for example, men in the 65–74 age group had a heart disease death rate of 2170 per 100,000. This rate had fallen to 1178 by 1993. A decline of similar magnitude occurred with women during the same time frame: from 1082 to 589.3. Clearly, older Americans have been included in the overall decline in heart disease mortality that became evident from approximately 1970 onward. The very old have also benefitted from a decline in the death rate due to heart disease, although not to so large an extent. The remarkable reduction in heart disease mortality in the later adult years has not altered the fact that risk of death from this cause still increases with age. For every person who dies of heart disease between the ages of 15 and 24, more than 200 die at age 75 and beyond (with substantial increments at intervening ages).

It is a different story with cancer. Unfortunately, the overall decline in the cancer death rate that was first noted in 1989 does not apply to elderly adults (Parker, Tong, Bolden, & Wingo, 1997). It is clear that the same major factor contributes both to the decline in overall cancer death rates for the general population and the elevated rate and number of cancer deaths among elders: the use of tobacco products. Americans have been smoking less in recent years, thereby reducing mortality from carcinoma of the lung and respiratory system. Nevertheless, more people are entering their later adult years and more are bringing with them a history of smoking that produces cancer or precancerous conditions. Between the ages of 60 and 79, 1 man in 15 and 1 woman in 26 develops cancer of the respiratory system—an incidence about four times greater than what is found between the ages of 40 and 59. Furthermore, the increase in smoking among women since World War II is now expressing itself in rising lung cancer mortality. As Cunningham (1997, p. 3) observes: "American women have the highest death rates in the world from cancer of the lung and bronchus, a sorry commentary on history's most technologically advanced society."

Life-Style Deaths

Smoking is an even more powerful contributor to death in the later adult years than what is revealed by lung cancer statistics alone. Many deaths that are attributed primarily to heart, cerebrovascular, and chronic obstructive pulmonary disease have been hastened by the effects of tobacco products, as have the development of some tumors in other organ systems, especially the oral cavity and digestive system. A realistic assessment of the causes of death in American elders requires serious attention to the role of tobacco products.

"Life-style" deaths include other major causes in addition to smoking. Cirrhosis of the liver is alcohol's equivalent of tobacco's lung disease. It takes many years of substance abuse for the liver to become dysfunctional, therefore cirrhosis becomes an increasingly prevalent cause of death in the later adult years.

The lethal effects of alcohol are also expressed through its role in accidents and suicide. People who have not been drinking are among the victims of those who have, as in motor vehicle fatalities. Accidental death rates increase substantially throughout the later adult years. Falls become a more common type of fatal accident. For example, African-American women have an accidental death rate of 28.7 per 100,000 when they are in the 45- to 54 year-old range. Those who survive to age 75 have an accidental death rate of 94.9, which doubles at age 85. African-American males have the highest accidental death rate throughout their lives, rising to a peak of 235.7 at age 85 and above (U. S. Bureau of Census, 1996). (Fortunately, in recent years the death rate for accidents has been declining for African-Americans and whites and males and females.)

Young drivers involved in fatalities are more likely to have been drinking, driving too fast, and operating unsafe vehicles; elderly drivers are more likely to have been inattentive and insufficiently responsive to road conditions. Whatever the type of accident, elders are at a higher risk for disability and death.

Suicide rates increase steadily for white men starting in the fifth decade. The oldest white males (85+) are also those with the highest rate of completed suicides in the entire age × race × gender configuration. This rate has been increasing for more than a decade. The suicide rate is much lower for both African-American and white women throughout the life-course, including the most advanced years. From the statistical standpoint, suicide makes a different type of contribution to the total death rate among youths and elders. Suicide has been among the five leading causes of death for young people in the United States for many years, although the rate is but a fraction of that for elders. By contrast, the very high rate of suicide for elderly white males is exceeded by even higher rates for heart disease, cancer, and other medical conditions. Most who die young in the United States are victims of life-style deaths such as accident, homicide, HIV infection, and suicide. Homicide and HIV infections are infrequent causes of death among elders; accident and suicide are important *preventable* causes of death, but account for a smaller percentage of all deaths.

Overall, people in their later adult years now have more years ahead of them than in any previous time in history. When their lives do end it is usually the result of conditions with which they have lived for many years, some of which are directly linked to life-style (for example, drinking, smoking, diet, exposure to noxious substances, and stress in occupational/residential settings). It is common for death to be the outcome of multiple causative pathways, for example, a respiratory infection that overtaxes a weakened cardiovascular system in a person who is somewhat depressed over the loss of loved ones and/or functional capacities. Death may also be hastened by lack of access to effective medical and psychosocial care. As compared with the past, there is less likelihood of elders dying in great numbers from contagious disease. People are more likely to cope as well as they can with chronic conditions that eventually transition into a terminal process.

Within this general picture there is the crucial matter of the elderly person's attitude toward life and death. Some people endure hardships and limitations without losing their will to live; others are sorely tempted to end their suffering by direct or indirect suicide. We must, then, enter the realm of attitudes and values.

Individual and Societal Attitudes toward Death in the Later Adult Years

In this section we focus on elderly men and women who are not in particular jeopardy for their lives, so far as this judgment can be made about anybody. They are engaged in living, but aware that they will not be living forever. We would be wise to bring the usual caveats with us: (1) there are marked individual differences in the death attitudes among elderly people, that have developed from (2) gender and cohort-related experiences over many years, and which are (3) subject to influence by the situations in which they find themselves at the moment. "Age" does not "cause" a particular configuration of attitudes; it serves instead as a useful index of how much life experience people bring to their views of dying and death.

Some Life History Influences on the Death Attitudes of Elderly People

Without losing sight of these caveats, it is possible to identify some fairly common biographical experiences that have influenced the death-related attitudes held by elderly men and women today.

Death Has Been in Their Lives in Many Ways for a Long Time. Today's elders were more likely than later cohorts to have been born into large families and to live in rural areas. Children growing up on the farm knew pigs and chickens as animals to be raised and slaughtered rather than as packaged bacon, pork, and thighs, breasts, and wings at the supermarket. Youth also had more exposure to death within their family circle: more people dying younger and less often shielded from their view by the intervention of health care professionals. A sibling would be lost to diphtheria or scarlet fever. A mother would die of "childbed fever," or some time later of an opportunistic infection. The shining youth on whom the family pinned its hopes would be taken by "consumption." Accidents (other than motor vehicle) were more common than today, and the victims, human or animal, lay where they fell until somebody in the family or neighborhood carted them away. Graveyards, local and stark, were seldom transfigured into "memorial parks."

A man in his late 80s speaks of his childhood on a potato farm:

Life was hard, hard for everybody I knew. But that's only what you expected, and there were good times, too. Some deaths were hard, but, you see, so was life—so, what the hell!

A woman of like age recalls that

So many of us went out horizontal. I'm talking about the influenza. My sisters and I, we'd sit on the porch and whisper about who might be next. Then we'd just sit silent. Did we know about death? How could we not know about death?

Feelings about Death Were Not to Be Explored and Discussed.   Many of today's elders developed a realistic attitude toward the basic facts of death through their direct exposure to the dying and the dead. Nevertheless, the implicit (and sometimes explicit) rules of discourse constricted the type and extent of communication on this subject (Luborsky & McMullen, Chapter 3, this volume). Popular religion and sentiment sanctioned such bromides as "Mother is in a better place." "Jack was out of his suffering." If one had to speak about a death, it was advisable to draw on the available cliches that emphasized acceptance of the inevitable, often enhanced by the assertion that whatever happens is part of God's plan, and the faith that "We will all meet in the next life." Such stereotyped discourse converted the death of an unique individual into a normative event. These statements inhibited open discussion of how one actually felt about losing a loved one and any fears or doubts raised by the death. Over many years the children who would become today's elders were instructed to bury their personal feelings about death and "be strong."

We are listening again to the woman who had spoken about the influenza epidemic (post-World War I).

I grew up knowing I was not supposed to say very much, period! 'Children should be seen not heard.' God and the grown-ups knew all about death and the next life. Open my mouth? Not me! (*If you did, what would have happened?*) "Oh, 'You don't understand, child!' Or 'Where is your faith, child?,' Or just 'That will be enough!'"

Many a person would continue the journey through adulthood with unanswered questions and unresolved feelings because of societal rules that limited death discourse. In turn, they tended to impose these rules on their children. Half a century or more after their formative experiences with death discourse, some elders are motivated to review and revise their attitudes—but have nobody available who is willing to converse with them on this subject. As a gerontology student discussed her interview assignment, she burst out with:

I didn't realize how I had been shutting off Grandmom every time she started to talk about . . . that stuff. I thought she was being morbid, I guess, but, really, *I* didn't want to hear it! This last week-end I had to listen because Grand-

mom was one of my interviews. I listened, so she talked, and now we know
each other a lot better. I had no idea what she'd been through!

Dying Is a Frightening and Hopeless Ordeal. Fear of dying is distinguishable
from fear of death. A person may come to terms with personal mortality, yet
have many concerns about the terminal phase of life. Death may even be sought
as a release from the anguish of dying, as in suicide. However, in practice it is
not unusual for apprehensions about dying and death to merge into a global
anxiety that includes fears of failure, dependency, separation, pain, and the unknown.

It is probable that fear of dying has been with us through the millennia,
but taking different forms in various ecological and sociocultural contexts (Luborsky & McMullen, Chapter 3, this volume). What form did it take
as nineteenth-century America gave way to the twentieth century? We were
then a rapidly industrializing society. Rural, agrarian, situated America was
on its way to the centralized, urbanized, everywhere-is-anywhere uptempo culture we know today. Mass culture was being shaped by the emerging power
of media and technology. Automobile, telephone, assembly line, and radio were
among the devices of our massification, our identities soon to be marked and
tracked by Social Security numbers. Even in Kansas we were not in Kansas any
more.

People born into this historical period were likely to experience the opportunities and temptations of an expanded and more open life scenario—but
also the dislocations, uncertainties, and sharp edges of technologically fueled
change that had outstripped society's integrative and meliorative resources.
There was more opportunity than ever to fly high, and more risk to fall without a safety net. Even before the stress of the Dust Bowl and The Great Depression, many individuals and families already were struggling desperately
to "make it."

Not infrequently, death was seen as a failure to thrive in "the heartless
city," or to adjust to the forces that were operating even in small town America. Youth seeking brighter lives in the city would sometimes end up as burnt-
out alcoholics, or hollow-eyed semiinvalids, awaiting the release of death
within a few years of entering the fray. Entire families would sometimes collapse under the oppressive and hazardous living conditions experienced by
immigrant generations in the crowded tenements. When the working poor
went to their early graves it was often with a sense of having failed in life. For
some of the winners, these deaths demonstrated their own superiority, the survival of the fittest. Death was not just the end of life; it was the way society
disposed of its weaklings and others who were considered to be without value.

A man now looking healthy and vigorous in his eighth decade remembers:

what really killed my Father. He knew his heart was bad and he knew that he
couldn't bring home that much more money no matter how many hours he
worked, and that was plenty. He wasn't a man to say much. Then one night

he was screaming at Mother, like we'd never heard before. . . . 'Don't you spend an extra penny! Don't you spend an extra penny!' He wanted her to bury cheap as she could. Mother had to promise him that. Then she said, 'But why are you screaming?' Father said, 'I'm screaming because I can scream and I will scream whenever I want to scream. What else can I do!' There was quiet then a moment. Then Mother said in her funny voice, 'Well—you're a pretty good screamer, that 's something!' Father said, 'Yeah' and the screaming was over for a while.

In this tenement scene going back many decades, the father was still struggling for a sense of self and value before death would prove him to have been a failure.

Father did work until the day he dropped, and he dropped just a few minutes before quitting time. I don't know for sure, but they probably docked him those few minutes on his final paycheck.

It was also not a particularly good time to go through the dying process. Medicine had already embarked on its aggressive, cure-oriented, and somewhat depersonalized course. Actual cures were still in short supply, however, and relatively little was being done to provide comfort for those who were en-route to become medical as well as personal failures. A person who was perceived as incurable was likely to be abandoned by the medical profession, whether to what was euphemistically called "home care" or to the large wards of public and charitable hospitals (Rosenberg, 1995). It would not be until 1959 that Herman Feifel would confront the American public with his identification of our "death taboo," but this phenomenon had been evident for many years. Health care professionals as well as the public tended to avoid both "death talk" and the people who were actually suffering through terminal illness or the grief of bereavement. If the doctors would not or could not tell the truth, who could? If the doctors would not comfort the dying person by the bedside, who would?

Dying took on a particularly horrific aspect because several common pathways to death were marked by symptoms that were painful both to experience and to witness. These were deaths through contagious diseases and other infections that would later be brought under control through public health advances and antibiotics. Tuberculosis ("consumption") was perhaps the most compelling example. One could live with tuberculosis for several years, perhaps to pull through, perhaps to die. There was ample time, then, to experience both physical symptoms and a sense of foreboding that nevertheless left a space for hope. Often people infected with tuberculosis were moved to a sanitarium where their companions would be other patients in similar states of illness and barely concealed terror. This, of course, entailed separation from family and familiar surroundings; they had been "put away" (Smyer & Allen-Burge, Chapter 14, this volume).

Those whose illnesses proved terminal and who remained in their own homes often were the source of extreme stress to their loved ones. The coughing fits were alarming, especially when bloody pieces of lung tissue were expelled. The emaciation characteristic of the advanced stages gave the sufferer a skeletal aspect. Throughout the ordeal, the dying person might remain lucid, except for feverish periods in which thoughts became excited and difficult to control. For many victims, tuberculosis was a horrible death to experience, and for many survivors, a horrible death to witness. It is not surprising that family members—and health care professionals—could not bring themselves to linger at the side of the person with advanced tuberculosis.

There can be little doubt that life-long fears of dying in anguish and isolation were intensified by the prevalence of tuberculosis and other contagions against which the medical arts of the time were only occasionally effective. Among today's elders there are many who recall hushed conversations and anxious faces, and some with all too vivid memories of direct witness to the death of a family member from tuberculosis. Fear of dying as an unbearable ordeal was intensified by the code of silence. The reality of dying with tuberculosis and other contagious diseases was so distressing that people avoided talking about it "like the plague." This avoidance in turn kept feelings locked inside and not readily subject to review, and added the vivid paintbrush of the imagination to what was already sufficiently horrible—which, in turn, made it even less likely that people would attempt to breach the taboo against open and honest communication. *For today's elders, then, there is often an "anxiety closet" with memories of loved ones who died in suffering and despair.*

"This is my health insurance policy," confided a veteran of World War I, as he produced a bulky pistol. "I can take death, but nobody can tell me I got to take dying."

Unresolved Griefs from the Past Influence the Course of Life and Rise to Meet New Griefs. The relatively high mortality rate in the early years of this century translates into a higher probability of multiple past bereavements for today's elders. "Grief counseling" was not known as such in those days, nor were most family constellations prepared to recognize and respond to the mute sorrows and acting-out behaviors of bereaved children. These children often carried with them bereavement wounds that had not healed well. The effects were individual and varied. Rando (1984) has described some of the major forms of unresolved grief:

- *Absent grief.* "It is as if the death never occurred at all. It requires either that the mourner completely deny the death or . . . remain in the stage of shock" (Rando, 1984, p. 59).
- *Inhibited grief.* "there is a lasting inhibition of many of the manifestations of normal grief, with the appearance of other symptoms such as somatic complaints in their place."

- *Delayed grief.* "for an extended period of time, up to years, especially if there are pressing responsibilities or mourners feel they cannot deal with the process at that time. A full grief reaction may eventually be initiated by another loss or by some event related to the original loss."
- *Conflicted grief.* Common patterns include "extreme anger and extreme guilt . . . abnormally prolonged and often associated with a previous dependent or ambivalent relationship with the deceased."
- *Chronic grief.* "the mourner continuously exhibits intense grief reactions that would be appropriate to the early stages of loss. Mourning fails to draw to its natural conclusion and it almost seems that the bereaved keeps the deceased alive with grief."
- *Unanticipated grief* "occurs after a sudden, unanticipated loss and is so disruptive that recovery is usually complicated . . . mourners are unable to grasp the full implications of the loss. Their adaptive capabilities are seriously assaulted and they suffer extreme feelings of bewilderment, anxiety, self-reproach, and depression that render them unable to function normally in any area of their lives."

Unresolved grief may take several of these forms in the same person, deriving from losses at various developmental periods, for example, death of a sibling in childhood, death of a parent in adolescence, death of a spouse at midlife. Some people have brought a a heavy burden of unresolved grief with them into the later adult years (Qualls, Chapter 11, this volume). Both the prospect and the reality of additional bereavements tend to intensify the impact of the past losses.

All Problems Notwithstanding, These Are the Survivors. It is useful to keep in mind the obvious fact that today's elders are those who have survived all the hazards to life from infancy onward. They have had some luck on their side. Their numbers include the girl who stayed home from work at the shirt factor one day to take care of her sick brother—the day that the factory went up in flames and many others died with their lungs full of smoke. Included also are the children whose bodies proved resistant to scarlet fever and tuberculosis, the soldiers who were about to be sent to the front a day before Armistice was declared, and patients who were treated by physicians who actually did wash their hands.

There is also little doubt, however, that many of today's elders owe their survival to their own hardiness and resourcefulness. In focusing now on death, dying, and bereavement we would not want to forget the life-affirming qualities that have contributed to the fact that we do have so many people with us in their advanced years. Among today's elders are many who would reward oral historians with their survival stories.

Attitudes toward Death Among Elderly Adults

We have explored some of the background influences on today's elders. It is time now to consider their attitudes specific to death, dying, bereavement, and suicide, keeping in mind the marked individual differences among elderly people, as well as the existence of several cohorts (sometimes categorized as the young–old, 64–74; old–old, 75–84; and very old–old, 85+). We will proceed by raising a few key questions and offering what answers can be given on the basis of available data.

Do We Become More or Less Anxious about Death with Advancing Adult Age?

This question perhaps could be answered if we had a reasonable body of longitudinal data with which to work. Unfortunately, the fairly numerous studies of death anxiety have been limited almost exclusively to cross-sectional samplings, while the major longitudinal studies of aging have rarely included assessments of death anxiety and related variables. We can speculate about age *changes*, then, but are limited to data on age *differences* (Cavanaugh & Whitbourne, Chapter 2, this volume).

Three basic hypotheses have been formulated about age-related changes in death anxiety (Kastenbaum, in press).

1. We become more anxious with age because the tide of mortality exerts an inexorably increasing pull on us.
2. We become less anxious with age because we perceive death as less of a threat.
3. We develop an orientation toward death early in our lives and it is this characteristic level of anxiety that we bring with us into the later adult years.

The last of these hypotheses implies another possibility that might be useful to articulate:

4. We develop the level and type of death anxiety that is characteristic of our cohort and it is this historically shaped orientation that we bring with us into the later adult years.

There is nothing inherently implausible about any of these hypotheses. Each hypothesis may have a domain to which it provides the most useful guide. Interaction effects and moderating variables may also influence the outcome. For example, the extent to which people scan the future could shape their orientations toward death. A 60 year old in good health might already have decline and death in sight because he or she has always looked many years ahead, whereas an 80 year old with multiple physical problems might not think much about the diminishing distance from death because he or she has characteristically taken life pretty much one day at a time. We cannot assume a close parallel between subjective and objective distance from death. Personal cognitive style is one of many mediating variables that contribute to elders' views of their present relationship to death, and this connection is best understood individual by individual.

The available (cross-sectional) data indicate that elderly people tend to report a lower level of death anxiety than do the young and middle-aged (DePaola et al., 1994). Most often, the age comparisons reveal lower death anxiety scores for elders, with occasionally no differences. DePaola et al.'s own investigation confirmed previous results, but, in addition, examined individual differences and added a useful new finding: those who were most anxious about death were also those who were most anxious about their own aging. The researchers drew the inference that "both fear of death and anxiety about growing older may the the results of a third, unmeasured factor, such as fear of losing one's identity or sense of control" (DePaola et al., 1994, p. 213).

This suggestion is consistent with clinical observations (Weisman & Kastenbaum, 1968). Heightened death anxiety with age is most likely to occur in conjunction with (1) episodes of acute physical symptomatology, (2) perceived lack of social support, (3) failure of characteristic coping strategies; and (4) fear of rejection or punishment by God. When people feel helpless and overwhelmed, it is not unusual for this sense of catastrophe to be symbolized through death imagery. The death imagery vanishes along with the elevated anxiety when the stress is alleviated and a sense of control is reinstated. The alert clinician pays attention to heightened death anxiety, then, but does not ignore the total context within which this sense of panic has emerged.

The general finding of relatively low death anxiety among elders seems to be associated with two self-reflections: the sense of having lived a full and rewarding life and the acceptance of their mortal vulnerability. These two related views contrast sharply with attitudes that are often found with young adults who are still seeking their identities and achievements and who are still swaddled in the (brittle) illusion of indestructibility. After his second heart attack, a man in his late 60s expressed his philosophy succinctly:

Death can't take my life away from me. All that good stuff really happened. Death can only take what's left over.

We can err in either direction when listening to elders expressing their views of life and death. We can mistake a depressed and withdrawn attitude for serene acceptance, and we can also mistake equanimity in the face of death for a lack of interest in continued survival or even an eagerness to exit. This latter misinterpretation can be especially dangerous in critical end-of-life decision-making situations. A person's philosophical acceptance of death can be used as part of the rationalization for withholding treatment. Many an elder, however, is both prepared for death to some extent but also very much connected to life. "I could die in my sleep tonight, and that would be all right," a youthful-looking nonogenarian told me at a spring training baseball game. "But I'd rather wake up tomorrow and see if the Cubs can pull one out tomorrow." (Note: He did, and the Cubs lost again.)

There Is Less Acceptance of Suicide But a Higher Rate of Completed Suicide

There is a cultural heritage, shared by the United States and a number of other countries, that regards a suicidal act as a sinful, weak, or criminal action. This judgmental attitude has been reduced over the course of the twentieth century in favor of the view that the suicidal person is attempting a desperate solution to problems that are experienced as overwhelming. Older adults are included in this attitudinal shift, but surveys find that in this age group there is still a residue of moral disapproval. As we have already seen, the rate of completed suicides is at its highest among elderly white men. Furthermore, suicidologists estimate that the odds of a suicide attempt proving lethal is at least five times greater among elderly as compared with younger adults (McIntosh, 1992). Case histories suggest that some elders who had previously disapproved of suicide have changed their minds when their own situations deteriorated (Kastenbaum, 1994b), but the general relationship between suicidal attitudes and actions among elders has not been determined.

Many Elders Express a Pragmatic, Task-Oriented Attitude toward Death-Related Issues

There are three assumptions that often interfere with intergenerational communications about death-related issues:

1. The aged person knows all about death because he or she is so close to it.
2. We should not talk about death with elderly people because it would upset them.
3. We should not talk about death with elderly people because it would upset us.

Sociocultural stereotypes include the image of the aged person as sage or wizard (Chinen, 1992). More specifically, it is sometimes assumed—without foundation—that elders have a more authoritative understanding of death because of their proximity to it. This is a difficult proposition to justify from either an empirical or an epistemological perspective (Kastenbaum, 1993). Furthermore, not all elders are sages or saints (Kastenbaum, 1994a), and being more thoroughly enveloped by the shadow of death does not guarantee exceptional insight or depth.

The other two assumptions go in a different direction. "Talking about it would upset *them* so much!" and "It would upset *me* so much!" are based on the assumption that elders are self-deceived and emotionally frail: they have shielded themselves from acknowledgment of mortality. Presumably they would collapse if the truth were spoken. As we have seen, the historical vectors go in the other direction. Today's elders are more likely than younger adults to have borne direct witness to dying and death. Furthermore, they are the survivors of difficult times, so it is unlikely they are inherently more vulnerable emotionally than younger adults. It is also rather condescending to hold that "I can deal with mortal issues, but Mother and Grandfather cannot."

The potential listener's fear of drowning in a whirlpool of death anxiety is seldom what happens when elders are given the opportunity to discuss death-related issues with adult children or other people significant to them. The conversation often is focused on practical arrangements and elements of life's business that need to be considered and resolved. When all involved have had ample opportunity to listen, speak their minds, and come to consensus, the "death talk" is likely to be put away until such time as there may be a new development to deal with. When elders do seem to be going on and on about death, it is usually because everybody else seems dedicated to not listening; the elderly person may quickly perceive that this is not a welcome topic and become an obedient follower of the rule of silence.

End-of-Life Issues

In recent years this apt phrase has earned currency: end-of-life issues are what many elders would discuss if given the opportunity and encouragement. A nontautological definition is elusive, but we can understand by "end-of-life issues" the most salient concerns for which resolution is sought prior to death. Discussion of end-of-life issues usually centers on the individual. However, these concerns often encompass family relationships and friends, and may also include business associates and have even broader implications (e.g., when legal precedents or societal customs are challenged).

End-of-life issues vary from individual to individual and family to family, but most commonly occur within three contexts:

1. *Management of the final phase of life.* This includes the choice of traditional or hospice care, the opportunity to make an advance directive, the resolution of core relationships and development of a final scenario, and the alternative of ending one's life prematurely.
2. *After-death body disposition and memorial services.* This includes the choice of cremation or traditional burial as well as type of funeral and memorial service.

3. *Distribution of assets.* This includes both the formal disposition of resources in one's estate and the informal passing of items to others.

An elder may choose to exercise influence over any, all, or none of these domains. The decisions may be made with or without consultation and either well in advance of the events or at the last possible minute. At one extreme there are elders with strong vested power within the family and the determination to shape events in accord with their own values and desires. At the other extreme are elders with but weak leverage within the family system who are resigned to going along with whatever plan others seem to favor and those who have no intimate support group. All persons involved have the implicit choice between making a choice or becoming recipients of whatever default processes of end-of-life management happen to prevail at the moment.

The Hospice Option

One choice point is between traditional medical management and hospice care. In general, traditional medical management involves more in-hospital time and continued use of diagnostic testing and interventions aimed at extending life. Hospice care is *palliative,* focused on control of pain and other symptoms and providing a sense of comfort for patient and family, often in the home rather than an institutional setting (Appleton & Henschell, 1995; Saunders, 1997). Every year many people reach this choice point without realizing it because knowledge of hospice benefits has not fully penetrated public awareness. Others recognize that they do have the option of requesting hospice care as a Medicare benefit.

Who becomes a hospice patient? Most hospice patients are in their middle or later adult years, simply because fewer people are dying young. Most of those who select the hospice option are afflicted with cancer, AIDS, or a progressive neurological condition (most frequently, amyotropic lateral sclerosis, also known as Lou Gehrig disease). Although heart disease is the major cause of death in the United States, few people with life-threatening heart conditions enter hospice care. This disparity is indicative both of the achievements and the limitations of hospice programs in their present form. Hospice care in its modern form was introduced in the 1960s with the urgent mission of alleviating the pain experienced by terminally ill cancer patients. Attention was also given to the control of other symptoms such as nausea, sleep disturbances, and confusion. Hospice did not exclude people with other types of illness, but the program was designed primarily to protect the quality of life for people who were moving inexorably toward death over a period of time. The hospice philosophy encompasses all terminal conditions: interpersonal support, symptom control, and sensitivity to the individual's beliefs and values are priorities regardless of the nature of the illness. In practice, though, the coverage of hospice expenses through federal or private insurance programs is limited by the requirement that a physician certifies the patient's life expectancy as being no greater than 6 months. Many physicians deplore this requirement, noting that predicting survival is not and cannot be an exact science. The unwelcome task of placing one's signature on an estimate of survival becomes even more difficult in conditions in which length of survival is inherently less predictable, as is the case with some forms of heart and cardiovascular disease.

What is required to make an informed choice between traditional and hospice forms of terminal care? The following points are worthy of consideration:

- *How well is the individual informed about the nature and prognosis of his or her condition?* The answer to this question includes the individual's readiness to deal with the communications received from health care professionals. An important cohort factor is the reluctance of some elderly people to raise questions and concerns in a clear and persistent manner. The physician may be regarded as an authority figure who should not be challenged or even "bothered" by patient's questions.

- *What are the options at this particular point in the illness?* It is not sufficient to have a general understanding of the condition. One must also have accurate and adequate information about the available treatment/management options. In turn, this requires up to date knowledge on the part of the health care professionals and their willingness to disclose the options with the patient's well-being in mind rather than being influenced by the financial implications for the physician and the health care system in which they are embedded.

- *What are the patient's expectations, fears, and hopes?* Some elderly men and women are haunted by memories or tales of people who have suffered greatly during the dying process. This can produce so much anxiety that the individual becomes depressed, reluctant to deal with end of life issues, and even suicidal. Others may have one particular concern that dominates their thinking, for example, fear of becoming dependent, or worry about how the surviving spouse will get along in their absence. Discovering the type of scenario the person anticipates, fears, and desires as life comes to an end can be invaluable in helping to reach decisions about management options.

- *What is the communication pattern within the patient's social support network?* There are still many families within which communications about dying and death are taboo (Book, 1996). Furthermore, there are also families within which intergenerational communications are strained and distorted, although in general adult children and their parents often report having a satisfactory relationship (Peterson, 1993). Even within reasonably adequate family communication systems, the prospect of an elder's death may constitute a zone of anxiety that becomes isolated behind a curtain of silence. Consequently, the elders at risk for death may lack the opportunity to articulate their concerns and wishes and to receive adequate feedback from others. The decision-making process usually operates most effectively when the entire family and social support group allows itself to become involved.

- *Availability of family members to participate actively in terminal care.* Typically, hospice programs rely on services provided by family members and volunteers as well as a core of paid professionals. In a model scenario, there will be a family member who is willing and able to serve as the primary caregiver, as well as other relatives, friends, or neighbors who are available to supplement and relieve the primary caregiver. Hospice professionals offer advice, counseling, and supervision to the primary caregiver in addition to providing some services directly. The entire management plan is built around an existing interpersonal support system, which in turn is supported by the hospice team. It has become increasingly evident in recent years that some people who would benefit from hospice care do not have a primary caregiver available. For example, the household may consist of an aged person with terminal cancer and an equally aged and rather infirm spouse who is willing but not able to shoulder the caregiving burden. Hospice organizations have been exploring alternative arrangements to find a way to provide care (especially home care) without the social anchor of a primary caregiver within the family. There are many possible solutions to the challenge of identifying a suitable primary caregiver, but the key to these solutions is to assess the situation ahead of time and discuss the possibilities in an open and constructive manner (Aldwin & Gilmer, Chapter 5, this volume).
- *Availability of a quality hospice care program.* The hospice movement has earned a glowing reputation for effectiveness in symptom relief and sensitivity to the full range of human needs of patient and family alike. Nevertheless, hospice organizations are not immune to both internal and external problems. Unfortunately a few organizations have proved to be "hospice" in name only. As in any choice of health care provider, the consumer is well advised to inquire through those who have used the services. Helpful guides to evaluating and selecting such programs are available through The American Hospice Foundation.

Hospice care has provided comfort to many terminally ill people and their families. It has become clear that social support during the last phase of life is every bit as important as the hospice pioneers believed—and the more stressful the illness, the more essential is the quality of support (Dobratz, 1995). The success of hospice in symptom relief has also contributed to medical and nursing education in general. Health care professionals who are committed to the relief of pain have learned to consult hospice experts and their writings. Hospices have also demonstrated the ability to provide empathic care for people with a broad spectrum of religious beliefs. This pattern was established by the first modern hospice (St. Christopher's, Sydenham, Great Britain) and has been widely emulated. The religious orientations of patients and families are respected and no attempts are made for "deathbed conversions," although many hospice staff and volunteers do express a religious faith that helps to sustain their own efforts (Schneider & Kastenbaum, 1993).

Nevertheless, terminally ill elders cannot benefit from hospice care systems unless they overcome two major barriers that still exist throughout the world: (1) family reluctance to face the reality of terminal illness and enter into the decision-making process; (2) physician reluctance to approve of hospice care for their patients until very late in the terminal process, thereby depriving them of much of the benefits they might have received. Again, an open communication process is a key to obtaining the services that are most in accord with one's values and life-style.

Whether traditional or hospice care is selected, it is important to recognize that terminally ill people have the right to state-of-the-art management for the relief of pain and other symptoms. The anguish of the dying process was witnessed by many of those who have become today's elders. This ordeal does not have to be repeated in a time when effective procedures are available and health care personnel need only make use of these procedures.

The Advance Directive Option

The second major choice point concerns the establishment of an *advance directive for medical care*. Such directives were all but unknown until 1968 when a document known as *the living will* was introduced to the public. This document made its appearance only a few months after the opening of St. Christopher's Hospice in Great Britain, and 6 years before the first hospice was established in the United States (New Haven, Connecticut). The living will soon became a touchstone for the professional and public dialogue on end-of-life issues that is still with us today (Binstock, Chapter 15, this volume). Future historians may judge that the living will was important chiefly for its stimulation of death-related discourse in a population that had avoided this topic for many years. Actually, relatively few people completed living wills, and even fewer had their documents consulted and honored at the time of death.

It is useful to revisit the original living will document both for what it accomplished and for the limitations that soon became apparent. Here is the basic version as offered by an organization known as Concern for Dying.

This statement would be signed in the presence of a notary public and possibly additional witnesses. The individual could also designate a person who would have the durable power of attorney for health care decisions should he or she be incapacitated and unable to affirm the intentions conveyed in the living will. Furthermore, people establishing living wills could (but seldom did) add more specific language to make their intentions clear (Scofield, 1989).

My Living Will To My Family, My Physician, My Lawyer and All
Others Whom It May Concern

Death is as much a reality as birth, growth, maturity, and old age—it is
the one certainty of life. If the time comes when I can no longer take part
in decisions for my own future, let this statement stand as an expression
of my wishes and directions, while I am still of sound mind.

If at such a time a situation should arise in which there is no reasonable
expectation of my recovery from extreme physical or mental disability, I
direct that I be allowed to die and not be kept alive by medications, ar-
tifical means or "heroic measures." I do, however, ask that medication be
mercifully administered to me to alleviate suffering even though this may
shorten my remaining life.

This statement is made after careful consideration and is in accordance
with my strong convictions and beliefs. I want the wishes and directions
here expressed caried out to the extent permitted by law. Insofar as they
are not legally enforceable, I hope that those to whom this Will is addressed will regard themselves as morally bound by these provisions.

The living will was remarkable for its time by its reversal of the power relationship between patient and physician. Ralph Nader and others had re-
minded the public that manufacturers and merchandisers do not hold all the
cards. The rising consumer consciousness started with the purchase of auto-
mobiles and other material goods and eventually penetrated into the health
care arena. The living will literally embodied the message that consumers of
health care services had their rights, too. Although couched in nonconfronta-
tional language, this document did increase tension between the patients and
those health care providers who were not prepared to relinquish control.

People who welcomed the living will (including a growing number of
health care professionals) also were jolting the prevailing assumption that pro-
longation of life was of the highest priority. More specifically, people usually
assumed that other people held this belief. The request "that I be allowed to
die" generated a sense of liberation for some people, but uneasiness or even
anger for others. People started talking about a "right to die," and this issue is
even more salient today with the surfacing of the physician-assisted death controversy, as will be touched on below.

What were the limitations of the living will? A major problem was the absence of a foundation in law. There was nothing illegal about the living will,
but there was also no legal obligation for a physician or hospital to behave in

accordance with this document. It was a poignant request that relied on the understanding and good will of others—the others in some cases turning out to be harried emergency room physicians or fatigued medical residents who had had no prior relationship with the patient. A related problem was the concern of some physicians and many administrators and their lawyers that compliance with a living will could be the basis for a malpractice suit or even criminal indictment. There were also practical problems in the implementation of the living will. How was the physician to know—right now—that this person had made a living will? The document had to be readily available, and this availability could not be taken for granted. How was the physician to interpret the patient's request in light of the particular circumstances? Did the patient really want the physician to withhold antibiotics for an infection that might respond to treatment during the terminal process? Did the patient want the physician to provide intravenous fluids but not nutrition? There was often a gap between the general guidelines given in the living will and the specific decisions that had to be made in the terminal care situation. Living wills were sometimes ignored, then, because their instructions seemed incomplete, contradictory, or ambiguous.

Three developments have altered the situation that has just been described. One of these developments has been the justice system's growing consensus that a competent adult has the right to refuse medical treatment. Another was the introduction of legislation to support a person's intention to restrict the type of biomedical procedures used when a person is critically ill with little or no prospect of recovery. Perhaps surprisingly, measures of this kind—often called "natural death acts"—were approved by most state legislatures throughout the nation within a relatively short time. Still another development was the enactment of federal legislation known as the *Patient Self-Determination Act (PSDA)*. This has been the law of the United States since December 1, 1991.

The PSDA targets health care agencies. It requires that patients receive information on their right to accept or refuse treatment and to formulate advance directives. The agencies are asked to provide patients being admitted to a hospital with clear and adequate information about their opportunity to express their preferences for medical management should a critical situation arise. By implication, patients are to be familiarized with a broad spectrum of possible situations and with the treatments/options available for each situation. For example, the situation in which a person has irreversible brain damage with loss of cognitive processes and ability to relate to others may occur with or without the presence of terminal illness, and the patient may or may not choose to exercise different options for these similar but not identical situations. Patients may come with an advance directive document already completed or they may indicate their preferences at the time of admission. These preferences are intended to be honored by the medical establishment unless subsequently altered by the patient. Patients are also given the opportunity of choosing to donate their organs (although it is standard practice not to use tissues or organs from aged people). If there is to be an advance directive, the patient is expected to designate a person who will function as his or her proxy in the role of attorney for medical decisions. This person often is not a lawyer, but simply a trustworthy person who knows the patient's mind and will see that these intentions are carried out as far as possible.

In practice, health care organizations differ appreciably in the attention given to implementation of the PSDA. The patient's knowledge of treatment options may receive careful or perfunctory attention. The decision-making process may be given reasonable time and discussion or hurried over as part of the admission work-up. The various situations that might arise are seldom identified, and the management options are usually compressed into brief generic statements such as "I want my life to be prolonged as long as possible, no matter what my quality of life," or "I do not want my life prolonged if I will be permanently unconscious."

Enactment of the PSDA has not dramatically improved communication and understanding of the management options available to a person who is terminally ill or facing a possible catastrophic medical situation (Miles, Koepp, & Weber, 1996). Many adults of all ages are not well prepared to make the decision (especially during the anxiety accompanying hospital admission), and many health care agencies have been giving less than wholehearted support to the process. Furthermore, there is still a major loophole in the regulatory apparatus: failures to honor an advance directive are not penalized (King, 1996).

Nevertheless, the PSDA does provide the opportunity to express one's wishes and intentions for the type of care to be received should a critical situation arise. Learning about the options and reflecting on one's own values while still in good health is a sensible course of action. Gerontologists could provide a valuable service to the elders in their lives by helping them to become better informed on this subject and, when possible, to enlist the interest of family members as well.

Developing a Final Scenario

Most people have definite ideas about how they do and do not want their lives to end. For example, terminally ill cancer patients hoped that the last three days of their lives would be experienced (1) without suffering, (2) in the company of the person or persons who were most important to them, while (3) they themselves could still do something useful for others (Kastenbaum, 1997). As one of these mostly elderly people said for most of the others: "I want my last days to be wonderfully ordinary." A crucial part of the final scenario for most people is the process of separation from family and friends. Asked to imagine acceptable and unacceptable endings to their lives, many people focus on the quality of their interactions with others as the end approaches. The final months, weeks, and days often are seen as opportunities to affirm love, resolve conflicts, and set their minds in order.

Clinicians and researchers are now calling renewed attention to the uniqueness of each person's final passage, an uniqueness that encompasses the individual's prior life experiences and the existing network of supportive relationships, and the particular biomedical and sociohistorical context within which a life is ending. The stage theory of dying (Kübler-Ross, 1969) remains popular with the general public and the teacher or health care professional with a limited knowledge of the actual dying process, but has been largely set aside by those who are aware of this model's flaws, limitations, and lack of verification (Niemeyer, 1997). Instead, attention is directed to the way in which an individual's total life course has prepared the way for end-of-life events and experiences and to the possibilities and limits within this unique situation. Weisman's (1974) concept of an "appropriate death"—the death that a person would choose if given the opportunity—is being given precedence over the model of a more or less mechanical shifting through gear stages that have little relationship with ongoing events in physical condition, social interaction, and personal cognitions (Dixon & Hultsch, Chapter 8, this volume).

Recent contributions provide useful examples of the varied ways in which dying elders and their families construct the final scenario (Byock, 1997; Callahan & Kelley, 1993) and interpret the deathbed scene (Kastenbaum, 1992). The perspectives of the dying person, each family member, and each service provider do not automatically converge into a coherent and integrated view of what is happening and what should be happening. Respecting each person's perspective and keeping communication channels open often prove more valuable than applying a ready-made model of the dying process.

Suicide and Assisted Death

It is not unusual for a person faced with progressive loss of functioning to think of "ending it all." The increasing risk of suicide for aging white men has already been noted, but some women and members of other racial groups also take their own lives. Canetto's (1992) studies have led to her theory that the surplus of male suicides in the later adult years is related to (1) the be-a-man-and-shoot-yourself image in our society; (2) a more limited repertoire of coping strategies, as compared with women; and (3) a relatively greater loss of social esteem and life structure upon retirement. According to this view, women are not as shaken to find themselves dealing with problems and limitations in their later adult years, and they are more skilled in alleviating their troubles through social support.

At higher risk are elders who live alone, have suffered a major interpersonal loss, lack a supportive social system, and/or are facing a terminal decline. Use of alcoholic beverages is often a contributing factor in suicides at all ages, therefore a pattern of increased use may be a warning sign. What are the indicators of possible suicide risk in specific elderly individuals? These indicators include the following:

- Sad, dejected, or emotionally flat mood.
- Lack of eye contact.
- Restlessness, constant motor activity.
- Loss of appetite and weight.
- Insomnia or oversleeping.
- Preoccupied by physical complaints.
- Stooped, withdrawn, fatigued.
- Careless in grooming and dress.
- Inattention, "losing the thread" of the conversation.
- Loss of interest in activities.
- Loss of interest in other people.

Physicians must be sensitive to the ambiguities in this picture. Is this person primarily depressed, or is the dysphoria secondary to physical problems? Unfortunately, there are still relatively few geriatric physicians in the United States. There is a pressing need for physicians and other service providers to improve their ability to evaluate the total picture presented by elderly clients and develop a management plan that does justice to both the physical and the psychosocial elements. It is also useful to realize that suicide prevention often begins when a straightforward communication interaction occurs. A question such as "Are you thinking about suicide?" usually elicits a frank reply. Further discussion can reveal whether the individual has also formulated a detailed suicide plan (e.g., stockpiling medications or cutting a length of hose to attach to the exhaust pipe). One might go so far as to suggest that all service providers who work with elders should attend workshops in suicide prevention and reflect on their own related thoughts and feelings. The lack of solid interpersonal contact is a contributing factor to many elder suicides; offering open communication and a helping hand is a contributing factor to prevent completion of the self-destructive impulse.

Furthermore, the alert applied gerontologist will also recognize suicidal plans that are constructed many years in advance of the proposed action. No reliable statistics are available on this point, but some middle-aged adults already have their suicidal plan in readiness for the time when they decide that aging is upon them, a fate preperceived as worse than death.

The "right to die" controversy, with us for some years, has taken a new turn recently. The statements and actions of Dr. Jack Kevorkian have fueled a national debate that is actually only our own version of an international controversy over the merits of physician-assisted death. To some extent the issues have been obscured by the use of descriptors (euthanasia, suicide, murder, deliverance) that import divisive emotional connotations. It is more useful to stick to assisted death if we are to examine the situation with a minimum of prejudice. Assisted death occurs when a physician complies with a patient's request to end his or her life because of intractable suffering. Kevorkian's usual approach has been to provide the patient with the means of ending life by his or her own hand. The death is therefore cocreated. This final episode is preceded by discussions with the patient and his or her significant others to be sure that this is what they want.

At present there is no jurisdiction in the United States in which assisted death is clearly legal. Voters in Oregon narrowly approved such a provision in 1994, but it was appealed by its opponents and is scheduled to be reconsidered again. Two federal courts subsequently made rulings favorable to assisted death in their jurisdictions, thereby creating a patchwork situation in which the legality of this action varies from one place to another. The most recent significant judicial response has been the June 26, 1997 decision by the United States Supreme Court that upholds the right of states to enact laws that make it a crime for physicians to give life-ending drugs to mentally competent terminally ill adults who have made this request. This decision does not rule out the possibility of states enacting laws that make it legal for physicians to assist death. The issue was judged primarily on the basis of state versus federal rights, and so leaves the future open to the influence process and new legislation. Furthermore, the Supreme Court ruling does not affect the accepted practice of providing sufficient medication to relieve the pain of a terminally ill person, even if this medication also has the effect of shortening the individual's life. This practice is becoming known as "slow euthanasia."

The primary arguments in favor of assisted death include the right of individuals to make choices regarding their own bodies and the relief of suffering. This approach resonates with the woman's right to make abortion decisions and everybody's right to withhold informed consent. The primary arguments against assisted death include the following:

- Many people who seek assisted death have been receiving inadequate care for the relief of their suffering. Better pain management and a hospice-type approach would enable these people to live with a higher quality of life.
- Depression is a common feature. Recognize and relieve the depression and many people will no longer seek assisted death.
- Assisted death has dangerous potentials for pushing us further along "the slippery slope." If we countenance assisted death for a suffering terminally ill person, in all probability this will lead to assisted death for people who have many years of life ahead of them.
- Physicians should never kill people.

A recent study by Kaplan (in press) examined the medical status of people whose deaths were assisted by Kevorkian. It was found that most of these people were neither terminally ill nor in severe pain. Moreover, the preponderance of women in this sample (the opposite of the national suicide statistics) suggests that the availability of assisted death may be attracting some people who would not otherwise take the initiative to end their lives. The assisted deaths of people who were not terminally ill has intensified the slippery slope controversy in The Netherlands, where the proassisted death regulations have never been without determined opposition (Meijburg, 1995–1996).

Whatever side one takes in the assisted death controversy, it is crucial to involve all affected people in open and sustained discussion of their needs and the available options. There is a difference between reaching a difficult decision after discussion and seizing upon death as the only solution to problems that nobody is willing to face head on.

Recovering from Grief

A long life often turns many valued companions into memories. As we have already noted, today's elders experienced the loss of family members and friends in their youth. New bereavements are likely to be encountered as other survivors drop out of one's social convoy (Antonucci, 1993). Part of the long-lived person's survival spirit has been the ability to move ahead after losing people who had been loved, admired, and depended on. The old losses have not been forgotten, and the new losses hurt—but many elders have developed ways of integrating multiple bereavements into their lives. One would not want to underestimate either the burden of sorrow and yearning experienced by multiply-bereaved elders or their capacity to keep going.

Spousal bereavement is the type of loss that has been most extensively studied. Lieberman's (1996) recent study confirms and extends earlier investigations in finding that many elders are able to take their lives in a positive new direction after experiencing loss, loneliness, doubt, and confusion immediately after the death of a spouse. Social support is a major variable. Newly widowed persons usually are more responsive to receiving support from people who were already in their lives and therefore expected to honor their implicit obligations to comfort. Peer support has also been observed to be very helpful either as supplement or, when necessary, substitute, for family support. The Widow-to-Widow Program (Silverman, 1986) has demonstrated that sharing experiences of spousal loss in an informal group setting can be effective in reducing the sense of isolation and helplessness and in confirming one's own abilities to cope with the situation. There are now many other peer support programs across the nation, often associated with church or other community agencies through which widowed people of all ages assist the grief recovery process.

It has become clear that grief and mourning are interpersonal as well as intrapersonal processes. Moos (1995) has made the case for considering not only the bereaved person's responses, but also the changes that occur within the family's communication patterns. For example, at the same time that the bereaved person is experiencing somatic symptoms (shortness of breath, tightness in throat, etc), the family as a whole may be demonstrating its grief through changes in who speaks to whom and in what way—and even in who may been reconnected or cut off from core interactions. A family systems approach seems to be especially promising in understanding and, when indicated, intervening in bereavement situations (Stephens & Franks, Chapter 12, this volume).

The death of a child is often devastating both because of the intense parent–child bond and the assumption that in the natural course of events our children will outlive us. When a grandchild dies, elders must cope both with their own grief and that of their adult children. The death of an adult child can lead to a depressive reaction in which the sorrow of the loss is intensified by a sense of being abandoned to face a now more uncertain future. Health care professionals who have learned to recognize depressive features in elderly adults usually also learn to explore the possibility of one or more bereavements as major contributing factors (Qualls, Chapter 11, this volume).

It is important to note that the resiliency of many elders to the loss of a loved one does not necessarily protect them from serious harm. This resiliency is usually a potential that fully actualizes itself only after a difficult transitional period after the death. Depression, anxiety, and vulnerability to physical illness often increase during the first year of bereavement. This can be a high stress period. People may suffer from impairments in physical functioning, attention, and memory while also withdrawing to some extent from social activities. Both symptomatic major depression syndromes and subsyndromal symptomatic depressions may persist into the second year of bereavement. Until the individual's resiliency has the opportunity to reassert itself there is increased risk for a wide variety of negative consequences from the changes in physical, mental, emotional, and social patterns. For example, there is more vulnerability to accidents, fraudulent schemes, attentuation or loss of existing relationships, and serious physical complications. The effect of bereavement-related stress on the immune system has been identified as one major pathway for the development or intensification of biomedical problems (Zisook, Schuchter, Sledge, & Judd, 1994).

Recently there has been a welcome shift in thinking about recovery from grief. First, the biomedical dimensions of grief are becoming much better defined and understood (Whitbourne, Chapter 4, this volume). Second, these medical advances have not obscured the growing realization that grief is basically a human process that should not be treated entirely as a set of symptoms to be managed. Rather, grief is inherent to the capacity for attachment, the experience of love, and the achievement of maturation and wisdom. Third, the grief-work hypothesis (Freud, 1959) is now being counterbalanced by the observation that many people are better able to go on with life by keeping some form of attachment to those they have lost (Stroebe, 1992–1993). There seems to be a core of truth in Freud's analysis of a painful, repetitive process through which the bereaved person works to detach from the lost loved one. Failure to "work through" grief in this manner can trap the bereaved person in the stress of the past, inhibiting recovery and return to life. Nevertheless, there is also a core of truth in the proposition that to live a whole live requires acceptance of all that one has experienced, including memories of the beloved. Looked at in this way, recovery from bereavement has much in common with the overall pattern of human development throughout the adult years—being true to our past, present, and future selves (Labouvie-Vief & Diehl, Chapter 9, this volume).

REVIEW QUESTIONS

1. What are the major causes of death for older men and women? How have these changed over the past few decades?

2. What attitudes and behaviors do people show in the period preceding death? How are these influenced by one.s life history?

3. What are the key end-of-life issues for older people? How does hospice fit into these issues?

4. What are the major personal and ethical issues concerning suicide, assisted death, and euthanasia?

5. How do people cope with grief?

References

Antonucci, T. (1993). Attachment across the lifespan. In R. Kastenbaum (Ed.), *Encyclopedia of adult development* (pp. 40–44). Phoenix: Oryx Press.

Appleton, M., & Henschell, T. (1995). *At home with terminal illness: A family guide to hospice in the home.* Englewood Cliffs, NJ: Prentice-Hall.

Baudrillard, J. (1993). *Symbolic exchange and death* (I. G. Grant, trans.). Thousand Oaks, CA: Sage.

Book, P. L. (1996). How does the family narrative influence the individual's ability to communicate about death? *Omega, Journal of Death and Dying, 33,* 323–342.

Byock, I. (1997). *Dying well.* New York: Riverhead.

Callahan, M., & Kelley, P. (1993). *Final gifts.* New York: Bantam.

Canetto, S. (1992). Gender and suicide in the elderly. In A. A. Leenaars, R. W. Maris, J. L. McIntosh, & J. Richman (Eds.), *Suicide and the older adult* (pp. 80–97). New York: Guilford.

Chinen, A. B. (1993). Fairy tales as commentary on adult development and aging. In R. Kastenbaum (Ed.), *Encyclopedia of adult development* (pp. 154–157). Phoenix: Oryx Press.

Cunningham, M. P. (1997). Giving life to numbers. *Cancer, 47,* 2.

DePaola, S. J., Neimeyer, R. A., Lupfer, M. B., & Fiedler, J. (1994). Death concern and attitudes toward the elderly in nursing home personnel. In R. A. Neimeyer (Ed.), *Death anxiety handbook* (pp. 201–261). Washinton, D. C.: Taylor & Francis.

Dobratz, M. C. (1995). Analysis of variables that impact psychological adaptation in home hospice patients. *The Hospice Journal, 10,* 75–88.

Feifel, H. (Ed.) (1959). *The meaning of death.* New York: McGraw-Hill.

Freud, S. (1959). Mourning and melancholia. *Collected papers* (Vol. 4). New York: Basic Books. (Original work published 1919)

Glaser B. G., & Strauss. A. L. (1968). *Time for dying.* Chicago: Aldine.

Kaplan, K. (in press). Psychosocial versus biomedical risk factors in Kevorkian's first 47 assisted deaths. *Omega, Journal of Death and Dying.*

Kastenbaum, R. (1992). *The psychology of death* (rev. ed.). New York: Springer.

Kastenbaum, R. (1993). Last words. *The Monist, an International Journal of General Philosophical Inquiry, 76,* 270–290.

Kastenbaum, R. (1994a). Saints, sages, and sons of bitches. *Journal of Geriatric Psychiatry, 27,* 61–78.

Kastenbaum, R. (1994b). Alternatives to suicide. In L. Tallmar & D. Lester (Eds.), *Now I lay me down: Suicide in the elderly* (pp. 196–213). Philadelphia: St. Charles Press.

Kastenbaum, R. (1997). *Death, society, and human experience* (6th ed.). Boston: Allyn & Bacon.

Kastenbaum, R. (In press). Death and dying. In J. E. Birren (Ed.), *The Encyclopedia of mental health.* New York: Academic Press.

Kastenbaum, R., & Herman, C. (1997) Death personifications in the Kevorkian era. *Death Studies, 21,* 115–130.

King, M. P. (1996). *Making sense of advance directives.* Washington, DC: Georgetown University Press.

Kübler-Ross, E. (1969). *On death and dying.* New York: Prentice-Hall.

Lieberman, M. (1996). *Doors close, doors open.* New York: C. P. Putnam's Sons.

McIntosh, J. (1992). Epidemiology of suicide in the elderly. In A. A. Leenaaars, R. W. Maris, J. L. McIntosh, & J. Richman (Eds.), *Suicide and the older adult* (pp. 15–35). New York: Guilford Press.

Meijburg, H. H. V. D. K. (1995–1996). How health care institutions in The Netherlands approach physician assisted death. *Omega, Journal of Death and Dying, 32,* 179–196.

Miles, S. H., Koepp, R., & Weber, E. P. (1996). Advance end-of-life treatment planning: A research review. *Archives of Internal Medicine, 156,* 1062–1067.

Moos, N. L. (1995). An integrative model of grief. *Death Studies, 19,* 337–364.

Neimeyer, R. (1997) Knowledge at the margins. *The Forum Newsletter.* (Association for Death Education and Counseling), *23*(2), 2, 10.

Parker, S. L., Tong, T., Bolden, S., & Wingo, P. A. (1997). Cancer statistics, 1997. *Cancer, 47,* 5–27.

Peterson, C. C. (1993). Adult children and their parents. In R. Kastenbaum (Ed.), *Encyclopedia of adult development* (pp. 1–5). Phoenix: The Oryx Press.

Rando, T. (1984). *Grief, dying, and death: Clinical interventions for caregivers.* Champaign, IL: Research Press.

Rosenberg, C. E. (1995). *The care of strangers.* Baltimore and London: The Johns Hopkins Press.

Saunders, S. (1997). Hospices worldwide: A mission statement. In C. Saunders & R. Kastenbaum (Eds.), *Hospice care on the international scene* (pp. 3–12). New York: Springer.

Schneider, S., & Kastenbaum, R. (1993). Patterns and meaning of prayer in hospice caregivers. *Death Studies, 17,* 471–485.

Scofield, G. (1989). The living will. In R. Kastenbaum & B. Kastenbaum (Eds.), *Encyclopedia of death* (pp. 175–176). Phoenix: Oryx Press, pp. 175–176.

Silverman, P. (1986). *Widow to widow*. New York: Springer.

Stroebe, M. S. (1992–1993). Coping with bereavement: A review of the grief w̲
pothesis. *Omega, Journal of Death and Dying, 26*, 19–42.

U. S. Bureau of the Census (1996). African-American male suicide rates. Current population report, p. 27.

Weisman, A. D. (1974). *The realization of death*. New York: Jason Aronson.

Weisman, A. D., & Kastenbaum, R. (1968). *The psychological autopsy: A study of the terminal phase of life*. New York: Behavioral Publications.

Zisook, S., Schuchter, S. R., Sledge, P. A., & Judd, L. L. (1994). The spectrum of depressive phenomena after spousal bereavement. *Journal of Clinical Psychiatry, 55*, 29–36.

Additional Readings

Attig, T. (1996). *How we grieve: Relearning the world*. New York: Oxford University Press.

Corless, I. B., Germino, B. B., & Pittman, M. (Eds.). (1994). *Dying, death, and bereavement: Theoretical perspectives and other ways of knowing*. Boston: Jones and Bartlett.

Jaffe, C. (1997). *All kinds of love: Experiencing hospice*. Amityville, NY: Baywood.

Kübler-Ross, E. (1995). *Death is of vital importance: On life, death and life after death*. Barrytown, NY: Station Hill Press.

Wass, H., & Neimeyer, R. A. (1995). *Dying: Facing the facts*. Washington, DC: Taylor & Francis.

7

Basic Cognitive Processes

Elizabeth A. L. Stine-Morrow and Lisa M. Soederberg Miller

> The brain is wider than the sky,
>   For, put them side by side,
> The one the other will include
>   With ease, and you beside.
>
> The brain is deeper than the sea,
>   For, hold them, blue to blue,
> The one the other will absorb,
>   As sponges, buckets do.
>
> The brain is just the weight of God,
>   For, lift them, pound for pound,
> And they will differ, if they do,
>   As syllable from sound.
>   —Emily Dickinson

One of the most important challenges in later adulthood is to maintain functional capacity in everyday life in spite of almost inevitable and profound age-related declines in basic cognitive processes. To be sure, such deterioration is pervasive enough that some theorists (Salthouse, 1991; Blanchard-Fields & Hess, 1996) equate the term "cognitive aging" with "the study of age-related declines." Nevertheless, many older adults meet the challenge to age successfully (Rowe & Kahn, 1987; Baltes & Baltes, 1990) by developing compensatory strategies, taking advantage of knowledge structures hewn over a lifetime, and relying on social supports. Thus, aging well may be viewed as a skill that entails finding contexts and domains in which the impact of declines in basic processes is minimized.

Lest the reader find this vision of aging dispiriting, one should consider the life-span context of these changes. It is important to remember that the nature of the human mind at any age is to be limited (James, 1890; Miller, 1956) so that at any one moment our capacity for attending, comprehending, and remembering is finite. Yet it is also our nature to transcend these limits in the practice of everyday life (through the development of domain knowledge and skill, for example), so that ultimately "the brain is wider than the sky." The point here is that skilled aging is a dance of limits and transcendence that starts at the beginning of life rather than at the end. To be sure, it is a dance that accelerates in intensity in old age as the extremes of both what limits us (basic processing capacity) and what enables us to transcend these limits (e.g., knowledge) are reached, but it is nonetheless a dance that has been moving apace for sometime.

Our goal in this chapter is to explore the nature of this dance and to consider its impact on everyday function. Toward this end, we will (1) consider how cognitive psychologists conceptualize the structure and function of human cognition, (2) review several theories of how cognition may change with age, (3) describe age-related neurological changes that could give rise to changes in cognitive function, (4) explore some of the age-related changes in specific domains of function (i.e., sensation and perception, attention, learning, memory, and language), and (5) examine the extent to which these changes in basic processing components contribute to change in performance in real-world domains.

Models of Human Cognition

There are two dominant metaphors that are currently used in cognitive psychology to describe the human mind. The older metaphor, the "multistore model," rests on the comparison of the mind with the computer (cf. Lachman, Lachman, & Butterfield, 1979). Like a computer, the mind is assumed to have a "random access memory," a limited-capacity short-term memory that holds and transforms the information at any given point in time, as well as a "hard drive," which stores the data and programs to which the limited-capacity buffer has access (Waugh & Norman, 1965; Atkinson & Shiffrin, 1968). New data and programs can be entered into the buffer via a keyboard (i.e., the senses) to be stored ultimately on the hard drive. In more recent renditions of this model, the limited-capacity buffer has been called *working memory* (WM; Baddeley, 1986) to accentuate the function of this buffer in transforming information. The larger capacity knowledge store, known as *long-term memory* (LTM) is virtually unlimited in capacity. Most basic cognitive processes can be conceptualized within this metaphor. So for example, "attention" is the selection of information from the sensory array for processing within working memory; "memory" is the encoding of information from WM into LTM with appropriate directories so that it can later be retrieved; understanding discourse is characterized as constructing a segment-by-segment representation in WM such that the important elements of meaning are stored in LTM.

In an extension of this model to account for the superior memory performance of experts operating in their domain of skill, Ericsson and Kintsch (1995) proposed the existence of a *long-term working memory*, a mechanism through which the expert can very quickly store and retrieve intermediate products of processing in LTM. In their theory, this is accomplished via the construction of "retrieval structures" in LTM that allow the expert to effectively increase WM capacity by off-loading storage tasks that might otherwise strain processing resources. Evidence for such an extension comes in part from the finding that experts appear to be able to tolerate an interruption in skilled performance with little or no deterioration in performance—as though the intermediate products of such performance were completely available in WM (even though such products would be expected to exceed its usual empirical limits).

A more contemporary metaphor compares the mind with the brain (McClelland & Rumelhart, 1985; cf. Feldman & Ballard, 1982, for a review). Like a brain, the mind is hypothesized to consist of a set of interrelated units (i.e., neural connections), some subset of which is activated at any point in time. Activation spreads through the network, and in so doing makes some nodes more (excitatory processes) or less (inhibitory processes) available. In this model, LTM can be thought of as the entire neural net (or as stable patterns of activation within the net), and WM can be thought of as the subset of activated nodes, and/or as the amount of activation itself. In one contemporary rendition, Just and Carpenter (1992) describe WM as "the pool of operational resources that perform the symbolic computations and thereby generate the intermediate and final products" (p. 122). Thus, the limiting factor in human cognition within this model is the amount of activation available (Just & Carpenter, 1992, p. 124).

Theories of Cognitive Aging

Not surprisingly, the field of cognitive aging has to some extent followed the lead of cognitive psychology in developing theories to explain the changes in basic processes in late life. In the 1970s and early 1980s the dominant approach used to account for age differences in cognition involved localizing the loss within the multistore model (e.g., Poon et al., 1980). The logic was that since there are some domains of function in which age deficits are pronounced and others in which they are minimal or nonexistent, it must be that only some parts within the model are "broken." The task of the cognitive aging researcher, then, was to find an experimental manipulation that could dissociate age-sensitive from age-insensitive processes, as evidenced by a significant statistical interaction between age and the manipulated variable (Kausler, 1991). Using this methodological approach, age deficits have been localized to a specific component in memory, e.g., as LTM processing, and not STM processing (Craik, 1977); as encoding, rather than storage or retrieval (Smith, 1980); as retrieval, rather than encoding (Burke & Light, 1981); or as effortful processes, rather than automatic processes (Hasher & Zacks, 1979). The consequent catalog of "broken parts" was not only unparsimonious but also offered no developmental explanation and prediction for what would and would not show age sensitivity (Salthouse, 1982).

Fortunately, a pattern emerged: regardless of the particular processes being dissociated, age differences appeared to be greatest under conditions that produced the lowest levels of performance for the younger group (e.g., Fozard, Vercruyssen, Reynolds, Hancock, & Quilter, 1994). In other words, taking the younger group's performance as an indicator of task complexity, older adults seemed to show differential declines whenever the task was complex—a relationship termed the "Complexity Hypothesis" (Cerella, Poon, & Williams, 1980). In fact, plotting reaction time (RT) (Cerella et al., 1980) or accuracy of memory performance (Verhaeghen & Marcoen, 1993) of the old as a function of that of the young [a "Brinley plot" (Brinley, 1965)] typically shows a very high correlation (often 0.9 or better for RT and 0.8 or better for memory). Thus, rather than age deficits in cognitive function being explicable in terms of a finite number of deteriorating processes, they appeared to be due to a decline in some general processing resource; rather than being specific, declines seemed to be general (e.g., Cerella, 1990; Salthouse, 1996; Verhaeghen & Marcoen, 1993).

Scholarly debate over this point has been heated at best and rancorous at worst. Arguments on both sides are compelling. Theories of generalized deficit are criticized for masking interactions. Thus, even though large portions of variance in the average performance of the old are explicable simply by knowing the average performance of the young, there is nonetheless residual variance that can be accounted for only by Age × Task interactions—which presumably reflect localized loss (Fisk, Fisher, & Rogers, 1992). Furthermore, Monte Carlo simulations in which data sets are generated from Brinley functions with different slope parameters show that such data sets can easily be fit with a Brinley function with a single slope parameter, further suggesting that Brinley plots can mask subtle—but real—age interactions (Perfect, 1994). Counterarguments revolve around the undebatably large portion of age variance explained by Brinley functions; so the argument is that even though there may be subtle localized loss, it is important to understand this generalized loss first (Salthouse, 1996). This debate may ultimately come down to a glass-half-full–half-empty (or data-set-half-explained–half-unexplained) distinction, and the contemporary literature in cognitive aging comprises research of both approaches.

In spite of the controversy, the attention of many researchers has turned to trying to characterize what the generalized mechanism might be. Explanations for the nature of this resource have centered on three metaphors: space (i.e., the computational capacity of working memory), time (i.e., the speed with which operations in WM are performed), and energy (i.e., the attentional capacity or mental energy available for transformations). These three metaphors grew out of the multistore approach but dove-tail nicely with the neural net approach. In laying the groundwork for formal theorizing, Salthouse (1988) argued that cognitive aging could be conceptualized as an increase in the complexity of the structure of the neural net (reflecting the growth of knowledge with experience) with a concomitant decline in the processing resources that operate on the network; declines could be modeled as a decrease in the number of nodes that could be activated at any point in time (space), as the speed with which activation could spread from one node to another (time), or as the total amount of activation available to operate on the network (energy). Most contemporary theories of age-related change in basic cognitive processes can be understood in these terms.

Front Lobe

Working Memory

WM is based on the space metaphor such that aging is thought to bring about the reduction in the capacity for processing operations. Very often, research in this area relies on an individual-differences approach, the assumption being that WM capacity varies within as well as between age groups and that age differences in cognitive performance in a number of domains can be explained in terms of these individual differences in WM. The WM construct is typically measured using some sort of memory span task. In the computation span task (Salthouse & Babcock, 1991), for example, subjects are presented with a series of simple arithmetic problems (e.g., $5 + 6 = ?$, $4 + 3 = ?$, $8 + 9 = ?$). They select the correct answer for each, and then, at the end of the series, report the last digit of the problem (e.g., 6, 3, 9). Such tasks require the subject to simultaneously transform and store information. Older adults very often show lower levels of performance on these tasks, and more importantly such deficits are predictive of deficits in other sorts of cognitive performance, e.g., reasoning accuracy (Salthouse, 1992), text recall (Stine & Wingfield, 1987), and performance on procedural assembly tasks (Morrell & Park, 1993). In spite of the moderate success of WM as an explanation of age deficits, it appears to be closely related to processing speed under some conditions.

Slowing Hypothesis

The idea that aging brings a slowing in basic cognitive processes and that it is this slowing that causes age-related change in a variety of other functions has been with us for some time (cf. Birren, 1974). In fact, older adults are very often found to be proportionally slower on a variety of tasks such that the Brinley plots that we discussed earlier typically yield slopes of about 1.5 (cf. Cerella, 1990), suggesting that cognitive processes slow about one and a half times from young to later adulthood, representing a "broad phenomenon . . . not simply attributable to specific and independent processing deficits" (Salthouse, 1996, p. 407).

Recent work has focused on examining the generality of slowing across cognitive domains, and the use of relatively simple measures of perceptual speed to explain age differences in more complex behaviors (Salthouse, 1996). The letter comparison and pattern comparison tasks are such indices that have begun to receive wide use in the literature. Used by Salthouse and Babcock (1991), these measures can account for a large proportion of the age-related variance in WM. Given the critical role of WM for complex behaviors such as memory, problem solving, and language processing already demonstrated in the literature, the inference is that the more fundamental cause of age deficits for all of these domains is slowing, an idea that is receiving increasing empirical support (Bryan & Luszcz, 1996; Park et al., 1996; Salthouse, 1994; Salthouse & Coon, 1994).

Even though there is now considerable evidence that cognitive slowing is a general phenomenon causing age differences in a wide array of cognitive tasks, it appears that the rate of slowing itself may vary across domains. For example, in their meta-analysis, Lima, Hale, and Myerson (1991) showed that the Brinley slope for nonlexical tasks was much steeper than that for lexical tasks, suggesting some degree of domain specificity in the extent of slowing. But there does not appear to be even limited general slowing within each of these two domains. Mayr and Kliegl (1993) argued that nonlexical tasks may vary in terms of both *sequential complexity*, related to simple processing steps, and *coordinative complexity*, related to the coordination of processing steps [see also Salthouse's (1996) distinction between *limited time* and *simultaneity mechanisms*]. Operationalizing this distinction in terms of processing individual items in an array vs. the interrelationships among items in the array, they show that elderly subjects' performance is more affected in rule verification and identification tasks by an increase in coordinative complexity than in sequential complexity. They attribute this difference to the simultaneous demands of processing, storage, and retrieval within working memory that are characteristic of coordinative complexity, but not sequential complexity. This is similar to a view expressed by Park et al. (1996), who found that speed measures were very good predictors of memory performance, but that this was most true for a memory task that was presumably less resource consuming (location memory) and less so for one that was more resource consuming (free recall of a random word list). In fact, as the criterion memory task became more difficult, WM indices became relatively better predictors of performance—and were more powerful in explaining age differences. The result is that as cognitive tasks become more resource consuming, speed measures apparently begin to lose some of their predictive power.

Ironically, it appears that the quest for a generalized mechanism of loss has come full circle. Although a slowing in basic processing mechanisms seems to provide good explanatory power for a wide range of aging phenomenon, more recent data suggest that there are indeed process-specific rates of slowing. Thus, the field is back to casting about for a developmental theory that can account for a new generation of distinctions that amount to "localizing the loss." That is, what makes the nonlexical domain, coordinative complexity, and the simultaneity mechanism (in contrast to the lexical domain, sequential processing, and the limited time mechanism, respectively) more vulnerable to the effects of aging?

Inhibition Deficit Hypothesis

Hasher and Zacks (1988; Zacks & Hasher, 1994) argued that a critical function of WM is to inhibit task-irrelevant information. That is, any cognitive task occurs in some context in which there is some information that is off-target (e.g., a dripping faucet while you read) or in which information that was relevant to the task has ceased to be relevant (e.g., in your novel, you expected the murderer to be in the closet, but new evidence suggests otherwise); fluid cognitive performance requires us to ignore irrelevant information and discarded expectations so as to construct a veridical representation of reality. According to Hasher and Zacks, aging brings a decreased ability to suppress such extraneous material. Indirectly, the inhibition deficit theory may be considered a resource theory since presumably the irrelevant information that remains in WM reduces functional capacity and the mental energy that is available to be allocated where it is needed. Numerous studies in attention and language have provided support for such a conceptualization of age deficits (Hartman & Hasher, 1991; Hamm & Hasher, 1992; McDowd & Filion, 1992). However, some data do not (e.g., McDowd & Filion, 1995; Hartman, 1995), and in an interesting recent review, Burke (1997) questions the logic of some of the predictions that have been made from inhibition deficit theory and points out a number of findings that seem to run counter to what should happen if elderly adults really have an inhibition deficit.

Self-Initiated Processing and Environmental Support

Craik and Jennings (1992) argued that aging brings a decrease in the ability to engage in "self-initiated" processing. The implication is that elderly adults are most likely to have difficulty in cognitive tasks that are ill-structured or in which there is little environmental support. The corollary to this, of course, is that older adults are expected to take special advantage of environmental support so that age differences are reduced under these conditions.

Selective Optimization and Successful Aging

Although much of the theoretical development in cognitive aging has focused on explaining deficits, there is increasing recognition that aging can also bring a certain degree of "worldly competence." Over a decade ago, Rowe and Kahn (1987) argued that it was not sufficient for us to have a "gerontology of the usual," that to truly understand the great potential of aging, we must look to those who do it successfully—since most of us do not want to age in the average way, but in the best way. They note that in spite of age-related declines being the rule in a variety of domains "on the average," good health, mental stimulation, and an integrated social network can make "declines on the aver-

age" irrelevant. An approach to successful aging that is of particular importance to cognitive aging is "selective optimization" (Baltes & Baltes, 1990), i.e.,
selecting out some subset of possible skills and strengthening those through
intense practice. Thus, there is a growing literature examining the effects of experience on preserving abilities into late life (e.g., Meinz & Salthouse, 1997).

Recapitulation

It is clear that there is no shortage of ideas about possibilities for the causes of
age-related change in cognition. Having considered these different theories and
perspectives, we briefly review what is known about age differences in brain
structure and function in an attempt to show that much of the theorizing from
the cognitive perspective can be grounded in biological change. We will then
proceed to examine age differences in particular domains of functioning in an
effort to see where these theories apply.

The Aging Brain and Cognition

As Whitbourne (Chapter 4, this volume) notes, there are numerous structural
changes in the aging brain. A growing literature relates this change in structure to change in brain function and to the capacity for carrying out basic cognitive operations. For example, asymmetries in the size of the right and left lateral ventricle (as measured by a CT scan) have been found to correlate with
patterns of memory performance for faces and words (Berardi, Haxby, De Carli,
& Schapiro, 1997), prompting the investigators to attribute age-related declines
in language to localized atrophy of the left hemisphere.

Several technologies also provide a window directly into brain function, e.g.,
positron-emission tomography (PET) and event-related potentials (ERPs). PET
imaging requires that participants ingest innocuous radioactive material, which
gradually emits positrons that are detected. The resulting three-dimensional image depicts activity, such as glucose metabolism, cerebral blood flow, and neurotransmitter binding, that indicates cognitive activity. This technique has been
used to show age-related reductions in regional cerebral blood flow, metabolic
rates for oxygen, and the number of dopaminergic receptors (Jagust, 1994).

The measurement of ERPs is another noninvasive technique that records
electrophysiological responses to sensory stimuli using scalp electrodes. The
resulting small amplitude brain waves are averaged and time-locked to a sensory stimulus. The primary advantages of this technique are that it is sensitive
to the rate, intensity, and duration of the stimulus presentation but not to the
participant's cognitive state (e.g., drowsiness, alertness). The latency between
the stimulus presentation and a particular wave peak is measured. Although
there is significant variability among individuals in peak amplitudes, the latencies are fairly consistent (after consideration of age, height, and gender).

The P300 evoked potential (named for its 300-msec latency), which occurs in response to infrequent (novel) stimuli, is thought to represent an attentional component of cognition. P300 latencies are correlated with performance on short-term memory tasks such as the digit span (Polich, Howard, & Starr, 1983) and digit symbol (Emmerson, Dustman, Shearer, & Turner, 1989) and are sensitive to age differences even when there is age constancy in the task performance itself. For example, Verleger and colleagues (Verleger, Neukater, Kompf, & Vieregge, 1991) found that although there were no age differences in accuracy on a signal detection task, older adults had significantly longer P300 latencies. Some researchers argue that data from P300 studies can be used to isolate the component causes of behavioral slowing (Bashore, 1993; Strayer, Wickens, & Braune, 1987).

Domains of Functioning

Sensation and Perception

To the extent that information processing begins with sensory processes, it is important to explore the nature and extent of age-related changes in sensory–perceptual abilities [cf. Whitbourne (Chapter 4, this volume) for a review]. These changes can mediate older adults' performance on various cognitive tasks. Lindenberg and Baltes (1994), for example, reported that sensory declines accounted for 93.1% of the age-related variance in cognitive performance among adults aged 70 and over.

Most older adults face the challenge of maintaining functioning in the face of degraded sensory input. Of course, older adults compensate for these declines with external supports such as corrective eye wear and hearing aids, but equally important are the cognitive strategies of compensation. For example, language processing may perhaps be expected to show gross deterioration as a function of sensory declines, but it does not. The prosodic contour of speech [i.e., patterns of word stress (pitch, timing, loudness), intonation contour, and timing] differentially enhances the performance of elderly listeners (Stine & Wingfield, 1987; Wingfield, Lahar & Stine, 1989; Wingfield & Lindfield, 1995). Older adults also can take special advantage of sentence context to understand individual words in noisy environments (Cohen & Faulkner, 1983) or to process degraded visual input (Madden, 1988). Thus, elderly can often use "top-down" strategies to compensate for "bottom-up" input that is degraded due to impoverished sensory processes.

Attention

Orienting.   Orienting is the most basic of attentional processes in that it involves simply tuning sensory receptors toward something and away from something else. It can be either involuntary, as when a sudden noise occurs, or under conscious control, and both types cooccur with a general arousal response including changes in skin conductance, heart rate, blood flow, and breathing (cf. Plude, Schwartz, & Murphy, 1996).

Orienting has been found to be less selective in older adults. McDowd and Filion (1992) recorded subjects' orienting response using changes in skin conductance. The researchers asked young and old participants to listen to a prerecorded radio broadcast during which tone bursts sounded at irregular intervals throughout. They asked half the participants to ignore the presentation of tones and asked the other half to attend to the tones by counting them and by judging whether they all sounded the same. The researchers reasoned that if older adults have more difficulty inhibiting the allocation of attention, then their orienting responses should be similar for both the "attend" and "ignore" conditions. Younger adults, on the other hand, should show a diminished orienting response in the "ignore" condition. As predicted, younger adults showed a smaller orienting response over trials, particularly for the "ignore" condition, while older adults showed the same level of skin conductance for both conditions. These findings thus supported the claim that the ability to inhibit unattended information declines with age (cf. Hasher & Zacks, 1988).

Sustained Attention.   Sustained attention, sometimes referred to as vigilance, is the ability to actively maintain the allocation of resources over an extended period of time. Typically, participants are asked to detect changes in a stream of stimuli that is presented over a period of time. Performance is assessed in terms of the number of correct detections overall as well as the vigilance decrement, defined as the rate of decline in performance over time. Giambra and Quilter (1988) used the Mackworth Clock Task in which participants attempted to detect the occurrence of double jumps in the second hand of a clock. They found no age differences in either overall sensitivity or in the vigilance decrement. Parasuraman, Nestor, and Greenwood (1989), on the other hand, found some evidence of age differences using a cognitive task that required subjects to monitor a continuous presentation of digits for the occurrence of zeros, which occurred infrequently. Because the stimuli were presented rapidly, and in some conditions included stimuli that were degraded, this task demanded more focused attention than did the Mackworth Clock Task. Parasuraman found that accuracy was lower for older adults overall and that the vigilance decrement was higher relative to that of the young, but only when the stimuli were most degraded. When stimuli were not degraded, older adults showed no vigilance decrement. More recently, researchers have identified two factors that appear to moderate age effects in vigilance. Mouloua and Parasuraman (1995) found age deficits only when the event rate was high or when targets appeared in uncertain locations (i.e., were not precued). Thus, the general picture painted from this research is that sustained attention is resistant to the effects of aging provided the visual attention system is not overtaxed by a rapid event rate, spatial uncertainty, or degradation of the stimulus array.

Selective Attention.   Selective attention refers to the ability to select relevant information from a stimulus array. As the number of distracter items (i.e., irrelevant information) increases, performance declines (Madden & Plude, 1993). Rabbitt's (1965) seminal work on selective attention demonstrated that the cost associated with greater amounts of irrelevant information is higher for older than for younger adults. In this study, subjects were asked to sort cards into piles according to two different criteria: either they sorted according to two letters on the card or they sorted according to eight letters. To manipulate the amount of irrelevant information, cards had zero to eight distracting letters (that were not relevant to the sort). Rabbitt found that even though older adults were not differentially slowed by an increasing number of targets, they were particularly hindered by a large number of distracters, and consequently argued that these data showed evidence for age-related declines in the ability to ignore irrelevant information. A great deal of work on distractibility has since been done to elaborate on these findings. McDowd and Birren (1990) concluded in their review that irrelevant information is distracting for older adults only when it must be processed with the relevant information, that the process of ferreting out what is relevant from the irrelevant is age sensitive, and that older adults suffer declines in visual search only when the component tasks are challenging.

Age differences in selective attention can be considered within Treisman and Gelade's (1980) Feature Integration Theory, which proposes that visual information processing consists of feature extraction and feature integration. Feature extraction is assessed in "feature search" tasks in which targets differ from nontargets on all dimensions (e.g., a red X amid a group of green Os). When search time is plotted as a function of the number of distracters, the resulting slope indicates the degree of attentional selectivity employed (cf. Plude & Doussard-Roosevelt, 1990). In the feature search task just described, this slope is typically zero, indicating perfect selectivity (or "pop out") such that search time does not increase as a function of display size. Feature integration, on the other hand, is studied using "conjunction search" in which participants identify targets that share features with the distracters (e.g., a red X amid red Os and green Xs and Os). In this case, the slope relating search time with display size is positive, indicating a cost associated with feature integration processes.

Using a card-sorting task similar to that developed by Rabbitt (1965), Plude and colleagues (Plude & Hoyer, 1986; Plude & Doussard-Roosevelt, 1989) found age differences in the slope for conjunction search tasks, indicating older adults were slower in feature integration. Nevertheless, older adults showed the phenomenon of pop out just as the young in the feature search tasks, showing age constancy in feature extraction.

Ellis, Goldberg, and Detweiler (1996) proposed a two-stage model to specifically explore the nature of age differences within visual search processes and found evidence of a stage-specific decrement in encoding during visual attention rather than a central slowing of processing and response execution. Their model supports the notion that younger adults use a type of parallel processing including both feature learning (the ability to differentiate between the target and distracter) and priority learning (that differentially weights attention to targets and away from distracters). Older adults, on the other hand, use a serial processing approach that contains more feature learning and less priority learning.

Other research supports the notion that a failure to inhibit irrelevant information is responsible for age differences in selective attention. Negative priming occurs when the distracter in one trial becomes the target in a subsequent trial such that response latency is increased relative to a condition in which distracters are unrelated to targets. In other words, negative priming is an increase in processing time that occurs when information that was once inhibited must be immediately activated. The extent to which older adults are less efficient inhibitors would be evident in a reduction in negative priming. This has, in fact, been demonstrated: older adults do not show negative priming (Hasher, Stoltzfus, Zacks, & Rympa, 1991), suggesting that compromised inhibitory processing in old age may be responsible for age decrements in selective attention.

However, as noted earlier there are several anomalies in the literature for which the inhibition framework cannot account, and this is particularly salient in dealing with phenomena related to selective attention. For example, Stoltzfus and colleagues (Stoltzfus, Hasher, Zacks, Ulivi, & Goldstein, 1993) show that there is no correlation between negative priming and interference; i.e., if older adults fail to inhibit in a Tipper task, then they should also be more susceptible to interference from the flanking items, but this does not appear to be the case. In a more recent study, McDowd and Filion (1995) explored age differences in the time course of inhibition relative to those in facilitation. Using negative priming as an index of inhibitory processes and repetition priming as an index of facilitation, they showed that while facilitation was maintained into a three-second interval for both young and old, inhibition was diminished by this time for the old but not for the young. Furthermore, there was a negative correlation between the two types of priming. McDowd and Filion thus concluded that these processes may draw on the same pool of resources, and that older adults, who have limited resources, give priority to facilitation and, therefore, may show diminished inhibition as a consequence. These data are interesting because they suggest that selection among older adults may be accomplished differently from the way it is among younger adults.

Divided Attention.   Divided attention is required when we try to perform two tasks simultaneously. In the laboratory, researchers measure performance on one task as a function of increasing processing demands on another task. Thus, to the extent that attentional resources are being consumed by one task, performance declines are evident on another. For example, in a dichotic listening task, subjects are simultaneously presented with two auditory messages and are asked to recall one of the channels first. The channel recalled first typically has fewer errors than the second, which must be held in memory while the first channel is reported. Older adults typically show poorer performance, particularly for the second channel, though the data are not clear as to whether age differences are unique to divided attention per se or are attributable to general processing resource declines (cf. Hartley, 1992).

Nevertheless, the literature as whole is not uniform in showing age-related declines in tasks designed to tap divided attention. McDowd and Craik (1988) explored possible factors responsible for these discrepancies. Based on the mental energy metaphor, they argued that when relatively easy, or automatic, tasks are used, age differences should be minimal. These researchers manipulated the depth of cognitive processing required by the component tasks and found that task complexity explained more variance than did the divided-attention manipulation, and in fact, elderly performance was parsimoniously explained as an example of proportional slowing. Divided attention, Craik and McDowd suggest, is simply a more complex task (see also Plude & Doussard-Roosevelt, 1990, for a similar conclusion).

Therefore, the data suggest that divided attention itself may not be a problem for older adults. To the extent that older adults are found to have particular problems with divided attention tasks, this may be simply due to the overall difficulty. Consistent with this notion, a factor analytic approach to the components of attention failed to find support for a separate factor of divided attention (Stankov, 1988). The implication is that if the component tasks are not overly resource consuming, elders would not be expected to have any more difficulty than the young in doing two things at once.

Compensation.   Although age differences have been found in some areas of attention, there are some factors that can serve to offset declines. For example, differences in visual search can be mitigated by the presence of prior knowledge. Clancy and Hoyer (1994), for example, used a visual search task in which knowledge in medical technology could be applied. The researchers had a group of young and middle-aged adults who were knowledgeable in bacterial morphology and a control group (young and middle-aged adults who were not) perform a choice-reaction time task in which subjects had to determine whether an illustration of a bacterium (the probe) was present in a three-panel display. Participants were also given the name of a bacterium prior to the probe (the prime) that could either be informative about the upcoming trial (valid) or uninformative (invalid or neutral). Subjects were to respond as quickly as they could as to whether the probe was present in the subsequent display. In addition to this skilled search task, participants also performed a standard letter search in which they indicated whether a letter probe was present in a three-item display as a control task. The researchers reasoned that if knowledge can partially offset age-related declines in visual search, then the presence of related primes in the skilled search task should be of greater benefit to the older subjects than to the younger adults. Although they failed to find a differential benefit for valid primes within the skilled search task, they did find evidence of the benefits of knowledge when looking at performance differences between the skilled search and the standard letter search. That is, age differences among medical technologists were found in the control task but these differences disappeared in the skilled task where the middle-aged adults could draw on their knowledge. Thus, knowledge appears to offer one way in which age differences in attentional performance can be attenuated.

Learning

Deficits in processing resources appear to have implications for the ability to form new associations in old age. In a comprehensive examination of the processing mechanisms underlying the learning of new associations, Salthouse (1994) engaged younger and older adults in tasks of associative learning and memory. Individual differences in processing speed were measured as well as the particular kinds of errors (e.g., forgetting a previously learned association) made during learning. Using path analysis to model performance, Salthouse showed that 40–80% of the age-related variance in associative learning could be accounted for with speed measures. The causal path was indirect, however (cf. Salthouse, 1994, Figure 5). Speed was related to the ability to form associations at encoding (i.e., memory accuracy at Lag 0), which in turn was predictive of accuracy on subsequent memory trials as well as to forgetting in the associative learning task. Thus, age-related slowing seemed to produce a less durable memory trace that caused the older adults to take more trials to learn the associations. Age also had independent effects on forgetting, however, suggesting that age-related forgetting may be attributable to factors outside of slowing as well.

Under some conditions, associative learning may show preservation. Spieler and Balota (1996) tested younger and older adults in a primed naming task in which participants named both the prime and target out loud. Both younger and older adults were faster at naming the target over repeated trials when it was preceded by the same prime than they were when the target was preceded by a different prime. This facilitation in naming provides evidence of an association that is formed between the prime and target, even though no conscious recollection of the material is required. The fact that older adults showed the same facilitation as the young suggests that they indeed had learned the association and that under conditions in which retrieval requirements are minimized, older adults can demonstrate this learning of new associations. Interestingly, in a subsequent experiment, in which participants named only the target (and not the prime), younger adults showed implicit learning whereas older adults did not. Spieler and Balota argue that the act of naming both the prime and target in the first experiment may have allowed the older adults to rely on motoric forms of associative learning that enhanced the encoding process. Thus, these data suggest that although there are age deficits in the ability to encode new associations that are a consequence of age-related slowing, these deficits may be offset through motoric support.

Another factor that may facilitate elders in learning new associations is a deliberate shift away from elders' usual tendency to respond more accurately at the cost of speed. Strayer and Kramer (1994) had young and elderly participants practice a memory search task (i.e., subjects held a set of up to six words in memory and were then presented two items and had to indicate whether they were among the words held in memory) over a period of 9 days and found that older adults were generally slower to acquire this task and that their asymptotes for their response times were higher. By manipulating the instructions to emphasize speed or accuracy, Strayer and Kramer were able to show that elders' poorer performance was due in part to their more conservative approach in learning the task, a strategy that was already known to be detrimental to performance among the young.

Memory

The extent of age differences in memory performance seems to depend on the type of memory structure involved. Episodic memory, for example, is an internal diary or record of autobiographical information that has been contrasted to semantic memory, a repository of factual information. To be sure, these two aspects of memory are not entirely independent; episodic memory is dependent on semantic memory to the extent that the potential benefits of the encoding situation depend on relevant knowledge (cf. Craik & Jennings, 1992; Backman, 1991). In general, aging entails a greater loss of episodic memory relative to semantic memory (cf. Craik & Jennings, 1992; Park et al., 1996; Smith & Earles, 1996). Other distinctions that have been used to account for age-related memory change are ones between implicit and explicit memory and between retrospective and prospective memory.

Implicit versus Explicit Memory.   Traditionally, memory research has focused on explicit memory, the conscious and deliberate retrieval of specific information. Implicit memory, on the other hand, involves retrieval of information without conscious recollection. This is often operationalized by facilitation of performance on one task that is dependent on a specific preceding experience. In this way, it is an indirect test of memory, not requiring subjects to refer back to that prior experience. Age differences are more common in explicit memory than implicit memory, which requires less effortful processing. For example, Light and Singh (1987) gave subjects a study list followed by a list of word stems. Participants were asked to complete the stems with words they just studied (an explicit memory task) or with whatever words came to mind (an implicit memory task). Age differences were greater in the explicit memory condition. Although age differences are sometimes found on tests of implicit memory (e.g., Chiarello & Hoyer, 1988), the bulk of the evidence is consistent with Light and Singh (1987) suggesting relative preservation of implicit memory (Howard, 1996; Schacter, Kihlstrom, Kaszniak, & Valdiserri, 1993).

Prospective versus Retrospective Memory. In contrast to remembering something about an event that has happened, memory can also involve remembering to do something in the future. This ability, called prospective memory, shows minimal, if any, age-related declines (see Maylor, 1993a, for a review). Age differences tend to be found in prospective memory, however, to the extent that self-initiated processes are required. Thus, prospective memory tasks can be distinguished as either time based, which require self-initiated processing to remember to carry out a specific task at a specific time (e.g., taking medication at 4 P.M.) or event based, which contain cues of the event itself (e.g., getting gasoline when the gauge approaches "empty"). Age differences tend to be greater in the former than in the latter (Einstein, Holland, McDaniel, & Guynn, 1992).

Prospective memory tasks can also require self-initiated processing to the extent that they contain retrospective memory demands. For example, Einstein and colleagues (1992) asked subjects to memorize a list of words and also told them to press a key when a certain word appeared during a memory task. Difficulty was manipulated by increasing the number of words to remember from one to four. There were no age differences in prospective memory for the one-word condition; age differences occurred only when subjects had to remember the four words. Because age differences in retrospective memory for the four words (indexed by a subsequent surprise recall test) could completely account for age differences in performance on the prospective memory task, these data suggest that prospective memory in and of itself remains intact with age, and that age-related difficulty arises primarily when older adults forget what it was they were trying to remember.

However, the data are not completely consistent. Age differences have been found in event-based prospective memory when performance is assessed over time. Maylor (1993b) presented subjects with faces of famous people and asked them to name them. For the prospective component of the task, they were asked to remember to make a circle when they saw a beard and a cross when they saw someone smoking a pipe. This was repeated three times with a filler task administered in between each block of trials. The results showed that older adults were just as proficient as the young on the initial trial, but that their prospective memory performance deteriorated over subsequent blocks. Thus, the data suggest preservation of prospective memory relative to retrospective memory (Einstein et al., 1992; Maylor, 1993a), however, as with many areas of cognition, age differences are most evident when task demands increase.

Compensation. Under what circumstances are age differences in memory mitigated? The environmental support hypothesis suggests that age-related decrements in performance are influenced by the extent to which memory processes are supported by external events. These supported processes mitigate demands on processing resources in contrast to those that are self-initiated and therefore resource consuming (Craik & Jennings, 1992). Thus, conditions that improve memory for the young are not necessarily optimal for the old. For example,

Bryan and Luszcz (1996) found that although younger adults benefited from increased rehearsals during a free recall task, older adults did not. They argued that cognitive slowing may limit the ability of elders to effectively rehearse the lists. Interestingly, even though time allocated to rehearsal increased with the number of rehearsals permitted for both younger and older adults, older adults did not allocate differentially more time (somewhat of a violation of the Complexity Hypothesis). This is consistent with the notion that without environmental support, older adults may have difficulty with self-initiated processing that would be needed to take advantage of the extra practice. This may be why older adults are sometimes found to show less benefit from mnemonics (e.g., Baltes & Kliegl, 1992; Craik & Jennings, 1992).

Rather, older adults appear to do their best in memory performance under conditions that optimize support so as to enable the productive allocation of resources to the task. For example, the finding that age differences are more reliable on recall tasks than on recognition tasks (e.g., Schonfield & Robertson, 1966, Craik & McDowd, 1987, Rabinowitz, 1984) can be attributed to the greater environmental support available at retrieval in a recognition task. Similarly, environmental support at encoding that guides resource allocation can differentially benefit older adults. Park, Smith, Morrell, Puglisi, and Dudley (1990) presented younger and older adults with pictures of two objects that were either unrelated to each other (e.g., a spider and a cherry) or were related semantically (e.g., a spider and an ant) or perceptually (e.g., a spider eating a cherry). Consistent with the notion that age differences are minimized when environmental support promotes the effective allocation of processing resources, age differences were largest in the unrelated condition, so that older adults benefited more from the integrated conditions.

Language

Change and Stability in Basic Language Processes. The literature on language processing and aging reveals both areas of preservation and decline [cf. Stine, Soederberg, & Morrow (1996) for a review]. On the one hand, cognitive slowing seems to have strong effects on the ability to construct a representation of meaning from discourse, and therefore compromises the consequent memory trace. This principle has been empirically demonstrated in a very interesting study by Hartley, Stojack, Mushaney, Annon, and Lee (1994). These researchers measured the processing time required to understand or remember a single idea unit (or "proposition") in connected text using three different methodologies: threshold reading time, in which the experimenter controlled the reading time of single sentences so as to determine the minimum time needed for effective processing (i.e., perfect recall), self-paced reading of paragraphs for comprehension, and self-paced reading for recall. The results are highly informative about the way in which cognitive slowing impacts language processing. First, even though these measures represented very different approaches to the processing speed construct, they were moderately intercorrelated ($r =$

0.44–0.55), suggesting that processing time for an idea unit in text has some measure of construct validity (these measures also showed good test–retest reliability). Second, older adults produced longer estimates of processing time from the threshold measure than did younger adults but not for either self-paced estimate, suggesting that the cognitive processes underlying the construction of meaning operate more slowly in the older reader, but that on average, these readers do not allocate more time to the text. Third, in plotting memory performance as a function of reading time for each age group, Hartley et al. (1994) were able to show that age differences in memory performance *increased* as processing time increased suggesting that the quality of processing time is diluted for older readers; i.e., both younger and older adults showed better memory performance as more time was allocated to the text, but the "rate of return" was shallower for elderly readers. Finally, in a regression analysis, recall performance was negatively related to threshold reading time and positively related to self-paced reading time, showing that good text memory is best among adults who *can* process information quickly, but nonetheless allocate extra time.

Slowing has also been implicated in the ability to understand spoken discourse. For example, older adults' memory for language is especially compromised when the speech is presented at a very fast rate (Wingfield, Poon, Lombardi, & Lowe, 1985; Stine, Wingfield, & Poon, 1986). Furthermore, age differences in working memory span measures can often account in large part for age differences in language measures (e.g., Stine & Wingfield, 1987).

Such resource limitations make it especially difficult to extract the meaning of discourse when the syntactic structure of the language is complex (e.g., Kemper, 1987; Kemper, Rash, Kynette, & Norman, 1990). These deficits, too, can be accounted for in terms of working memory limitations (Norman, Kemper, & Kynette, 1992).

On the other hand, there are also areas of language competence that are preserved in later adulthood. For example, word-level comprehension seems to remain remarkably stable (e.g., Burke, White, & Diaz, 1987; Light, Valencia-Laver, & Zavis, 1991), as does the ability to create a mental model of the situation suggested by the discourse, e.g., the ability to keep track of a character moving through the spatial array described by the discourse or the ability to track the emotional dynamics of a character (Morrow et al., 1997; Soederberg & Stine, 1995).

Compensation. It should be noted that even though the effects of diminished processing resources on discourse processing can be readily demonstrated in the laboratory, this is one domain in which older adults often show memory performance that is equivalent to that of the young (e.g., Hultsch & Dixon, 1984). Thus, it would appear that older adults compensate for declines in basic processing mechanisms in the rich context of language, and in fact this has been empirically demonstrated in a variety of ways. For example, as mentioned earlier, in speech processing older adults rely on the intonational contour of the language (e.g., Wingfield, Wayland, & Stine, 1992). Also, in the case where the speaker is visible, older listeners depend more on the lip movements that are redundant with the speech (i.e., the "visible speech") (Thompson, 1995). In reading, older adults can adopt reading strategies so as to minimize the burden on working memory, e.g., by organizing more frequently, taking time early in the text to build a mental model, and allocating extra processing time as the text demands it (Stine-Morrow, Loveless, & Soederberg, 1996; Morrow et al., 1997). Furthermore, older adults appear to be differentially facilitated in on-line organization while they read by the availability of knowledge (Miller & Stine-Morrow, 1998). In fact, under conditions of low knowledge, older readers had to spend much more time than younger readers for organization to produce high levels of subsequent recall, but under conditions of high knowledge, older readers showed reading time allocation patterns comparable to those of the young—and achieved the same high level of recall performance. It appears that the ability to build retrieval structures so as to make use of a long-term working memory (Ericsson & Kintsch, 1995) is intact in later adulthood and affords some measure of compensation in the on-line processing of discourse. Thus, even though processing limitations can have an impact on everyday discourse processing, they do not necessarily have to be given the availability of linguistic redundancy, a base of crystallized knowledge, and the flexibility of a processing system that allows elders to circumvent limitations in basic mechanisms.

Implications for Everyday Cognition

As the field of cognitive aging matures, there is an understandable impatience on the part of consumers, government agencies, and researchers for theories and empirical data that address age-related changes in cognitive performance and adaptations that are required in everyday life. This yearning for an answer to the "So what?" question has given rise to an exciting alliance between human factors and the psychology of aging (Fisk & Rogers, 1997), and hence to a subfield, "applied cognitive aging" (Park, 1992).

Not surprisingly, the declines we have seen in basic processing mechanisms do impact on everyday functioning. For example, older adults often have difficulty understanding medication instructions (e.g., Morrow et al., 1996). It is not clear whether there are age differences in the rates of adherence errors (Park & Jones, 1997), but given the larger number of medications taken by the average elder, even an equivalent rate means that the absolute number of errors is larger; such cognitive lapses in the context of medication can, of course, have significant consequences. Thus, one approach taken to this topic has been to develop different sorts of instruction formats (e.g., verbal vs. pictorial) in an attempt to find a format that enhances comprehension among elderly adults (e.g., Morrell, Park, & Poon, 1990).

Another area of everyday functioning that has been linked to basic cognitive processes is driving (e.g., Ball & Rebok, 1994). Per mile, elderly are involved in more traffic accidents than any other adult age group (elders, however, tend to self-select out of the driver's seat when they feel they cannot drive, so per capita, elders, in fact, have relatively few accidents), but there are wide individual differences in driving capability, so considerable research is being devoted to determining the critical cognitive characteristics that make for a safe or unsafe (elderly) driver. One construct that has been found to be particularly useful is the "useful field of view" (UFOV), which is the spatial area within which a driver can orient to a stimulus. The size of the UFOV varies with the situation (e.g., it is smaller under conditions of divided attention or when the number of targets to be monitored increases) and tends to be smaller (and reduced more by distraction) among elderly drivers. The UVOF, which has been related to a slower speed in attentional processing, lower ability to divide attention, and a lower ability to discriminate between targets and distracters, has been found to be a strong predictor of crash frequency. One implication of this work is that someday a cognitively based screening instrument could be developed that would be a better predictor of safe driving than either age or simple sensory tests alone. Another implication suggested by preliminary work is that the UFOV can be enhanced by training. Thus, such work targets a specific cognitive intervention that could enable elderly drivers to safely stay on the road for a longer period of time.

The field of applied cognitive aging has particular relevance for the workplace. Airline piloting, for example, is receiving increasing attention by cognitive aging researchers, in part because the existence of an aging workforce would be expected to have special implications for a job that by its nature requires multiple demands on attention (cf. Morrow & Leirer, 1997). Piloting is changing in that the airspace is becoming more crowded, thus exacerbating attentional demands. An increase in the use of automation also means that pilots who have been in the job for some time have to relearn certain flying skills. Another skill that is tapped in piloting is language comprehension in that pilots must process and respond to directions from air traffic controllers. Thus, many of the principles we have reviewed with respect to attention, learning, and language would be expected to apply. In fact, laboratory research and research using flight simulators tend to show that older pilots make more errors when attention is divided. This research also suggests, however, that pilot experience can offset age-related deficits in basic processes (Morrow & Leirer, 1997).

So it appears that age-related change in basic cognitive processes that we have discussed are not just isolated laboratory phenomena, but rather basic mechanisms that can impact our ability to perform everyday tasks, such as taking medicine or driving effectively. As we have seen in the different domains of cognition, successful aging is very often possible through a combination of environmental support flexibility, and adaptive strategy change.

Acknowledgment

Preparation of this chapter was supported by NIA grant R01 AG13935 to EALS.

REVIEW QUESTIONS

1. Discuss contemporary theories of cognitive aging with respect to their focus on deficit and compensation. To what extent are these theories mutually exclusive and to what extent are they compatible?

2. How are event-related potentials measured and what can they tell us about aging brain function? From the information given in the chapter, which theory of cognitive aging is most consistent with age-related changes in event-related potentials?

3. A number of domains of cognitive functioning are discussed. For any one domain, (a) describe some of the empirical data that suggest age-related deficits in that domain of functioning, (b) discuss whether we are able to compensate for these losses in any way, and (c) consider which theory(ies) of cognitive aging can best account for functioning in this domain.

4. How does aging impact the ability to function in everyday cognitive tasks? Cite specific examples.

References

Atkinson, R. C., & Shiffrin, R. M. (1968). Human memory: A proposed system and its control processes. In K. W. Spence & J. T. Spence (Eds.), *Advances in the psychology of learning and motivation* (Vol. 2). New York: Academic Press, 89–195.

Backman, L. (1991). Recognition memory across the adult life span: The role of prior knowledge. *Memory and Cognition, 19,* 63–71.

Baddeley, A. D. (1986). *Working memory.* New York: Oxford University Press.

Ball, K., & Rebok, G. (1994). Evaluating the driving ability of older adults. *Journal of Applied Gerontology, 13,* 20–38.

Baltes, P. B., & Baltes, M. M. (1990). Psychological perspectives on successful aging: The model of selective optimization with compensation. In P. B. Baltes & M. M. Baltes (Eds.), *Successful aging* (pp. 1–34). New York: Cambridge University Press.

Baltes, P. B., & Kliegl (1992). Further testing of limits of cognitive plasticity: Negative age differences in a mnemonic skill are robust. *Developmental Psychology, 28,* 121–125.

Bashore, T. (1993). Differential effects of aging on the neurocognitive functions subserving speeded mental processing. In J. Cerella, J. Rybash, W. Hoyer, & M. L. Commons (Eds.), *Adult information processing: Limits on loss* (pp. 37–76). San Diego: Academic Press.

Berardi, A., Haxby, J., De Carli, C., & Schapiro, M. (1997). Face and word memory differences are related to patterns of right and left lateral ventricle size in healthy aging. *Journal of Gerontology: Psychological Sciences, 52B,* 54–61.

Birren, J. E. (1974). Translations in gerontology—From lab to life. *American Psychologist, 29,* 808–815.

Blanchard-Fields, F., & Hess, T. M. (Eds.). (1996). *Perspectives on cognitive change in adult-hood and aging.* New York: McGraw-Hill.

Brinley, J. F. (1965). Cognitive sets, speed and accuracy of performance in the elderly. In A. T. Welford & J. E. Birren (Eds.), *Behavior, aging, and the nervous system* (pp. 114–149). Springfield, IL: Charles C Thomas.

Burke, D. M. (1997). Language, aging, and inhibitory deficits: Evaluation of a theory. *Journal of Gerontology: Psychological Sciences, 52B,* 254–264.

Burke, D. M., & Light, L. L. (1981). Memory and aging: The role of retrieval processes. *Psychological Bulletin, 90,* 513–546.

Burke, D. M., White, H., & Diaz, D. L. (1987). Semantic priming in young and older adults: Evidence for age constancy in automatic and attentional priming. *Journal of Experimental Psychology: Human Perception and Performance, 13,* 79–88.

Bryan, J. & Luszcz, M. (1996). Speed of information processing as a mediator between age and free-recall performance. *Psychology and Aging, 11,* 3–9.

Cerella, J. (1990). Aging and information processing rate. In J. E. Birren & K. W. Schaie (Eds.), *Handbook of the psychology of aging* (3rd ed., pp. 201–221). New York: Academic Press.

Cerella, J., Poon, L. W., & Williams, D. M. (1980). Age and the complexity hypothesis. In L. W. Poon (Ed.), *Aging in the 1980's.* Washington, DC: American Psychological Association.

Chiarello, C., & Hoyer, W. (1988). Adult age differences in implicit and explicit memory time course and encoding effects. *Psychology and Aging, 3,* 358–366.

Cohen, G., & Faulkner, D. (1983). Word recognition: Age differences in contextual facilitation effects. *British Journal of Psychology, 74,* 239–251.

Craik, F. I. M. (1977). Age differences in human memory. In J. E. Birren & K. W. Schaie (Eds.), *Handbook of the psychology of aging* (pp. 384–420). New York: Van Nostrand Reinhold.

Craik, F. I. M., & Jennings, J. M. (1992). Human memory. In F. I. M. Craik & T. A. Salthouse (Eds.), *The handbook of aging and cognition* (pp. 51–110). Hillsdale, NJ: Erlbaum.

Craik, F. I. M., & McDowd, J. (1987). Age differences in recall and recognition. *Journal of Experimental Psychology: Learning, Memory, and Cognition, 13,* 474–479.

Einstein, G., Holland, L., McDaniel, M., & Guynn, M. (1992). Age-related deficits in prospective memory: The influence of task complexity. *Psychology and Aging, 7,* 471–478.

Ellis, R. D., Goldberg, J. H., & Detweiler, M. C. (1996). Predicting age-related differences in visual information processing using a two-stage queuing model. *Journal of Gerontology: Psychological Sciences, 51B,* 155–165.

Emmerson, R. Y., Dustman, R. E., Shearer, D. E., & Turner, C. W. (1989). P3 latency and symbol digit performance correlations in aging. *Experimental Aging Research, 15,* 151–159.

Ericsson, K. A., & Kintsch, W. (1995). Long-term working memory. *Psychological Review, 102,* 211–245.

Feldman, J. A., & Ballard, D. H. (1982). Connectionist models and their properties. *Cognitive Science, 205,* 205–254.

Fisk, A. D., Fisher, D. L., & Rogers, W. A. (1992). General slowing alone cannot explain age-related search effects: Reply to Cerella (1991). *Journal of Experimental Psychology: General, 121,* 73–78.

Fisk, A. D., & Rogers, W. A. (1992). Toward an understanding of age-related memory and visual search effects. *Journal of Experimental Psychology: General, 120*, 131–149.

Fisk, A. D., & Rogers, W. A. (Eds.). (1997). *Handbook of human factors and the older adults.* New York: Academic Press.

Fozard, J. L., Vercruyssen, M., Reynolds, S. L., Hancock, P. A., & Quilter, R. E. (1994). Age differences and changes in reaction time: The Baltimore Longitudinal Study of Aging. *Journal of Gerontology: Psychological Sciences, 49*, P179–P189.

Giambra, L., & Quilter, R. (1988). Sustained attention in adulthood: A unique, large-sample, longitudinal and multicohort analysis using the Mackworth Clock-Test. *Psychology and Aging, 3*, 75–83.

Hamm, V. P., & Hasher, L. (1992). Age and the availability of inferences. *Psychology and Aging, 7*, 56–64.

Hartley, A. A. (1992). Attention. In F. I. M. Craik & T. A. Salthouse (Eds.), *The handbook of aging and cognition* (pp. 3–49). Hillsdale, NJ: Erlbaum.

Hartley, J. T., Stojack, C. C., Mushaney, T. J., Annon, T. A. K., & Lee, D. W. (1994). Reading speed and prose memory in older and younger adults. *Psychology and Aging, 9*, 216–223.

Hartman, M. (1995). Aging and interference: Evidence from indirect memory tests. *Psychology and Aging, 10*, 659–669.

Hartman, M., & Hasher, L. (1991). Aging and suppression: Memory for previously relevant information. *Psychology and Aging, 6*, 587–594.

Hasher, L., Stoltzfus, E. R., Zacks, R. T., & Rympa, B. (1991). Age and inhibition. *Journal of Experimental Psychology: Learning, Memory, and Cognition, 17*, 163–169.

Hasher, L., & Zacks, R. T. (1979). Automatic and effortful processes in memory. *Journal of Experimental Psychology: General, 108*, 356–388.

Hasher, L., & Zacks, R. T. (1988). Working memory, comprehension and aging: A review and a new view. *The Psychology of Learning and Motivation, 22*, 193–225.

Howard, D. V. (1996). The aging of implicit and explicit memory. In F. Blanchard-Fields & T. M. Hess (Eds.), *Perspectives on cognitive change in adulthood and aging* (pp. 221–254). New York: McGraw-Hill.

Hultsch, D. F., & Dixon, R. A. (1984). Memory for text materials in adulthood. In P. B. Baltes & O. G. Brim (Eds.), *Life-span development and behavior* (Vol. 6, pp. 77–108). New York: Academic Press.

Jagust, W. J. (1994). Neuroimaging in normal aging and dementia. In M. L. Albert & J. E. Knoefel (Eds.), *Clinical neurology of aging* (2nd ed., pp. 190–213). New York: Oxford University Press.

James, W. (1890). *The principles of psychology.* New York: Holt.

Just, M. A., & Carpenter, P. (1992). A capacity theory of comprehension: Individual differences in working memory. *Psychological Review, 99*, 122–149.

Kausler, D. H. (1991). *Experimental psychology, cognition, and human aging.* (2nd ed.). New York: Springer-Verlag.

Kemper, S. (1987). Syntactic complexity and elderly adults' prose recall. *Experimental Aging Research, 13*, 47–52.

Kemper, S., Rash, S., Kynette, D., & Norman, S. (1990). Telling stories: The structure of adults' narratives. *European Journal of Cognitive Psychology, 2*, 205–228.

Lachman, R., Lachman, J. L., & Butterfield, E. C. (1979). *Cognitive psychology and information processing: An introduction.* Hillsdale, NJ: Erlbaum.

Light, L. L., & Singh, A. (1987) A. Implicit and explicit memory in young and older adults. *Journal of Experimental Psychology: Learning, Memory, and Cognition, 13*, 531–541.

Light, L. L., Valencia-Laver, D., & Zavis, D. (1991). Instantiation of general terms in young and old adults. *Psychology and Aging, 6,* 337–351.

Lima, S. D., Hale, S., & Myerson, J. (1991). How general is general slowing? Evidence from the lexical domain. *Psychology and Aging, 6,* 416–425.

Lindenberg, U., & Baltes, P. B. (1994). Sensory functioning and intelligence in old age: A strong connection. *Psychology and Aging, 9,* 339–355.

Madden, D. J. (1988). Adult age differences in the effects of sentence context and stimulus degradation during visual word recognition. *Psychology and Aging, 3,* 167–172.

Madden, D., & Plude, D. (1993). Selective preservation of selective attention. In J. Cerella, J. Rybash, W. Hoyer, & M. L. Commons (Eds.), *Adult information processing: Limits on loss* (pp. 273–302). New York: Academic Press.

Maylor, E. (1993a). Minimized prospective memory loss in old age. In J. Cerella, J. Rybash, W. Hoyer, & M. L. Commons (Eds.), *Adult information processing: Limits on loss* (pp. 529–551). New York: Academic Press.

Maylor, E. (1993b). Aging and forgetting in prospective and retrospective memory tasks. *Psychology and Aging, 8,* 420–428.

Mayr, U., & Kliegl, R. (1993). Sequential and coordinative complexity: Age-based processing limitations in figural transformations. *Journal of Experimental Psychology: Learning, Memory, and Cognition, 19,* 1297–1320.

McClelland, J. L., & Rumelhart, D. E. (1985). Distributed memory and the representation of general and specific information. *Journal of Experimental Psychology: General, 114,* 159–188.

McDowd, J. M., & Birren, J. E. (1990). Aging and attentional processes. In J. E. Birren & K. W. Schaie (Eds.), *Handbook of the psychology of aging* (3d ed., pp. 222–238). San Diego: Academic Press.

McDowd, J. M., & Craik, F. I. M. (1988) Effects of aging and task difficulty on divided attention performance. *Journal of Experimental Psychology: Human Perception and Performance, 14,* 267–280.

McDowd, J. M., & Filion, D. L. (1992). Aging, selective attention, and inhibitory processes: A psychophysiological approach. *Psychology and Aging, 7,* 65–71.

McDowd, J. M., & Filion, D. L. (1995). Aging and negative priming in a location suppression task: The long and short of it. *Psychology and Aging, 10,* 34–47.

Meinz, E. J., & Salthouse, T. A. (1998). The effects of age and experience on memory for visually presented music. *Journal of Gerontology: Psychological Sciences, 53B,* P60–P69.

Miller, G. A. (1956). The magical number seven, plus or minus two: Some limits on our capacity for processing information. *Psychological Review, 63,* 81–96.

Miller, L. M. S., & Stine-Morrow, E. A. L. (1998). Age and the effects of knowledge on on-line reading strategies. *Journal of Gerontology: Psychological Science 53B,* P223–P233.

Morrell, R. W., & Park, D. C. (1993). The effects of age, illustrations, and task variables on the performance of procedural assembly tasks. *Psychology and Aging, 8,* 389–399.

Morrell, R. W., Park, D. C., & Poon, L. W. (1990). Effects of labeling techniques on memory and comprehension of prescription information in young and old adults. *Journal of Gerontology: Psychological Sciences, 45,* P166–P172.

Morrow, D. G., & Leirer, V. (1997). Aging, pilot performance, and expertise. In A. D. Fisk & W. A. Rogers (Eds.), *Handbook of human factors and the older adults* (pp. 199–230). New York: Academic Press.

Morrow, D. G., Leirer, V. O., Andrassy, J. M., Tanke, E. D., & Stine-Morrow, E. A. L. (1996). Medication instruction design: Younger and older adult schemas for taking medication. *Human Factors, 38,* 556–573.

Morrow, D. G., Stine-Morrow, E. A. L., Leirer, V. O., Andrassy, J. M., & Kahn, J. (1997). The role of reader age and focus of attention in creating situation models from narratives. *Journal of Gerontology: Psychological Sciences, 52B*, P73–P80.

Mouloua, M., & Parasuraman, R. (1995). Aging and cognitive vigilance: The effects of event rate and spatial uncertainty. *Experimental Aging Research, 21*, 17–32.

Norman, S., Kemper, S., & Kynette, D. (1992). Adults' reading comprehension: Effects of syntactic complexity and working memory. *Journal of Gerontology: Psychological Sciences, 47*, P258–P265.

Parasuraman, R., Nestor, P., & Greenwood, P. (1989). Sustained-attention capacity in young and older adults. *Psychology and Aging, 4*, 339–345.

Park, D. C. (1992). Applied cognitive aging research. In F. I. M. Craik & T. A. Salthouse (Eds.), *Handbook of cognition and aging*. Hillsdale, NJ: Erlbaum.

Park, D. C., & Jones, T. R. (1997). Medication adherence and aging. In A. D. Fisk & W. A. Rogers (Eds.), *Handbook of human factors and the older adult* (pp. 257–287). New York: Academic Press

Park, D. C., Smith, A. D., Lautenschlager, G., Earles, J. L., Frieski, D., Zwahr, M., & Gaines, C. L. (1996). Mediators of long-term memory performance across the life span. *Psychology and Aging, 11*, 621–637.

Park, D. C., Smith, A. D., Morrell, R., Puglisi, J., & Dudley, W. (1990). Effects of contextual integration on recall of pictures by older adults. *Journal of Gerontology: Psychological Sciences, 45*, P52–P57.

Perfect, T. J. (1994). What can Brinley plots tell us about cognitive aging? *Journal of Gerontology: Psychological Sciences, 49*, P60–P64.

Plude, D. J., & Doussard-Roosevelt, J. A. (1989). Aging, selective attention, and feature integration. *Psychology and Aging, 1*, 4–10.

Plude, D., & Doussard-Roosevelt, J. (1990). Aging and attention: Selectivity, capacity, and arousal. In E. A. Lovelace (Ed.), *Cognition and aging* (pp. 97–133). Amsterdam: Elsevier.

Plude, D., & Hoyer, W. (1986). Age and the selectivity of visual information processing. *Psychology and Aging, 1*, 4–10.

Plude, D., Schwartz, L., & Murphy, L. (1996). In F. Blanchard-Field & T. M. Hess (Eds.), *Perspectives on cognitive change in adulthood and aging* (pp. 165–191). New York: McGraw-Hill.

Polich, J., Howard, L., & Starr, A. (1983). P300 latency correlates with digit span. *Psychophysiology, 20*, 665–669.

Poon, L. W., Fozard, J. L., Cermak, L. S., Arenberg, D. & Thompson, L. W. (Eds.) (1980). *New directions in memory and aging*. Hillside, N. J.: Erlbaum.

Rabbitt, P. (1965). Age decrements in the ability to ignore irrelevant information. *Journal of Gerontology, 20*, 233–238.

Rabinowitz, J. C. (1984). Aging and recognition failure. *Journal of Gerontology, 39*, 65–71.

Rowe, J. W., & Kahn, R. L. (1987). Human aging: Usual and successful. *Science, 237*, 143–149.

Salthouse, T. A. (1982). *Adult cognition*. New York: Springer-Verlag.

Salthouse, T. A. (1988). Initializing the formalization of theories in cognitive aging. *Psychology and Aging, 3*, 1–16.

Salthouse, T. A. (1991). *Theoretical perspectives on cognitive aging*. Hillsdale, NJ: Erlbaum.

Salthouse, T. A. (1992). Working-memory mediation of adult age differences in integrative reasoning. *Memory and Cognition, 20*, 413–423.

Salthouse, T. A. (1994). Aging associations: Influence of speed on adult age differences in associative learning. *Journal of Experimental Psychology: Learning, Memory, and Cognition, 20,* 1486–1503.

Salthouse, T. A. (1996). The processing-speed theory of adult age differences in cognition. *Psychological Review, 103,* 403–428.

Salthouse, T. A., & Babcock, R. L. (1991). Decomposing adult age differences in working memory. *Developmental Psychology, 27,* 763–776.

Salthouse, T. A., & Coon, V. E. (1994). Interpretation of differential deficits: The case of aging and mental arithmetic. *Journal of Experimental Psychology: Learning, Memory, and Cognition, 20,* 1172–1182.

Schacter, D. L., Kihlstrom, J., Kaszniak, A., & Valdiserri, M. (1993). Preserved and impaired memory functions in elderly adults. In J. Cerella, J. Rybash, W. Hoyer, & M. L. Commons (Eds.), *Adult information processing: Limits on loss* (pp. 329–350). San Diego: Academic Press.

Schonfield, D., & Robertson, B. A. (1966). Memory storage and aging. *Canadian Journal of Psychology, 20,* 228–236.

Smith, A. D. (1980). Age differences in encoding, storage and retrieval. In L. W. Poon, J. L. Fozard, L. S. Cermak, D. Arenberg, & L. W. Thompson (Eds.), *New directions in memory and aging* (pp. 23–45). Hillsdale, NJ: Erlbaum.

Smith, A., & Earles, J. (1996). Memory changes in normal aging. In F. Blanchard-Fields & T. M. Hess (Eds.), *Perspectives on cognitive change in adulthood and aging* (pp. 192–220). New York: McGraw-Hill.

Soederberg, L. M., & Stine, E. A. L. (1995). Activation of emotion information in text among younger and older adults. *Journal of Adult Development, 2,* 253–270.

Spieler, D. H., & Balota, D. A. (1996). Characteristics of associative learning in younger and older adults: Evidence from an episodic priming paradigm. *Psychology and Aging, 11,* 607–620.

Stankov, L. (1988). Aging, attention, and intelligence. *Psychology and Aging, 4,* 59–74.

Stine, E. A. L., Soederberg, L. M., & Morrow, D. G. (1996). Language and discourse processing through adulthood. In F. Blanchard-Fields & T. M. Hess (Eds.), *Perspectives on cognition in adulthood and aging* (pp. 255–290). New York: McGraw-Hill.

Stine, E. A. L., & Wingfield, A. (1987). Process and strategy in memory for speech among younger and older adults. *Psychology and Aging, 2,* 272–279.

Stine, E. A. L., Wingfield, A., & Poon, L. W. (1986). How much and how fast: Rapid processing of spoken language in later adulthood. *Psychology and Aging, 1,* 303–311.

Stine-Morrow, E. A. L., Loveless, M. K., & Soederberg, L. M. (1996). Resource allocation in on-line reading by younger and older adults. *Psychology and Aging, 11,* 475–486.

Stoltzfus, E. R., Hasher, L., Zacks, R. T., Ulivi, M. S., & Goldstein, D. (1993). Investigations of inhibition and interference in younger and older adults. *Journal of Gerontology: Psychological Sciences, 48,* P179–P188.

Strayer, D. L., & Kramer, A. F. (1994). Aging and skill acquisition: Learning-performance distinctions. *Psychology and Aging, 9,* 589–605.

Strayer, D. L., Wickens, C., & Braune, R. (1987). Adult age differences in the speed and capacity of information processing: 2. An electrophysiological approach. *Psychology and Aging, 2,* 99–110.

Thompson, L. A. (1995). Encoding and memory for visible speech and gestures: A comparison between young and older adults. *Psychology and Aging, 10,* 215–228.

Treisman, A. M., & Gelade, G. (1980). A feature-integration theory of attention. *Cognitive Psychology, 12,* 97–137.

Verhaeghen, P., & Marcoen, A. (1993). More or less the same? A memorability analysis on episodic memory tasks in young and older adults. *Journal of Gerontology: Psychological Sciences, 48,* P172–P178.

Verleger, R., Neukater, W., Kompf, D., & Vieregge, P. (1991). On the reasons for the delay of P3 latencies in healthy elderly subjects. *Electroencephalography and Clinical Neurophysiology, 79,* 488–502.

Waugh, N. C., & Norman, D. A. (1965). Primary memory. *Psychological Review, 72,* 89–104.

Wingfield, A., Lahar, C. J., & Stine, E. A. L. (1989). Age and decision strategies in running memory for speech: Effects of prosody and linguistic structure. *Journal of Gerontology: Psychological Sciences, 44,* P106–P113.

Wingfield, A., & Lindfield, K. C. (1995). Multiple memory systems in the processing of speech: Evidence from aging. *Experimental Aging Research, 21,* 101–121.

Wingfield, A., Poon, L. W., Lombardi, L., & Lowe, D. (1985). Speed of processing in normal aging: Effects of prosody and linguistic structure. *Journal of Gerontology, 40,* 579–585.

Wingfield, A., Wayland, S. C., & Stine, E. A. L. (1992). Adult age differences in the use of prosody for syntactic parsing and recall of spoken sentences. *Journal of Gerontology: Psychological Sciences, 47,* P350–356.

Zacks, R. T., & Hasher, L. (1994). Directed ignoring: Inhibitory regulation of working memory. In D. Dagenbach & T. H. Carr (Eds.), *Inhibitory mechanisms in attention, memory, and language* (pp. 241–264). New York: Academic Press.

Additional Readings

Blanchard-Fields, F., & Hess, T. M. (Eds.). (1996). *Perspectives on cognitive change in adulthood and aging.* New York: McGraw-Hill.

Craik, F. I. M., & Salthouse, T. A. (Eds.). (1992). *Handbook of cognition and aging.* Hillsdale, NJ: Erlbaum.

Light, L. L. (1991). Memory and aging: Four hypotheses in search of data. *Annual Review of Psychology, 42,* 333–376.

Park, D. C., Smith, A. D., Lautenschlager, G., Earles, J. L., Frieski, D., Zwahr, M., & Gaines, C. L. (1996). Mediators of long-term memory performance across the life span. *Psychology and Aging, 11,* 621–637.

Salthouse, T. A. (1996). The processing-speed theory of adult age differences in cognition. *Psychological Review, 103,* 403–428.

8

Intelligence and Cognitive Potential in Late Life

Roger A. Dixon and David F. Hultsch

The area of psychological research focusing on the study of cognitive development in adulthood is often referred to as the field of "cognitive aging." It is a particularly active and vibrant domain of research that is at the crossroads of novel trends and emerging disciplines. Recent collections and reviews highlight the significance of several challenging issues. For example, fundamental theoretical issues are addressed (Dixon & Hertzog, 1996). These include directionality (of aging-related changes) and explanation (why cognition changes as it does). Methodological issues are also prominent (Hertzog & Dixon, 1996). These include how best to measure cognitive performance and potential in older adults and how best to evaluate the profiles of cognitive change with aging. In addition, newly developing and promising areas of research are emerging with regularity. These include topics such as metamemory and memory self-efficacy (e.g., Cavanaugh, 1996), social cognition (Blanchard-Fields, 1996), practical cognition (e.g., Berg & Klaczynski, 1996), collaborative cognition (e.g., Dixon, 1996), and brain and cognition (e.g., Woodruff-Pak, 1997).

Both long-standing and novel issues in cognitive aging are addressed in this chapter. The first focus of attention is on intellectual development, a topic that has received widespread attention for many decades. The subsequent focus is on recent research in several areas of perennial interest in cognitive aging. Derived in part from new perspectives on intellectual development, new aspects of potential cognitive growth have been identified and studied. These processes include wisdom, creativity, and compensation.

Issues considered in the study of cognitive aging go to the heart of our view of both the human life course, in general, and of individual aging adults, in particular. Personal expectations about aging are based in part on personal perceptions of cognitive skills—how adaptive they are and how they are believed to change during the adult years (e.g., Cavanaugh, 1996; Hertzog & Dixon, 1994). Similarly, one of the prominent themes in societal stereotypes of aging is that of cognitive decline (e.g., Hummert, Gartska, Shaner, & Strahm, 1994). Notably, however, some stereotypes of aging include processes believed to improve or grow into and throughout late life (e.g., Heckhausen & Krueger, 1993). Some of these potential growth-like processes (such as wisdom) have substantial cognitive components (e.g., wisdom). Whether cognitive aging should be characterized as consisting of gains or losses (or both) has been the topic of much debate for many decades (Baltes, 1987; Dixon, 1998; Salthouse, 1991; Uttal & Perlmutter, 1989).

Although it may be used in different ways and to accomplish different goals, cognition is no less important in late adulthood than in early adulthood. It contributes to—or detracts from—one's sense of achievement, self-esteem, self-efficacy, life planning, life management, and further life potential. There- fore, it is instructive to compare the basic stories told about cognitive devel- opment during the first 20 or so years of life, on the one hand, and during the remaining 40 or 50 years of life, on the other. Obviously, the stories told of in- fant, child, adolescent, and even early adult cognitive development are gener- ally optimistic ones. Cognition during these years is progressing and growing, and cognitive potential is being realized. For normal individuals, there are some differences in the level of performance attained and in the rate at which growth occurs, but virtually no differences in the direction of change. Cognition im- proves from early infancy.

After early adulthood, however, the story of cognitive development evi- dently changes. The term "evidently" is used because there is some contro- versy about the range and causes of aging-related changes in cognition. There is, however, little remaining controversy regarding the fact that there is sub- stantial and necessary cognitive decline (Salthouse, 1991). Nevertheless, an im- portant theme in cognitive aging is one of individual differences in profiles and causes of change. Increasingly, researchers are attending to questions con- cerning issues such as whether people differ in when they start to decline, whether processes differ in rate of decline, what processes are maintained and for how long, how normal decline differs from that associated with various brain-related diseases (e.g., Alzheimer's disease), and the extent to which this decline affects their everyday lives. A common proposal is that individual dif- ferences in cognitive development are greater in late life than in early life. Re- search in intellectual development is ideally suited to investigating such indi- vidual differences (Hertzog & Dixon, 1996).

Intelligence

Cognition can be viewed from several related perspectives. From one such per- spective, the focus is on cognition as intelligence, as an intellectual ability. Com- plementary approaches to cognition are covered in other chapters in this and other books (Blanchard-Fields & Hess, 1996; Craik & Salthouse, 1992; Kausler,

1991; Salthouse, 1991). There is a long tradition of research on intelligence, and a surprisingly long history of research on intellectual aging.

Research on the aging of intellectual abilities [*brain/mind*] typically uses procedures adapted from research on *psychometric intelligence*. This means that intelligence is measured by one or more tests. These tests may be composed of more than one *scale* or subtest. Each subtest measures a relatively unique aspect of intelligence. There are a variety of statistical means through which the uniqueness of the subtests can be evaluated. In addition, however, the subtests typically should be linked both conceptually and empirically. ◁

A good test of psychometric intelligence, then, might include clusters of subtests or scales. The subtests within each of these clusters should be related to one another. The conceptual relatedness could be evaluated by similarity of the content of the items or by the cognitive processes required to solve them. For example, a test in which one must complete a picture of a common item is similar in this way to a test in which one must construct a picture from a randomly arranged set of pieces. The empirical relatedness could be evaluated by giving both of these tests to many people and then examining the statistical correlation (an index of how related the performance on each of these tasks is) between the two. A relatively high correlation would suggest that people who score high on one of the tests also score relatively high on the other. In this way, evidence for the conceptual and empirical linkage of the two tests can be gathered.

A psychometric test of intelligence contains many items, usually incorporated into separate scales. Developing and using the test demand that close attention be paid to the content of the items as well as their conceptual and empirical linkage to other items in the test. The degree to which the scales function as a unit and the extent to which they relate to other scales are also assessed in the development of the test. Psychometric intelligence tests are often evaluated, as well, by how well they predict intelligent behavior in real life. For all of these reasons, then, psychometric tests of intelligence have proven to be valuable indicators of intellectual abilities. They are sometimes criticized, however, for attending primarily to cognitive products and being apparently unrelated to cognitive performance in everyday life.

Psychometric tests of intelligence allow the investigator to summarize a person's intellectual ability by using a single or small set of numbers. If the investigator uses one of the standard psychometric tests, then summarizing across all the scales would result in a single score. One summary score is the *intelligence quotient*, or *IQ*. The IQ is an index of intelligence obtained by dividing an individual's mental age by his or her chronological age and then multiplying this quotient by 100. Suppose the mental age of a child is assessed by an intelligence test to be 11 and his or her chronological age is 10. Performing the mathematical operations results in an IQ of 110, which is roughly within the average range. The IQ, however, is not designed to be employed with adults. One reason is that the divisor (chronological age) continues to increase

Conceptual → imaginary → mental conception
Empirical → practical experience → Relying on or derived from observation or experiment

with advancing age, but the dividend (mental age) should not be expected to continue to increase past a certain mature peak. Another reason the IQ is of questionable value for adults is that it is a single indicator, and intelligence, like other aspects of cognition, is quite likely multidimensional.

Contemporary psychometric approaches to adult intellectual development employ multidimensional theories of intelligence. Therefore, they also use intelligence tests in which performance on multiple scales or dimensions may be tested. Using multiple scales of intelligence allows the investigator to examine the extent to which dimensions of intelligence change similarly or differently across adulthood. The psychometric approach to intellectual aging has a long and illustrious history. We turn now to a brief review of the major developments in this approach.

Development of Research on Intelligence

Mental testing—or the testing of intelligence— began in the nineteenth century (Dixon, Kramer, & Baltes, 1985). Much of the early interest was in developing means to measure mental functioning for particular purposes. Intelligence was frequently viewed as practical or useful in everyday life. Consequently, intelligence testing was done to measure how adaptive one's intelligence was. Abercrombie (1839), for example, described the "intellectual power" of the well-regulated mind as being contemplative, attentive, regulated, selective, active, practical, goal-directed, and inquiring.

William James (1890), who is one of the major early figures in psychology, argued that intelligence played a critical role in human adaptation. Intelligence was crucial in helping humans to survive and adapt in a complex environment. In general, one of the reasons for the success of humans is that, despite some limitations in physical strength, endurance, and speed, they have been able to develop and use their intellectual power to assist in survival. Therefore, intelligence is directed at problems of living, whether these be everyday, mundane, or abstract problems.

Research on intelligence grew dramatically in the early part of this century. We note two aspects of this growth. First, it became understood that intelligence developed and changed over time. Second, more and more attention came to be focused on just how intelligence should be measured and conceptualized. Some of the contemporary approaches to the study of intellectual aging have their roots in tests developed during the first half of the twentieth century. David Wechsler's work, in which 11 scales were collected into two general dimensions of intelligence, was developed during this period (Wechsler, 1939). Thurstone's intelligence test, which has been adapted in one of the leading current studies of adult intellectual development, also first appeared during this period (Thurstone, 1938). Research began to address not just readiness for schooling or for the military but group differences. Age-related differences between infants and children were studied frequently (e.g., Bayley,

1955). In addition to these developmental interests were a series of controversial studies in which racial groups were compared, and immigrants were compared to nonimmigrants. In particular, the ability of intelligence tests to measure intelligence in diverse groups fairly was called into question. If unfairly applied, intelligence test results could be misinterpreted to indicate that one group (especially one that is disadvantaged in its experience of the culture represented in the test) was intellectually inferior to another (especially one that has the advantage of having grown up in the culture of the test-maker). Immigrants who would be tested for their intelligence soon after their arrival in the United States might not perform well on the intelligence test. The reason for their failure, however, might be related less to how intelligent they are than to the fact that they were not exposed to the kinds of questions being asked, the kinds of answers required, and the actual content of the intelligence test.

[handwritten margin note: UNFAIRLY TEST]

This issue of cultural fairness in intelligence testing continues to be an important ethical and political concern (Gould, 1981; Sternberg, 1997). An important and provocative lesson is that intelligence tests are not necessarily valid for all groups. In intellectual aging work, this implies the possibility that intelligence tests that are developed for use with young adults may not be equally valid for use with very old adults. How has intellectual testing been applied to the study of human aging?

Patterns of Intellectual Aging *[handwritten: older Adult]*

A typical expectation about intellectual aging is that intelligence increases until early adulthood and then declines through late adulthood. This results in a inverted U-shaped curve. Botwinick (1977) referred to this curve as a "classic" pattern, partly because it was so frequently supported in the literature. Interestingly, however, even the earliest theories and research did not lead to the unequivocal conclusion that intelligence inevitably and universally declined after early adulthood. Contemporary research has confirmed the prescient early theorists, who operated without the benefit of modern technology, contemporary theories, or even much research data. Several examples illustrate this point.

For example, issues of age fairness and late life potential and plasticity were identified early. Kirkpatrick (1903) noted that age-fair intelligence tests were crucial to identifying patterns of intellectual aging. Almost a century ago, he also speculated that adults could be trained to perform better on intelligence tests; recently, several researchers (e.g., Schaie, 1996) reported that this was indeed possible. Another important issue raised almost 100 years ago is the potentially close connection between the aging body and the aging mind. For example, Sanford (1902) noted that intellectual decline was likely associated with the inevitable physical decline that accompanies late life. Thus, Sanford anticipated some aspects of contemporary theories focusing on the roles of physiological, neurological, and sensory factors (e.g., Baltes & Lindenberger, 1997). Could older adults overcome such inevitable changes? Sanford speculated that

[handwritten: assume to be true]

some maintenance of performance levels is possible if aging adults made an effort to maintain them by, for example, continuing challenging activities. This idea, too, has recently been the target of considerable research (e.g., Gold, Andres, Etezadi, Arbuckle, Schwartzman, & Chaikelson, 1995; Hultsch, Hertzog, Small, & Dixon, in press). Still, in the first half of the century, Weisenburg, Roe, and McBride (1936) attended to the question of whether all adults developed in the same pattern, and whether all intellectual abilities changed in the same way. They reported a wide range of ages in adulthood at which performance on intelligence tests peaked. This implies that individuals may differ in peak age, rate of growth and decline, overall degree of decline, and perhaps even final performance level. If some individuals decline relatively early in adulthood, and if their decline is sharply downward, others may decline relatively late and quite gradually, and perhaps not even noticeably. This prediction, too, proved to be uncannily accurate.

One final similarity between early and recent research on intellectual development may be noted: The study of intellectual aging has long been viewed as a research topic with important and immediate practical implications. That is, how well society understands the characteristics of intellectual aging may have a direct impact on the welfare of individuals and of the society. For example, in the early 1920s, R. M. Yerkes set out to enhance the recruitment and training of excellent military officers. Shortly after World War I, it was clear that each side in a war would want people in charge who were intellectually competent if not intellectually superior. How would the best people be selected and promoted to sensitive and influential positions? How could the best officers be identified and retained? Were older officers less competent than younger officers? Yerkes found that older officers performed worse on an intelligence test than did younger adults. Nevertheless, he argued that many older officers had accumulated valuable experience and had command of specific relevant domains of knowledge. It could take years for younger officers to acquire similar levels of knowledge. Yerkes believed that this actually put older adults at an advantage in the intellectually demanding role of planning and executing war. Thus, even when a great deal is at stake, some observers opted for (older) adults possessing age-related experience and a seasoned mind over (younger) adults who might be able to learn novel information more quickly.

In sum, many early researchers identified remarkably contemporary concerns in the study of intelligence and aging. Moreover, several early leaders commented on the implications of intellectual development for continued cognitive potential throughout life.

The Wechsler Adult Intelligence Scale (WAIS). David Wechsler's first contribution to the study of intellectual development was in 1939, when he published a book entitled *The Measurement of Adult Intelligence*. In this book he used what was to become the Wechsler Adult Intelligence Scale (WAIS) to study adults of different ages. This cross-sectional study revealed age differences, with patterns similar to those we have described above. In later work (e.g., Wechsler, 1958, 1997) he elaborated on these results and, perhaps more importantly, refined his intelligence test.

The WAIS is now one of the major tests of intelligence, and the WAIS-III is especially relevant for testing adults (Wechsler, 1997). It is also used in assessment of intellectual functioning in special populations, such as those suffering from Alzheimer's disease. It is useful for assessment because there are norms of performance for a wide range of ages and groups with similar clinical profiles (Spreen & Strauss, 1998). Because of its general importance to our understanding of intellectual aging, we discuss the WAIS in detail.

The recent versions of the WAIS have both practical and clinical applications. One of its main features is that it is multidimensional. This means that it represents more than one aspect of intelligence. Furthermore, it is therefore possible to examine potentially differing patterns of change in more than one dimension across life. The WAIS has numerous separate scales, divided into two sets, the *Verbal Scales* and the *Performance Scales*. Generally, the verbal scales require the use of words to understand and perform. In addition, they are not administered under conditions in which the individual must perform at a particularly fast pace. Although these characteristics do not favor old adults, the use of language and the deemphasis on speed of performance may allow the older participant to perform relatively well. In contrast, the performance scales involve symbols and symbol manipulation, and relatively little use of words and language. They are also typically administered under requirements of speeded performance. That is, the measure of performance is not so much how many tasks are completed correctly, but how quickly the tasks are solved. Relatively unique symbols and tasks must be performed as quickly as possible. Both of these characteristics may actually penalize the older adult, who is often less adept at performing unique tasks and is slowed by physiological changes.

The WAIS was used extensively to investigate patterns of intellectual performance across adulthood. Combining all scales, the expected pattern is observed. There is some increase in performance until the 20s, and then decline thereafter. The curves for the Verbal and Performance Scales, however, are somewhat different. Although both peak in early adulthood and then decline, their peaks and rates of decline are different. The peak for the Verbal Scales is later (late 20s) than the peak for the Performance Scales (late teens or early 20s). This suggests that the abilities measured by the Verbal Scales may be maintained longer than the abilities measured by the Performance Scales. Put another way, the Performance Scales test abilities that are more sensitive to aging loss. This pattern has been observed repeatedly in research using the WAIS (Botwinick, 1977; Kausler, 1991). Unfortunately, however, the WAIS, and the tests used by earlier investigators, are not linked explicitly to a theory of adult intellectual development. This means that understanding *why* the changes occur as they do is mostly speculative. To describe the age differences is an important task in life-span human development. To interpret, understand, or explain these differences is equally critical (Dixon & Hertzog, 1996; Light, 1991; Salthouse, 1991).

A good theory may provide guidance in answering the more challenging explanatory questions. Why does the peak for the Verbal Scales occur later in life than the peak for the Performance Scales? Why is the rate of decline apparently slower for the Verbal Scales than for the Performance Scales? Why are verbal abilities maintained longer in adulthood than performance abilities? Viable answers to these intriguing questions are now available.

Crystallized and Fluid Intelligence

Beginning in the 1960s, John Horn and Raymond Cattell began developing an alternative view of the classic aging pattern. Most of their work was cross-sectional, and some was cited as contributing to the classic aging pattern. Horn and Cattell collected a variety of intelligence tests data from adults of varying ages. Rather than interpreting the scores from each of the tests, or even collapsing across categories of tests (such as Verbal and Performance), Horn and Cattell conducted complicated statistical analyses. In these analyses they sought to empirically assess whether there was indeed more than one category (or factor) of intelligence. If so, this would support the notion that intelligence in adulthood was multidimensional. This empirical support for this fact would then allow Horn and Cattell to investigate three major issues. First, how many and what were the dimensions of intelligence? Second, what were the age-related patterns of performance on these dimensions. Third, to what explanatory processes could these empirically derived dimensions be linked?

In their research, Horn and Cattell (1966; Horn, 1982) identified two major dimensions of intelligence. These dimensions of intellectual abilities were called *fluid intelligence* (Gf) and *crystallized intelligence* (Gc). Fluid intelligence reflected the level of intellectual competence associated with casual learning processes. This learning is assessed by performance on novel, usually nonverbal tests. Crystallized intelligence, on the other hand, reflects intellectual competence associated with intentional learning processes. This variety of learning is assessed by measures of knowledge and skills acquired during school and other cultural learning experiences. Most verbal tests are examples of this.

How is this perspective an alternative to the classic aging pattern? Because crystallized intelligence indexes lifelong accumulation of cultural knowledge, it should show a pattern of maintenance or increase during the adult years. According to the theory, fluid intelligence is more dependent on physiological functioning, including the neurological system. The physiological and neurological base declines with advancing age (e.g., Medina, 1996). If this neurological base is impaired, the ability to perform associated intellectual skills is undermined. Horn and Cattell have therefore provided the WAIS classic aging pattern with two contributions. First, they provided a firmer empirical basis for the verbal–performance distinction. Roughly speaking, crystallized intelligence corresponds to the verbal scales and fluid intelligence corresponds to the performance scales. Second, they have provided potential explanations for the common observation of differential decline across the two dimensions.

Seattle Longitudinal Study

Longitudinal research in intellectual aging has been carried out in a number of locations (Schaie, 1983). Although longitudinal investigations have the advantage of examining *age changes* rather than simply *age differences*, they have their associated limitations as well (see Hultsch, Hertzog, Dixon, & Small, 1998; Schaie, 1983). For example, *selective sampling* and *selective attrition* factors plague longitudinal designs, but are now manageable with contemporary design features and statistical techniques (e.g., Hultsch et al., 1998; Schaie, 1996). Individuals who volunteer to participate in longitudinal studies are committing considerable time and effort often over a period of many years. The sample of people who would volunteer for such a long-term commitment is generally positively selected on a number of dimensions that may be relevant to intellectual performance. Those who continue in such studies are also positively selected. Indeed, they often perform initially on the intelligence tests at a higher level than those who drop out. In this way, a volunteer longitudinal sample is somewhat selective at the outset, and those who continue are more positively selected than the dropouts. Because of this bias, simple longitudinal designs may underestimate the extent of age-related declines.

In 1956, K. Warner Schaie began a carefully designed and exhaustive longitudinal and cohort-sequential study of intelligence in adulthood. Schaie administered the Primary Mental Abilities (PMA) test and additional measures related to intelligence. His initial sample was some 500 adults living in the community. This sample was carefully constructed to be representative, and ranged in age from 20 to 70 years. Testing was done at 7-year intervals: 1956, 1963, 1970, 1977, 1984, and 1991. At each occasion, new participants were added and then followed in subsequent occasions. Thus, there was a sequence of longitudinal studies. Because of the location of all the testing, Schaie's study has become known as the Seattle Longitudinal Study (Schaie, 1996).

Schaie applied special techniques for comparing longitudinal samples to new cross-sectional samples. In doing so, he was able to estimate that until the age of 50 a substantial portion of the age differences observed in cross-sectional studies was not due exclusively to aging-related decline. Instead, much of the observed age differences in cross-sectional studies was due to cohort effects. That is, observed age differences may be related to cultural and historical changes. Indeed, Schaie (1990) reported such a phenomenon when he noted that historical analyses indicate that successive generations have performed at higher levels on intelligence tests. Notably, the patterns suggest that the historical increases may be greater for older than for younger cohorts. If so, future studies may find reduced age differences between younger and older participants. Such a trend can provide only more pressure to utilize the productive potential of older adults.

Throughout his career, Schaie (1994, 1996) emphasized that there are considerable individual differences in degree of decline and age at onset of decline. Indeed, up to age 70 there are some individuals who do not decline at all. Some individuals show modest gains for all of the intellectual abilities he evaluates. Nevertheless, a prominent conclusion is that the age at which each ability peaks and the patterns of decline thereafter are quite different. For example, those abilities associated with fluid intelligence have earlier peaks and longer declines than those abilities associated with crystallized intelligence. He also pointed out that the patterns vary for women and men. For example, one finding was that women generally decline earlier on fluid intelligence, whereas men generally decline earlier on crystallized intelligence. Not only is there diversity in how dimensions of intelligence develop, there is diversity in how men and women develop in different dimensions. Because of this diversity, Schaie (1994, 1996) underscored the warning that an overall index of ability such as the IQ score should not be used in research on intellectual development in adulthood.

Schaie eventually began to study issues of intervention or application. As the Seattle Longitudinal Study progressed, he realized that he could address a unique question with profound implications for both theory and application. The issue is the age at which substantial cognitive decline actually begins. Whether substantial decline begins earlier or later in life should influence social policy problems such as mandatory retirement (e.g., Perlmutter, 1990; Schaie, 1994). Schaie's studies suggested that such decline is not observed on average for all dimensions of intelligence until about the late 60s (Schaie, 1996). These results may be surprising to even the most optimistic theorist and practitioner, for they imply that the overall profile of intellectual aging is one of maintenance. In fact, in one analysis, Schaie (1990) reported that over 70% of 60 year olds and over 50% of 81 year olds declined on only one ability over the previous 7 years. Thus, intellectual declines occur with aging, but not appreciably until quite late in life, and then not uniformly across dimensions of intelligence.

Schaie also discovered some tentative answers to frequently asked questions about risk and protection factors. Everyone would like to know what they can do to increase the probability that their cognitive aging will by characterized by maintenance and growth, and to minimize the probability that it will instead be characterized by decline and decay. By analyzing the differences among individuals in decline versus growth patterns, Schaie (1996) cited several factors that may lead to reducing the risk of cognitive decline in late life. These protective factors include (1) avoiding chronic illnesses, especially cardiovascular disease, or life-styles that lead to these diseases; (2) pursuing high levels of education and having professions that involve high complexity and higher than average incomes; (3) continuing to be active in reading, travel, culture, and further education; (4) being married to a spouse with high and similar cognitive skills; and (5) feeling generally satisfied with life (Schaie, 1996). Of course, these factors were not linked causally or directly to maintenance of intellectual functioning, so the above list should not be interpreted too literally. Therefore, it is not yet a list of "dos and don'ts" for maintaining high levels of cognitive performance into late adulthood. Nevertheless, such hypotheses highlight the close link between research on cognitive aging and questions of application and real life. Overall, it can safely be said, however, that the above factors cannot hurt your chances of maintaining intellectual functioning, and they may help.

Cognitive Potential In Late Life

Schaie (1990, 1996) sprinkles his reports with detectable notes of optimism. Things may not get decisively better, but not everything declines precipitously for everyone either. The balance between the gains and losses of cognitive aging continues to be an issue of vigorous and compelling debate (e.g., Baltes, 1987; Dixon, 1998; Salthouse, 1991; Schaie, 1996; Uttal & Perlmutter, 1989).

Plasticity and Potential

Under what circumstances can older adults experience gains in cognitive performance? Whereas early researchers speculated about this matter, recent researchers have produced useful empirical information. Some evidence regarding potential is revealed in intervention research, such as training older adults to perform better on challenging cognitive tasks. For example, this literature supports four principal theses. First, many normal older adults can improve their performance on intelligence tests simply by having the opportunity for some self-directed practice (e.g., Baltes & Willis, 1982). Second, healthy older adults can benefit from specific training on how to perform cognitive tasks (e.g., Verhaegen, Marcoen, & Goosens, 1992). Third, selected older adult who have experienced severe or pathological decline can benefit from specific and aggressive interventions (e.g., Camp & McKitrick, 1992). Fourth, there may be some conditions in which training higher levels of performance on intelligence tests can lead to better performance in some cognitive tasks of everyday life (e.g., Neely & Bäckman, 1995; Willis, Jay, Diehl, & Marsiske, 1992)

Overall, some interventions work to improve performance or even reverse losses associated with aging. Theoretically, this implies that some degree of normally observed decline in intellectual aging may be due to disuse. Older adults decline partly because they no longer have the experience or the social and cultural context that will help them maintain some intellectual abilities. Recall that several very early observers had produced prescient speculations remarkably consistent with this empirical generalization. The implication is not, however, that there is no real decline, or that simply providing mental exercises or social support will overcome observed decline. Intellectual decline is real, but there is some degree of plasticity available to many older adults. This conclusion does support the contention that potential for improvement may be present in many older adults.

The "potential for potential" in late life is of interest not only to theorists and researchers interested in gerontology. It is also of interest—or should be of interest—to politicians, policy-makers, aging workers, and just about everyone who knows someone who is nearing the retirement years, or who plans to reach old age themselves. Why should so many people be interested in the fact that aging individuals retain the potential for cognitive maintenance and growth? One reason is that, as noted in an earlier chapter in this volume, our population is increasingly an aging one. More and more people are getting older, more and more people are reaching retirement age and beyond, and more and more people may be feeling that they are being closed off from making useful contributions at an age in which they feel quite competent and potentially useful. Many recent books have addressed precisely this issue, and its many varieties of implications, as the titles of several of them indicate: *Late Life Potential* (Perlmutter, 1990), *Successful Aging* (Baltes & Baltes, 1990), *Promoting Successful and Productive Aging* (Bond, Cutler, & Grams, 1995), and *Compensating for Psychological Deficits and Declines: Managing Losses and Promoting Gains* (Dixon & Bäckman, 1995). These and similar recent contributions explore the possibility that there is considerable cognitive potential in late life, as well as how such potential can be actuated or preserved.

Some authors have also focused on the social policy implications of late life potential. For example, Achenbaum (1990) suggested that North American society may have to place a greater emphasis on adult education. In particular, training and retraining programs may have to be instituted so that potentially competent workers are not placed on the sidelines, simply because of their age. A critical issue, however, is how and who will fund such training and retraining programs. Numerous other policy issues can be specified, but most have the same fundamental theme: How do we take advantage of increasing numbers of adults who are getting older but not substantially less competent? This is a challenge for policy-makers to address at the beginning of the twenty-first century. If not, the number of individuals who are prematurely discarded or discounted—whose skills and potential contributions will be forever lost—will grow.

In the following sections we discuss three forms of continued cognitive potential in late life. These forms are *wisdom, creativity,* and *compensation.* First, however, what do people generally believe about late-life potential?

Beliefs about Cognitive Potential and Aging

The guarded optimism about the potential for further cognitive growth into late adulthood (Sinnott, 1996; Uttal & Perlmutter, 1989) stems at least partly from em-

pirical research. Such relevant research includes the successes researchers have
had in enriching the cognitive abilities of older adults through intervention. The
optimism also stems, however, from many anecdotes of highly achieving older
adults and the common observation that numerous older adults successfully ne-
gotiate the everyday complexities of contemporary life (Bieman-Copland, Ryan,
& Cassano, in press; Dixon, 1995; Simonton, 1990, 1994). Beliefs about changes
in potential with aging have cognitive and developmental bases. They reflect
both general stereotypes of aging and the believer's own personal experiences
with, and expectations for, aging. In a sense, they are related to metacognition
about aging, implicit theories about aging, and sense of self-efficacy concerning
aging (e.g., Cavanaugh, 1996; Hertzog & Dixon, 1994).

Heckhausen and colleagues are among those who have studied this phenomenon. She found that healthy young, middle-aged, and older adults shared
some expectations about the course of adult cognitive development (Heckhausen, Dixon, & Baltes, 1989). Overall, the profile of aging-related changes
was one of an increasing proportion of losses and a decreasing proportion of
gains. For example, she found that many desirable cognitive skills (such as
speed, thinking clearly, and curiosity) were viewed as peaking relatively early
in adulthood, and then declining throughout middle and late adulthood. Correspondingly, many undesirable characteristics (such as rigidity, forgetfulness,
and confusion) were viewed as beginning later in adulthood, and becoming
increasingly typical of middle and late life. Taken together, these results would
seem to support a pessimistic view of cognitive aging, for they emphasize the
losses associated with aging.

Nevertheless, there was a glimmer of optimism in Heckhausen's results
(Heckhausen et al., 1989). At least two characteristics were viewed as being
both desirable and continuing to grow through old age. These characteristics
were "wisdom" and "dignity." Other studies have found similar results (e.g.,
Hummert et al., 1994). In later studies, Heckhausen found that older adults
view undesirable aging-related changes as being uncontrollable. However, she
also found that many older adults believed they were experiencing fewer of
these losses than were others their own age and that they had more control
over the undesirable changes than did typical late-life adults (Heckhausen &
Krueger, 1993).

This analysis of beliefs about aging should convey how complexly they
may be intertwined with actual performance, observations of self and others,
general and specific self-efficacy beliefs, and even stereotypes. We turn now to
one of the prominently mentioned processes representing cognitive potential
in late life, that of wisdom.

Wisdom

The study of wisdom is as old as the study of thought or philosophy. Although
philosophers have struggled with the concept of wisdom for centuries, psy-

chologists and other researchers in human development have addressed it only more recently. In the field of gerontology, wisdom is naturally of considerable interest. There are relatively few processes that are generally thought to improve substantially with advancing age. Wisdom is one such process.

Many provocative questions have been addressed. What is wisdom and how does one know if someone is wise? What are the signs of wisdom and how might it be recognized? Until the late 1980s only a few researchers had attempted to study the aging of wisdom (e.g., Baltes & Smith, 1990; Baltes & Staudinger, 1993; Clayton & Birren, 1980; Sternberg, 1990). One early psychologist, G. Stanley Hall (1922), thought that wisdom was one of the desirable characteristics of late adulthood. For Hall, wisdom included taking perspective, synthesizing significant factors of life, and moving toward higher levels. Other observers have portrayed wisdom as good or sound judgment regarding the conduct of life. Good judgment about a life problem would probably involve consideration of a variety of aspects of the situation: personal strengths and weaknesses, talents and emotions, health and physical abilities, as well as social and cultural considerations may be considered.

Recent investigators have explored empirically whether wisdom does indeed develop in late life and, if so, whether it is in fact an important aspect of successful aging. The first step is to define wisdom in a way that allows for empirical study. It is clear from common conceptions of wisdom that it involves good judgment about life problems. As pointed out by Kekes (1983), the life problems that bring out wisdom are those for which there may be multiple considerations and even multiple solutions, each with a variety of repercussions. For example, it is likely to require some wisdom to deal with a life problem such as deciding whether to leave college and get a job or whether to marry or divorce somebody. These are everyday problems with many uncertainties associated with them—this is what makes them complex and difficult. Solving such problems well (or wisely) is important because the implications for the individual's (and family's) future are significant.

Wise decisions would therefore involve several ingredients (Baltes & Staudinger, 1993). First, there would be some analysis of the problem. This would include knowledge about (1) the individual and his or her talents and weaknesses, (2) the situation or problem with which they are faced, and (3) the context of this problem, especially with respect to the individual's life-span development. In cognitive psychology this kind of knowledge—knowledge about something—is known as *declarative knowledge*.

Second, wisdom would involve some knowledge about how to solve the problem. This would include strategies and procedures that typically work for a particular kind of problem. In cognitive psychology this kind of knowledge—knowledge about how to do something—is known as *procedural knowledge*. Third, wisdom would involve good judgment about what to do in particular situations. In this way, the declarative knowledge would be combined with the procedural knowledge and decisions or suggestions would result. Because of the uncertainty associated with many life problems, it is likely that even these judgments would be qualified. That is, good judgments may be characterized less by absolute recommendations than by qualified suggestions. Such tentative suggestions would be dependent on new developments in the life course, new information obtained, or other changing aspects of the context.

Is wise advice therefore inherently wishy-washy? Probably not, for the wisest way to solve some life problems could be known with certainty. Solving a problematic life situation by turning to addictive drugs is not a wise decision. A wise person would be unlikely to give a wishy-washy answer to someone seeking advice about whether to begin taking heroin as an escape from a given set of life problems. This fact makes the measurement of wisdom difficult.

How can wisdom be measured? Some researchers have presented a variety of life problems in the form of personal vignettes to adults of all ages (Smith, & Baltes, 1990). They then asked them to indicate how they would go about giving advice to the character in the vignette. Wisdom is measured by analyzing the responses given to these problems. Two kinds of problems have been used. Smith and Baltes (1990) used *life-planning* problems. In these problems, individuals learn about a problem in the life of a character and are asked to indicate what the character should do and consider in planning the future. Staudinger, Smith, and Baltes (1992) used *life-review* problems. In these problems, a similar vignette is presented in which a character experiences a life event that causes him or her to look back over their life. The individual solving the problem is asked to describe the aspects of life that the character might remember, and how the character might explain or evaluate his or her life.

Would older adults do better at these tasks than younger adults? Or would just wise older adults do better than younger adults? These questions are critical in evaluating the results of the life-planning and life-review wisdom studies. Results from both studies indicate a substantial *similarity* between young, middle-aged, and older adults in how they respond to these problems. Obviously, an initial expectation would have been that if wisdom is associated with aging, then older adults would do better than younger adults. That this was not found may reflect on (1) the adequacy of the measures of wisdom and (2) the definition of wisdom being used. Future research will further refine the measures and theories of wisdom and aging (e.g., Simonton, 1990; Sternberg, 1990). One avenue to explore is whether the development of wisdom occurs only for a select few older adults. If this is true, then it would be unlikely that a group of normal older adults would perform at a particularly high level. Some results from these studies appear to be promising. For example, middle-aged and older adults who were selected to be tested on the basis of having been nominated by a peer performed slightly better than did comparison groups on some indicators related to wisdom (Baltes & Staudinger, 1993). Wisdom, like intelligence, may require some training and effort to maintain.

Creativity

Creativity is the "ability to innovate, to change the environment rather than merely adjust to it in a more passive sense" (Simonton, 1990, p. 320). If the popular stereotype about wisdom is that it "grows" with age, the stereotype about creativity may be that it declines during adulthood. Are people more creative in their 20s than in their 60s? Think about all the creative people you know of—scientists, poets, artists, novelists, actors, musicians, and so forth. Are younger individuals typically better than older individuals in the same field? Are their most creative products generated during their early years in the field? Or are creative people always creative, regardless of their age? Many researchers have investigated these issues. For example, some adults believe that aging is accompanied by an increase in conservatism and cautiousness and a decrease in creative achievement and productivity (e.g., Heckhausen et al., 1989; Hummert et al., 1994). Unlike research on wisdom, there are clear results about the development of creativity during adulthood.

In 1953 Lehman published an influential but controversial volume entitled *Age and Achievement*. In this volume he plotted creative productivity as a function of age. After examining the historical records in numerous domains of productivity, he found that there was an increase in creative output in early adulthood, followed by a decline. Although there were numerous criticisms of his methods and interpretations (e.g., Dennis, 1954, 1956; Lehman, 1956), recent reviewers argue that Lehman's basic results are correct. More recently, Simonton (1990, 1994) noted that across a wide range of studies a robust age-related function can be observed, but that there are some important qualifications. One relevant qualification is that in some cases the life-span trajectories have two peaks, one in early adulthood and one in late adulthood. The one in late adulthood can be thought of as the "second-wind phenomenon." That is, in some cases there may be a general decline in creative output until a second wind hits about retirement age.

A second important qualification to Lehman's model is that both the age at peak performance and the steepness of the decline in creative productivity vary according to domain. This means that peak creativity in some domains may occur much earlier in life than in other domains. For example, in fields such as pure mathematics, lyric poetry, and theoretical physics the peaks are in the late 20s or early 30s. In contrast, in fields such as history, philosophy, novel writing, and general scholarship, the peaks are in the 40s or 50s, and the declines are not very steep. For a number of fields—including psychology— the peak of creative output is in the late 30s or early 40s.

What about the argument that creativity should not be measured simply by amount of creative output—a quantitative measure. Instead, it should be measured by quality of output—a focus on the truly creative part of productivity. Would this shift in emphasis result in a different profile across the life span? As Simonton (1994) has elegantly shown, the answer to this intriguing question is "no." Separating the truly creative productions from the less inspired pieces results in virtually identical patterns across the life course. This implies that the quantity of creative output is highly related to the quality of that output. This relationship holds throughout the life course or the career of an individual. Specifically, those who begin their careers with a great deal of productive output can continue this output throughout their careers. People who are less precocious may also have careers characterized by a stable quality-to-quantity ratio of productivity.

There are several reasons that some careers can be curtailed or can become substantially less productive. As Simonton (1990, 1994) noted, these include declining physical health, increasing family responsibilities, and accumulating administrative activities. Declining physical health can, of course, make concentrated effort more laborious or even less frequent. Both increasing family responsibilities and administrative duties can reduce the amount of time available for productive and creative work. Few administrators in universities, for example, are able to maintain full and energetic scholarship programs. However, with seniority some compensatory mechanisms may be available. For example, highly accomplished senior researchers may be called upon to perform full-time administrative duties (e.g., Chair of a Department at a University), but they may be able to employ several highly qualified and ambitious post-doctoral fellows, as well as numerous graduate students, to carry on their scholarly program. These younger collaborators become, in this way, human compensatory mechanisms for senior creative scholars.

Overall, Simonton's (1990, 1994) research has generated three general statements about the life course of creativity. First, there is age-related decline in creativity in the late years of life. However, this decline is rarely so substantial as to turn a creative person into a noncreative person. For most creative individuals, their lives end before their potential for creative production is exhausted. Second, how creative or productive older adults are depends more on their early-life creativity than on their age. Simonton argued that people who are exceptionally creative in early adulthood are often quite prolific throughout their careers. Indeed, they may continue to produce excellent creative products into very late life. Third, there is no evidence to suggest that the decline in creative output occurs because of a corresponding decline in cognitive skills. Even individuals who enter new arenas of interest in mid or late life have the opportunity to have productive new careers. Creativity, then, may be one area in which potential in late life may be actuated. At least, it may be possible to contend that creative people may continue to be creative across their careers.

Compensation

[handwritten annotation: A psychological mechanism by which feeling of inferiority, frustration, or failure in one field are counterbalanced by achievement in another]

Compensation is a promising new concept in the field of cognitive aging. It refers to a set of mechanisms through which an individual may continue to perform difficult or complex skills, although they are experiencing some loss in relevant abilities required to perform that task. Aging involves decline in

[handwritten annotation: An unconscious psychological mechanism by which one tries to make up for imagined or real deficiencies in personality or physical ability]

fundamental sensory, motor, neurological, and cognitive abilities. Many of these abilities are components of higher-level skills. Some of these skills may be maintained into late life. One mechanism through which such maintenance can occur is compensation. Adults may be able to compensate for declines they experience in even very basic components; they may continue to perform even complex skills (composing, writing novels, driving) at competent, if not creative, levels.

Several forms of compensation have been identified (Bäckman & Dixon, 1992; Dixon & Bäckman, 1995; Salthouse, 1995). For older adults all forms of compensation begin with the experience of a mismatch between their available abilities and the requirements they either place on themselves (as personal expectations) or accept as given by the community in which they operate. The term "community" can refer to a wide range of environmental demands, such as those accruing as a function of professional requirements, social and interactive obligations, familial responsibilities, sensory and physical contexts, and so forth. The important point is that by using one or more of the forms of compensation, the gap between their ability and their expected level of performance can be closed. In this way, a satisfactory level of performance for a given skill can be attained, and an individual's potential can be maximized. Compensation can occur in normal aging, but also as a form of recovery from brain injury or other pathogenic neurological conditions (e.g., Dixon & Bäckman, in press; Wilson & Watson, 1996). Compensation is also a viable concept in recovery from a wide range of social and personal deficits and losses, many of which are quite pertinent to gerontology (see Dixon & Bäckman, 1995).

What are the forms of compensation applicable to aging in general and cognitive aging in particular? Scholars offer somewhat different perspectives on these forms (e.g., Marsiske, Lang, Baltes, & Baltes, 1995; Salthouse, 1995), but the convergence and overlap are impressive (Dixon & Bäckman, 1995). Four forms appear to cover most of the situations in which compensation might occur in late life. The first form is perhaps the simplest. It reflects *investing time and effort* when there is a deficit in learning or performing a target skill. For example, an individual whose work environment is becoming increasingly computerized, and whose understanding of hardware and specific applications is lagging behind, may compensate for the gap between his or her environmental demands and skill level by putting more time and effort into acquiring the requisite skills. This deliberate and effortful upgrading of skill levels such that it matches the requirements of the community can result in successful compensation.

The second form of compensation, *substitution*, originates in a deficit that is the result of important components of skills declining with age, and therefore contributing ineffectively to overall skill performance (e.g., Salthouse, 1995). Compensation as substitution occurs when other components of the skill are correspondingly improved, such that the overall skill performance level is maintained. That is, the global skill is supported by new, emerging components after the original components decline. One well-known example concerns aging typists who can no longer tap their fingers as fast as they might have as younger adults, and who can no longer respond to visual stimuli (e.g., to-be-typed characters) as quickly as they might have in earlier years (Salthouse, 1995). Finger tapping and reaction time are components of the global skill of typing, in that speeded typing cannot be accomplished without some contribution from these abilities. As Salthouse observed, however, some successful older typists compensated for these decrements by possibly developing a substitutable mechanism, namely, eye–hand coordination. That is, they compensated for slower speeds of reaction and tapping by looking further ahead in the to-be-typed text so that their fingers had more time to prepare for the upcoming characters. In this way, their overall performance (typing rate) could be maintained into late life.

A third compensatory process, *selection and optimization*, involves optimizing one's development overall by selecting different paths or goals when the original one is blocked or unattainable (e.g., Marsiske et al., 1995). If the deficit is too great to overcome through investment of time and effort, and if no substitutable components are available, then this form of compensation might be invoked. Essentially, the deficit in the global skill is accepted, and alternative skills and performance domains are emphasized. For example, an aging typist for whom substitution is unavailable might become an office manager, combining "people" or supervisory skills with declarative and procedural knowledge about the office and business. In this way, one has selectively optimized their development by choosing an alternative path, after the original trajectory was blocked.

A fourth category reflects processes in which one *adjusts goals and criteria of success*. Specifically, individuals may accommodate to deficits by modifying their goals (e.g., Brandtstädter & Wentura, 1995) or lowering their criteria of what constitutes successful performance (Dixon & Bäckman, 1995). For example, older adults may modify their goals or personal expectations of performance such that it is no longer necessary to perform at quite the same level or with quite the same speed as they did when they were younger. Given no other available form of compensation, older typists might decide that their personally required typing rate can be adjusted downward, focusing perhaps instead on maintaining accuracy. A complication, of course, is that employers or senior colleagues may not concur with the lowered performance goals. For some everyday, social, and life skills, however, such changing expectations may indeed be a viable form of compensating for increasing limitations and performance decrements (Brandtstädter & Wentura, 1995). Managing one's changing resources efficiently may involve devaluing and disengaging from some blocked goals, while selecting new and feasible goals. Some aging-related losses may be compensated by rearranging priorities or constructing palliative meanings (i.e., selecting positive interpretations) (Brandtstädter & Wentura, 1995).

Compensation may be an important mechanism of successful aging, a means of realizing and maintaining cognitive potential into late life (Baltes & Baltes, 1990; Dixon, 1998). It is perhaps not an achievement that will garner awards from historians or critics (as would the creative products of a renowned composer), and it may not be a success that brings the respect accorded to the wise sage. It is, however, a practical and functional process associated with both elite levels of technical and artistic performance and everyday life skills such as driving, working, and leisure activities (Dixon, 1995).

Conclusion

Intelligence and cognitive potential in late life are concepts linked by historical and conceptual features. They have been of concern since the earliest days of speculative and empirical research on aging. Concerns about declining intelligence have sparked interest in exceptions to the rule, the possibility that the declining competence according to laboratory and psychometric tests does not necessarily mean that potential is lost with aging. Notably, these ideas are as linked in contemporary research in cognitive aging as they were in the works of the earliest observers. While demonstrating substantial decline in fluid aspects of intelligence, Schaie (1996) underscored individual differences and speculated about practical implications. Researchers in wisdom and creativity have sought to clarify the concepts and measurement of these domains, and to specify the life-span trajectories of relevant indicators. Especially with creative output, the results are suggestive of continued potential into late life. Regarding wisdom, researchers continue to work at finding suitable measures and samples with which to explore a domain that is generally believed to be one of the few growing in late life. If there is a decline in skills of various sorts, it may also be possible for older adults to compensate, thus preserving an overall level of satisfactory performance. Accompanying aging are inevitable limits and decrements in the biological and neurological substrates. Nevertheless, many older adults can lead rewarding and productive lives, in social, professional, and cognitive realms. How this happens—and what it means for individuals, families, and social policy—are topics for much further research in gerontology.

Acknowledgments

Preparation of this chapter was supported by grants from the National Institute on Aging (AG08235) and the Natural Sciences and Engineering Research Council of Canada. We appreciate John Cavanaugh's helpful comments on an earlier version of this chapter.

REVIEW QUESTIONS

1. What are the main advantages of conducting longitudinal research on intellectual aging? Name several main findings from Warner Schaie's Seattle

Longitudinal Study that likely would not have been discovered using standard cross-sectional designs. Are there any disadvantages to conducting longitudinal studies?

2. According to the chapter, many older adults can improve their performance on cognitive tasks if given appropriate practice or training. Are there any limitations in the extent to which older adults can improve their cognitive performance? [*Hints:* Consider whether improvements due to training should be observed for all cognitive tasks or for all older adults. Consider whether the maximum levels of performance may be different for younger and older adults.]

3. Do you think intelligence in the general population is better or worse at the beginning of the twenty-first century than it was at the beginning of the twentieth century? Is intelligence of older adults now better or worse than a century ago? Explain your answers.

4. Think of a real-life example of older adults compensating for aging-related deficits. List at least one example from each of the forms of compensatory mechanisms.

5. Try to think of someone you know—or know of—who is wise. What are the characteristics of this person that lead you to think of them as wise? Give at least one example of something they have done or said that was wise. How well do the characteristics of wisdom described in the chapter capture the wisdom displayed by this person?

6. What is the role of intelligence in creativity? Are creative people more intelligent than individuals who do not produce celebrated creative products? If so, is creativity just another form of intelligence? If not, how important is intelligence in generating creative products or following creative careers?

References

Abercrombie, J. (1839). *Inquiries concerning the intellectual powers and their investigation of truth.* Boston: Otis, Broaders.

Achenbaum, W.A. (1990). Policy challenges of late life potential. In M. Perlmutter (Ed.), *Late life potential* (pp. 121–142). Washington, DC: The Gerontological Society of America.

Bäckman, L., & Dixon, R.A. (1992). Psychological compensation: A theoretical framework. *Psychological Bulletin, 112,* 259–283.

Baltes, P.B. (1987). Theoretical propositions of life-span developmental psychology: On the dynamics between growth and decline. *Developmental Psychology, 23,* 611–626.

Baltes, P.B., & Baltes, M.M. (Eds.). (1990). *Successful aging: Perspectives from the behavioral sciences.* New York: Cambridge University Press.

Baltes, P.B., & Lindenberger, U. (1997). Emergence of a powerful connection between sensory and cognitive functions across the adult life span: A new window to the study of cognitive aging? *Psychology & Aging, 12,* 12–21.

Baltes, P.B., & Smith, J. (1990). Toward a psychology of wisdom and its ontogenesis. In R.J. Sternberg (Ed.), *Wisdom: Its nature, origins, and development* (pp. 87–120). New York: Cambridge University Press.

Baltes, P.B., & Staudinger, U. (1993). The search for a psychology of wisdom. *Current Directions in Psychological Science, 2,* 1–6.

Baltes, P.B., & Willis, S.L. (1982). Enhancement (plasticity) of intellectual functioning in old age: Penn State's Adult Development and Enrichment (ADEPT) Project. In F.I.M. Craik & S.E. Trehub (Eds.), *Aging and cognitive processes* (pp. 353–389). New York: Plenum.

Bayley, N. (1955). On the growth of intelligence. *American Psychologist, 10,* 805–818.

Berg, C.A., & Klaczynski, P.A. (1996). Practical intelligence and problem solving: Searching for perspectives. In F. Blanchard-Fields & T.M. Hess (Eds.), *Perspectives on cognitive change in adulthood and aging* (pp. 323–357). New York: McGraw-Hill.

Bieman-Copland, S., Ryan, E.B., & Cassano, J. (1998). Responding to the challenges of late life: Strategies for maintaining and enhancing competence. In D. Pushkar, W. Bukowski, A. Schwartzman, D. Stack, & D. White (Eds.), *Improving competence across the lifespan* (pp. 141–157). New York: Plenum.

Blanchard-Fields, F. (1996). Social cognitive development in adulthood and aging. In F. Blanchard-Fields & T.M. Hess (Eds.), *Perspectives on cognitive change in adulthood and aging* (pp. 454–487). New York: McGraw-Hill.

Blanchard-Fields, F., & Hess, T.M. (Eds.). (1996). *Perspectives on cognitive change in adulthood and aging.* New York: McGraw-Hill.

Bond, L.A., Cutler, S.J., & Grams, A. (Eds.). (1995). *Promoting successful and productive aging.* Thousand Oaks, CA: Sage.

Botwinick, J. (1977). Intellectual abilities. In J.E. Birren & K.W. Schaie (Eds.), *Handbook of the psychology of aging* (pp. 580–605). New York: Van Nostrand Reinhold.

Brandtstädter, J., & Wentura, D. (1995). Adjustment to shifting possibility frontiers in later life: Complementary adaptive modes. In R.A. Dixon & L. Bäckman (Eds.), *Compensating for psychological deficits and declines: Managing losses and promoting gains* (pp. 83–106). Mahwah, NJ: Erlbaum.

Camp, C.J., & McKitrick, L.A. (1992). Memory interventions in Alzheimer's-type dementia populations: Methodological and theoretical issues. In R.L. West & J.D. Sinnott (Eds.), *Everyday memory and aging: Current research and methodology* (pp. 155–172). New York: Springer.

Cavanaugh, J.C. (1996). Memory self-efficacy as a moderator of memory change. In F. Blanchard-Fields & T.M. Hess (Eds.), *Perspectives on cognitive change in adulthood and aging* (pp. 488–507). New York: McGraw-Hill.

Clayton, V.P., & Birren, J.E. (1980). The development of wisdom across the life span: A re-examination of an ancient topic. In P.B. Baltes & O.G. Brim (Eds.), *Life-span development and behavior* (Vol. 3; pp. 103–135). New York: Academic Press.

Craik, F.I.M., & Salthouse, T. (Eds.). (1992). *The handbook of aging and cognition.* Hillsdale, NJ: Erlbaum.

Dennis, W. (1954). Review of *Age and achievement. Psychological Bulletin, 51,* 306–308.

Dennis, W. (1956). *Age and achievement:* A critique. *Journal of Gerontology, 9,* 465–467.

Dixon, R.A. (1995). Promoting competence through compensation. In L.A. Bond, S.J. Cutler, & A. Grams (Eds.), *Promoting successful and productive aging.* (pp. 220–238). Thousand Oaks, CA: Sage.

Dixon, R.A. (1996). Collaborative memory and aging. In D.J. Herrmann, C. McEvoy, C. Hertzog, P. Hertel, & M.K. Johnson (Eds.), *Basic and applied memory research: Theory in context* (pp. 359–383). Mahwah, NJ: Erlbaum.

Dixon, R.A. (1998). The concept of gains in cognitive aging. In N. Schwarz, S. Sudman, B. Knäuper, & D. Park (Eds.), *Cognition, aging, and self-reports* (pp. 71–92). Philadelphia, PA: Psychology Press.

Dixon, R.A., & Bäckman, L. (Eds.). (1995). *Compensating for psychological deficits and declines: Managing losses and promoting gains.* Mahwah, NJ: Erlbaum.

Dixon, R.A., & Bäckman, L. (In press). Principles of compensation in cognitive neurorehabilitation. In D.T. Stuss, G. Winocur, & I.H. Robertson (Eds.), *Cognitive neurorehabilitation: A comprehensive approach.* Cambridge: Cambridge University Press.

Dixon, R.A., & Hertzog, C. (1996). Theoretical issues in cognition and aging. In F. Blanchard-Fields & T.M. Hess (Eds.), *Perspectives on cognitive change in adulthood and aging* (pp. 25–65). New York: McGraw-Hill.

Dixon, R.A., Kramer, D.A., & Baltes, P.B. (1985). Intelligence: A life-span developmental perspective. In B.B. Wolman (Ed.), *Handbook of intelligence: Theories, measurements, and applications* (pp. 301–350). New York: Wiley.

Gold, D.P., Andres, D., Etezadi, J., Arbuckle, T., Schwartzman, A., & Chaikelson, J. (1995). Structural equation model of intellectual change and continuity and predictors of intelligence in older men. *Psychology and Aging, 10,* 294–303.

Gould, S.J. (1981). *The mismeasure of man.* New York: Norton.

Hall, G.S. (1922). *Senescence: The last half of life.* New York: Appleton.

Heckhausen, J., Dixon, R.A., & Baltes, P.B. (1989). Gains and losses in development throughout adulthood as perceived by different adult age groups. *Developmental Psychology, 25,* 109–121.

Heckhausen, J., & Krueger, J. (1993). Developmental expectations for the self and most other people: Age grading in three functions of social comparisons. *Developmental Psychology, 29,* 539–548.

Hertzog, C., & Dixon, R.A. (1994). Metacognitive development in adulthood and old age. In J. Metcalfe & A.P. Shimamura (Eds.), *Metacognition* (pp. 227–251). Boston, MA: M. I. T. Press.

Hertzog, C., & Dixon, R.A. (1996). Methodological issues in research on cognition and aging. In F. Blanchard-Fields & T.M. Hess (Eds.), *Perspectives on cognitive change in adulthood and aging* (pp. 66–121). New York: McGraw-Hill.

Horn, J.L. (1982). The theory of crystallized and fluid intelligence in relation to concepts of cognitive psychology and aging in adulthood. In F.I.M. Craik & S. Trehub (Eds.), *Aging and cognitive processes* (pp. 237–278). New York: Plenum.

Horn, J.L., & Cattell, (1966). Refinement and test of a theory of fluid and crystallized intelligence. *Journal of Educational Psychology, 57,* 253–270.

Hultsch, D.F., Hertzog, C., Dixon, R.A., & Small, B.J. (1998). *Memory change in the aged.* New York: Cambridge University Press.

Hultsch, D.F., Hertzog, C., Small, B.J., & Dixon, R.A. (in press). Use it or lose it: Engaged lifestyle as a buffer of cognitive decline in aging? *Psychology and Aging.*

Hummert, M.L., Garstka, T.A., Shaner, J.L., & Strahm, S. (1994). Stereotypes of the elderly held by young, middle-aged, and elderly adults. *Journal of Gerontology: Psychological Sciences, 49,* P40–P49.

James, W. (1890). *The principles of psychology* (2 vols.). New York: Dover.

Kausler, D. (1991). *Experimental psychology, cognition, and human aging* (2nd ed.). New York: Springer.

Kekes, J. (1983). Wisdom. *American Philosophical Quarterly, 20,* 277–286.

Kirkpatrick, E.A. (1903). *Fundamentals of child study: A discussion of instincts and other factors in human development with practical applications.* New York: Macmillan.

Lehman, H.C. (1953). *Age and achievement.* Princeton, NJ: Princeton University Press.

Lehman, H.C. (1956). Reply to Dennis' critique of *Age and achievement. Journal of Gerontology, 11,* 128–134.

Light, L.L. (1991). Memory and aging: Four hypotheses in search of data. *Annual Review of Psychology, 42,* 333–376.

Marsiske, M., Lang, F.R., Baltes, P.B., & Baltes, M.M. (1995). Selective optimization with compensation: Life-span perspectives on successful human development. In R.A. Dixon & L. Bäckman (Eds.), *Compensating for psychological deficits and declines: Managing losses and promoting gains* (pp. 35–79). Mahwah, NJ: Erlbaum.

Medina, J.J. (1996). *The clock of ages.* Cambridge: Cambridge University Press.

Neely, A. S., & Bäckman, L. (1995). Effects of multifactorial memory training in older adults: Two 3½ year follow-up studies. *Journal of Gerontology: Psychological Sciences, 50,* 134–140.

Perlmutter, M. (Ed.). (1990). *Late life potential.* Washington, DC: Gerontological Society of America.

Salthouse, T. (1991). *Theoretical perspectives on cognitive aging.* San Diego: Academic Press.

Salthouse, T.A. (1995). Refining the concept of psychological compensation. In R.A. Dixon & L. Bäckman (Eds.), *Compensating for psychological deficits and declines: Managing losses and promoting gains* (pp. 21–34). Mahwah, NJ: Erlbaum.

Sanford, E.C. (1902). Mental growth and decay. *American Journal of Psychology, 13,* 426–449.

Schaie, K.W. (1983). The Seattle Longitudinal Study: A twenty-one-year exploration of psychometric intelligence in adulthood. In K.W. Schaie (Ed.), *Longitudinal studies of adult psychological development* (pp. 64–135). New York: Guilford Press.

Schaie, K.W. (1990). Intellectual development in adulthood. In J.E. Birren & K.W. Schaie (Eds.), *Handbook of the psychology and aging* (3rd ed.; pp. 291–309). New York: Academic Press.

Schaie, K.W. (1994). The course of adult intellectual development. *American Psychologist, 49,* 304–314.

Schaie, K.W. (1996). *Intellectual development in adulthood: The Seattle Longitudinal Study.* Cambridge: Cambridge University Press.

Simonton, D.K. (1990). Creativity and wisdom in aging. In J.E. Birren & K.W. Schaie (Eds.), *Handbook of the psychology of aging* (3rd ed., pp. 320–329). San Diego: Academic Press.

Simonton, D.K. (1994). *Greatness: Who makes history and why.* New York: Guilford Press.

Sinnott, J. (1996). The developmental approach: Postformal thought as adaptive intelligence. In F. Blanchard-Fields & T.M. Hess (Eds.), *Perspectives on cognitive change in adulthood and aging* (pp. 358–383). New York: McGraw-Hill.

Smith, J., & Baltes, P.B. (1990). Wisdom-related knowledge: Age/cohort differences in response to life-planning problems. *Developmental Psychology, 26,* 494–505.

Spreen, O., & Strauss, E. (1998). *A compendium of neuropsychological tests: Administration, norms, and commentary* (2nd ed.). New York: Oxford University Press.

Staudinger, U.M., Smith, J., & Baltes, P.B. (1992). Wisdom-related knowledge in a life review task: Age differences and the role of professional specialization. *Psychology and Aging, 7,* 271–281.

Sternberg, R.J. (Ed.). (1990). *Wisdom: Its nature, origins, and development*. New York: Cambridge University Press.
Sternberg, R.J. (Ed.). (1997). Special issue: Intelligence and lifelong learning. *American Psychologist, 52*, 1029–1139.
Thurstone, L.L. (1938). *The primary mental abilities*. Chicago: University of Chicago Press.
Uttal, D.H., & Perlmutter, M. (1989). Toward a broader conceptualization of development: The role of gains and losses across the life span. *Developmental Review, 9*, 101–132.
Verhaegen, P., Marcoen, A., & Goossens, L. (1992). Improving memory performance in the aged through mnemonic training: A meta-analytic study. *Psychology and Aging, 7*, 242–251.
Wechsler, D. (1939). *The measurement of adult intelligence*. Baltimore: Williams & Wilkens.
Wechsler, D. (1958). *The measurement and appraisal of adult intelligence* (4th ed.). Baltimore: Williams & Wilkens.
Wechsler, D. (1997). *Wechsler Adult Intelligence Scale—third edition*. San Antonio, TX: The Psychological Corporation.
Weisenburg, T., Roe, A., & McBride, K.E. (1936). *Adult intelligence: A psychological study of test performance*. London: Commonwealth Fund.
Wilson, B.A., & Watson, P.C. (1996). A practical framework for understanding compensatory behavior in people with organic memory impairment. *Memory, 4*, 456–486.
Woodruff-Pak, D.S. (1997). *The neuropsychology of aging*. Malden, MA: Blackwell.

Additional Readings

Blanchard-Fields, F., & Hess, T.M. (Eds.) (1996). *Perspectives on cognitive change in adulthood and aging*. New York: McGraw-Hill.
Bond, L.A., Cutler, S.J., & Grams, A. (Eds.). (1995). *Promoting successful and productive aging*. Thousands Oaks, CA: Sage.
Craik, F.I.M., & Salthouse, T.A. (Eds.). (1992). *The handbook of aging and cognition*. Hillsdale, NJ: Erlbaum.
Dixon, R.A., & Bäckman, L. (Eds.). (1995). *Compensating for psychological deficits and declines: Managing losses and promoting gains*. Mahwah, NJ: Erlbaum.
Salthouse, T.A. (1991). *Theoretical perspectives on cognitive aging*. San Diego: Academic Press.
Schaie, K.W. (1996). *Intellectual development in adulthood: The Seattle Longitudinal Study*. Cambridge: Cambridge University Press.
Simonton, D.K. (1994). *Greatness: Who makes history and why*. New York: Guilford.
Sternberg, R.J. (Ed.). (1990). *Wisdom: Its nature, origins, and development*. New York: Cambridge University Press.

9

Self and Personality Development

Gisela Labouvie-Vief and Manfred Diehl

Stories of midlife excursions and transformations abound in myth and literature. Often, such stories suggest that throughout history, self and personality
in adulthood were associated with important reorganizations, symbolized by
images of death and rebirth. These images hint at giving up youthful ideal-
izations and facing life realistically. Yet, from this symbolic "death" individuals emerge not with a sense of ultimate defeat but with an increased sense of
integration (e.g., Campbell, 1988; Labouvie-Vief, 1994).

Scientific views of adulthood often portray a more sober picture; they are
informed less by patterns of symbols, stories, and myth and more by cooler rational perspectives. Growing into mature and late adulthood often has been
framed in terms of theoretical models that have idealized youthful tendencies—
the belief in the power of cognition, conscious control, stability, coherence and
harmony, perfection, independence, and masculinity. Yet as rationalism's hold
on modern science is loosening, the view of adult development as bringing
important transformations is definitely in ascendancy, and theorists and
researchers are eager to record not only the inevitable decline and disillusion-
ment that come with growing older, but also the gains and progressions
(Labouvie-Vief, 1982a).

Interest in transformational views of personality have become widespread
in modern culture and constitute a movement that unites many disciplines beyond psychology per se. This interest is part of a wide ranging revision of a
traditional model of individuals as it is visible in philosophy, natural science,
religion, and literature. According to that traditional view, development was
to be described in terms of rational processes. Rational processes were believed
to transcend spatial, temporal, and subjective conditions, rather than being tied
to the embodied and contextual nature of thinking. However, current scientific
trends are focusing more on integrating the rational and contextual dimensions
of existence, and although such integration is part of a broad interdisciplinary
movement, it also has affected psychology—and specifically, the ways psychologists view self and personality. In fact, the addition of "self" to "person-

238

ality" when talking about changes related to patterns of motivation and their organization over time reflects in many ways such integrative trends.

In the current chapter, we will examine recent issues in self and personality using such an integrative framework. In the first section, we will review several of the general ways in which thinking and talking about personality have been affected by contemporary reconceptualizations of human nature. In particular, we will focus on how theorists' and researchers' conceptualizations of self and personality development during adulthood have changed over the last two or three decades or so. In the three sections to follow, we will then offer a review of major theoretical issues and research from the perspective of different traditions. Specifically, we will concentrate on theories rooted in (1) the psychoanalytic tradition and its more recent developments in self- and object-relations theory, (2) the cognitive-developmental tradition, and (3) the trait-theoretical tradition.

Self and Personality: Contemporary Assumptions

In her book *Culture and Commitment*, Margaret Mead (1970) proposed that modern life has profoundly changed our experience of the life course. Mead (1970) suggested that in relatively simple societies the life structure for individuals was clear and predictable. In contrast, contemporary societies display profound differences in how the life course is structured and experienced. Urbanization, the emergence of a global community, and the graying of the world population all have effected a wide-ranging revision of how we conceptualize the nature of human beings. Many disciplines, from philosophy, mathematics, and physics to art, literature, and religion, have participated in this process, and, as a result, views of human nature and development are being revised as well (see Labouvie-Vief, 1996). In particular, these revised views of human nature and development are exemplified in the debates about the stability vs. plasticity of human abilities and behavior, the role of contextual influences, and the transactions between individual and context across the life span.

Stability versus Change and Plasticity

In simpler, more isolated societies of the past, suggests Mead (1970), what impressed individuals is the repeatability of the life course: Basic core patterns repeat themselves from generation to generation. However, in complex societies that involve the confrontation of multiple cultural and racial components, demands are made on individuals with regard to continuous change. For example, among immigrant families, the parents no longer are the "experts" in how to live life; rather, the younger generation teaches the older generation about new ways. Thus as different generations grow up in contexts that are quite different, information between generations flows in two ways rather than just one and roles may be reversed to adjust to new challenges.

Similar cultural changes have dramatically changed notions of development in this century. Original concepts often emphasized a tightly regulated developmental course that primarily reflected biological regulation and that culminated in biological maturation. In contrast to these early models, current discussions of psychological development highlight the openness, multidimensionality, and multidirectionality of developmental trajectories, and emphasize that even in later stages of development, a considerable capacity exists for positive change. Thus earlier theories of development, such as Freud's psychoanalytic theory or Piaget's cognitive-developmental theory, assumed that individuals were fairly fixed in later life. Indeed, Freud believed that interventions such as psychotherapy were not to be recommended for adults older than about 40 years of age. In contrast, following the lead of Bloom (1964), more recent positions have criticized this stability position and have emphasized that the potentials for change and plasticity need to be examined across the whole life span and into old age (Baltes, 1987; Baltes, Lindenberger, & Staudinger, 1998).

Along with an interest in continued change, notions of development also have begun to embrace the historical and cultural dimensions of change and development. Such contextual views of change over the life span are currently predominant in research on human development. By examining the association of change in context with change in personality characteristics, theorists and researchers now propose less monolithic views of development. Instead, the emphasis is on how diverse contexts channel individuals into different developmental trajectories, and how changes in context are associated with turning points in individual characteristics (Caspi, 1987; Labouvie-Vief & Chandler, 1978).

Individualism versus Relatedness

With the rediscovery of context also came a new awareness that classical models of mind and self have idealized the individual; the fact that we are profoundly related to others at all points of the life span did not receive similar attention and was, in fact, treated as a "problematic" aspect that we ideally overcome. Thus, positive development often was described in terms of characteristics and values such as individuality, autonomy, independence, achievement motivation, and identity; in contrast, values such as relatedness, compassion, and dependence were seen as less important and indeed as less mature (Gilligan, 1982; Guisinger & Blatt, 1994). And since these two sets of values are often thought to be associated with gender, women's development did not really fit older, more "masculine" models (Gilligan, 1982). In contrast, many theories have begun to account for the profound ways in which humans are interrelated (e.g., Bowlby, 1969, 1988; Erikson, 1982). Indeed, such interrelatedness must constitute a basic, biologically based propensity in a species that is neotenous and has a long period of extrauterine development. Failure to be in relation to others, in turn, is associated with not only a host of psychological disorders (Helgeson, 1994), but also biological ones such as depressed immunocompetence (Bakan, 1966; Guisinger & Blatt, 1994). As a consequence, a number of more recent models of development have emphasized the need for a balance between autonomy and dependence of relatedness as attributes of mature adults, whether male of female (e.g., Erikson, 1982; Guisinger & Blatt, 1994).

Coherence of the Individual

The changed views of context and relations also have affected how we look at the single individual, not just the individual in relationship to other individuals. An assumption often made in the past was that personality characteristics emanate from some inner structures such as an ego or some other central processor that gives coherence and unity to self and experience. However, many recent theories emphasize that different, and sometimes vastly contradictory experiences and attributes may be activated by different contexts or relationships. Thus individuals are no longer seen as having a single coherent mind, self, and personality. Instead, human mind, self, and personality are seen as dynamic and multidimensional entities, which combine in themselves contradictions and conflicts in ways that define the unique individuality of a person (Fischer & Ayoub, 1994; Markus & Wurf, 1987; Mitchell, 1988).

Growth versus Decline

Past models of human development have made it difficult (if not impossible) to develop a unified theory of the total life course. Strongly influenced by biological models of development and maturity, most past theories associated growth and gain with early life, whereas adulthood and later life were seen solely in terms of loss and decline. Yet, as suggested by Labouvie-Vief (1980, 1981; see also Baltes, 1987), losses are not unique to later life. Indeed, from the beginning, the process of human development is characterized by the interweaving of gains with losses, and often gains in development are related to losses in a direct gain–loss relationship. Thus, what is often called decline or regression can result from the operation of developmental processes that are usually related to progressive development or growth.

Several principles demonstrate this trade-off between growth and decline. For example, as development proceeds, old structures often become displaced or function with less efficiency. Another principle is that of selective depletion, a principle widely important in evolutionary processes. Much as evolution is based on an oversupply of organisms out of which only the "fittest" are selected, so a similar mechanism operates in developing systems. For example, the progressive maturation of the brain during the first stages of life does involve not only growth and refinement, but actually profound losses as well. Originally, neurons are supplied in abundance, but as workable networks are established, many neurons are "weeded out" through a process of selective death. Third, development typically involves increasing degrees of specialization, or the trading off of potential for realized structure. Thus, smooth functioning at the system or collective level can be traded off for specialization at the individual level.

In Labouvie-Vief's (1981) work, these trade-off processes have been conceptualized as being proactive and progressive. In addition, Baltes (1987) has added to these progressive trade-off processes reactive ones that may reflect processes of aging proper (see also Baltes et al., 1998). Thus as in the process of growing older, psychological and social resources decline, individuals actually may evolve highly adaptive and resilient compensatory strategies. In addition, individuals who experience a loss of capacity may compensate by selecting one area of functioning and may focus an increased amount of attention and energy on it. Such selective optimization is at times associated with extraordinary and highly evolved skills. Even so, however, Baltes suggests that the process of aging does place a limit on this ability to compensate, and even with optimal training and allocation of attention and energy, elderly individuals usually do not achieve at youthful levels.

In this section we have summarized several common threads that are woven into diverse ways of talking about adult development and later life. All of these common themes and issues are part of a broad and pervasive transformation of the life course that affects the modes of inquiry in all developmental disciplines. This "new look" contrasts past views of development with an emphasis on context, change, continued growth, and the complexity and multidimensionality of self and personality. In the sections to follow, we will focus on three theoretical traditions in the study of self and personality and discuss recent developments and future directions.

Psychodynamic Approaches to Self and Personality

Contemporary psychodynamic formulations of self and personality derive from Freud's (1911/1957) original formulation of psychoanalytic theory. Interestingly, psychoanalytic theory itself represented a significant movement in the redefinition of mind and self. Pointing out that emotions and relationships with others are not derived processes, but the very ground on which the self is built, Freud's theory was a bold move, advocating that researchers take the study of the mind out of the transcendent and make it part of the natural world. Still, in retrospect it is clear that Freud's theory maintained many traditional rationalist assumptions, which were modified by psychoanalytic theorists to come.

Beyond Ego and Culture

One of the first individuals to propose an extension of Freud's theory was his colleague Carl Gustav Jung. Jung (1933) and some of his students (e.g., Neumann, 1973) suggested that Freud's view of development was particularly pertinent for the first part of life, when in the interest of cultural adaptation and socialization the individual must develop a strong ego that suppresses aspects of the self, including contrasexual and aggressive tendencies not valued by most societies. However, Jung also pointed out that this form of development encouraged the formation of fairly rigid dualisms between mind and body, thinking and emotion, conscious and unconscious, outer experience and inner experience, good and evil, masculine and feminine, and so forth—dualisms that were part of becoming a competent and well-controlled member of culture. In contrast to this emphasis on socialization during early life, Jung (1933) suggested that around the middle of life, development shifts to individuation. Jung proposed that during middle age, individuals have an opportunity to explore and accept unconscious motives, to integrate contrasexual aspects and tendencies, and to integrate the dualisms formed in early development. In this way, they begin to transcend a narrow self-identification with ego and superego. Indeed, Jung suggested that during the middle years the dynamic of development shifts to the "Self," a structure that comprises both the id and the ego and that establishes an active dialogue between these structures. As a consequence of these processes, older individuals may become guided by a more genuine dialectic relationship between ego processes and the deeper patterns of human experience expressed by the self. Jung felt that such core patterns of experience indicate deep longings and desires that are often unconscious, yet that constitute part of our collective human heritage. These patterns, (called "archetypes" by Jung, 1933) are expressed in stories and symbols worldwide, and they express universal aspects of the human experience, such as birth and death, success and failure, growth and decline, or masculinity and femininity.

Jung's ideas often have stood at the periphery of academic concerns. Yet more recently, the notion of important aspects of self and personality that are organized by symbols and stories has become an accepted and vigorous topic of inquiry (McAdams, 1995). Similarly, the notion that adulthood can bring a transcendence of dualistic tendencies, a more comfortable relationship between conscious and unconscious, and a reorganization of rigid gender polarization all have constituted active and informative areas of inquiry. However, the claim that the reorganizations that Jung proposed represent normative and universal aspects of human experience (e.g., Levinson, Darrow, Klein, Levinson, & McKee, 1978) has not really been borne out by empirical research, as further discussed below and in the section on cognitive perspectives. To date, most of the empirical evidence suggests that the reorganizations proposed by Jung are aspects of rather exceptional and advanced development—albeit aspects that, as Jung suggested, can lead to an upsurge of creativity and well being (Labouvie-Vief, Chiodo, Goguen, Diehl, & Orwoll, 1995a).

Jung's suggestion that the essence of mature development was to be able to step back from cultural regulation mechanisms, to look through them as it were and discern a broader self than that defined by a cultural mask, also became an influential component of other theories of mature development. One of those is that of Erik Erikson who called attention to cultural mechanisms. Erikson's theory implicitly proposed a generalization of the Freudian notion of 'identification'. For Freud, processes of identification took place in the 'phallic' period as a result of the internalization of parental attributes and rules. However, Erikson suggested that the parent-derived inner required further development and expansion.

Erikson proposed that the self defines itself through successively widening circles of relations. For example in adolescence, identification is no longer primarily concerned with parental introjections, but includes attempts to differentiate oneself from one's primary origins and to fit into broader institutional and cultural patterns of norms and ideologies. At advanced adult levels, the individual still becomes more invested in the active shaping of culture through generative behavior and investments. In particular, generative individuals are those who create and tend to cultural patterns that can guide younger generations, making them the "caretakers" of culture (Erikson, 1982; Gutmann, 1994). From this stage of generativity, finally, the wise elder's identification moves on to encompassing enduring patterns that define mankind and the human condition in general.

In his book, *The Wisdom of the Ego*, George Vaillant (1993) also suggested that processes of identification can be arranged on a developmental continuum ranging from less to more complex. Earlier forms of identification are built on relatively immature forms of introjection and imitation—they are relatively inflexible, wholesale adoptions of parental ideals and characters. However, as individuals mature, processes of identification are carried by more complex processes that involve more flexible, differentiated, and choice-determined decisions about the nature of the "I." Thus, like Jung, Vaillant's work suggests that the ego and the superego indeed continue to take on a new structure that is more self-determined on the one hand and more informed by generic human concerns on the other.

Midlife Crisis (turning point = traumatic change in a person's life

The notion introduced by Jung (1933) that there are major reorganizations around midlife has been the focus of much interest. Research related to the concept of a midlife crisis, however, has not been extremely supportive of this notion. For example, there is little evidence that upheavals and dramatic change are related to a unique period of adulthood. Although some individuals do experience a crisis, those individuals who do may suffer from general problems of psychopathology (Rosenbaum & Farrell, 1981). Thus, some researchers in the field have tended to conclude that the idea of a midlife crisis has been over-stated.

However, there is some fairly good evidence that many individuals experience some reorganization of self and values across the adult life span. Why, then, should it be difficult to find clear evidence? There are two major reasons. One is the issue raised by Block (1995a; Labouvie-Vief, DeVoe, & Bulka, 1989a) discussed in the next section—i.e., the general bias in many current assessments toward stability. To the extent that many psychological tests and questionnaires are insensitive to transformations of meaning, they are useless for the assessment of important changes. Another major issue to be considered is that the major dynamic driving changes associated with midlife may not be so much period or age dependent, but rather may follow general cognitive changes. As discussed in the next section, there is a considerable body of neo-Piagetian research that suggests that individuals around the middle of adulthood show the most complex understanding of self, emotions, motivations—in general, attributes that fall under the rubric of "personality." At the same time, this literature suggests that more significantly than age, independent measures of cognitive complexity are the strongest predictors of higher levels of complexity. Thus, phenomena usually associated with a midlife crisis may be the result of general gains in cognitive complexity from early to middle adulthood.

Abigail Stewart (1996) reported a series of studies examining changes related to midlife in several well-educated samples of women. A sizable number of the women reported that they would make changes to their lives if they could; most of these cases were women who had "traditional role regrets." That is, they wished they had pursued educational and work opportunities rather than having focused on traditional feminine role aspects. Not all of those who had role regrets made adjustments to their lives—but those who did were better off at midlife in terms of psychological adjustment, and in fact they did as well as those women who had no role regrets at all. Thus, Stewart suggests that rather than talking about the notion of a midlife crisis, it is perhaps more appropriate to talk about a midlife correction. That is, individuals are likely to examine and reevaluate their roles and dreams, and those with strong enough psychological, social, and material resources may go on and apply a correction, if necessary.

The Duality of the Self

Although both Jung and Erikson pushed the boundaries of Freud's theory, many recent criticisms suggest that one of their core concepts—that of the basic duality of the self—was not sufficiently developed, and that both maintained a bias toward autonomy, individuality, and masculinity. That adult development should be seen as the full conjoining of two fundamental developmental lines has been emphasized by several theorists. For example, Bakan (1966) called these two fundamental developmental lines agency versus communion; others have called them an orientation toward separateness versus connection (e.g., Gilligan, 1982; Miller, 1976), power and achievement versus intimacy and love (McAdams, 1985), or individuation and attachment (Franz & White, 1985). These orientations have often been associated with masculinity and femininity, an association that pervades symbolic constructions of reality in stories, myth, religion, and other domains. Indeed, this association even undergirds many of the prominent theories of gender and development. Yet, as Jung was the first to point out, these dualities are inherent in all humans, regardless of gender, and in part become gender associated as a result of socialization pressures (e.g., Gutmann, 1994). However, both Jung and Gutmann suggest that these lines are integrated in configurations that include a consolidated self that combines autonomy and productivity with healthy relatedness.

A considerable body of evidence does, indeed, indicate that early in the life span men and women are routed into somewhat different developmental pathways. For example, throughout the school age period boys come increasingly to deal with conflict in ways that are externalizing, whereas girls become more likely to use defenses that internalize conflict and direct feelings of aggression inward. Similarly, in the literature on adult development, Labouvie-Vief, Hakim-Larson, and Hobart (1987) and Diehl, Coyle, and Labouvie-Vief (1996) reported that women's predominant coping strategies were based on self-doubt and turning against the self, whereas men were more likely to use strategies of externalization and dissociation. Perhaps as a consequence of these patterns, men and women evidence different patterns of vulnerability/resilience for psychological disorders with age. For example, much interest has been directed to gender differences in aggression, which increase for men from childhood to adulthood, whereas the prevalence of unipolar depression in women persists into adulthood and is generally twice that of men (McGrath, Keita, Strickland, & Russo, 1990).

Profound differences also exist in how men and women subjectively experience their successes in the academic domain and intellectual domain. Despite few objective differences in intellectual status between men and women, women on average continue to attain lower levels of achievement than men (e.g., Tomlinson-Keasey & Blurton, 1992). As noted earlier, however, these different orientations may be particularly characteristic of the early half of the life span, whereas the second half brings a relaxation of the demands for "sex-appropriate" behaviors (Gutmann, 1994).

As reviewed by Labouvie-Vief (1994), some individuals around the middle of adulthood do appear to experience such integrative changes. Accordingly, some women around midlife claim domains they have avoided thus far, moving from a stance of interiority to one of openness, assertiveness, and power. In turn, some men integrate their "feminine" aspects, accepting their vulnerability and nurturance. However, many studies have not carefully ruled out alternative interpretations. For example, Gutmann's discussions suggest that some men, rather than integrating notions of feminine power, become threatened and enfeebled by a sense of overpowering, "masculine" women.

Another problem is that postulated midlife changes have not yet been differentiated from cultural/cohort changes. Since over the course of this century, gender roles have become less polarized, it is possible that movements toward integration are easier for more recent cohorts.

Long-Term Continuities *earlier & later*

One of the controversial assertions of psychodynamic theory is the claim that structures of the self are critically formed in early life and that these early formed structures determine an individual's personality and style of adaptation for the remainder of his or her life course. The prime example for this position is John Bowlby's (1969) attachment theory, which has recently been extended into the domain of adult personality development (Hazan & Shaver, 1994). Attachment theory developed as an outgrowth of psychoanalytic theory, but was reworked by Bowlby (1969) into an ethological theory that also incorporated principles of control theory. From the beginning, Bowlby (1969) stated that attachment is an integral part of human behavior "from the cradle to the grave," thus emphasizing the lifelong relevance of the attachment relationship. For example, Kahn and Antonucci (1980) noted in the context of social support research that "the attachment relationships in infancy may be both a prototype and a precursor of supportive interactions in adulthood" (p. 258). This is because the attachment relationship a child forms in his or her interactions with the primary caregiver (usually a parent) results in a prototypical internal working model (Bowlby, 1980) of close relationships. This internal working model integrates basic beliefs about the self, others, and the social world in general, and is thought to affect the formation and maintenance of close relationships for the remainder of an individual's life course (Bowlby, 1988; Hazan & Shaver, 1994).

Considerable support for the importance of attachment styles in adulthood have been provided by Collins and Read (1990), Hazan and Shaver (1987), and Kobak and Sceery (1988). In addition, individuals (usually, young adults) with different attachment styles have been found to differ in (1) their experience of positive or negative emotions in relationships (Simpson, Rholes, & Nelligan, 1992), (2) their reports of perceived quality of family climate and family functioning (Feeney, Noller, & Callan, 1994), and (3) their communication and modulation of emotion in the marital relationship, marital adjustment, and marital satisfaction (Feeney et al., 1994; Kobak & Hazan, 1991).

There is also some evidence that attachment styles continue to account for a significant amount of the variance in individuals' social activities, self-esteem, and adjustment in later periods of adulthood. Results from a Swedish study with older adults (Andersson & Stevens, 1993), for example, indicated that the quality of parental care as well as current attachment relationships were significantly related to participants' feelings of self-esteem, anxiety, and loneliness. Yet, it appeared that intervening relationship experiences profoundly affected the degree to which long-term continuities remained effective into old age. In addition, Labouvie-Vief and Diehl (1996) and Diehl, Brady, Bourbeau, and Labouvie-Vief (1998) provided evidence that attachment styles, assessed both in terms of current relationship and in terms of retrospective reports of the family of origin, were significantly related to coping and defense processes in young, middle, and late adulthood. Thus, there is some evidence that adults with different attachment styles differ with regard to certain personality characteristics and that these relations extend into later adulthood and old age. However, it also must be noted that to date, most studies dealing with adults have relied on retrospective accounts and have used paper and pencil self-report questionnaires as assessment procedure. Thus, the degree to which these accounts do rely on factual recall versus transformed memories and may be a result of the particular assessment procedure is not known at the current time.

In sum, in this section we have reviewed a number of approaches and avenues of research that have originated out of psychodynamic formulations about personality and its development over the life course. In general, this class of theories has offered a rich set of hypotheses and has spawned many fruitful areas of investigation. In that process, many original notions—such as those relating to the midlife crisis, or the transformation of gender roles, had to be modified as a result of actual empirical research. Yet, there is considerable evidence to suggest that adulthood is, indeed, the focus of significant transformations of self and personality-related processes, and that these processes are, to a considerable extent, influenced by aspects of early experience.

Cognitive Approaches to Self and Personality

To talk about cognitive approaches to self and personality may be somewhat surprising. As Riegel (1977) pointed out in his historical review of the field of psychogerontology, the domains of personality and cognition developed rather separately, and cross-communication and cross-fertilization were relatively rare before about 1970. With a rising interest in contextual approaches to development, however, cognitively based approaches to self and personality processes have become increasingly popular.

Ego Level

One of the first important approaches in personality research influenced by cognitive formulations was the ego level approach proposed by Loevinger (1976; Hy & Loevinger, 1996). Loevinger's work was influenced not only by psychodynamic formulations of personality, but also by some important theoretical work that had called attention to the role of cognitive processes in personality organization and coping (Harvey, Hunt, & Schroeder, 1961). Loevinger further developed this notion into the proposition that processes of emotion regulation and ego functioning could be ordered along a sequence of levels ranging from relatively low complexity, differentiation, and reflective awareness to ones with high complexity, differentiation, and reflective cognition. According to Loevinger (1976), at low levels of functioning, ego processes are dominated by impulsivity and the need to please others, but at more advanced levels this impulsive organization gives way to a mode of regulation in which a person's inner life is subordinated to social norms and conventions. However, at even more complex levels, the individual evolves a way of speaking about self and emotion that is able to acknowledge conflict between impulse and norm, self and society, and inner and outer experiences. Thus, in the process of progressive ego development, a cognitively complex language replaces a youthful one that characterizes ego processes within the need for physical or emotional comfort, good–bad dichotomies, and shows little tolerance of intrapersonal and interpersonal conflict.

Several theoretical models of coping and defense have proposed similar cognitive reorganizations of self and emotion processes. Haan (1977) and Vaillant (1977, 1993), for example, distinguished forms of less and more mature coping and defense processes that also can differ in conceptual complexity. According to these taxonomies, the younger or less mature person uses more polarizing defenses such as denial, repression, or projection. In contrast, the more mature individual copes by means of strategies such as sublimation, suppression (i.e., flexible temporal modulation of affect by deciding to deal with a conflict at another, more appropriate moment), and constructive (as opposed to hostile) humor.

The notion that use of defense strategies is related to age/development has been supported in several empirical studies and with a variety of assessment methods. Research based on the Defense Mechanisms Inventory (Ihilevich & Gleser, 1986), for example, has consistently shown that throughout adulthood, the endorsement of projection and turning against object decreases with age, whereas the endorsement of principalization and reversal has been shown to increase (Diehl et al., 1996; Labouvie-Vief et al., 1987). Similarly, McCrae (1982) showed that older adults were consistently less inclined than younger persons to rely on the immature strategies of hostile reaction and escapist fantasy as coping mechanisms, a finding that parallels the age-related decreases in projection and turning against object reported by Diehl et al. (1996). In McCrae's (1982) research this decrease in less mature coping strategies was, however, not accompanied by a simultaneous increase in more mature coping mechanisms. Folkman, Lazarus, Pimley, and Novacek (1987) reported similar findings with the "Ways of Coping" questionnaire. These authors found that compared to younger individuals, older adults used more distancing and positive reappraisal to cope with stressful situations. Such findings suggest that there are continuous developmental changes in ego processes throughout adulthood and into old age.

Neo-Piagetian Approaches

Another major influence on formulations of self and personality processes has come out of Neo-Piagetian approaches to adulthood. These various approaches arose out of a critique of the Piagetian model of maturity. Although Piaget, like Freud, was interested in establishing that cognition was, first and foremost, based on organic processes, his view of mature adulthood nevertheless was modeled on classical, modernist notions of reason. Thus he highlighted qualities such as objective, scientific reasoning and judgment and disregarded modes of thinking that were rooted in the subjective, symbolic, and emotive (see Labouvie-Vief, 1996). Yet, as some research suggests, these forms of reasoning may come to maturity in a unique form that blends objective analysis with the need for subjective meaning and significance (Blanchard-Fields, 1986; Labouvie-Vief, 1994).

To be sure, Piaget's work already addressed the significance of cognitive advances for changes in the area of self, emotion, and personality. For example, in *Intelligence and Affectivity* (Piaget, 1980) he suggested that during early childhood, emotions are tied to the concrete, sensory here-and-now. In later childhood, however, individuals can use symbols and language to think about and regulate their emotions. And by adolescence, Piaget suggested, individuals are able to structure their emotions along collective ideals and norms, and to project themselves into the future by means of a life plan and an identity. According to Piaget, however, for many individuals, especially those at early life stages, the worlds of reason and emotion remain mostly separate. In turn, trends toward integration of reason and emotion become apparent throughout the college years.

In modern philosophy, such forms of thinking that blend a concern with objectivity and deep knowledge of emotions, subjective viewpoints, and interpersonal processes are often referred to as hermeneutics (Gadamer, 1976). Following this tradition, Labouvie-Vief (1994) proposed to term this form of thinking hermeneutic reasoning. In this form of thinking, the two concepts of the objective and the subjective are interdependent concepts that codefine and complement each other. Thus subjectivity informs objectivity and gives it personal meaning; yet at the same time, objective reasoning processes transform subjectivity, transmuting it to more stable processes. This form of thinking brings, then, a new form of rationality that aims at reconnecting rational thought with the organismic, evolutionary, and spiritual-communal ground of life. It also brings a new sense of self and reality, in which the individual evolves a deeper sense of self that is more attuned with the symbolic and affective dimensions of life, yet is able to adhere to a vision of objective conduct under a new concept of "passionate rationality" (see Belenky, Clinchy, Goldberger, & Tarule, 1986).

Thus far, research appears to suggest that such forms of complex thinking continue to evolve at least until midlife (King & Kitchener, 1994; Labouvie-Vief et al., 1989a, 1995a). In turn, older individuals as a group often display lower levels of thinking. There is some evidence that such lower levels are a result of the cognitive restrictions of late adulthood. However, it is not clear at this time whether older individuals' lower levels truly reflect developmental change. An alternative interpretation is that they reflect a cohort/generational component. Thus, recent cohorts have tended to grow up in settings that emphasize more diversity and openness in thinking; to the extent that this is so, older individuals' lower levels may reflect styles they adopted in early life and maintained without significant change. Clearly, to clarify this issue, more complex sequential designs will be needed (see Schaie, 1983, 1996).

Self, Emotions, and Wisdom

What is the significance of such changes in thinking for the broader domain of adult self, personality, and emotion? To be sure, individuals do not necessarily resolve these issues by building complex epistemological theories! Nevertheless, most adults do appear to evolve a "naive epistemology" that allows them to examine the meanings and adequacy of a number of everyday constructs. One of those is the construct of emotion. Labouvie-Vief (1982a), for example, has argued that the adolescent understanding of truth as certain and computable may be a significant factor in her or his defense structure. Since that structure is based on a dualism between objective and subjective processes, it does not involve a mechanism by which such defensive cognitive distortions can be analyzed and they remain, therefore, uncorrected. In turn, the movement to a model of knowledge that is more historically situated may bring a more integrated structure that, by analyzing its own subjectivity, provides a more powerful device for self-regulation and correction (Blanchard-Fields, 1986; Kitchener, 1983; Pascual-Leone, 1984).

Research has pointed out that for young children, emotions are a rather direct bodily experience, but as they grow up, they come to see emotions more and more in terms of processes such as evaluating, deciding, delaying, and controlling. By adolescence and young adulthood, individuals master a cultural language of emotions that emphasizes such processes of valuation and control—not unlike the Freudian notion of the superego (Labouvie-Vief, Hakim-Larson, DeVoe, & Schoeberlein, 1989b).Yet, there is little sense of a self that transcends these culturally valued controls.

In contrast, research by Labouvie-Vief and co-workers (e.g., Labouvie-Vief et al., 1989a) suggested that as individuals move through adulthood, they begin to redefine their emotions in relation to the cultural context that shaped their unique emotional repertory. The search is for a self that transcends the cultural language of emotions and that attempts to differentiate the self from that institutional/cultural language. In that process of searching for the "real self," a more spontaneous emotion language emerges—one that both acknowledges the reality of one's emotions as bodily expressions and that at the same time is comfortable with transforming and regulating them. Indeed, a unique feature of individuals who display that language is their concern with the "objectivity" of their emotions!

This conclusion is also supported by Blanchard-Fields (1996) who showed that older adults' thinking about emotional conflicts is better integrated than younger adults' thinking. For example, older individuals were better able to differentiate their (emotionally influenced) interpretations from a body of objective data that they evaluated; they also were less likely to view others' behavior in static terms, but were more likely to explain it in terms of contextual factors. Evidence such as this suggests that older adults may become experts at dealing with emotionally relevant information (Adams, Labouvie-Vief, Hobart, & Dorozs, 1990; Jepson & Labouvie-Vief, 1992). Thus. adolescents and college students process text primarily by focusing on literal features, as they attend to the structure of actions and events depicted in the text. However, for mature and older adults the primary interest is not in this literal action-event structure, but rather in what it reveals about underlying emotional and motivational patterns of the human condition. To that extent, the mature adults' interest in text becomes more abstract and symbolic: A narrative does not refer to the concrete here and now of protagonists and their actions, but rather is seen as being indicative of human actions in general (Jepson & Labouvie-Vief, 1992).

The research discussed above suggests that as individuals move into mature adulthood, they are better able to relate the process of thinking back to a set of subjective processes, such as intentions, values, and biographical understanding. Kohlberg (1984), Loevinger (1976, 1993), and Kegan (1982) have suggested that the youthful and/or conventional self remains fused with an interpersonal and institutional matrix. Thus the ability to experience distinctness and an individuated self remains limited at a younger age. The capacity to maintain a more autonomous sense of selfhood emerges at the final stage, when self and other can be understood as entities that transcend interpersonal and institutional meanings. Thus, both a more authentic sense of selfhood and a deeper capacity for intimacy can result.

Labouvie-Vief and collaborators (Labouvie-Vief et al., 1995a; Labouvie-Vief, Diehl, Chiodo, & Coyle, 1995b) developed a framework within which to examine such changes. In this research, younger or less mature individuals framed descriptions of self and others in terms of a conventional perspective: self and others were described in terms of an organized, codified, and abstract set of role expectations. At a more advanced level, institutional values became susceptible to doubt and criticism: for example, individuals acknowledged that such values can be "carried too far." Instead of a language of fixed roles and obligations, a dynamic perspective evolved in which descriptions of self and others were conveyed in a vivid language describing the unique and evolving experience of individuals within the context of their particular life histories. Lives now were understood in the context of multiple frames—cultural, social, and psychological, for example. There was a keen insight into the psychological dynamics that are at the root of human diversity, yet an understanding that such diversity appears to be regulated by a common human heritage.

Just as the self becomes viewed more from the perspective of historical patterns and general emotional transformation, so do the representations of others become more complex and elaborated. In our research, individuals' representations of their parents were studied as a prototype of other-representations (Labouvie-Vief et al., 1995b). Younger individuals and those over the age of 60 primarily described their parents in the interpersonal context of their roles as providers of emotional and financial support to the self, or, to a lesser extent, in the institutional context of their societal position. Few youthful individuals represented their parents as autonomous individuals in their own right. In contrast, around midlife there was a peak of responses that indicated an appreciation for the unique individuality of parents: Participants described their parents not just as carriers of parental and other social roles, but showed an awareness of the conditions that had shaped the parents and made them become the persons they were.

These results are consistent with views that suggest that a restructuring of representations of one's parents is part of the reorganizations in self often associated with middle adulthood discussed earlier in this chapter. Overall, however, it is also notable that relatively few individuals displayed the higher levels of parent-representations. The finding that higher levels of self- and other-representations are quite rare in the population and that they tend to be concentrated in the middle age period is also replicated by many other studies (Labouvie-Vief et al., 1995a,b). One reason for the fact that older individuals display lower levels may be that levels of self-representation are related to intellectual variables; thus, older individuals' lower scores may constitute part of an age-related resource restriction. However, as already noted, generational/cohort differences also need to be ruled out. All of the above proposals indicate that over the life course rational processes on the one hand, and processes related to self and emotions on the other, become profoundly interconnected. This ability to bridge the tensions between the universal and the contextual, the theoretical and the pragmatic, and the rational and emotional is often referred to as wisdom (Labouvie-Vief, 1994). The notion that wisdom consists of a balanced and integrated form of knowing is, in fact, an ancient one. It is embodied in myth and literature, such as Euripides' tragedy *The Bacchae*. This play shows the tragic conflict that arises out of an unbalanced form of rationalism as represented in the King, and an unbridled and ecstatic feeling of orientation as represented by the god Dionysius and his entourage of women. Although most work on wisdom appears to adopt some vision of integration of these two views, the specific way in which this vision is implemented, however, differs from approach to approach (see Sternberg, 1992).

This form of wisdom is somewhat different from more cognitive definitions of wisdom such as that of Baltes and his colleagues (see Chapter 8). In that model, wisdom is defined as expert knowledge with regard to important but uncertain matters of life and can be characterized by several components, such as exceptional insight into human development and life matters, good judgment, and an understanding of how to cope with difficult life problems

(Baltes, Smith, & Staudinger, 1992). However, other researchers on the issue of "wisdom" do not agree with Baltes' definition of wisdom, which leads to a form of educated subjectivism. Instead, several authors (Kitchener & King, 1981; Labouvie-Vief, 1994) have suggested that from this more abstract form of subjectivism, the individual again begins to search for a set of "objective" criteria. These criteria are, however, more procedural and dynamic in nature: even though a person may, in principle, not know what is good evidence, the individual has a general procedure for distinguishing solid evidence from less trustworthy evidence by examining the process through which knowledge has been gained. With this understanding, the individual also realizes that objectivity and subjectivity are not dualistic categories, but rather influence and inform each other. Rationality and the search for objectivity thus are transformed into a new mode of thinking (Labouvie-Vief, 1994).

Indeed, the work by Labouvie-Vief on emotions and the self (e.g., Labouvie-Vief et al., 1989, 1995a,b) suggests that the most mature individuals are those who are concerned about presenting self and emotions in an "objective" form. Thus, for example, coping strategies of mature and older individuals are often specifically aimed at making sure that one's own subjective biases are understood and checked—say, as a result of discussing it with friends who can provide a more "objective" viewpoint. Indeed, this wider definition of "wisdom," then, goes beyond awareness of relativism, pragmatic constraints, and contextualism. Instead, it transcends the merely local and looks, as it were, through and beyond the contextual to more universal aspects of the human condition.

As already noted, much of the research above is predicated on the assumption that changes in individuals' cognitive-developmental organization provide a driving force to the development of self, emotion, and personality. However, it is also important to point out that many emotional changes in later life are not necessarily driven by such continued gains in cognitive complexity. For example, it is possible that later adulthood may bring a more general bias for emotion-based responses, as noted by Blanchard-Fields (1997) and Carstensen (1992; Carstensen & Turk-Charles, 1994). In our own research, too, we noted that older adults showed a preference for psychological explanations when they were asked to summarize the gist of different texts. However, they did so in styles that differed in complexity and elaboration. Some adults would give summaries that involved complex back-and-forth references between the textbase and some psychological process they thought the text symbolized. In fact, in Adams' (1986) study, such responses peaked in middle-aged adults. Other responses were rather global and undifferentiated, affectively-laden responses such as "The trouble is that nobody believes in God anymore," and it was this type of response that was most frequent in the older group.

The observation that emotion-based language sometimes is rather global and undifferentiated suggests that even though older adults may use a more emotion-based language, this emotional language may not necessarily imply the ability to reason about emotions in complex and coordinated ways. Thus mechanisms other than emotional understanding may play a role. Brandstädter and Greve (1994) and Carstensen Gross, and Fung (1997) suggest that awareness of time and mortality is a major factor by which an increasing acceptance of emotions is ushered in, even though this awareness may be stimulated by events that are not related to age (e.g., illness). However, although such realization may affect a switch in the preferred processing system as implied by Carstensen's work, such a simple switch must be distinguished from the kinds of processes of cognitive-affective integration with which our work has been concerned. Furthermore, it is also possible that certain cognitive restrictions, particularly in the domains of fluid intelligence and of processing resources, may limit some older individuals' ability to modulate and understand complex emotions (see Labouvie-Vief & Diehl, 1996; Labouvie-Vief et al., 1995a,b). Thus conceivably, an increase in emotion-based language might reflect less complex emotion regulation strategies. This core question will form an important area of inquiry for future research.

Trait Approaches to Self and Personality

Trait approaches to self and personality constitute a third major area of inquiry into stability and change through adulthood. In comparison to the cognitive and psychodynamic approaches, the trait approach appears less ideally suited for the study of change and transformation across the life span. This is because trait theorists believe that an individual's personality can be defined as a limited number of basic behavioral tendencies that the individual has and consistently displays. These basic tendencies may be inherited or acquired and may or may not be malleable over the course of development. Behavioral tendencies and temperament traits that are usually examined by trait theorists include extraversion/introversion, emotional lability (i.e., neuroticism), shyness, conscientiousness, rigidity/flexibility, hostility, and others. Trait theorists assume that over the course of the life span, these basic tendencies interact with external influences to produce characteristic adaptations that show a high degree of stability (Costa & McCrae, 1994). An important consequence of this assumption of stability/continuity is that the structure of individuals' personality can be assessed using self-report questionnaires or objective ratings from others.

From Stability to Change and Transformation

Historically, the trait-theoretical approach has centered around two major questions: (1) How many basic traits are required to allow a comprehensive description of individuals' personality? and (2) Do these characteristics display change or stability across the life span? One major research project is that of Costa and McCrae (1992), who developed an assessment instrument to measure five general personality factors (i.e., Neuroticism—N, Extraversion—E, Openness to Experience—O, Agreeableness—A, and Conscientiousness—C). Costa and McCrae (1992) claim that this description yields an exhaustive classification of personality traits that exhibits remarkable stability throughout the life span, and that after the age of 30 individuals' personality is "set like plaster" (Costa & McCrae, 1994, p. 21). In support of their position, Costa and Mc-Crae (1994) have provided considerable evidence indicating moderate to high stability over a 30-year period. In terms of mean level differences, these authors have shown (Costa & McCrae, 1992) that there are small but fairly consistent adult age differences: older individuals score lower on Neuroticism, Extroversion, and Openness to Experience, whereas Agreeableness and Conscientiousness show small increases across the adult age groups.

Cross-sectional studies, of course, cannot rule out that observed age differences reflect changes related to cohort and generation rather than age-related processes. However, in a 6-year longitudinal study, Costa and McCrae (1988) also found declines in self-reported neuroticism, although when participants were rated on neuroticism by their spouses, these same men were judged as *increasing* in neuroticism. Costa and McCrae's notion that adult personality in essence is characterized by stability is supported by other studies as well. Using data from the Kelly Longitudinal Study, Conley (1984) showed substantial mean correlations for indicators of neuroticism and introversion–extraversion over a 45-year period (Leon, Gillum, Gillum, & Gouze, 1979).

In a subsequent study, Conley (1985) reported that individual differences on some traits remain rather stable even if they are measured with different methods, such as spouse ratings. Other longitudinal studies that have documented considerable stability in personality functioning are the Duke University Studies of Normal Aging (Siegler, George, & Okun, 1979), the Bonn Longitudinal Study of Aging (Schmitz-Scherzer & Thomae, 1983), and the Seattle Longitudinal Study (Schaie, 1995; Schaie & Willis, 1991). Although different measures of personality functioning were used in these studies, all three research programs showed remarkable stability (i.e., very limited change over time) in participants' self-reported personality descriptions.

Personality and Context

Although the studies discussed above suggest that adult personality can be characterized by a fair amount of stability, high retest correlations by no means preclude the potential for change. For example, it is important to note that, in general, the test–retest correlations accounted only for 35%–50% of the variance, leaving half of the variance unaccounted for. Thus contextualists have looked at this evidence and have suggested that it is entirely compatible with the notion that personality development is influenced by changes in context. This is especially true since, as noted by Bloom (1964), the contexts in which personality evolves themselves tend to remain rather stable. In addition, Bloom also suggested that in evaluating stability coefficients, one needs to take into account the time interval that has lapsed—thus, with longer intervals elapsing between measurement points, one is more likely to find evidence for instability.

Contextual investigations of personality have gained great popularity in recent years. In general, these studies have focused on several questions. One question has focused on variations in stability with different time periods and time intervals. For example, using data that covered a time span of 50 years, Haan, Millsap, and Hartka (1986) found that consistency indexes were largest for adjacent age periods but were considerably smaller when examined over the entire time span. In addition, consistency coefficients varied by age period, suggesting that personality stability may be considerably reduced during periods of the life course that are characterized by extensive transitions and role changes. For example, the transition to parenthood in young adulthood and family and work-related transitions (e.g., retirement) in later adulthood represent such periods in individuals' life course.

That both stability and change characterize personality development even in advanced old age has been shown by Field and Millsap (1991) for the Berkeley Older Generation Study. Although Field and Millsap (1991) found moderate rank order stability for the traits satisfaction, extraversion, agreeableness, and intellect, they also showed significant mean level changes in some of these traits over a 14-year period as study participants grew into old age. For example, more than one-third of the participants increased significantly over time in agreeableness, and both men and women and old-old and oldest-old participants declined significantly in extraversion. Field and Millsap (1991) concluded that these findings do not support the common stereotype that personality "rigidifies" in old age.

Taken together, these studies contribute in two major ways to the literature on personality development. First, in combination with the long-term findings reported by Conley (1984, 1985), these results document that the consistency coefficients tend to decline as the testing interval increases, resulting in only a modest degree of stability in personality components when individuals are examined over long periods of time. Second, these studies also suggest that periods that are characterized by life course transitions and changes in important social roles (e.g., work and family) are accompanied by considerably less personality stability than is found elsewhere in the life span (see also Kogan, 1990). Thus, these studies provide evidence for the hypothesis that interindividual stability in personality varies at different portions of the life span (Moss & Susman, 1980).

One of Bloom's (1964) suggestions was that personality be studied specifically in association with changes in context. This suggestion has been incorporated into some longitudinal work about adult personality changes. For example, working with the parents of the participants of the Berkeley Growth Study, Maas and Kuypers (1974) investigated this proposition over a 40-year interval. In general, this study showed that although there was considerable stability in personality, this stability also was matched by stability in context.

There was, however, one group of mothers whose personality development was characterized by a great deal of instability. In their 30s, these women were judged as least well adjusted. They were unhappy in their marriages and felt critical of their husbands. Forty years later, these individuals had dramatically altered their lives. They were either divorced or widowed and had established lives that were extremely well balanced, moving between their own active interests and contact with their adult children.

A third set of studies has examined how different life paths or contexts chosen during early adulthood are associated with patterns of change in middle and late adulthood. These questions have been addressed in an exemplary fashion in the context of several longitudinal studies of women's personality development during adulthood. Most notably, Helson and her colleagues (Helson, Mitchell, & Moane, 1984; Helson & Moane, 1987; Helson, Stewart, & Ostrove, 1995) have adopted a process approach and have examined the interplay between social context and personality development for several samples of adult women. In this research, the lives of women who had chosen a typically feminine social clock (FSC) project was dominated by the adaptation to the roles of wife and mother, which was frequently accompanied by a withdrawal from social life, the suppression of impulse and spontaneity, a more negative self-image, and decreased feelings of competence. Twenty percent of the women who adhered to the FSC relinquished this life structure and were divorced between the age of 28 and 35. In contrast, women who had entered careers by 28 were less respectful of norms and more rebellious toward what they experienced as constrictive pressures. Although these women did not score lower on femininity or on well-being, they were more independent and self-assertive than their FSC counterparts (Helson et al., 1984). Long-term follow-up of these women showed that those who continued to stay in career paths into middle adulthood showed greater confidence, initiative, forcefulness, and intellectual independence than women who did not.

In another study, Helson et al. (1995) examined how different ego-identity patterns were related to women's personality characteristics and life outcomes in three different longitudinal samples. In particular, Helson et al. (1995) distinguished four ego-identity groups depending on whether individuals had an integrated or unintegrated identity and whether they had actively searched for an identity or had accepted a foreclosed identity. Across the three samples, results were consistent in showing that unintegrated accepters showed less initiative than other women, that unintegrated searchers had less impulse control, and that integrated accepters scored higher on support of norms and traditional values. These relations showed high consistency across time. Moreover, in the three cohorts, identity status showed different relations to life outcomes such as marital status, family status, and work. Overall, Helson and her colleagues (see also Helson & Moane, 1987; Helson & Wink, 1992) have shown that women's personality structures changed not only in systematic and normative ways in early and middle adulthood (Helson, 1993; Helson & Stewart, 1994), but that the observed changes were often related to specific changes in social roles and transitions in social contexts, thus creating distinctly different life paths for individuals with different personalities (VanManen & Whitbourne, 1997; York & John, 1992).

Levels of Organization

five up
abardson

The work discussed so far has more and more relinquished the notion that traits are stable aspects of personality that do not change across the life span, and has instead examined contexts and life patterns that are associated with individual differences and changes in traits. However, several even more recent approaches are beginning to doubt the ubiquitous importance of traits, and note that the very concept of traits is limited when personality organization is the focus of inquiry.

BIG FIVE M-of Personality

For example, recent critics of the "Big Five" model of personality have pointed out several limitations of this approach. First, in a comprehensive critique, Jack Block (1995a) has meticulously documented the inconsistencies and the subjectivity in the use of the lexical approach by different researchers. Second, Block has also questioned the inconsistent and often very subjective use of factor analysis, specific rotation methods, and the labeling of the derived factors to describe particular factor structures (Block, 1995a). Taken together, Block (1995b) has drawn two major conclusions based on his review of the relevant literature. First, he concluded that from the beginning the trait perspective has been inherently biased in its measurement approach toward the stability of traits, thus neglecting contextual influences and age-related factors that may contribute to variability in personality development. Second, he also concluded that presently advocates of the "Big Five" factor model present conclusions in support of the five-factor approach (FFA) far stronger than seems to be warranted (Block, 1995b). In contrast to the proponents of the FFA, Block (1995a,b) has argued in favor of a perspective in personality research that incorporates (1) the sociocultural context in which personality development occurs and (2) the notion of age-period specific variability across individuals' life course (Caspi, 1987).

"Big 5"
supports
Five –
Factor
approach
(FFA)

Thus, Block (1995a,b) has argued in favor of a perspective that focuses on change as well as on stability in personality development. Block's position and concerns regarding the FFA have been shared by other personality theorists (Emmons, 1995; McAdams, 1992). Winter (1996), for example, has come to the conclusion that although "the five-factor theory is a promising development, it is hardly the final word even in trait psychology" (p. 471).

From a developmental perspective, a particularly important aspect is that changes in conceptual organization also are associated with changes in the very meaning and coordination of traits. For example, Loevinger (1993) noted that within the "Big Five" model, conscientiousness has the meaning of norm fitting and well socialized behavior. However, in her own model, this form of conscientiousness describes relatively low level, conformist expressions of this characteristic. In contrast, at more mature levels "conscientiousness" implies the ability to examine standards and norms from a more autonomous perspective. However, such distinctions are lost in measurement instruments that collapse such developmental variance into a single category or scale.

Similarly, our review of cognitive theories of adulthood suggests that the meaning individuals at different life stages impart on test items may change quite profoundly with age or cognitive complexity. However, to the extent that tests rely on "Yes–No" answers or simple scaling of agreement/disagreement with items, no room is left for different constructions of meaning. This issue has been raised by Labouvie-Vief et al. (1989) in the context of examining coping strategies across the life span. Although some researchers (e.g., Lazarus, 1991) have argued against generalized age differences in coping strategies, others have reported consistent patterns of strategies of coping and defense. One reason for this ambiguity may be that current codings of coping strategies confound strategies of different levels of complexity and cognition-affect integration within a single category. In earlier research on self-regulation strategies, Labouvie-Vief et al. (1987, 1989) already noted that the same strategy can have very different meanings depending on the developmental level at which it appears. For example, turning to others may imply that an individual attempts to dissipate anxiety through aligning with "others in the same boat"—a less mature strategy, or that the person seeks out others in an attempt to consider alternative choices and raise his or her level of objectivity—a more mature strategy.

The above concerns are also expressed in the work of McAdams (1995), who proposed that aspects of personality can be represented at different levels of organization. For example, at the most basic level we can think of personality as being a collection of independent traits. However, at more complex levels, we can think about how these traits are coordinated in terms of core motivational mechanisms and, finally, in terms of how these are interwoven across time through such techniques as narratives. Indeed, this notion of levels of organization finds support from research that indicates that after first developing a vocabulary of trait terms that are treated as independent, individuals come more and more to develop complex organizational networks of traits, indicating how trait aspects become modulated over time and across situations. Similarly, the work by Labouvie-Vief et al. (1989, 1995a) discussed earlier suggests that early in life individuals may primarily describe self and others in terms of simple emotions and traits, whereas at later stages of adulthood, descriptions are much more likely to be in terms of complex motivations that are discussed from a contextual and biographical perspective.

Another aspect in which traditional traits are static is that they assume that individuals' standing on a particular trait is relatively fixed. Jung (1933) already addressed this issue of a more dynamic view in his theory of introversion and extraversion. Rather than seeing these characteristics as stable categories, Jung suggested that they are poles of functioning whose relationship to each other becomes reorganized in development. For example, early in life, extroverted individuals may suppress their introverted tendencies and vice versa, creating a relatively polarized and dualistic structure. However, in later life, suggests Jung, individuals can move more freely and flexibly back and forth between the poles. Several more recent researchers (see Ogilvie & Rose, 1995) have begun to echo these early conceptualizations and suggested that we study the dynamic back-and-forth movement between characteristics.

Conclusions

In this chapter, we have reviewed recent approaches to the study of self and personality development in adulthood and later life. Although historically several approaches have concerned themselves with this topic, the approaches nevertheless have shared a number of similar assumptions. In the past, the core assumption has been that the most important ontogenetic developments happen early in the life span, whereas in adulthood and later life development was seen as being limited, showing mostly a picture of stability. However, based on new research there is now a general consensus that during adulthood important transformations continue to take place.

We traced such transformations from three different perspectives. From that of psychodynamically influenced theories, core questions have been concerned with the role of midlife reorganizations in the adult life course, the role of gender organization, and the role of early childhood experiences. In all of these areas, the picture over time has affirmed that adulthood is not a period of stasis, but one in which earlier life patterns are reassessed and a sense of growth and plasticity is maintained. In particular, in areas such as identity development and coping and defense, research has demonstrated considerable change throughout adulthood.

Cognitive-developmental approaches have added to those of psychodynamic notions and have elaborated some cognitive mechanisms related to reorganizations in self and personality. Thus evidence indicates that from young to middle adulthood, individuals reorganize their sense of reality, including how they see themselves and others and their own and others' emotions. In part, these patterns may complement the ones discussed by psychodynamic theories, although the specific ways in which they interface has not yet been studied extensively. Even within trait approaches, notions of stable personality patterns that are set in stone relatively early in life are giving way to investigations that trace the ups and downs of personality as individuals move through different contexts and encounter different experiences.

Indeed, as the field has been influenced by more developmentally oriented views, the traditional roles of psychodynamic processes, cognitive mechanisms, and traits as relatively separate domains of theoretical and empirical inquiry have become less distinct and more intermingled. Thus, many newer studies are beginning to mix traditional models of personality to bring them to bear on integrative questions about the self and personality development. Indeed, this may be the specific reason that more and more, rather than finding references to personality, we find researchers referring to the self—that totality, as Jung suggested, that coordinates all those motivational and cognitive processes that make up the person as a whole.

REVIEW QUESTIONS

1. What are the major theories about self and personality changes in adulthood and later life?

2. What are major theoretical assumptions of recent theories about self and personality?

3. What does the notion of a midlife crisis refer to?

4. What is empirical evidence re the midlife crisis?

5. What basic orientations appear to differentiate men and women?

6. What evidence concerns the role of early experience in personality development?

7. What are major trends in coping and defense strategies across the adult life span?

8. What do Neo-Piagetian approaches to adult cognition propose?

9. What evidence supports the notion of transformations of self and emotions in adulthood?

10. What is the evidence concerning change and stability of traits across adulthood?

11. What is the role of context in adult personality?

12. Discuss several core criticisms of the trait approach to personality.

References

Adams, C. (1986). *Qualitative changes in text memory from adolescence to mature adulthood.* Unpublished doctoral dissertation, Wayne State University, Detroit, MI.

Adams, C., Labouvie-Vief, G., Hobart C. J., & Dorozs M. (1990). Adult age group differences in story recall style. *Journal of Gerontology, 25,* 17–27.

Andersson, L., & Stevens, N. (1993). Associations between early experiences with parents and well-being in old age. *Journal of Gerontology: Psychological Sciences, 48,* P109–P116.

Bakan, D. (1966). The duality of human existence. Chicago, IL: Rand McNally.

Baltes, P.B. (1987). Theoretical propositions of life-span developmental psychology: On the dynamics between growth and decline. *Developmental Psychology, 23,* 611–626.

Baltes, P.B., Lindenberger, U., & Staudinger, U. M. (1998). Life-span theory in developmental psychology. In W. Damon (Series Ed.) & R.M. Lerner (Vol. Ed.), *Handbook of child psychology: Vol. 1. Theoretical models of human development* (5th ed.). New York: Wiley.

Baltes, P.B., Smith, J., & Staudinger, U. M. (1992). Wisdom and successful aging. In T. Sonderegger (Ed.), *Nebraska Symposium on Motivation 1991: Psychology and aging* (Vol. 39, pp. 123–167). Lincoln, NE: University of Nebraska Press.

Belenky, M. F., Clinchy, B. M., Goldberger, N. R., & Tarule, J. M. (1986). *Women's ways of knowing*. New York: Basic Books.

Blanchard-Fields, F. (1986). Reasoning on social dilemmas varying in emotional saliency: An adult developmental perspective. *Psychology and Aging, 1,* 325–333.

Blanchard-Fields, F. (1996). The role of emotion in social cognition across the adult lifespan. In K. W. Schaie (Chair), *Cognitive and affective aspects of emotion*. Symposium conducted at the 1996 Emotion and Adult Development Conference, The Pennsylvania State University.

Blanchard-Fields, F. (1997). The role of emotion in social cognition across the adult life span. In K. W. Schaie & M. P. Lawton (Eds.), *Annual review of gerontology and geriatrics* (Vol. 17, pp. 325–352). New York: Springer.

Block, J. (1995a). A contrarian view of the five-factor approach to personality description. *Psychological Bulletin, 117,* 187–215.

Block, J. (1995b). Going beyond the five factors given: Rejoinder to Costa and McCrae (1995) and Goldberg and Saucier (1995). *Psychological Bulletin, 117,* 226–229.

Bloom, B. S. (1964). *Stability and change in human characteristics*. New York: Wiley.

Bowlby, J. (1969). *Attachment and loss: Attachment* (Vol. I). New York: Basic Press.

Bowlby, J. (1980). *Attachment and loss: Depression* (Vol. III). London: Hogarth Press.

Bowlby, J. (1988). *A secure base: Parent-child attachment and healthy human development*. New York: Basic Books.

Brandstädter, J., & Greve, W. (1994). The aging self: Stabilizing and protective processes. *Developmental Review, 14,* 52–80.

Campbell, J. (1988). *The power of myth*. New York: Doubleday.

Carstensen, L. L. (1992). Social and emotional patterns in adulthood: Support for socioemotional selectivity theory. *Psychology and Aging, 7,* 331–338.

Carstensen, L. L., & Turk-Charles, S. (1994). The salience of emotion across the adult life span. *Psychology and Aging, 9,* 259–264.

Carstensen, L. L., Gross, J. J., & Fung, H. H. (1997). The social context of emotional experience. In K. W. Schaie & M. P. Lawton (Eds.), *Annual review of gerontology and geriatrics* (Vol. 17, pp. 325–352). New York: Springer.

Caspi, A. (1987). Personality in the life course. *Journal of Personality and Social Psychology, 53,* 1203–1213.

Collins, N. L., & Read, S. J. (1990). Adult attachment, working models, and relationship quality in dating couples. *Journal of Personality and Social Psychology, 58,* 644–663.

Conley, J. J. (1984). Longitudinal consistency of adult personality: Self-reported psychological characteristics across 45 years. *Journal of Personality and Social Psychology, 47,* 1325–1333.

Conley, J. J. (1985). Longitudinal stability of personality traits: A multitrait-multimethod-multioccasion analysis. *Journal of Personality and Social Psychology, 49,* 1266–1282.

Costa, P. T., Jr., & McCrae, R. R. (1988). Personality in adulthood: A six-year longitudinal study of self-reports and spouse ratings on the NEO personality inventory. *Journal of Personality and Social Psychology, 54,* 853–863.

Costa, P. T., Jr., & McCrae, R. R. (1992). *Professional manual: Revised NEO Personality Inventory (NEO PI-R) and NEO Five-Factor Inventory (NEO-FFI)*. Odessa, FL: Psychological Assessment Resources.

Costa, P. T., Jr., & McCrae, R. R. (1994). Set like plaster? Evidence for the stability of adult personality. In T. F. Heatherton & J. L. Weinberger (Eds.), *Can personality change?* (pp. 21–40). Washington, DC: American Psychological Association.

Diehl, M., Brady, A., Broubeau, L., & Labouvie-Vief, G. (1998). Adult attachment styles: Their relation to family context and personality. *Journal of Personality and Social Psychology*.

Diehl, M., Coyle, N., & Labouvie-Vief, G. (1996). Age and sex differences in strategies of coping and defense across the life span. *Psychology and Aging, 11*, 127–139.

Emmons, R. A. (1995). Levels and domains in personality: An introduction. *Journal of Personality, 63*, 341–364.

Erikson, E. (1982). *The life cycle completed*. New York: Norton.

Feeney, J. A., Noller, P., & Callan, V. J. (1994). Attachment style, communication and satisfaction in the early years of marriage. *Advances in Personal Relationships, 5*, 269–308.

Field, D., & Millsap, R. E. (1991). Personality in advanced old age: Continuity or change? *Journal of Gerontology: Psychological Science, 46*, P299–P308.

Fisher, K. W., & Ayoub, C. (1994). Affective splitting and dissociation in normal and maltreated children: Developmental pathways for self in relationships. In D. Cicchetti & S. L. Toth (Eds.), *Rochester symposium on developmental psychopathology: Vol. 5. Disorders and dysfunctions of the self* (pp. 147–222). Rochester, NY: Rochester University Press.

Folkman, S., Lazarus, R. S., Pimley, S., & Novacek, J. (1987). Age differences in stress and coping processes. *Psychology and Aging, 2*, 171–184.

Franz, C. E., & White, K. M. (1985). Individuation and attachment in personality development: Extending Erikson's theory. *Journal of Personality, 53*, 224–255.

Freud, S. (1957). Formulations regarding the two principles in mental functioning. In J. Rickman (Ed.), *A general selection from the works of Sigmund Freud* (pp. 43–44). Garden City, NY: Doubleday.

Gadamer, H. G. (1976). *Philosophical hermeneutics* (D. E. Linge, Trans). Berkeley, CA: University of California Press.

Gilligan, C. (1982). *In a different voice*. Cambridge, MA: Harvard University Press.

Guisinger, J.S., & Blatt, S.J., (1994). Individuality and relatedness. *American Psychologist, 49*, 104–111.

Gutmann, D. (1994). *Reclaimed powers: Men and women in later life*. Evanston, IL: Northwestern University Press.

Haan, N. (1977). *Coping and defending: Processes of self-environment organization*. New York: Academic Press.

Haan, N., Millsap, R., & Hartka, E. (1986). As time goes by: Change and stability in personality over fifty years. *Psychology and Aging, 1*, 220–232.

Harvey, O. J., Hunt, D. E., & Schroeder, H. M. (1961). *Conceptual systems and personality organization*. New York: Wiley.

Hazan, C., & Shaver, P. R. (1987). Romantic love conceptualized as an attachment process. *Journal of Personality and Social Psychology, 52*, 511–524.

Hazan, C., & Shaver, P. R. (1994). Attachment as an organizational framework for research on close relationships. *Psychological Inquiry, 5*, 1–22.

Helgeson, V.S. (1994). Relation of agency and communion to well-being: Evidence and potential explanations. *Psychological Bulletin, 116*, 412–428.

Helson, R. (1993). Comparing longitudinal studies of adult development: Toward a paradigm of tension between stability and change. In D. C. Funder, R. D. Parke, C. Tomlinson-Keasey, & K. Widaman (Eds.), *Studying lives through time: Personality and development* (pp. 93–119). Washington, DC: American Psychological Association.

Helson, R., Mitchell, V., & Moane, G. (1984). Personality and patterns of adherence and nonadherence to the social clock. *Journal of Personality and Social Psychology, 46,* 1079–1096.

Helson, R., & Moane, G. (1987). Personality change in women from college to midlife. *Journal of Personality and Social Psychology, 53,* 176–186.

Helson, R., & Stewart, A. J. (1994). Personality change in adulthood. In T. F. Heatherton & J. L. Weinberger (Eds.), *Can personality change?* (pp. 201–225). Washington, DC: American Psychological Association.

Helson, R., Stewart, A.J., & Ostrove, J. (1995). Identity in three cohorts of midlife women. *Journal of Personality and Social Psychology, 69,* 544–557.

Helson, R., & Wink, P. (1992). Personality change in women from the early 40s to the early 50s. *Psychology and Aging, 7,* 46–55.

Hy, L.-X. & Loevinger, J. (1996). *Measuring ego development* (2nd ed.). Mahwah, NJ: Erlbaum.

Ihilevich, D., & Gleser, G. C. (1986). *Defense mechanisms: Their classification, correlates, and measurement with the Defense Mechanisms Inventory.* Owosso, MI: DMI Associates.

Jepson, K., & Labouvie-Vief, G. (1992). Symbolic processing in youth and elders. In R. West & J. Sinnott (Eds.), *Everyday memory and aging: Current research and methodology* (pp. 124–137). New York: Springer-Verlag.

Jung, C. G. (1933). *Modern man in search of a soul* (W. S. Dell & C. F. Baynes, Trans.). New York: Harcourt, Brace & World.

Kahn, R.L., & Antonucci, T.C. (1980). Convoys over the life course: Attachment , roles, and social support. In P.B. Baltes & O.G. Brim, Jr. (Eds.), *Life span development and behavior* (Vol. 3, pp. 253–286). New York: Academic Press.

Kegan, J. (1982). *The evolving self.* Cambridge, MA: Harvard University Press.

King, P. M., & Kitchener, K. S. (1994). *Developing reflective judgement: Understanding and promoting intellectual growth and critical thinking in adolescents and adults.* San Francisco: Jossey-Bass.

Kitchener, K. S. (1983). Cognition, metacognition, and epistemic cognition: A three-level model of cognitive processing. *Human Development, 26,* 222–232.

Kitchener, K. S., & King, P. M. (1981). Reflective judgment: Concepts of justification and their relationship to age and education. *Journal of Applied Developmental Psychology, 2,* 89–116.

Kobak, R., & Hazan, C. (1991). Attachment in marriage: Effects of security and accuracy of working models. *Journal of Personality and Social Psychology, 60,* 861–869.

Kobak, R., & Sceery, A. (1988). Attachment in late adolesence: Working models, affect regulation, and representations of self and others. *Child Development, 59,* 135–146.

Kogan, N. (1990). Personality and aging. In J.E. Birren & K.W. Schaie (Eds.), *Handbook of the psychology of aging* (3rd ed., pp. 330–346). San Diego, CA: Academic Press.

Kohlberg, L. (1984). *Essays on moral development. Vol. 2: The psychology of moral development.* San Francisco: Harper & Row.

Labouvie-Vief, G. (1980). Beyond formal operations: Uses and limits of pure logic in life span development. *Human Development, 23,* 141–161.

Labouvie-Vief, G. (1981). Proactive and reactive aspects of constructivism: Growth and aging in a life-span perspective. In R. M. Lerner & N. A. Busch-Rossnagel (Eds.),

Individuals as producers of their development: A life-span perspective (pp. 197–230). New York: Academic Press.

Labouvie-Vief, G. (1982a). Growth and aging in life span perspective. *Human Development, 25,* 38–88.

Labouvie-Vief, G. (1982b). Dynamic development and mature autonomy. *Human Development, 25,* 161–191.

Labouvie-Vief, G. (1994). *Psyche and Eros: Mind and gender in the life course.* New York: Cambridge University Press.

Labouvie-Vief, G. (1996). Emotion, thought, and gender. In C. Magai & S. H. McFadden (Eds.), *Handbook of emotion, adult development, and aging* (pp. 101–117). San Diego, CA: Academic Press.

Labouvie-Vief, G., & Chandler, M. J. (1978). Cognitive development and life-span developmental theory: Idealistic versus contextual perspectives. In P. B. Baltes (Ed.), *Life-span development and behavior* (Vol. 1, pp. 181–210). New York: Academic Press.

Labouvie-Vief, G., Chiodo, L. M., Goguen, L. A., Diehl, M., & Orwoll, L. (1995a). Representations of self across the life span. *Psychology and Aging, 10,* 404–415.

Labouvie-Vief, G., DeVoe, M., & Bulka, D. (1989a). Speaking about feelings: Conceptions of emotion across the life span. *Psychology and Aging, 4,* 425–437.

Labouvie-Vief, G., & Diehl, M. (1998). *Cognitive complexity and maturity of coping and defense: Two dimensions of cognitive-emotional adult development.*

Labouvie-Vief, G., Diehl, M., Chiodo, L. M., & Coyle, N. (1995b). Representations of self and parents over the life span. *Journal of Adult Development, 2,* 207–222.

Labouvie-Vief, G., Hakim-Larson, J., & Hobart, C. J. (1987). Age, ego level, and the life-span development of coping and defense processes. *Psychology and Aging, 2,* 286–293.

Labouvie-Vief, G., Hakim-Larson, J., DeVoe, M., & Schoeberlein, S. (1989b). Emotions and self-regulation: A life-span view. *Human Development, 32,* 279–299.

Lazarus, R. S. (1991). *Emotion and adaptation.* New York: Oxford University Press.

Leon, G.R., Gillum, B., Gillum, R., & Gouze, M. (1979). Personality stability and change over a 30–year period: Middle to old age. *Journal of Consulting and Clinical Psychology, 47,* 517–524.

Levinson, D. J., Darrow, C.N., Klein, E.B., Levinson, M.H., & McKee, B. (1978). *The seasons of a man's life.* New York: Ballantine.

Loevinger, J. (1976). *Ego development: Conceptions and theories.* San Francisco: Jossey-Bass.

Loevinger, J. (1993). Measurement of personality: True or false. *Psychological Inquiry, 4,* 1–16.

Maas, H. S., & Kuypers, J. A. (1974). *From thirty to seventy.* San Francisco: Jossey-Bass.

Markus, H., & Wurf, E. (1987). The dynamic self-concept: A social psychological perspective. *Annual Review of Psychology, 38,* 299–337.

McAdams, D. P. (1985). *Power, intimacy, and the life story: Personological inquiries into identity.* New York: Dorsey Press.

McAdams, D. P. (1992). The five-factor model in personality: A critical appraisal. *Journal of Personality, 60,* 329–361.

McAdams, D. P. (1995). What do we know when we know a person? *Journal of Personality, 63,* 365–396.

McCrae, R.R. (1982). Age differences in the use of coping mechanisms. *Journal of Gerontology, 37,* 454–460.

McGrath, E., Keita, G. P., Strickland, B. R., & Russo, N. F. (1990). *Women and depression:*

Risk factors and treatment issues. Washington, DC: American Psychological Association.

Mead, M. (1970). *Culture and commitment*. Garden City, NY: Doubleday.

Miller, J. B. (1976). *Toward a new psychology of women*. Boston, MA: Beacon.

Mitchell, S. A. (1988). *Relational concepts in psychoanalysis*. Boston: Harvard University Press.

Moss, H. A., & Susman, E. J. (1980). Longitudinal study of personality development. In O.G. Brim, Jr., & J. Kagan (Eds.), *Constancy and change in human development* (pp. 530–595). Cambridge, MA: Harvard University Press.

Neumann, E. (1973). *The origins and history of human consciousness*. Princeton, NJ: Princeton University Press.

Ogilvie, D.M., & Rose, K.M. (1995). Self-with-other representations and a taxonomy of motives: Two approaches to studying persons. *Journal of Personality, 63,* 643–680.

Pascual-Leone, J. (1984). Attentional dialectic and mental effort: Toward an organismic theory of life stages. In M. L. Commons, F. A. Richards, & C. Armon (Eds.), *Beyond formal operations: Late adolescent and adult cognitive development* (pp. 182–215). New York: Praeger.

Piaget, J. (1980). *Experiments in contradiction* (D. Coleman, Trans.). Chicago, IL: University of Chicago Press.

Riegel, K.F. (1977). History of psychological gerontology. In J.E. Birren & K.W. Schaie (Eds.), *Handbook of psychology of aging* (pp. 70–102). New York: Van Nostrand Reinhold.

Schaie, K.W. (1983). What can we learn from the longitudinal study of adult psychological development? In K.W. Schaie (Ed.), *Longitudinal studies of adult psychological development* (pp 1–19). New York: Guilford.

Schaie, K. W. (1995). *Intellectual development in adulthood: The Seattle Longitudinal Study*. New York: Cambridge University Press.

Schaie, K.W. (1996). *Intellectual development in adulthood: The Seattle Longitudinal Study*. New York: Cambridge University Press.

Schaie, K. W., & Willis, S. L. (1991). Adult personality and psychomotor performance: Cross-sectional and longitudinal analyses. *Journal of Gerontology: Psychological Sciences, 46,* P275–P284.

Schmitz-Scherzer, R., & Thomae, H. (1983). Constancy and change of behavior in old age: Findings from the Bonn Longitudinal Study on Aging. In K. W. Schaie (Ed.), *Longitudinal studies of adult psychological development* (pp. 191–221). New York: Guilford.

Siegler, I. C., George, L. K., & Okun, M. A. (1979). Cross-sequential analysis of adult personality. *Developmental Psychology, 15,* 350–351.

Simpson, J. A., Rholes, W. S., & Nelligan, J. S. (1992). Support seeking and support giving within couples in an anxiety-provoking situation: The role of attachment styles. *Journal of Personality and Social Psychology, 62,* 434–446.

Sternberg, R. J. (1992). *Wisdom: Its nature, origin, and development*. New York: Cambridge University Press.

Stewart, A. J. (1996). *Personality in middle age: Gender, history and mid-course corrections*. Murray Award Lecture presented at the American Psychological Association, Toronto, Canada.

Tomlinson-Keasey, C., & Blurton, E. U. (1992). Gifted women's lives: Aspirations, achievements, and personal adjustment. In J. Carlson (Ed.), *Cognition and educational practice: An international perspective* (pp. 151–176). Greenwich: JAI Press.

Vaillant, G. E. (1977). *Adaptation to life.* Boston, MA: Little, Brown.

Vaillant, G. E. (1993). *The wisdom of the ego.* Cambridge MA: Harvard University Press.

VanManen, K.J., & Whitbourne, S.K. (1997). Psychosocial development and life experiences in adulthood: A 22-year sequential study. *Psychology and Aging, 12*(2), 239–246.

Winter, D. G. (1996). *Personality: Analysis and interpretation of lives.* New York: McGraw-Hill.

York, K. L., & John, O. P. (1992). The four faces of eve: A typological analysis of women's personality at midlife. *Journal of Personality and Social Psychology, 63,* 494–508.

Additional Readings

Block, J. (1995). A contrarian view of the five-factor approach to personality description. *Psychological Bulletin, 117,* 226–229.

Brandstädter, J., & Greve, W. (1994). The aging self: Stabilizing and protective processes. *Developmental Review, 14,* 52–80.

Costa, P. T., Jr., & McCrae, R.R. (1994). Set like plaster? Evidence for the stability of adult personality. In T.F. Heatherton & J.L. Weinberger (Eds.), *Can personality change?* (pp. 21–40). Washington, DC: American Psychological Association.

Funder, D. C., Parke, R. D., Tomlinson-Keasey, & K. Widaman (Eds.). (1993). *Studying lives through time: Personality and development.* Washington, DC: American Psychological Association.

Gergen, K. J. (1991). *The saturated self: Dilemmas of identity in contemporary life.* New York: Basic Books.

Labouvie-Vief, G. (1994). *Psyche and Eros: Mind and gender in the life course.* New York: Cambridge University Press.

Loevinger, J. (1976). *Ego development: Conceptions and theories.* San Francisco, CA: Jossey-Bass.

McAdams, D. P., & Emmons, R. A. (Eds.). (1995). Levels and domains in personality [Special issue]. *Journal of Personality, 63*(3).

Pervin, L. A. (1996). *The science of personality.* New York: Wiley.

10

Clinical Assessment of Older Adults

Barry Edelstein and Kimberly Kalish

[handwritten annotations: "the act or result of judging", "the worth or value of something someone"]

Introduction

Knowledge of assessment is important for gerontologists, regardless of whether they will actually participate in the process. For the nonclinician, merely becoming a good consumer of assessment methods and instruments is valuable for at least some of the following reasons: One can (1) determine the appropriateness of assessment methods and instruments for older adults, (2) appreciate the importance of the various characteristics (psychometric properties) of assessment instruments for clinical practice and research, (3) more fully participate in the gathering of information related to psychosocial problems of older adults, (4) make informed requests for specialized assessment to answer very specific questions, and (5) gain a better understanding of what is discussed in interdisciplinary and multidisciplinary team meetings. For the clinician who will assess older adults, knowledge of the unique characteristics and problems of older adults that can influence the assessment process is invaluable.

In the following sections we will discuss conceptual issues, including the meaning and utility of assessment, traditional versus behavioral assessment, and why knowledge of assessment is important for clinician, researcher, and consumer. We will then discuss measurement (psychometric) issues, multidimensional assessment, factors that can influence assessment process and outcome, assessment methods, and the assessment process. Finally, we will present a case study to illustrate the assessment process.

What does it mean to assess? Assessment enables us to talk about the behavior or other characteristics of individuals in meaningful ways. Assessment is a process that assists us in measuring, understanding, and predicting behavior. Psychological assessment involves the gathering of psychological information about individuals through a variety of methods (e.g., interviews, self-report, physiological recordings) with the use of a variety of assessment instruments (e.g., tests, structured interviews, polygraphs). Though the specific objectives of assessment are numerous and varied, many of them might be sub-

269

sumed under the following (noncomprehensive) categories: (1) evaluation of intervention process or outcome, (2) diagnostic determination, (3) description of behavior patterns (overt and covert), (4) identification of psychological strengths and weaknesses, and (5) prediction of future behavior.

The distinction between assessment and testing is important; the average person probably thinks of testing as synonymous with assessment. Testing has traditionally involved the administration, scoring, and interpretation of tests. Today a distinction is made between tests, as assessment instruments, and assessment as a more general problem-solving process (see Maloney & Ward, 1976). A distinction is therefore made between assessment, a process that can employ several assessment methods, and assessment instruments. Assessment methods might include interviews, direct observation of behavior, recording of emotionally related physiological events, self-report of psychological information, and reports of behavior by significant others. Assessment instruments include, for example, self-report inventories and questionnaires, checklists listing behaviors to be observed, video cameras, and polygraphs. Testing, therefore, is only one form of self-report assessment wherein individuals might be asked to respond to questions about their thoughts and overt behaviors. In the remainder of this chapter, we will use the term assessment in its broadest sense, to include a variety of assessment methods and instruments.

A second important distinction in psychological assessment is between behaviors and inferences drawn from the behaviors, or between more *traditional* and *behavioral assessment*. More traditional approaches to assessment tend to focus on the measurement of intangible constructs (e.g., personality traits, personality states, motives, attitudes, defenses). These constructs are inferred from the behavior of the examinee as exhibited on a test, in an interview, etc. The traditional or psychodynamic clinician tends to seek underlying "signs" that would offer clues to an individual's behavior. In contrast, behaviorally oriented clinicians tend to view the behavior they observe as samples of the examinee's behavior. The relative emphasis placed on directly measured behavior versus the inferences one draws from such behavior regarding the characteristics of individuals (e.g., evidence of underlying traits, schemas, psychopathology, predilections) is often viewed as the principal distinction between behavioral and traditional assessment. Behavioral assessment may focus primarily on the frequency, duration, and intensity of a set of problem behaviors. One might, for example, be interested solely in a description of an individual's behavior (e.g., he walked with a limp; she struck the nurse three times over a 2-minute period; he made statements of hopelessness). However, the distinction between behavioral and traditional assessment is not precise, as behaviorally oriented clinicians will often go beyond direct observation and use more traditional instruments. The major difference between behavioral and more traditional assessment when traditional assessment instruments are used is how the obtained information is used. If the information is used to describe behavior, then one might consider the assessment process to be behavioral. If the emphasis is on inferences regarding internal states or hypothetical constructs, then the assessment process is likely to be considered traditional. Overall, one's conceptual orientation will frequently determine not only the assessment method and instrument used, but also the interpretation of the obtained information.

Psychometric and Other Considerations

The goal of assessment is to describe or evaluate an individual's behavior with regard to present or future functioning. How well an assessment instrument accomplishes this is, to a large degree, dependent on its psychometric or measurement properties. Regardless of the assessment method (e.g., interview, direct observation of behavior, physiological recording), the particular "instrument" used for the assessment (e.g., structured interview, personality inventory, behavior checklist), or the conceptual approach to assessment (traditional vs. behavioral), the assessment instrument must reliably measure what it is intended to measure if it is to be considered a "good" assessment instrument. The adequacy with which this is accomplished is typically measured with respect to the assessment instrument's psychometric properties. The characteristics of greatest interest to psychologists are *validity* and *reliability*. A discussion of the many forms of reliability and validity is included in Cavanaugh and Whitbourne (Chapter 2, this volume). Interested readers are also referred to Edelstein, Staats, Kalish, and Northrop (1996) and Allen and Yen (1979) for more complete treatments of these factors.

Reliability refers to consistency or stability of measure of behavior

Measurement reliability (discussed in Cavanaugh & Whitbourne, Chapter 2, this volume) must be carefully considered when addressing older adult assessment instruments. *Test–retest reliability* could be influenced by disorders that are more common among older than younger adults. For example, dementia can result in inconsistent performance due to changes in mental status over time. It is important to distinguish such changes in performance from inherent reliability of an assessment instrument.

If one's assessment instrument is a behavior checklist used for direct observation of specific behaviors, *interobserver reliability* or *agreement* is important. Two or more observers using the same assessment instrument and observing the same behavior should arrive at the same results. Interobserver reliability can be affected by virtually any factor that might bias the observer (e.g., positive and negative biases, ageism) or otherwise affect his or her behavior (e.g., fatigue, inattention, changes in criteria). It is important to recognize the possibility of biases influencing behavioral observation data, particularly when population-based biases are likely, as they are with older adults.

272   Edelstein and Kalish

Validity – [handwritten: "The truthfulness" of a measure – a valid measure is one that measures what it claims to measure.]

Validity, as discussed in Cavanaugh and Whitbourne (Chapter 2, this volume), is particularly important for assessment instruments that purport to measure a construct (e.g., depression, independence) rather than a discrete behavior (e.g., falls, smiles, physical contacts). The *content validity* of an assessment instrument is of particular interest when evaluating an older adult, as the content areas sampled by a test might be inadequate for older adults. That is, a test may have been constructed for use with younger adults and not address subject matter of importance to older adults. For example, a measure of fears may not include fears that are likely among older adults (Kogan & Edelstein, 1997; e.g., fear of being a burden to others; fear of losing sensory functions). Even symptoms of common psychiatric disorders can vary with age. For example, depressed older adults tend to emphasize somatic and cognitive symptoms (Zarit, 1980). Symptoms of one disorder can be mistaken for another disorder with older adults. For example, depression can be mistaken for cognitive impairment since individuals who are depressed or cognitively impaired perform similarly on some psychological tests and share some of the same symptoms.

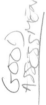

The results of assessment with a good assessment instrument should be interpretable in a consistent fashion by anyone who is trained to interpret the results. This is a particularly important characteristic for assessment instruments that encourage inferences about individuals based on their performance on an assessment instrument (e.g., aptitude, suicidality, capacity to live independently).

An instrument's *construct validity* must be carefully considered when assessing older adults. Instruments designed to measure constructs that apply for younger adults may not adequately capture the characteristics of older adults whose presentation of the construct (e.g., depression) may differ from that of younger adults. Factor structures of assessment instruments may vary among age and diagnostic groups making it difficult to develop hypotheses for older adults using tests developed with and for younger adults (Kaszniak, 1990). In light of the foregoing, the development of assessment instruments designed to measure particular constructs in general and how the construct of interest is conceptualized and operationalized must be carefully considered.

Finally, the *external validity* of assessment instruments should be considered when assessing older adults. It is not always possible to generalize the findings of one age group to another, of performance under one set of conditions to performance under other conditions, and of one's performance in one setting to performance in another setting. It is also important to avoid construing categories of individuals, conditions, and places as being functionally similar. For example, the category of "older adults" represents a heterogeneous group encompassing individuals varying in age by as much as 40 or more years. Older adults of age 60 perform quite differently on many tasks than older adults at age 85. Similarly, assessments performed in an institutional setting may not yield performance comparable to that obtained in a personal home.

In summary, it is necessary to be sensitive to the many ways in which the validity and reliability of assessment instruments can be compromised by inattention to development factors that contribute to the psychometric characteristics of an instrument.

Utility → *The fuclity of being suitable or adaptable to an end The fuclity or condition of being useful*

Perhaps the most important feature of assessment is its utility, that is, the extent to which it contributes to the desired, or at least a beneficial, outcome. The adequacy or merit of the assessment results cannot be judged independently of the purposes for which the assessment was accomplished. The assessment outcome must be judged in the context of how the information is used. For example, when assessing someone for the purpose of designing treatment interventions, the assessment should foster or lead to favorable treatment outcomes (Hayes, Nelson, & Jarrett, 1987). When assessing someone for the purpose of matching their functional skills to the demands of an environment, the assessment should foster or lead to a good (successful) match between the person and the environment, and ultimately a favorable outcome for the individual. In the latter case, assessment would involve establishment of an accurate and valid template of the environment and an accurate and valid measurement of the person's skill strengths and deficits as they pertain to the environmental demands. Ultimately, it is the practical value of assessment that must be emphasized in determining the value of assessment methods and instruments for any particular individual.

Multidimensional Assessment

Assessment can be more complicated with older adults than with younger adults and children. The problems of older adults are often multiple, multicausal, and multidimensional in nature (cf. Edelstein et al., 1996). Consequently, a thorough assessment frequently involves examinations of multiple domains or dimensions, each of which relates to the assessment question being addressed. These dimensions might include physical health status, medication regimen, psychological status, cognitive functioning, daily living skills (e.g., bathing, dressing, eating), stress-coping skills, social interactions, and economic/environmental resources (Fry, 1986; Gallagher, Thompson, & Levy, 1980; Martin, Morycz, McDowell, Snustad, & Karpf, 1985). A multidimensional approach can result in a more thorough and integrated characterization of the older adult than might be obtained through the assessment of a limited number of domains. Therefore, thorough assessment often involves the work of multiple disciplines, each of which is proficient in addressing one or more of the multiple dimensions. For example, a social worker might examine the economic and environmental resources, a psychologist the cognitive functioning, a nurse the daily living skills, and a physician the medication regimen of a client. The results of these assessments can then be addressed through interdisciplinary or multidisciplinary teams (see Zeiss & Steffen, 1996).

Multidimensional assessment is encouraged in the *Diagnostic and Statistical Manual of Mental Disorders* (*DSM-IV*; American Psychiatric Association, 1994), the standard diagnostic reference for mental health practitioners, and is the heart of comprehensive geriatric assessment (CGA). CGA is intended for frail older adults and places emphasis on functional status and quality of life. CGA characterizes a continuum of services ranging from screening to referral to specialized centers or clinicians who intervene and provide follow-up (Rubenstein, 1995). The Veteran's Administration has adopted CGA and offers such services at most of their medical centers under the name of geriatric evaluation and management programs (GEMs). Finally, multidimensional assessment is mandated by the Omnibus Reconciliation Act (OBRA, 1987), which requires that all older adults, whose services are funded by the federal government (through Medicaid or Medicare), have regular, comprehensive assessment of functional, medical, psychosocial, and cognitive status (Morris et al., 1994). We will briefly discuss a few representative dimensions of multidimensional assessment.

Assessment of Physical Health

Older adults have a higher incidence of medical and psychiatric disorders than do younger adults (Bressler, 1987). In many cases, older adults simultaneously experience multiple disorders, often requiring multiple medications. The interplay between physical disorders and psychiatric symptoms complicates the assessment process and requires specialized knowledge and skills. Physical diseases may present symptoms of psychiatric disorders (see Frazer, Leicht, & Baker, 1996 for a more complete discussion). For example, cancer of the pancreas, dementia, and hypothyroidism can each present with many of the symptoms of depression. Similarly, physical symptoms can be manifestations of psychiatric disorders. For example, sleep and appetite disturbances are often found in depression. To make the assessment process even more complicated, the medications used to treat a variety of medical and psychiatric disorders can cause psychiatric symptoms. The side effects of medications prescribed for older adults can include confusion or delirium, depression, anxiety, sexual dysfunction, sensory changes, urinary incontinence, psychosis, and mania, among others.

Assessment problem areas are typically prioritized based on patient complaints and existing physical conditions (Applegate, 1995). Initial assessment involves general observations and more focused identification of factors that offer clues to the patient's physical and psychological status. These factors might include, for example, personal grooming (clues for self-care, manual dexterity, mood), engagement in the interview (clues for mood, cognitive skills, language disorders), and gait (clues to neurological disorders, muscle weaknesses, medication side effects). A medical history may reveal risk factors (e.g., poor dentition, polypharmacy, inactivity) that can be markers for various problem areas (e.g., poor nutrition, toxic medication side effects and interactions, and muscle loss, respectively).

Physical examinations may explore a wide range of areas that pertain to potential "problems" that are more common among older adults. For example, changes in muscle strength, postural blood pressure changes, sensory changes or disorders, and the use of particular medications can place an older adult at risk for falls. See Whitbourne (Chapter 4, this volume) for a more comprehensive discussion of normal and pathological physical changes associated with aging.

Physicians may also order laboratory tests that can reveal clues to the presence and even causes of physical and psychiatric disorders. For example, an examination of blood chemistry can reveal vitamin deficiencies associated with dementia, abnormal thyroid hormone levels associated with symptoms of depression or anxiety, and urinary tract infections associated with delirium.

Mental Status/Cognitive Functioning

Estimates of cognitive impairment among older adults range from 5 to 10% among those 65 years and older and 25 to 48% among those over the age of 85 (Evans et al.,1989). Complaints of cognitive impairment are relatively common among older adults being seen by clinicians for evaluation (Alberts, 1994). Moreover, one of the most frequently asked professional referral questions is whether a client has depression, cognitive impairment, or both. Thus, assessment of mental status is a frequent activity of the geropsychologist.

Two forms of assessment fall under the rubric of mental status examination. One involves a relatively comprehensive assessment of multiple clinical domains (e.g., cognitive functioning, psychiatric symptoms, neuropathological symptoms). This form of mental status examination is an element of a typical psychiatric evaluation. The second form of mental status examination is more brief and circumscribed, intended primarily for screening for cognitive impairment in selected cognitive skill areas (e.g., orientation, memory, perceptual-motor skills). This latter form of mental status or cognitive assessment will be discussed here.

Assessment of cognitive functioning often initially involves administration of a brief cognitive screening instrument, perhaps the most commonly used being the Mini-Mental State Examination (MMSE; Folstein, Folstein, & Hugh, 1975). The MMSE requires approximately 10 minutes to administer and covers a wide range of cognitive and perceptual motor skills (e.g., memory, naming, set shifting, attention, figure copying).

Other commonly used brief screening instruments include the Blessed Dementia Scale (Blessed, Tomlinson, & Roth, 1968), Short Portable Mental Status Questionnaire (Pfeiffer, 1975), Cambridge Cognitive Examination (Roth et al., 1986), Dementia Rating Scale (Mattis, 1988), and Neurobehavioral Cognitive Status Examination (Kiernan, Mueller, Langston, & Van Dyke, 1987).

Though these brief screening instruments are efficient, standardized, and reliable, they have several limitations including their susceptibility to educational influences, less than optimal relevance for various ethnic groups, insensitivity to certain forms of cognitive impairment, and heavy reliance on language skills (see Alberts, 1994).

If cognitive impairment is suggested by the cognitive screening, additional neuropsychological assessment may be warranted. This might occur through the use of comprehensive neuropsychological assessment batteries such as the Halstead–Reitan (Reitan & Wolfson,1993) and Luria–Nebraska (Golden, Purisch, & Hammeke, 1985) comprising multiple tests, or through the selective use of neurological tests employed in the context of a problem-solving or hypothesis-testing approach to determining neuropsychological strengths and weaknesses (e.g., poor spatial abilities, but memory skills within normal limits). Information obtained from neuropsychological assessment may then be used to make recommendations regarding further assessment, develop a rehabilitation program, inform caregivers as to what can be expected regarding the individuals behavior deficits and excesses in the future, etc.

Psychological Functioning/Mental Health

Though clinical assessment of psychological functioning is discussed throughout this chapter, little of the assessment content is discussed due to space limitations. Interested readers are referred to psychological assessment texts (e.g., Anastasi & Urbina, 1997; Hersen & Bellack, 1998) for a more thorough treatment of this topic. For a thorough presentation of geriatric assessment instruments, see the *Geropsychology Assessment Resource Guide*, 1996 revision, published by the National Center for Cost Containment. We will offer a brief overview of the assessment of mental health that should enable the reader to gain a general sense of the process content of such assessment.

From the 1940s until recently, clinical psychologists typically performed clinical interviews followed by the administration of a large standard battery of tests when assessing clients. This approach was intended to provide information on the client's personality, psychopathology, intellectual functioning, and possible problems attributable to organic (brain) dysfunction. Those days of lengthy assessment batteries are virtually gone with a shift to a more strategic selection of assessment instruments and the pressure for greater efficiency

GEROPSYCHOLOGIST

imposed by managed mental health care systems. A clinical geropsychologist now typically begins the mental health assessment process with a general screening for clinical problems (e.g., clinical interview, mental status examination) followed by more strategic assessment focusing on the problem areas identified in the initial assessment. Numerous assessment instruments exist for measuring a wide range of psychological constructs and psychopathology, although the psychometric properties of many of these instruments have not been established for older adults (see Edelstein et al.,1996). Some of these instruments are relatively brief and circumscribed in their scope (e.g., Geriatric Depression Scale; Tennessee Self-Concept Scale; Assertion Inventory), whereas others are lengthy and much broader in scope [e.g., Minnesota Multiphasic Personality Inventory—2 (MMPI—2); 16PF; NEO-Personality Inventory]. Advantages of the shorter, more circumscribed instruments are the brief time required for administration and scoring and the ease of use when repeatedly evaluating therapeutic progress and outcome. Their potential disadvantage is that more skill is required of the clinician in selecting the appropriate instruments. The advantage of the broader instruments is that they concurrently assess a wide range of psychological or psychopathological constructs. Their principal disadvantage is the length of time required to administer and score them. For example, administration of the MMPI—2 can require an hour or more, with scoring sometimes requiring several hours depending on the scoring system or service used.

Let us consider an example. If a client reported symptoms consistent with depression during an initial clinical interview (e.g., depressed mood, recent weight loss, lack of interest in previously rewarding social activities, difficulty sleeping), one might then administer the Geriatric Depression Scale (GDS) and briefly interview a family member regarding the client's behavior over the past few weeks. In contrast, one might follow the clinical interview with the MMPI—2. An advantage of conducting a clinical interview and administering the GDS is the savings in time, as both could be accomplished within an hour. This is particularly economical if the person obtains a high score on the GDS suggestive of depression. A potential disadvantage of using an instrument designed to measure only depression (the GDS) is that time could conceivably be wasted if the person is not depressed. For example, the person could be experiencing an anxiety disorder that includes social avoidance and other related symptoms that overlap with depression. An advantage of administering the MMPI—2 is that it assesses multiple forms of psychopathology, with depression being one of many. A disadvantage of using the MMPI—2 is the length of time required to administer and score it.

In sum, the ultimate choice of clinical assessment methods and instruments is influenced by the time permitted for assessment, the assessment questions being addressed, and the skills and proclivities of the individual clinician. A multitude of instruments exist for the determination of mental health, but many remain unproven with older adults.

Adaptive Functioning

The functional status of older adults is typically characterized by their abilities to perform activities of daily living (ADLs). These include, for example, skills required to eat, toilet, groom, dress, and use a telephone. The oldest and most frequently used measure of ADLs is the Katz Index of Independence in the Activities of Daily Living (Hedrick, 1995; Katz, Ford, Moskowitz, Jackson, & Jaffee; 1963), addressing bathing, dressing, eating, transfer, toileting, and continence. This instrument was also developed with an eye to rehabilitation, and later revised (see Katz, Downs, Cash, & Gratz, 1970).

More complex or demanding skills, termed instrumental activities of daily living (IADL), involve higher levels of cognitive or physical functioning that are required for an individual's more independent functioning outside the home or an institution (e.g., meal preparation, money management). One of the more popular IADL inventories was developed by Lawton and Brody (1969; Lawton, Moss, Fulcomer, & Kleban, 1982). It measures eight activities, including ability to handle financial affairs, self-medicate, shop, prepare food, take care of a house, launder clothing, use transportation, and use the telephone. The instrument was originally developed for institutionalized individuals with an eye to rehabilitation, and later became popular for assessing community-dwelling adults (Kovar & Lawton, 1994).

Information obtained from an assessment of ADLs or IADLs is useful in determining, for example, an individual's current level of adaptive skills, a diagnosis, the need for assistive devices (e.g., wheelchair, hearing aid, specialized eating utensils), current service needs, the required level of nursing care, the appropriate community placement, the need for further more specialized assessment, and future needs predicted by cognitive decline (Kasniak, 1996).

Another area of functional competence is decision-making capacity, which may be called into question with regard to one's overall competence or more circumscribed decision-making abilities. Each state has legal standards that must be met in any determination of competence. Appelbaum and Grisso (1988) gleaned four skills from these standards that they recommended using when assessing an individual's capacity to make medical decisions: communicating a choice, understanding relevant information, appreciating the current situation and its consequences, and manipulating information rationally. Appelbaum and Grisso later developed an instrument for assessing medical decision-making capacity (Grisso & Appelbaum, 1998), although the instrument was developed primarily for use with psychiatric patients. To our knowledge, the only standardized instrument developed for the assessment of decision-making capacity of older adults is the Hopemont Capacity Assessment Interview developed by Edelstein, Nygren, Northrop, Staats, and Pool (1993) for assessing medical and financial decision-making capacity among nursing home residents. The instrument appears reliable and has been shown by Pruchno, Smyer, Rose, Hartman-Stein, and Henderson-Laribee (1995) to facilitate accurate prediction of decision-making capacity among long-term care residents.

Social Functioning

The relation between social factors (e.g., social support, social relationships) and physical and mental health is well documented (e.g., Burman & Margolin, 1992). "Aspects of older adults' social involvement have been found to predict mortality, morbidity, health behaviors, treatment compliance and rehabilitation outcomes, psychological health, perceived quality of life, risk of institutionalization, and adaptation to a variety of serious life stresses" (Rook, 1994, p. 142). In spite of their importance, there is little agreement regarding the best measures of social factors (Kane, 1995; Rook, 1994).

Rook (1994) has described three conceptual dimensions of social functioning for which measures have been developed: (1) social integration—social network ties, (2) relational content—functional content of interactions with network members, and (3) network evaluations—evaluations of quantitative and qualitative aspects of these interactions. Rook notes that simple measures of social integration (e.g., number of friends, marital status) can assist in identifying older adults who are at risk for health and mental health problems. Second, with regard to the relational aspects of interactions, both positive and negative social interactions should be assessed. Though positive social interactions (social support) have been associated with physical and emotional health (Oxman & Berkman, 1990; Baron, Cutrona, Hicklin, Russel, & Lubaroff, 1990) negative social interactions have been associated with diminished emotional and physical health (e.g., Pagel, Erdly, & Becker, 1987; Rook, 1990). Kane (1995) offered four reasons for including the assessment of social functioning in a comprehensive geriatric assessment:

AGING PROCESS

> to see if a patient has crossed some threshold of social isolation or inadequacy of social arrangements and resources so as to endanger his or her health and justify some intervention; to examine whether the patient's social situation is such that it may impede recovery or maximum well being; to examine the extent to which the patient's social arrangements suggest that he or she can live safely in the community; to allow health care providers to understand the social preferences and values that are important to the patient. (p. 93)

A variety of multidimensional assessment instruments have been designed to assess the foregoing and additional dimensions. Three of the more popular multidimensional assessment instruments are the Multidimensional Functional Assessment Questionnaire (MFAQ) of the Older Americans Resources and Services (OARS) Methodology (Duke University Center for the Study of Aging, 1978), the Comprehensive Assessment and Referral Evaluation (CARE; Gurland, Kuriansky, Sharpe, Simon, Stiller, & Birkett, 1977), and the Multilevel Assessment Instrument (MAI; Lawton et al., 1982). All of these measures have at least adequate psychometric characteristics, and although they differ in dimensions of functioning and content, they can meet the needs of most clinicians seeking indices of a variety of areas of functioning.

Factors Influencing Assessment Process and Outcome

The assessor's preconceived notions about the elderly, which may exist before the assessment process even begins, have potentially deterimental effects on the assessment process. Such preconceived notions may result in negative biases, positive biases, and ageism, all of which may prevent accurate assessment. Within this section, preconceived beliefs and attitudes regarding the elderly will be discussed. Included in these are biases, both positive and negative, and ageism. Bias of a clinician is a characteristic of that clinician's behavior that systematically prevents accurate assessment. Stereotypes can lead to positive or negative biases. Ageism differs from a negative bias only in that it is more extreme, resulting in not only attitudes but also behavioral discrimination.

Biases

Numerous clinician biases, positive and negative, can affect the process and outcome of psychological assessment.

Negative Biases.   There are many negative stereotypes of the elderly that contribute to negative biases and that are perpetuated daily by the media in the United States, a society that values physical beauty and youth (Butler, 1969; Rodeheaver, 1990). Some commonly held, yet inaccurate stereotypes about the elderly include the following: (1) with age comes senility; (2) older adults have increased mental illness, particularly depression; (3) the elderly are inefficient in the workplace; (4) older adults are frail and ill, (5) older adults experience economic hardship and are an economic burden; (6) older people are socially isolated; (7) the aged have no interest in sex or intimacy; (8) older adults are inflexible and stubborn; and (9) older adults should gracefully accept these changes (Butler, 1969; Feinson, 1991; Knight, 1996; Rodeheaver, 1990; Zarit, 1980). Biases resulting from these stereotypes have led to misdiagnosis of disorders (Gatz & Pearson, 1988; Goodstein, 1985). For example, an older man with a treatable depression, who reports symptoms such as lethargy, decreased appetite, and lack of interest in activities, may be overlooked for treatment due to a belief that such symptoms are attributable to "old age" or he is too old to change (Zarit, 1980). In fact, complaints such as anxiety, tremors, fatigue, confusion, and irritability are frequently attributed to "old age" or "senility" without sufficient assessment (Goodstein, 1985). In addition, Greene, Adelman, Charon, and Hoffman (as cited in Edelstein, et al., 1996) have reported that in-

terviewers of older adults have dominated conversations, behaved disrespect-
fully, exhibited less patience, and appeared less engaged than when interviewing younger individuals.

Positive Biases. Positive biases are often overlooked in discussions relative
to age biases. However, positive biases also work against accurate assessment
of older adults (Kimerling, Zeiss, Nezu, Follette, & Linehan, 1996; Zarit, 1980).
Some sterotypes that lead to positive biases are that older individuals have
more concern for others, are more responsible, place a higher value on friend-
ship and companionship, and are more calm and peaceful than their younger
counterparts (Braithwaite, 1986). Other positive biases are based on stereotypes
of the elderly being "cute," "childlike," or "grandparentlike" (Kimerling et al.,
1996). Positive biases may result in inflated estimates of the individuals' abilities or mental health due to sympathy for the older adults or a desire to make
allowances for them (Braithwaite, 1986). Such erroneous assessment results
could eventuate in ineffectual treatment or placement in an inappropriate living environment.

Ageism. "Ageism" is a term coined by Robert Butler in 1968; it is defined as
"a systematic stereotyping of and discrimination against people because they
are old" (p. 144, as cited in Achenbaum, 1985). Ageism may exist on many levels, from (1) discriminatory attitudes toward older adults by older adults themselves (Goodstein, 1985), (2) discriminatory behaviors against older adults by
individuals, such as prejudicial comments and poor treatment by service
providers (Braithwaite, 1986), and (3) discrimination of older adults by institutionalized practices and policies, such as mandatory retirement and age-
based promotions and raises (Cavanaugh, 1993). The prejudices held by inter-
viewers may impact assessment results for three reasons: (1) the assessor may
report poorer performance due to lowered expectations, (2) the older adult may
perform poorly in response to poor treatment by the assessor, or (3) older adults
may perform poorly due to personally held beliefs that because of their age
they cannot perform well (Rodeheaver, 1990). Because of the consequences of
age-related stereotypes on assessment results in older adults, it is important
that individuals involved in assessing older adults attend to their own preconceived ideas about the aged and make efforts to avoid biases in testing behaviors.

Environmental Conditions ⌐ *Influences* ⌐

When assessing older adults, one does not always have the luxury of choosing the ideal environment for the task. In fact, assessment may require walking down the hall of a nursing home and addressing questions to a pacing
older adult, or attempting to assess an older adult's ability to write a sentence
while the individual is lying on his or her bed, in a poorly lit room, surrounded

by distracting noises. When there is the opportunity to choose the environment in which assessment will occur, the considerations for an appropriate setting include (1) the relation between the assessment environment and the assessment question and (2) the relation between the environment and the individual's health and sensory deficits.

Relation between the Environment and the Assessment Question. When deciding where the client should be evaluated, some options may include the client's home, in his or her bed, at an outpatient office, or in the clinician's work environment. Depending on the assessment question, the setting may be critical in determining the quality of assessment results (Silver & Herrmann, 1991). For example, an assessment to determine the most appropriate living environment might be best conducted in the natural living environment. That is, if the assessor is trying to determine whether an older adult is capable of cooking his or her own meals, the assessment may be best performed in a kitchen, where the individual can exhibit cooking skills, rather than in a doctor's office, where the individual may be asked to discuss how a meal would be cooked. Although the appropriate environment may be beneficial in the assessment process, there are several measures of functional assessment that have been proven valid and reliable in assessing functioning when administered outside the target environment. Such instruments include, for example, the Instrumental Activities of Daily Living Scale (IADL; Lawton & Brody, 1969), the Multidimensional Functional Assessment Questionnaire (OARS; Duke University Center for the Study of Aging, 1978), and the Direct Assessment of Functional Status (Lowenstein et al., 1989).

Relation between the Environment and Health and Sensory Deficits. The second consideration, involving the characteristics of the environment, requires some knowledge about the physical strengths and weaknesses of the client. Older adults may be particularly sensitive to environmental conditions as a result of sensory and physical deficits (Schaie & Willis, 1986). Failure to accommodate for such deficits may result in inaccurate assessment results due to unnecessarily poor performance. Sensory and physical abilities in older adults will be discussed separately and with special attention to the environmental considerations that should be made when assessing older adults. Please note that the following symptoms of sensory and physical deficits may be common to some older adults, but are not inevitable consequences of aging.

Sensory Considerations. A variety of sensory deficits common to older adults may necessitate special environmental conditions. Hearing impairments may be compensated for by turning on a hearing aid, speaking in a steady, low-pitched voice, speaking into the client's "good" ear, using sound amplifying devices (Silver & Herrmann, 1991), reducing background noise (Herr & Mobily, 1991), and sitting face to face with the client. In addition, narrow rooms may improve hearing due to increased reverberations (Schaie & Willis, 1986).

TAT (Thematic Apperception Test) → TAT pictures are designed to be sufficiently vague to allow respondents to project their own meaningful story onto it → but most of these pictures are depressing pictures

Severe hearing impairments may require the investigator to rely on nonvocal forms of communication such as written words and hand gestures (Herr & Mobily, 1991). Hearing is important to assess because even mild impairment may result in comprehension and concentration problems (Herr & Mobily, 1991).

Visual impairments may be accommodated for by sitting closer to the client and ensuring that the client wears corrective lenses when appropriate (Silver & Herrmann, 1991). Because of the high prevalence of presbyopia (inability of the lens to adjust to close images) access to a magnifying lens can be helpful (Markson, 1991). Different types of visual impairments may require different types of compensatory techniques. For example, larger print will help visual acuity deficits, nonglare paper and adequate glare-free lighting can reduce glare, and solid, bold black lines, rather than multicolored drawings, can prevent assessment problems that could otherwise result from decreased color discrimination (Herr & Mobily, 1991).

Physical Health. The physical health of older clients may result in a variety of assessment complications. The effects of physical illness may complicate assessments for three primary reasons. The first is that symptoms of physical illness or side effects of medications prescribed to treat the physical illness may "look like" symptoms of a mental illness. For example, chronic obstructive pulmonary disease (COPD) may result in fatigue and sleep disturbances, and medications used to treat COPD often cause cognitive impairment, anxiety, and insomnia, which are symptoms of depression (Frazer et al., 1996). In fact, illnesses such as cancer, Parkinsonism, cardiovascular disease, and multiple sclerosis often present first as emotional problems rather than physical illness (Goodstein, 1985). A second complication is that physical illness and medications may result in a mental disorder. For example, the unpredictable nature of cardiovascular disease often results in anxiety disorders (Frazer et al., 1996) and betablockers, often used to treat hypertension, are known to cause symptoms of depression (Alessi & Cassel, 1991). Finally, physical illness and medications used to treat these illnesses may affect performance on performance-based tasks by influencing sensory abilities, dexterity, or cognition. For example, diabetes may affect vision, various neurological disorders may affect all senses (Segal, 1996), and arthritis may cause drawing or writing difficulties. In addition, medications such as antihistamines and antiparkinsonian drugs often result in impairment of cognition and memory (Storandt, 1995). Therefore, physical illness and medications may result in a psychological illness (e.g., older adults become depressed because they have to alter their life-style in response to a diabetes diagnosis) or may "look like" a psychological illness (the illness or medications may cause symptoms of depression such as loss of appetite or sleep disturbances) and it is often difficult to distinguish between the two. What is clear, however, is that several physical disorders are strongly associated with mental illness (Alessi & Cassel, 1991). It is therefore imperative that assessments of older adults be performed along with physical examinations or, at least, that the assessor be aware of physical diseases and medications.

Jerry Depression Scale → function

Assessment Methods

We have already discussed the importance of multidimensional assessment when evaluating the elderly. When assessing different dimensions (e.g., physiological, mental, social), there are many different methods with which to assess each dimension. In fact, using more than one method of assessment, termed "multimethod assessment," is often warranted. The term "multimethod" in this context refers to the practice of assessing a construct (e.g., depression, dementia, capacity) with more than one method. Such methods could include (1) interviews, (2) self-report questionnaires, (3) reports by others, (4) psychophysiological recording, (5) direct observation, and (6) task performance. For example, in an interview a woman may report feeling anxious. A psychophysiological examination may reveal considerable muscle tension, an elevated heart rate, and increased skin conductance. Direct observation of the woman's behavior may reveal wringing hands and pacing. In this example, three different types of information have substantiated the diagnosis of anxiety (American Psychiatric Association, 1994). Failure to examine a construct with more than one method of assessment may provide only part of the picture of the problem at hand, resulting in decisions with harmful ramifications, or perhaps resulting in less effective or ineffective interventions (Sattler, 1986). For example, assessing complaints of memory problems without actually assessing memory skills may result in misdiagnosis and treatment. That is, older adults with a dementia will have memory deficits but may or may not complain of memory problems. In contrast, an older adult with depression is likely to complain of memory problems, but actually exhibit no memory deficits (Kaszniak, 1990). This example illustrates that a self-report may be inconsistent with evidence obtained from a performance evaluation. Multiple methods of psychological assessment (e.g., self-report, behavioral observation) help to identify such discrepancies. Within this section, the primary methods of psychological assessment will be discussed. Keep in mind that no gold standards exist for many of the constructs in which clinicians are interested. Therefore, we believe these constructs are best characterized by a multidimensional combination of measures.

Interview

The clinical interview is the most widely used method of assessment (Edelstein & Semenchuck, 1996). It is a valuable and popular assessment method because it affords the interviewer the opportunity to gather information not only by attending to clients' responses, but also by observing their nonverbal behaviors (e.g., energetic, slow at responding, tearful). Some of the many functions served by an interview include (1) obtaining historical information about the client, (2) determining which additional assessment procedures are appropriate, (3) building rapport with the client, (4) obtaining a client's informed consent to participate in the assessment, and (5) evaluating the effects of treatment (Haynes, 1991). As interviews are often the first step in the assessment process in which the assessor has contact with the older adult, they set the tone for the rest of the assessment process. Therefore, sensitivity and rapport building are essential.

Interviewing any age group requires rapport-building skills, knowledge about the client and his or her potential problems (e.g., sensory deficits, bereavement issues), an interesting and engaging demeanor, flexibility during unstructured and semistructured interviews, the will to help the client to the best of his or her ability, and self-awareness about his or her own motivations and biases (Cormier & Cormier, 1991). In addition, due to the socially interactive nature of the interview, clients of any age may be reluctant to endorse symptoms or behaviors that they perceive as undesirable. However, when working with older adults, some specific obstacles may hinder the interview process. The following considerations and recommendations have been compiled for individuals interested in interviewing older adults: (1) when appropriate, plan brief interview sessions to avoid fatigue, (2) space stressful questions throughout the interview rather than asking them all at once, (3) explain the goals of the interview and "normalize" concerns—older adults are often wary of mental health professionals, (4) learn something about social history that may have impacted large cohorts of older adults (e.g., the Great Depression, the Jazz age), (5) be aware of sensory deficits and accommodate for them during the interview, (6) be aware of the impact of cognitive skills, physical health, and medication side effects on responses, (7) be aware that older adults may become anxious when they think they are being "tested" (e.g., they are at risk of losing rights such as driving or living independently), (8) be aware of your own biases, and (9) do not condescend (Knight, 1996; Lawton, 1986; Pruchno & Lawton, 1991; Schaie & Schaie,1977).

Self-Report

A self-report instrument includes any of a variety of instruments in which the client responds to questions designed to address the reason for referral of the client. The self-report structure is useful because the client may be the only person who can answer questions such as "How is your mood this week as compared to last week?" or "Do you enjoy your job?" or "How is your memory?" On the other hand, self-report data may be of questionable validity because the respondent may give innacurate reponses due to poor memory, misunderstanding of the question, a desire to make a particular impression on the interviewer, etc. There are several formats of self-report measures including checklists, true–false questions, sentence completion, multiple choice questions, rating scales, fill-in the blanks, computer-assisted assessments, and open-ended questions (Haynes, 1991). Although responses on self-report measures are subject to many of the same threats to reliability and validity as responses to interview questions, self-report measures also offer many benefits. Self-report measures are typically cost effective in terms of both administration and scoring time, and they have been developed to measure many clinically relevant constructs (see Corcoran & Fischer, 1987; Fischer & Corcoran, 1994). Many of these measures also permit repeated evaluations, enabling one to monitor treatment progress and outcome. Comparisons between a client's performance and those of other reference groups are also possible.

Few self-report measures are designed for or validated on older adults. That is, some self-report measures have items that assume certain symptoms that may not be appropriate for older adults. For example, older adults are more likely to report somatic symptoms to describe emotions (Zarit & Spore, 1990), tend to respond more cautiously (Edelstein & Semenchuk, 1996), and may be less likely to respond accurately to questions about sexuality (Yesavage, 1986) than younger adults. In addition, older adults tend to respond more conservatively than younger adults (Hertzog & Schear, 1989). Older adults may also be more hesitant to respond in the affirmative, more likely to skip items or respond "I don't know," and may take longer to choose their responses than younger adults (Hertzog & Schear, 1989; Okun, 1976; Sherbourne & Meredith, 1992). Older adults are also more likely than younger adults to experience anxiety during an assessment procedure (Poon, Rubin, & Wilson, 1989) and give socially desirable responses (Edelstein & Semenchuk, 1996).

Several self-report measures have been found to be psychometrically suitable for older adults. These include, for example, measures of depression [Center for Epidemiological Studies-Depression Scale (CES-D, Radloff, 1977) and Geriatric Depression Scale (GDS, Brink, Yesavage, Lum, Heersema, Adey, & Rose, 1982)], anxiety [State-Trait Anxiety Inventory (STAI, Speilberger, Gorsuch, & Lushene, 1970)], and coping [Ways of Coping Checklist (WCCL, Folkman & Lazarus, 1980)].

Report by Others

Report by others is an assessment method in which information about the older adult is obtained from people familiar with the client's behavior (e.g., family, friends, staff members). Multiple sources of information can be extremely helpful for formulating an accurate and complete picture of the client in the context of the client's daily life. This information is used to validate, clarify, or augment information obtained from other sources (e.g., the client, physician, or medical records) (Edelstein et al., 1996). Reports from others may also provide valuable information about the perceptions of family or staff toward the older adult (Morrison, 1988). They are particularly useful if the older adult is unlikely to report symptoms accurately, or at all, due to cognitive impairment (e.g., confusion, memory difficulties), lack of motivation (e.g., depression), or physical impairment (e.g., sensory deficits, inability to speak, lack of consciousness) (Kaszniak, 1996). Reports by others may be obtained through a variety of nonstandardized questions and standardized assessment instruments [e.g., The Geriatric Evaluation of Relative's Rating Instrument (GERRI; Schwartz, 1983); Cognitive Behavior Rating Scales (Williams, Klein, Little, & Haben, 1986, as cited in Kazniak, 1996)].

Information obtained from others must be viewed with the same cautious eye as information obtained from the client. Numerous threats to reliability and validity of reports by others can be found in the literature. Familial observers are untrained and may therefore miss important information (Schwartz, 1983). The biases previously mentioned may affect the accuracy of reports by others. Spouses may report fewer deficits than younger relatives (Kaszniak, 1996). Unfortunately, even the empirical literature is not as helpful as would be desired in sorting out the accuracy of reported information, as Kaszniak's review of this literature noted that findings were neither consistent nor conclusive.

Psychophysiological Assessment

Psychophysiological assessment examines the relation between psychological and physiological (e.g., changes in heart rate, muscle activity, brain waves, skin temperature) activity (Sturgis & Gramling 1988). Psychophysiological assessment information is used differently depending on the theoretical orientation of the assessor. For example, some clinicians use psychophysiological data to determine personality characteristics or types. They might, for example, use readings from the electroencephalogram (EEG) to infer levels of impulsivity and sensation seeking, or introversion and extroversion. Other clinicians might use psychophysiological data to determine the physiological responses to a set of conditions in a laboratory (Zuckerman, 1991). For example, an individual who complains of anxiety symptoms when presented with bees may be monitored for autonomic nervous system arousal when presented with the word "bee," a picture of a bee, an imaginary bee, or a real bee. One would expect physiological responses to occur in conjunction with verbal reports of different levels of anxiety in the presence of these different stimuli. If a substantial correlation is found between the subjective states of arousal and the physiological readings, then such readings can be used to assess treatment effects aimed at reducing arousal and subjectively reported anxiety in the presence of bees. Physiological measurement becomes complicated considering significant individual differences in the physical manifestation of various constructs (e.g., stress, anger) (Zuckerman, 1991). Thus, one individual's reported bee anxiety may be accompanied by increased heart rate and decreased galvanic skin response (i.e., sweaty palms), whereas another person may have a steady heart rate and dry palms, but an increase in muscle tension and rate of shallow breathing. Personal stress response patterns vary even within individuals and with age (Schaie & Schaie, 1977). In summary, psychophysiological measures can be quite sensitive to individual differences and may complement data obtained from other methods.

Psychophysiological assessment has been used for a wide range of clinical research with older adults. For example, the EEG has been used to examine various types of dementia (Marsh & Thompson, 1977) and may help differentiate dementia from uncomplicated depression. Depression without dementia does not result in an abnormal EEG, whereas dementia often results in an abnormal EEG (Adams, Parsons, Culbertson, & Nixon, 1996). In addition, the EEG results may be used to differentiate vascular dementia (VD) from dementia of the Alzheimer's type (DAT) (Adams et al., 1996). The EEG is also useful in determining whether an older adult is experiencing delirium. Delirium typically results in a slowed EEG reading (Leuchter, 1991). Seizure disorders are also diagnosed with the assistance of EEG readings (Leuchter, 1991).

Direct Observation

Direct observation can be an invaluable method of assessment. From the most structured and systematic naturalistic observation to the simple observation of behaviors during an interview, direct observation provides the most veridical evidence of overt behavior and, consequently, verification of self-reported overt behavior or reports by others. Direct observation is especially useful with clients for whom accurate verbal reports are precluded by cognitive or physical disabilities (Sattler, 1988). A potential benefit of direct observation, over many of the other forms of assessment methods discussed in this chapter, is that it can obviate the necessity of inferring information when overt behavior is the variable of interest (Haynes, 1991). For example, direct observation of eating is preferable to inferences about meal skipping based on weight loss. Weight loss can occur for numerous reasons, only one of which is meal skipping.

Direct observation may be naturalistic, occurring in the natural environment, or analogue, occurring in less than naturalistic settings (e.g., laboratories, offices). Naturalistic observations tend to be more externally valid and less internally valid, whereas analogue observations tend to be more internally valid and less externally valid. Naturalistic direct observation is often scheduled in circumscribed brief sessions throughout a period of time depending on the frequency and duration of the behavior of interest (e.g., four 30-minute sessions per day) known as *time sampling*. This is intended to yield a representative sample of behaviors throughout the day without requiring an observer to spend an entire day watching an individual. Observations are also made in specific intervals of time. For example, an observer might tally the number of times a nursing home resident curses in a 30-second period or self-injures per 2-minute period. There are a variety of structured behavior observation scales for older adults, for example, the Agitation Behavior Mapping Instrument (Cohen-Mansfield, Werner, Marx, & Freedman, 1991) and the Wandering Observational Tool (Hoeffer, Rader, & Siemsen, 1987), intended primarily for institutionalized older adults.

Naturalistic direct observation allows one to observe behaviors under varying conditions. As behavior patterns emerge, linking behaviors to particular conditions, one is in a better position to develop effective interventions. For example, if aggressive behavior is observed only when a certain staff member is on duty or only before meals, one may begin to isolate contextual variables (i.e., environmental antecedents or consequences) that are maintaining problem behaviors.

Overall, direct observation of overt behavior (analogue and naturalistic) offers numerous advantages over less direct methods (e.g., interview, self-report) with the potential inconvenience of being more time consuming and labor intensive.

Performance-Based Assessment

The final assessment method to be discussed is performance- based assessment, which requires the individual to perform specific tasks, such as memorizing a list of words, making an entry in a checkbook, or solving a puzzle. This method includes, for example, tests of mental state, memory, spatial ability, fine- and gross-motor functioning, ADLs, and subtests of standardized intelligence tests. An individual's performance on a task is then compared to his or her own performance on another occasion or to a normative sample (as previously discussed). Performance tasks are typically used to answer relatively specific assessment questions. For example, immediate- and delayed-recall tasks are used to assess memory in the process of determining whether an individual is experiencing dementia or depression. A neuropsychological assessment battery, comprised of many specific tasks, may help localize a lesion in the brain or determine the degree of impairment an individual is experiencing following a stroke or head injury. As with all assessment measures, performance tasks should be appropriate for older adults, whether designed specifically for older adults or demonstrated to be psychometrically sound for that population. For example, if one is interested in how an older adult performs on a test of motor speed relative to other older adults, then the performance should be compared to the motor speed of a comparably aged normative group, not a group of young college students. Cohort factors may play a role in appropriate performance-based assesssment. A computer-based task may require some additional explanation for older adults who may be less familiar with this technology than younger individuals who have grown up with computers. Some older adults may experience problems with performance-based assessments relative to younger individuals due to age-related changes (e.g., decreased performance speed, distractibility and interference, fatigue, sensory and physical deficits; see Aldwin & Gilmer, Chapter 5, this volume).

The Assessment Process

Though we have presented many of the elements of the assessment process in the preceding sections, it is important for the reader to have an appreciation for how these and other elements of this process come together. In this section we will briefly summarize the clinical assessment process and offer an example that illustrates several elements of the process. The elements to be discussed include clarify question, define the problem, obtain a medical and mental health history, examine environmental factors, determine need for other assessment methods, and putting it all together. Although these steps may be representative of assessment as practiced by many clinicians, they are not all inclusive and may be addressed in a nonlinear fashion.

Clarify Question

Individuals are often referred to psychologists to address an assessment question (e.g., Is this person depressed? Can this person live independently?). In most cases the assessment process is driven by the assessment question posed by the clinician or a referral source. Unfortunately the referral question is sometimes not sufficiently clear or circumscribed to permit one to proceed with the assessment process. Questions/statements such as "tell me what is going on with this person" or "is this person competent?" require clarification. In the first case, a more specific question is requested. One might merely ask the referral source to clarify what it is about this person's behavior that raised some questions. In the second example, the clinician may request clarification regarding the domains in which the person's competence (capacity) is being questioned. Does the referral question have to do with financial affairs, living independently in the community, or making medical decisions? Individuals may have the capacity to perform adequately in some domains but not in others or might be capable of performing simple tasks that require limited cognitive resources but lack the capacity to perform more complex tasks. For example, one might be competent to make decisions about day to day expenditures but not competent to organize a retirement plan or weigh the costs and benefits of various retirement packages.

Define the Problem

In contrast to the previous referral questions, clinicians are also asked to develop interventions for problem behaviors that require some form of initial assessment. For example, one might be asked to develop an intervention program for the aggressive behavior of a nursing home resident. The assessment task requires a clear and unambiguous definition of the presenting problem so there is no question about the nature of the problem and so that the referral source and the clinician are in complete agreement about what it is that requires intervention. The simplest way of accomplishing this is to have the referral source provide examples of the problem areas or behaviors.

Medical and Mental Health History

The medical and mental health history, obtained from as many sources as possible (e.g., patient, patient chart, family member), is critical in light of the interplay of medical and mental health factors and the relations between past and present mental health problems. A variety of chemicals (e.g., prescription and nonprescription drugs) and medical disorders can both produce and alter behaviors and reported symptoms. A thorough medical history can often expedite the assessment process and preclude erroneous assessment results based on incomplete information. For example, excessive caffeine intake and/or hyperthyroidism can produce symptoms of anxiety disorders. Failure to obtain a thorough medical history could lead one to seek sources of anxiety outside the individual, thus potentially resulting in an incomplete analysis of the factors contributing to the anxiety. Similarly, any recent changes in medical condition or medications may lead to changes in behavior and symptom complaints. A relevant mental health history can lead to a more efficient assessment process and sometimes preclude overlooking relevant mental health-related information.

Environmental Factors

A multitude of environmental factors can contribute to the presenting problem, some of which may not be obviously associated with it. A thorough analysis of the person's current social and physical environment can be quite helpful in developing an accurate conceptualization of the presenting problem and associated environmental factors and in developing a treatment program. For example, a person presenting with depression and the early stages of Alzheimer's disease might be experiencing depression as a reaction to the dementia or as a function of the recent death of a good friend or family member. The source of the depression may well dictate the nature or focus of the treatment.

Interview Client

The next step in the assessment process is typically a clinical interview of the client. This is more than an opportunity to query the client; it is an excellent opportunity to observe the behavior of the client in the context of the interview. Numerous factors can be considered, ranging from the overall appear-

ance (e.g., dress, cleanliness, unilateral muscle weaknesses) of the client to the
client's nonverbal and other motor behaviors (e.g., smiles, facial affective responses, tremors, gait, tics). This information can provide valuable clues regarding various psychiatric and neurological disorders. For example, inappropriate affect, an unkempt appearance, and inattention may all be associated
with schizophrenia, whereas tremors of the hands occurring at a particular frequency may be an indicator of Parkinson's disease.

Determine Need for Other Assessment Methods

The broad range of information obtained from the interview and a review of
the medical and mental health records are used to determine what additional
information is needed for more focused assessment and hypothesis testing (e.g.,
specific medical tests, personality assessment). In addition, it is necessary to
determine the best methods for obtaining that information. As previously
noted, multiple method assessment is desirable (e.g., direct observation, interview, self-report, performance-based assessment). For example, depression
may be suspected based on the client's facial affect, decreased psychomotor
activity, reported depressed mood, reported difficulty sleeping, and decreased appetite. If that is the case, one might request that the client complete
a self-report depression inventory and obtain reports of the client's behavior
at home (e.g., sleeping patterns, eating patterns, energy, initiative, mood,
crying episodes). When selecting self-report assessment instruments one must
consider the factors previously discussed including, for example, the physical
limitations of the client, the psychometric characteristics of the instruments,
time required to administer the instrument, and the environment in which the
instrument is to be administered.

Putting It All Together

What is done with all the assessment information once the assessment process
is completed? That depends on the clinician's conceptual orientation and the
objective of the assessment process. A thorough discussion of this process is
beyond the scope of this chapter, primarily because of the many theoretical approaches (see Prochaska & Norcross, 1994; Hersen, Kazdin, & Bellack, 1991)
and potential assessment objectives. Instead, we will focus briefly on one approach to this integrative process as conceived by behaviorally oriented clinicians and that is often overlooked in traditional assessment textbooks.

     When engaged in behavioral assessment of a problem behavior (e.g., ag-
gressive behavior resulting from cognitive impairment), there may be an additional series of steps taken once the preliminary assessment information is
obtained. A *functional analysis*, based on principles of operant conditioning, is
performed to determine whether and how environmental variables are con-

trolling or somehow influencing a person's behavior in any particular setting. The underlying assumption is that if one can identify the functional relations between stimuli (internal/cognitive and external/environmental) and the behavior of interest, the behavior of interest can be influenced by manipulating these stimuli. Thus, a functional analysis can be prescriptive in that the results may offer direction to the clinician who is attempting to either understand what factors are maintaining the behavior or alter the behavior in some way. The information used to conduct a functional analysis may be obtained with any of the assessment methods previously discussed (e.g., interview, direct observation). The functional relations addressed in this analysis are typically explored by examining the antecedents and consequences (e.g., reinforcement, punishment) of the behavior of interest. For example, to determine the controlling conditions under which a nursing home resident screams, one might begin by observing the antecedents and consequences of the screams. The resident may be more likely to scream when particular staff members approach the resident for a bath and during the bathing of the resident. The screaming could be controlled by a variety of antecedent and consequent conditions. For example, the resident may have a history of rather rough treatment by a particular staff member who is approaching the resident for a bath on a particular day. Screaming in the presence of this staff member may lead to bathing by a more favorable staff member, which terminates the screaming. Thus, the screaming is reinforced by withdrawal of the undesirable staff member. Alternatively, a frail resident may be frightened by being bathed for fear of drowning in the bathtub. Screaming may reduce the frequency with which the resident is bathed because the staff members avoid the aversive screaming of the resident. At the consequences end we may find that bath time is shortened when the resident screams and lengthened when the resident is quiet and compliant. Therefore, the resident's screaming is reinforced by early bath termination. This functional analysis reveals a variety of potential controlling variables, most of which can be manipulated to reduce the likelihood of screaming.

Such analyses are particularly appealing because the assessment process leads directly to possible interventions by revealing the controlling variables that can be manipulated as part of an intervention. Another advantage of the functional analysis is that the hypothesized relations between the ostensible controlling variables and the problem behavior can be tested via the manipulation of these variables. Therefore, if the manipulation does not work, one can reconsider the accuracy or completeness of the functional analysis and other potential controlling variables (e.g., physiological or other environmental factors).

Communicating Assessment Results

Following the clinician's analysis of the assessment information, a clinical report is typically drafted that brings together behavioral observations made prior, during, and subsequent to formal assessment, historical information obtained from various sources (e.g., significant others, the client, previous case histories), test results, and information about the assessment situation that could influence the validity or reliability of the assessment findings.

The typical psychological report includes the following sections:

1. Identifying information (e.g., name, gender, ethnicity, date of birth, age, date of assessment).
2. Reason for referral (e.g., determine whether this person is experiencing dementia, depression, or both).
3. Historical information (e.g., family history, patient psychiatric history, prior assessment findings).
4. Behavioral observations (e.g., physical appearance, behavior during assessment, attention to questions and tasks, response to successes and failures).
5. Assessment results (e.g., factors that might influence reliability or validity of findings, results of specific assessment instruments, patterns of findings including strengths and weaknesses).
6. Diagnostic impressions (e.g., dementia, schizophrenia).
7. Recommendations (e.g., answers to referral question, recommendations for intervention, recommendations for staff regarding problem behavior management).
8. Summary (e.g., reason for referral, review and integration of assessment results, strengths and weaknesses, diagnostic impressions, recommendations).

Information obtained from an assessment report can be used for a variety of purposes, but is typically used to answer questions addressed at the outset. Moreover, most residential/inpatient facilities routinely assess individuals on admission to the facility. The assessment information may be used for the determination of placement or treatment setting (e.g., nursing home, independent living setting, adult day center, respite program, psychiatric hospital). An older adult may also be assessed to determine decision-making and other functional capacities so that a guardian or other surrogate decision maker can be appointed when the individual lacks such capacities. Treatment options are also considered on the basis of assessment information. The decision to pursue medical, psychosocial, or both treatment approaches is made on the basis of assessment information. In addition, the specific type of treatment (e.g., psychodynamic psychotherapy, antidepressant medication, cognitive–behavioral therapy) is determined by the assessment results. Interventions aimed at enhancing skills (e.g., teaching how to compensate for visual impairment) or manipulating the environment (e.g., increasing lighting intensity) may all be prescribed by the results of a thorough assessment.

Case Example

One of the most commonly asked assessment questions, based on our survey of clinical geropsychologists, is whether a client is suffering from depression, dementia, or both. Below is a case example in which we briefly illustrate the assessment process.

Depression versus Dementia

You are the consulting psychologist for a nursing home. Judy, one of the residents, is referred to you by one of the nurses who isresponsible for Judy's care. The nurse is concerned that Judy appears apathetic at times and no longer attends social activities. Judy complains of difficulties with concentration and memory, and has experienced difficulty remembering the subject ofconversations. She is also disoriented at times and becomes frustrated and angry when this occurs. Last night, Judy walked into another resident's room and climbed into the resident's bed. When a staff member explained to Judy that she was in the wrong room and tried to move her, Judy become aggressive and then cried.

Your role

Client is referred

Define the problem

Operationalize the problem

Obtain concrete examples

Judy seems unhappy and withdrawn most of the time. Her daughter has expressed concern and reports that she has never seen her like this before. Now that Judy has begun to enter other residents' rooms and act aggressively, the nursing home staff are afraid for the safety of Judy and other residents.

Whose problem is it?

What led to the referral?

You peruse Judy's chart and find that she has a family history of Alzheimer's disease and there is no known history of mental illness. She has not had any recent changes in her medication. She has lost 8 pounds in the past 3 weeks, putting her just under her ideal weight range.

Medical and mental health history

After speaking with staff, you learn that 4 weeks ago Judy was given a new roommate after her roommate of 9 months died. Judy's new roommate is bedridden

Environmental or organismic changes

and noncommunicative. Judy's daughter tells you that she has not been able to visit as often because she is going through a custody battle with her ex-husband. She further reports that when she does visit, she notices that Judy's cognitive and emotional decline has been rapid.

When you interview Judy, you notice that her gait is slow and unsteady. She is still wearing her bedclothes and her hair is uncombed at 3 P.M. She has forgotten her glasses. She seems to hesitate and look around between steps. As you interview her, she is polite, but tearful. She reports that she is not interested in activities that she formerly enjoyed, she sleeps much more often, her appetite is almost nonexistent, she worries constantly about her daughter and grandchildren, her memory and concentration are markedly impaired, a source of great distress for her, and she reports feeling worthless and unhappy. You find that she frequently needs to be prompted to complete sentences because her sentences trail off or she stares out the window. She asks you to repeat questions several times because she reports having forgotten the question.

Observe appearance behavior

In light of Judy's symptoms (e.g., memory and concentration deficits and reports of depressed mood) you are uncertain whether Judy is experiencing depression or dementia. You decide to observe her behavior, administer a self-report measure of depression (GDS), and assess her memory using a few simple working, primary and secondary memory tasks. You observe Judy at various times during the day and find that she leaves her room only for meals, has difficulty finding her room when she returns, and becomes agitated and tearful when trying to locate her room. When other residents approach her, she either complains or does not respond at all; they quickly leave her alone.

Determining the appropriate assessment method

Direct observation

When you assess her memory, you find that Judy's performance is inconsistent, sometimes within normal

Performance-based assessment

limits, other times far below. Although she cries throughout the assessment process and reports feeling "frustrated and worthless," you find that Judy's memory is not as bad as she reports it to be. When you tell this to Judy, she shakes her head and tells you that the task she just completed was an easy one. Judy performs well on simple tests of short-term memory (e.g., recalling a series of numbers), but performs poorly on tests that require greater concentration (e.g., recalling and sorting a list of words by category). On follow-up tests, her rate of forgetting is within normal limits. Judy endorses 12 out of 15 depression items on the GDS.

Self-report measure

Based on Judy's reports, her performance, your observations, and reports from staff and family, you conclude that Judy is experiencing a major depressive episode. This conclusion is based on Judy's rate of decline (rapid), complaints of deficits (abundant), emotional reaction to deficits (marked distress), evaluation of accomplishments (minimized), and poor performance on concentration-based, but not simpler memory tasks. These symptoms are all indicators of depression. Had Judy been experiencing dementia, the rate of decline would have been slower and her complaints about her decline, as well as her emotional reaction to them, would probably have been inconsistent (sometimes complaining, other times not reporting any distress related to her decline).

Interpretation of results

You discuss your finding with Judy's treatment team with Judy present. You explain to Judy that her current life experiences (new roommate, concern for daughter) may have resulted in depression, which impacts concentration abilities, mood, and memory.

Communication of results

With the input of Judy, her daughter, and the treatment team, Judy is given an antidepressant medication with few side effects. She is also placed on a reinforcement schedule at the nursing home. That is, staff members are

Treatment recommendations

trained to provide enjoyable activities for Judy to participate in and to praise her when she participates. She is
also kept better informed by her daughter on the custody
proceedings and receives more visits from her grandchildren. Over the course of a month, Judy's GDS score   Posttest
drops to 2/15, her performance on concentration-based
tasks improve, her orientation is back to normal, she re-
gains her appetite, and resumes participation in activities.
She reports feeling much happier, although she still worries about her grandchildren.

REVIEW QUESTIONS

1. What is assessment and why is it important?

2. What are some of the objectives of assessment?

3. What is the difference between assessment and testing?

4. What is meant by the utility of assessment and why is it important?

5. What is multidimensional assessment and why is it important?

6. What are the components of multidimensional assessment?

7. Describe some of the factors that can influence the assessment process.

8. Discuss differences between multimethod and multidimensional assessment.

9. In what ways can physical health problems compromise the assessment process?

10. Discuss how one's conceptual approach to assessment can influence the selection of assessment instruments and methods.

11. Contrast norm-based and performance-based criterion-referenced assessment.

12. Distinguish between the different forms of reliabilty discussed in this chapter and discuss the importance of each.

13. Distinguish between the different forms of validity discussed in this chapter and discuss the importance of each.

14. List and describe the different methods of assessment.

15. How does behavioral assessment differ from more traditional forms of assessment?

16. What is the difference between functional assessment and functional analysis?

17. Describe the components of the assessment process beginning with the referral question and ending with the psychological report.

References

Achenbaum, W. A. (1985). Societal perceptions of aging and the aged. In R. H. Binstock & E. Shanas (Eds.). Handbook of aging and the sciences (2nd Ed.). (pp. 129–148). New York: Van Nostrand Reinhold.

Adams, R. L., Parsons, O. A., Culbertson, J. L., & Nixon, S. J. (1996). *Neuropsychology for clinical practice: Etiology, assessment, and treatment of common neurological disorders.* Washington, DC: American Psychological Association.

Alberts, M. S. (1994). Brief assessments of cognitive function in the elderly. In M. P. Lawton & J. A. Teresi (Eds.), *Annual review of gerontology and geriatrics: Assessment techniques* (pp. 93–106). New York: Springer.

Alessi, C. A., & Cassel, C. K. (1991). Medical evaluation and common medical problems. In M. Jenike J. Sadavoy, L. W. Lazarus, & L. L. Jarvik (Eds.), *Comprehensive review of geriatric psychiatry* (2nd ed., pp. 171–195). Washington, DC: American Psychiatric Press.

Allen, M. J., & Yen, W. M. (1977). *Introduction to measurement theory.* Belmont, CA: Wadsworth.

American Psychiatric Association (1994). Diagnostic and Statistical Manual of Mental Disorders (4th ed.). Washington, D.C.: Author.

Anastasi, A., & Urbina, S. (1997). *Psychological testing* (7th ed.). Upper Saddle River, NJ: Prentice-Hall.

Appelbaum, P., & Grisso, T. (1988). Assessing patients' capacities to consent to treatment. *New England Journal of Medicine, 319,* 1635–1638.

Applegate, W. B. (1995). The medical evaluation. In L. Z. Rubenstein, D. Wieland, & R. Bernabei (Eds.), *Geriatric assessment technology: The state of the art* (pp. 41–50). Milan Italy: Editrice Kurtis.

Baron, R. S., Cutrona, C. E., Hicklin, D., Russell, D. W., & Lubaroff. (1990). Social support and immune function among spouses of cancer patients. *Journal of Personality and Social Psychology, 59,* 344–352.

Blessed, G., Tomlinson, B. E., & Roth, M. (1968). The association between quantitative measures of dementia and of senile changes in the cerebral gray matter of elderly subjects. *British Journal of Psychiatry, 114,* 797–811.

Braithwaite, V. A. (1986). Old age stereotypes: Reconciling contradictions. *Journal of Gerontology, 41,* 353–360.

Bressler, R. (1987) Drug use in the Geriatric Patient. In L. Carstensen and B. Edeistein (Eds.), Handbook of Clinical Gerontology (pp. 152–174). New York: Pergamon Press.

Brink, T. L., Yesavage, J. A., Lum, O., Heersema, P., Adey, M., & Rose, T. L. (1982). Screening tests for geriatric depression. *Clinical Gerontologist, 1,* 37–43.

Burman, B., & Margolin, G. (1992). Analysis of the association between marital relationships and health problems: An interactional perspective. *Psychological Bulletin, 112,* 39–63.

Butler, R. N. (1969). Age-ism: Another form of bigotry. *The Gerontologist, 9,* 243–246.

Cavanaugh, J. C. (1993). *Adult development and aging* (2nd ed.). Pacific Grove, CA: Brooks/Cole.

Cohen-Mansfield, J., Werner, P., Marx, M. S., & Freedman, L. (1991). Two studies of pacing in the nursing home. *Journal of Gerontology: Medical Sciences, 46*, M77–M83.

Corcoran, K., & Fischer, J. (1987). *Measures for clinical practice: A sourcebook.* New York: The Free Press.

Cormier, W. H., & Cormier, L. S. (1991). *Interviewing strategies for helpers: Fundamental skills and cognitive behavioral interventions* (3rd ed.). Pacific Grove, CA: Brooks/Cole.

Duke University Center for the Study of Aging. (1978). *Multidimensional functional assessment: The OARS methodology* (2nd ed.). Durham, NC: Duke University Press.

Edelstein, B. A., & Semenchuck, E. M. (1996). Interviewing older adults. In L. L. Carstensen, B. A. Edelstein, & L. Dornbrand (Eds.), *The practical handbook of clinical gerontology* (pp.153–173). Thousand Oaks, CA: Sage.

Edelstein, B. A., Nygren, M., Northrop, L., Staats, N., & Pool, D. (1993). *Assessment of capacity to make financial and medical decisions.* Paper presented at the 101st annual meeting of the American Psychological Association, Toronto, Canada.

Edelstein, B., Staats, N., Kalish, K. D., & Northrop, L. E. (1996). Assessment of older adults. In M. Hersen & V. B. Van Hasselt (Eds.), *Psychological treatment of older adults: An introductory text* (pp. 35–68). New York: Plenum.

Evans, D., Funkenstein, H., Albert, M., Scherr, P., Cook, N., Chown, M., Hebert, L., Henekens, C., & Taylor, J. (1989). Prevalence of Alzheimer's disease in a community population of older persons. *Journal of the American Medical Association, 262,* 2551–2556.

Feinson, M. C. (1991). Reexamining some common beliefs about mental health and aging. In B. B. Hess & E. W. Markson (Eds.), *Growing old in America* (4th ed., pp. 125–135). New Brunswick, NJ: Transaction.

Fischer, J., & Corcoran, K. (1994). *Measures for clinical practice: A sourcebook* (2nd Ed.). New York: The Free Press.

Folkman, S. & Lazarus, R. S. (1980). An analysis of coping in a middle-aged community sample. *Journal of Health and Social Behavior, 21,* 219–239.

Folstein, M., Folstein, S., & McHugh, P. (1975). 'Mini-Mental State': A practical method for grading cognitive state of patients for the clinician. *Journal of Psychiatric Research, 12,* 189–198.

Frazer, D. W., Leicht, M. L., & Baker, M. D. (1996). Psychological manifestations of physical disease in the elderly. In L. Carstensen, B. Edelstein, & L. Dornbrand (Eds.), *The practical handbook of clinical gerontology* (pp. 217–235). Thousand Oaks, CA: Sage Publications.

Fry, P.S. (1986). *Depression, stress, and adaptations in the elderly: Psychological assessment and intervention.* Rockville, MD: Aspen Publishers.

Gallagher, D., Thompson, L. W., & Levy, S. M. (1980). Clinical psychological assessment of older adults. In L. W. Poon (Ed.), *Aging in the 1980's* (pp.19–40). Washington DC: American Psychology Association.

Gatz , M., & Pearson, C. G. (1988). Ageism revised and provision of psychological services. *American Psychologist, 43,* 184–189.

Golden, C., Purisch, A. D., & Hammeke, T. A . (1985). *Luria-Nebraska Neuropsychological Battery: Forms I and II: Manual.* Los Angeles: Western Psychological Services.

Goodstein, R. K. (1985). Common clinical problems in the elderly: Camoflaged by ageism and atypical presentation. *Psychiatric Annals, 15,* 299–312

Grisso, T., & P. Appelbaum (1998) (Eds). *Assessing competence to consent to treatment: a guide for physicians and other health professionals.* New York: Oxford Univ. Press

Gurland, B., Kuriansky, J., Sharpe, L., Simon, R., Stiller, P., & Birkett, P. (1977). The Comprehensive Assessment and Referral Evaluation (CARE): Rationale, development, and reliability. *International Journal of Aging and Human Development, 8,* 9–42.

Hayes, S. C., Nelson, R. O., & Jarrett, R. B. (1987). The treatment utility of assessment. *American Psychologist, 42,* 963–974.

Haynes, S. N. (1991). Behavioral assessment. In M. Hersen, A. E. Kazdin, & A. S. Bellack (Eds.), *The clinical psychology handbook* (2nd ed., pp. 430–464). Elmsford, NY: Pergamon.

Hedrick, S. C. (1995). Assessment of functional status: Activities of daily living. In L. Z. Rubenstein, D. Wieland, & R. Bernabei (Eds.), *Geriatric assessment technology: The state of the art.* Milan, Italy: Editrice Kurtis.

Herr, K. A., & Mobily, P. R. (1991). Complexities of pain assessment in the elderly: Clinical considerations. *Journal of Gerontological Nursing, 17,* 12–19.

Hersen,M., & Bellack, A. (1998) (Eds.), *Behavioral assessment: A practical handbook.* (4th ed.) New York: Allyn & Bacon.

Hersen, M., Kazdin, A., & Bellack, A. (1991). *The clinical psychology handbook* (2nd ed.). New York: Pergamon.

Hertzog, C., & Schear, J. M. (1989). Psychometric considerations in testing the older person. In T. Hunt & C. J. Lindley (Eds.), *Testing older adults: A reference guide for geropsychological assessments* (pp. 24–50). Austin, TX: Pro-Ed.

Hoeffer, B., Rader, J., & Siemsen, G. (1987). *An observational tool for studying the behavior of cognitively impaired nursing home residents who wander.* Poster presented at meeting of the Gerontological Society of America, Washington, DC.

Kane, R. A. (1995). Assessment of social functioning: Recommendations for comprehensive geriatric assessment. In L. Z. Rubenstein, D. Wieland, & R. Bernabei (Eds.), *Geriatric assessment technology: The state of the art* (pp. 91–110). Milan,Italy: Editrice Kurtis.

Kaszniak, A. W. (1990). Psychological assessment of the aging individual. In J. E. Birren & K. W. Schaie (Eds.), *Handbook of the Psychology of Aging* (3rd ed., pp. 427–445). San Diego, CA: Academic Press.

Kaszniak, A. W. (1996). Techniques and intruments for assessment of the elderly. In S. H. Zarit & B. G. Knight (Eds.), *A guide to psychotherapy and aging: Effective clinical interventions in a life-stage context* (pp. 163–219). Washington, DC: American Psychological Association.

Katz, S., Downs, T. D., Cash, H. R., & Grotz, R. C. (1970). Progress in development in the Index of ADL. *Gerontologist, 10,* 20–30.

Katz, S. C., Ford, A. B., Moskowitz, R. W., Jackson, B. A., & Jaffee, M. W. (1963). Studies of illness in the aged. The Index of ADL: A standardized measure of biological and psychosocial function. *Journal of the American Medical Association, 185,* 919–919.

Kiernan, R. J., Mueller, J .l., Langston, J. W., & Van Dyke, C. (1987). The Neurobehavioral Cognitive Status Examination: A brief but differentiated approach to cogniltive assessment. *Annals of Internal Medicine, 107,* 481–485.

Kimmerling, R. E. (Chair), Zeiss, A., Nezu, A. M., Follette, V. M., & Linehan, M. M. (1996). *Emotional reactions toward patients: The role in the training of behavior therapists.* Clinical roundtable presented at the 30th Annual Convention of the Association for Advancement of Behavior Therapy, New York, NY.

Knight, B. G. (Ed.). (1996). *Psychotherapy with older adults* (2nd ed.). Thousand Oaks, CA: Sage.

Kogan, J. N., & Edelstein, B. A. (1997). Fears of middle-aged and older adults: Relations to daily functioning and life satisfaction. Manuscript submitted for publication.

Kovar, M. G., & Lawton, M. P. (1994). Functional disability: activities and instrumental activities of daily living. In M. P. Lawton & J. A. Teresi (Eds.), *Annual review of geriatrics and gerontology*. NY: Springer Publishing.

Lawton, M. P. (1986). Functional assessment. In L. Teri & P. M. Lewinsohn (Eds.), *Geropsychological assessment and treatment: Selected topics* (pp. 39–84). New York: Springer.

Lawton, M. P., & Brody, E. M. (1969). Assessment of older people: Self-maintaining and instrumental activities of daily living. *The Gerontologist, 9*, 179–185.

Lawton, M. P., Moss, M., Fulcomer, M., & Kleban, M. H. (1982). A research and service-oriented multilevel assessment instrument. *Journal of Gerontology, 37*, 91–99.

Leuchter, A. (1991). Electroencephalography. In J. Sadavoy, L. W. Lazarus, & L. L. Jarvik (Eds.), *Comprehensive review of geriatric psychiatry* (pp. 273–283). Washington, DC: American Psychiatric Press.

Lowenstein, D. A., Amigo, E., Duara, R., Guterman, A., Hurwitz, D., Berkowitz, N., Wilkie, F., Weinberg, G., Black, B., Gittelman, B., & Eisdorfer, C. (1989). A new scale for the assessmnet of functional status in Alzheimer's disease and related disorders. *Journal of Gerontology, 44*, 114–121.

Maloney, M. P., & Ward, M. P. (1976). *Psychological Assessment*. New York: Oxford University Press.

Markson, E. W. (1991). Physiological changes, illness, and health care use in later life. In B. B. Hess & E. W. Markson (Eds.), *Growing old in America* (4th ed., pp. 173–186). New Brunswick, NJ: Transaction.

Marsh, G. R., & Thompson, L. W. (1977). Psychophysiology of aging. In J. E. Birren & K. W. Schaie (Eds.), *Handbook of the psychology of aging* (pp. 219–248). New York: Van Nostrand Reinhold.

Martin, D. C., Moryzc, R. K., McDowell, J., Snustad, D., & Karpf, M. (1985). Community-based geriatric assessment. *Journal of the American Geriatric Society, 33*, 602–606.

Mattis, S. (1988). Dementia rating scale (DRS). Odessa, FL: Psychological Assessment Resources.

Morris, J. N., Fries, B. E., Mehr, D. R., Hawes, C., Phillips, C., Mor, V., & Lipsitz, L.A. (1994). MDS Cognitive Performance Scale. *Journal of Gerontology: Medical Sciences, 49*, M174–M182.

Morrison, R. L. (1988). Structured interviews and rating scales. In A. S. Bellack & M. Hersen (Eds.), *Behavioral assessment: A practical handbook* (3rd ed., pp. 252–279). Elmsford, NY: Pergamon.

National Center for Cost Containment. (1996). *Geropsychology resource guide, 1996 revision* (NTIS No. PB96-144365).

Okun, M. (1976). Adult age and cautiousness in decision: A review of the literature. *Human Development, 19*, 220–233.

Oxman, T. E., & Berkman, L. F. (1990). Assessments of social relationships in the elderly. *International Journal of Psychiatry in Medicine, 21*, 65–84.

Pagel, M. D., Erdly, W. W., & Becker, J. (1987). Social networks: We get by with (and in spite of) a little help from our friends. *Journal of Personality and Social Psychology, 53*, 793–804.

Pfeiffer, E. (1975). SPMSQ: Short Portable Mental Status Questionnaire. *Journal of the American Geriatrics Society, 23*, 433–441.

Poon, L. W., Rubin, D. C., & Wilson, B. A. (Eds.)(1989). *Everyday cognition in adulthood and late life*. Cambridge, UK: Cambridge University Press

Prochaska, J., & Norcross, J. (1994). *Systems of psychotherapy: A transtheoretical analysis* (3rd ed.). Pacific Grove, CA: Brooks/Cole.

Pruchno, R., & Lawton, M. P. (1991). Gerontology. In C. E. Walker (Ed.), *Clinical psychology: Historical and research foundations* (pp. 361–392). New York: Plenum.

Pruchno, R. A., Smyer, M. A., Rose, M. S., Hartman-Stein, P. E., & Henderson-Laribee, D. L. (1995). Competence of long-term care residents to participate in decisions about their medical care: A brief objective assessment. *The Gerontologist, 35*, 622–629.

Radloff, L. W. (1977). The CES-D scale: A self-report depression scale for research in the general population. *Applied Psychological Measurement, 1*, 385–401.

Reitan, R. M., & Wolfson, D. (1993). *The Halstead-Reitan Neuropsychological Test Battery* (2nd ed.). Tucson: Neuropsychology Press.

Rodeheaver, D. (1990). Ageism. In I. A. Parham, L. W. Poon, & I. C. Siegler (Eds.), *Access: Aging curriculum content for education in the social and behavioral sciences* (pp. 7.1–7.43). New York: Springer.

Rook, K. S. (1990). Stressful aspects of older adults' social relationships: An overview of current theory and research. In M. A. P. Stephens, J. H. Crowther, S. E. Hobfoll, & D. L. Tennenbaum (Eds.), *Stress and coping in later-life families* (pp. 173–192). New York: Hemisphere.

Rook, K. S. (1994). Assessing the health-related dimensions of older adults' social relationships. In M. P. Lawton & J. A. Teresi (Eds.), *Annual review of gerontology and geriatrics: Focus on assessment techniques* (Vol. 14, pp. 142–181). New York: Springer.

Roth, M., Tym, E., Mountjoy, C., Huppert, F., Hendrie, H., Verma, S., & Goddard, R. (1986). CAMDEX: A standardized instrument for the diagnosis of mental disorder in the elderly with special reference to the early detection of dementia. *British Journal of Psychiatry, 149*, 698–709.

Rubenstein, L. Z. (1995). An overview of comprehensive geriatric assessment: Rationale, history, program models, basic components. In L. Z. Rubenstein, D. Wieland, & R. Bernabei (Eds.), *Geriatric assessment technology: The state of the art* (pp. 1–10). Milan, Italy: Editrice Kurtis.

Sattler, J. M. (Ed.). (1998). *Assessment of children* (Rev. and updated 3rd ed.). San Diego, CA: Jerome M. Sattler.

Schaie, K. W., & Schaie, J. P. (1977). Clinical assessment and aging. In J. E. Birren & K. W. Schaie (Eds.), *Handbook of the psychology of aging* (pp. 692–723). New York: Van Nostrand Reinhold.

Schaie, K. W., & Willis, S. L. (Eds.). (1986). *Adult development and aging* (2nd ed.). Boston, MA: Little, Brown.

Schwartz, G. E. (1983). Development and validation of the Geriatric Evaluation by Relative's Rating Instrument (GERRI). *Psychological Reports, 53*, 479–488.

Segal, E. S. (1996). Common medical problems in geriatric patients. In L. L. Carstensen, B. A. Edelstein, & L. Dornbrand (Eds.), *The practical handbook of clinical gerontology* (pp. 451–467). Thousand Oaks, CA: Sage.

Sherbourne, C. D., & Meredith, L. S. (1992). Quality of self-report data: A comparison of older and younger chronically ill patients. *Journal of Gerontology: Social Sciences, 47*, S204–211.

Silver, I. L., & Herrmann, N. (1991). History and mental status examination. In M. Jenike (Section Ed.), J. Sadavoy, L. W. Lazarus, & L. L. Jarvik (Eds.), *Comprehensive review of geriatric psychiatry* (pp. 149–169). Washington, DC: American Psychiatric Press.

Spielberger, C., Gorsuch, R, & Lushene, R. (1970). *STAI manual for the state-trait anxiety inventory*. Palo Alto, CA: Consulting Psychologists Press.

Storandt, M. (1995). General principles of assessment of older adults. In M. Strorandt & G. R. VandenBos (Eds.), *Neuropsychological assessment of dementia and depression in older adults: A clinician's guide* (pp. 7–32). Washington, DC: American Psychological Association.

Sturgis, E. T., & Gramling, S. (1988). Psychophysiological assessment. In A. S. Bellack & M. Hersen (Eds.), *Behavioral assessment: A practical handbook* (3rd ed., pp. 231–251). Elmsford, NY: Pergamon.

Yesavage, J. A., (1986). The use of self-rating depression scales in the elderly. In L. Poon, T. Crook, B. J. Gurland, K. L. Davis, A. W. Kazniak, C. Eisdorfer, & L. W. Thompson (Eds.), *Handbook for clinical memory assessment for older adults* (pp. 213–217). Washington, DC: American Psychological Association.

Zarit, S. H. (Ed.). (1980). *Aging and mental disorders: Psychological approaches to assessment and treatment.* New York: Free Press.

Zarit, S. H., & Spore, D. (1990). Mental health and aging. In I. A. Parham, L. W. Poon, & I. C. Siegler (Eds.), *Access: Aging curriculum content for education in the social and behavioral sciences* (pp. 5.1–5.51). New York: Springer.

Zeiss, A. M., & Steffen, A. M. (1996). Interdisciplinary health care teams: The basic unit of geriatric care. In L. Carstensen, B. Edelstein, & L. Dornbrand (Eds.), *The practical handbook of clinical gerontology* (pp. 423–450). Thousand Oaks, CA: Sage Publications.

Zuckerman, M. (1991). *Psychobiology and personality.* New York: Cambridge University Press.

Additional Readings

American Psychiatric Association (1994). *Diagnostic and statistical manual of mental disorders* (4th ed.). Washington, DC: American Psychiatric Association.

Carstensen, L., Edelstein, B., & Dornbrand, L. (1996). *The practical handbook of clinical gerontology.* Thousand Oaks, CA: Sage.

La Rue, A. (1992). *Aging and neuropsychological assessment.* New York: Plenum.

Lawton, M. P., & Teresi, J. A. (Eds.)(1994). *Annual review of gerontology and geriatrics: Focus on assessment techniques.* New York: Springer.

Mattis, S. (1976). Mental status examination for organic mental syndromes in the elderly patient. In L. Bellak & T. B. Karasu (Eds.), *Geriatric psychiatry* (pp. 79–121). New York: Grune & Stratton.

National Center for Cost Containment. (1996). *Geropsychology resource guide, 1996 revision* (NTIS No. PB96-144365).

National Center for Cost Containment. (1997). *Assessment of competency and capacity of the older adults: A practice guideline for psychologists* (NTIS No. PB-96-144365).

Poon, L. W. (1986). *Handbook for clinical memory assessment of older adults.* Washington, DC: American Psychological Association.

Rubenstein, L. Z., Wieland, D., & Bernabei, R. (Eds.)(1995). *Geriatric assessment technology: The state of the art.* Milano, Italy: Editrice Kurtis.

Storandt, M., & VandenBos, G. (1994). *Neuropsychological assessment of dementia and depression in older adults: A clinician's guide.* Washington, DC: American Psychological Association.

11

Mental Health and Mental Disorders in Older Adults

Sara Honn Qualls

James Johnston, age 73, lives in a mid-sized city with his wife of 51 years. Both are independent, although each has some health problems. James was diagnosed with Parkinson's disease, a neurological disorder that creates a shuffling gait, hand tremors, and some flatness of facial expressions. He has a history of depression for which he was hospitalized 15 years ago, but which is not evident currently. Upon recovery from the previous episode of depression, he retired from his job as a minister and began doing a lay ministry in which he visits elderly members of his congregation. Claire, age 74, is also quite active, having worked until recently as a receptionist. She had a hip replacement about 7 years ago, and began noting serious vision deterioration due to macular degeneration about 4 years ago. Last year, this couple moved from Manhattan, where they have lived for 40 years, to live near one son and his family. The decision to move was difficult, but their finances were insufficient to support them in New York City. Additionally, both James and Claire anticipate needing increasing amounts of care in their later years, which their son's family has offered to give. Adjusting to their new environment has been challenging, however. Claire has almost given up driving due to her vision impairment; James likely will be forced to quit driving in the near future. Claire's vision impairment also makes is harder for her to learn her way around unfamiliar places. James has enjoyed learning his way around, but finds himself more limited socially than he prefers. After decades as a minister in which his work took him into daily contact with others, he finds himself having few reasons for interaction. He finds it harder than expected to break into a "group" at the new church or the senior center. Both James and Claire reach out to members of their new church who need help, and thus create some social contact incidentally, but lack the sense of longevity that comes from decades of relating to families across the stages of their life cycle.

How can James and Claire adapt to their new environment and thrive as mentally healthy persons? This question can be addressed only after you have some foundational knowledge about normal aging. The field of mental health and aging presumes knowledge of normal as well as abnormal patterns of physiological, social, and psychological aging within various cultural contexts. Two questions focus our attention on the key issues in the field of mental health and aging. What characterizes mental well-being for older persons? When do aging processes create a condition that should be characterized as abnormal? Other chapters in this book will lay the foundation for your knowledge of "normal" aging across many domains of functioning (e.g., cognitive, emotional, social). In this chapter, the epidemiology and characteristics of the most prevalent mental disorders will be described, and strategies for assessment and treatment will be reviewed.

Mental Health and Well-being

The dividing line between mental health and mental disorder has never been simple. For example, is a low mood the same entity but less intense than clinical depression, or is clinical depression a disease or condition that can be diagnosed like medical conditions? How much distress must an individual feel and how much must functioning be impaired to classify a person as disordered, diseased, or in need of intervention? There is not a simple answer to this question. Indeed, the line between mental health and mental disorder changes over time as paradigms shift and empirical data inform our understanding of emotion, cognition, and behavior.

Unique issues related to defining mental disorders in older adults also arise. For example, although it may be normative for very old adults to experience some cognitive deterioration, is that "normal"? In other words, what is the relationship between mental health and age-correlated changes in physical well-being and social well-being? These questions require assumptions to be made about the definition and nature of mental health.

One way of conceptualizing mental health is simply as the absence of disorder or illness. Guidebooks such as the current *Diagnostic and Statistical Manual of Mental Disorders* (4th edition, American Psychiatric Association, 1994) identify the accepted set of disorders and syndromes that is usually used as the absolute guideline for legal, medical, and financial decision making. In many settings, mental health is a default condition; it is presumed in the absence of evidence of disorder or disease.

Others advocate more substantive definitions that identify key characteristics of mentally healthy persons. Jahoda (1958) provided six highly cited criteria for positive mental health (not specifically targeted to older persons): positive self-attitudes, growth and self-actualization, integration of the personality, autonomy, reality perception, and environmental mastery. These criteria appear to define optimal mental health. The vitality that would characterize a person meeting these criteria is the central characteristic of mental health in later adulthood as well as at any other age according to Erikson, Erikson, and Kivnik (1986). Although developmental tasks vary across the life span, at any age or stage, mentally healthy persons "have the ability to respond to other individuals, to love, to be loved, and to cope with others in give-and-take relationships" (Birren & Renner, 1980, p. 29).

With advanced age, the contexts in which positive mental health can be pursued are altered. As illustrated by the case of James and Claire, losses in physical health as well as changes in roles and familiar contexts alter, and often limit, the opportunities to meet needs that maintain positive well-being. As the balance of gains and losses shifts in favor of losses during old age, Baltes and colleagues suggest that reserve capacities are used more for maintenance than growth functions (Marsiske, Lang, Baltes, & Baltes, 1995). Compensatory mechanisms are put into place to make up for the lost functions so optimal aging can be achieved in specified domains of life (Baltes & Baltes, 1990). "Optimal aging refers to a kind of utopia, namely, aging under development-enhancing and age-friendly environmental conditions" (Baltes & Baltes, 1990, p. 8). Under less than utopian conditions, mental health problems can occur, as a function of the interplay among biological vulnerability, stressful life events, and psychological diathesis or stress (Gatz, Kasl-Godley, & Karel, 1996).

Gerontologists have tended to adapt theories to the experiences of older persons rather than generate new theories because older people are more similar to the general adult population than they are different. Whether the definition is drawn from the cognitive-behavioral, psychodynamic, or family systems models, for example, specific definitions of mental health flow directly from the theory one uses to conceptualize human beings. Regardless of definition, much less attention has been placed on identifying the prevalence and structure of positive mental health in later life than has been focused on learning about and treating the mental disorders. The remainder of the chapter provides an overview of a select subset of mental disorders.

Mental Disorders in Later Life

Margaret takes six pills with every meal and two at bedtime. Because her children worry about her health, they rotate weekend visit responsibility. Last weekend, when the oldest son visited, he found that Margaret's freezer was empty and the refrigerator had only moldy food. As he investigated further, he found her checking account in disarray with numbers entered haphazardly and incomplete entries. The most disturbing aspect of the visit was the odd conversations Margaret had with imaginary visitors. Her son wonders if this is normal for an elderly woman, or if something is wrong.

Lonnie's wife has had Alzheimer's disease for 7 years, during which he has watched her deteriorate from a bright, energetic leader in the community to a shell of a woman who cannot speak her own name. Lonnie provides her

daily needs: bathing, dressing, cooking, and sometimes feeding. He maintains
the house and stays in contact with her children from a previous marriage.
They rarely leave the house because she gets agitated in public places.

Last year when Jeanette was 58 and her only son, Jonathan, was 35, he died
of AIDS following a prolonged period of illness during which she served as
his primary caregiver. Jeanette reports that she is having trouble getting on
with life. She is not sleeping or eating well, has lost weight, and thinks about
Jonathan constantly. She prays for his soul at Mass every morning.

The Big Three: Delirium, Dementia, and Depression

A major challenge for health and mental health professionals is the differential diagnosis of delirium, dementia, and depression. The diagnostic challenge
results from the array of symptoms common to the three disorders. In particular, symptoms of lethargy, difficulty concentrating, and memory problems are
evident in all three disorders. A major cause for concern in this differential diagnosis is the importance of aggressively treating delirium and depression, because with treatment, each can be reversed, but with delays in treatment, long-
term negative consequences can accrue.

Delirium.   A delirium is "characterized by a disturbance of consciousness and
a change in cognition that develop over a short period of time" (American Psychiatric Association, 1994, p. 123). In addition to the changes in cognition (e.g.,
attention, memory, disorientation, language disturbance), delirium can also affect perception, the sleep–wake cycle, and affect. Typically, onset is rapid, but
the course of a delirium may fluctuate over the course of a day. The delirium
may be caused by one or more medical conditions (e.g., stroke, metabolic disturbances, cardiovascular disorders), medications, substance intoxication or
withdrawal, toxin exposure, or some combination of factors.

Older adults are particularly susceptible to delirium because of an increased likelihood of chronic illness and increased risk of over-the-counter and
prescription medication use. Medications are a risk factor for two primary reasons. The process for metabolizing medications becomes less efficient with age
thereby increasing the potential for drug toxicity (Salzman & Nevis-Olesen,
1992). In addition, the number of medications taken by older adults tends to
be quite high, thus increasing the likelihood of adverse drug reactions and interactions (e.g., the average nursing home patient is on 9.3 medications, Pollock et al., 1992).

In the community, the prevalence rate for delirium is relatively low
(0.4–1.1%) among adults over age 55 (Folstein, Bassett, Romanoski, & Nestadt,
1991). Due to increased risk of delirium in acutely ill patients, it is not surprising to find the prevalence of delirium is particularly high in hospitals. For
example, 8–50% of postoperative patients experience delirium (Tune, 1991).

The primary focus of assessment and treatment for delirium is on the phys-

Agnosia is the failure to identify familiar objects or people. (Elderly patients w/ dementia usually begin showing agnosia...)

Mental Health and Mental Disorders in Older Adults 309

iological cause, with attention also focused on ensuring safety and care during the active treatment phase. The case of Margaret, described above, depicts a prototypical picture of delirium. The significant symptoms appeared within the course of a week (between the children's visits). She is disoriented, hallucinating, and her cognitive abilities have deteriorated rapidly. Several hypotheses for the cause of the disorder are embedded in the case description: medication, medication interactions, or illnesses. Several other possibilities exist as well: a new illness (e.g., urinary tract infection, which are notorious causes of delirium in older persons), substance abuse, or toxin exposure. The most important step for the family is to seek immediate medical treatment. When treated, the cognitive impairment should resolve to premorbid levels.

APRAXIA/AGNOSIA → manifest a decline in motor skills.

Dementia. Dementias are characterized by "the development of multiple cognitive deficits manifested by both memory impairment (impaired ability to learn new information or to recall previously learned information) [and] one (or more) of the following cognitive disturbances: aphasia (language disturbance), apraxia (impaired ability to carry out motor activities despite intact motor function), agnosia (failure to recognize or identify objects despite intact sensory function), disturbance in executive functioning (i.e., planning, organizing, sequencing, abstracting)" (American Psychiatric Association, 1994, p. 134). Dementias are particularly devastating because they are characterized by progressive losses that are irreversible, and they destroy very basic cognitive, emotional, social, and personality functioning.

Dementias are found in 6–8% of persons over age 65, with the risk doubling approximately every 5 years such that about 30% of persons over age 85 are diagnosable with dementia (Cummings & Benson, 1992; Jorm, Korten, & Henderson, 1987; Skoog, Nilsson, Palmertz, Andreasson, & Svanbor, 1993). Multiple causes of dementia have been identified, although the neurodegenerative diseases make up the vast majority of dementias. The two most prevalent dementias are Alzheimer's disease (AD) and vascular dementias, which together account for about 90% of all dementias (Skoog et al., 1993). The cause of Alzheimer's disease is unknown, although certain subtypes appear to be genetically linked (Youngjohn & Crook, 1996). The pathophysiology of AD that occurs most dramatically in the hippocampus, cortex, and basal forebrain nuclei of the brain includes rapid cell death, unusual concentrations of amyloid protein that surrounds degenerating nerve cell endings to form neuritic plaques, and the formation of abnormal filaments within neurons that form neurofibrillary tangles. Reduced levels of acetylcholine are also present in the brains of persons with AD. Vascular dementias are produced by various dysfunctions within the vascular system that produce either occlusion or bleeding that permanently impairs brain tissue.

Although a specific prognosis regarding the timing and exact sequencing of decline is difficult to make with any precision, general patterns of declines in cognitive functioning can be outlined. The specific functioning that is lost by persons with dementia is determined by the sites of the brain that are most

APRAXIA – loss of impairment of the ability to execute complex & coordinate movements or execute voluntary movement in correct

Aphasia → refer to a deterioration in the ability to communicate w/ language

compromised. However, patterns of decline in cognitive functioning generally proceed from loss of complex functions toward loss of simple functions. One metric for describing the sequence of decline is provided by the Global Deterioration Scale (Table 11.1; Reisberg, Ferris, De Leon, & Crook, 1992). Although tremendous individual variability is evident, this scale describes the general direction of change.

The process of evaluating a person for dementia includes rigorous medical examinations to rule out all possible reversible conditions that might mimic or complicate the impairments characteristic of dementia (e.g., depression and delirium). Neuropsychological testing is helpful to determine the specific pattern of cognitive impairment, for the purpose of assisting with diagnosis, determination of decision-making capacity, and treatment planning. Functional evaluations (e.g., of skills necessary for daily life) and evaluation of the appropriateness and safety of the living environment are also important.

Interventions for dementia range from pharmacologic efforts to reduce the negative impact of the lower concentrations of acetylcholine in the brain to efforts to support the caregiver(s) whose role is increasingly important as the disease progresses (Stephens & Franks, Chapter 12, this volume). As is evident in the description of Lonnie's life, the caregiver usually experiences major changes in his or her life that increase the risk of mental disorder, social disruption, and in some cases, physical illnesses (Schulz, Visintainer, & Williamson, 1990). For many, the demands of caregiving constitute an unexpected career (Aneshensel, Pearlin, Mullan, Zarit, & Whitlatch, 1995) that is continuous and exhausting. Intervention programs to support caregivers have been well received by the caregivers who report significant benefit from the interventions which include education about the disease, practical problem-solving skills, anger management, and treatment of depression. Although the results of controlled intervention studies often do not show broad ranging effects on all aspects of the caregiver's well-being, the caregivers consistently report positive benefits in more focused areas. Recent data show that intensive intervention efforts with individuals and families help delay institutionalization (Mittelman et al., 1993). In addition to psychosocial interventions, many patients and families need to be referred for legal and financial advice to prepare for the phase when decision-making capacities and financial management skills will be compromised.

Depression.   Depression is a mood disorder that is characterized by depressed mood and/or "markedly diminished interest or pleasure in all, or almost all, activities most of the day" (American Psychiatric Association, 1994, p. 327) as well as a variety of other symptoms such as weight loss, insomnia or hypersomnia, psychomotor retardation or agitation, fatigue, feelings of worthlessness, guilt, diminished ability to think or concentrate, indecisiveness, and thoughts of death or suicide. The reason depression is a differential diagnostic challenge is that the symptoms and presentation of depression can be so similar to that of dementia and delirium. A disoriented, disheveled person

TABLE 11.1.
Global Deterioration Scale

Stage	Clinical Phase	Clinical Characteristics
1. No cognitive decline	Normal	No subjective complains of memory deficit No memory deficit evident on clinical interview
2. Very mild cognitive decline	Forgetfulness	Subjective complaints of memory deficit, most frequently in following areas: (a) forgetting where one has placed familiar objects and (b) forgetting names one formerly knew well No objective evidence of memory deficit on clinical interview No objective deficits in employment or social situations Appropriate concern with respect to symptomatology
3. Mild cognitive decline	Early confusional	Earliest clear-cut deficits appear, with manifestations in more than one of the following areas: (a) patient may get lost when traveling to an unfamiliar location, (b) co-workers become aware of patient's relatively poor performance, (c) word-finding and name-finding deficits become evident to intimates, (d) patient may read a passage of a book and retain relatively little material, (e) patient may demonstrate decreased facility in remembering names on introduction to new people, (f) patient may lose or misplace an object of value, and (g) concentration deficit may be evident on clinical testing Objective evidence of memory deficit is obtained only with an intensive interview conducted by a trained geriatric psychiatrist or neuropsychologist Decreased patient performance is apparent in demanding employment and social settings Denial begins to become manifest in the patient; mild to moderate anxiety accompanies symptoms
4. Moderate cognitive decline	Late confusional	Clear-cut deficit is apparent on careful interview; deficit manifests in the following areas: (a) decreased knowledge of current and recent events, (b) difficulty remembering one's personal history, (c) concentration deficit elicited on serial subtractions, and (d) decreased ability to travel, handle finances, and so on

(continued)

TABLE 11.1. (continued)
Global Deterioration Scale

Stage	Clinical Phase	Clinical Characteristics
		Frequently, no deficit is apparent in the following areas: (a) orientation to time and person, (b) recognition of familiar person and faces, and (c) ability to travel to familiar locations
		The patient is unable to perform complex tasks; denial is the dominant defense mechanism
		Flattening of affect and withdrawal from challenging situations occur
5. Moderately severe cognitive decline	Early dementia	Patient can no longer survive without some assistance
		Patients are unable during interview to recall a major relevant aspect of their current lives [e.g., their addresses or telephone numbers of many years, the names of close members of their families (such as grandchildren), or the names of the high schools or colleges from which they graduated]
		Frequently, some disorientation to time (date, day of week, season, etc.) or to place is present
		An educated person may have difficulty counting back from 40 by 4s or from 20 by 2s; persons at this stage retain knowledge of many major facts regarding themselves and others; they invariably know their own names and generally know their spouse's and children's names
		They require no assistance with toileting or eating but may have some difficulty in choosing the proper clothing to wear and may occasionally clothe themselves improperly (e.g., putting shoes on the wrong feet, etc.)
6. Severe cognitive decline	Middle dementia	They may occasionally forget the name of the spouse on whom they are entirely dependent for survival
		They will be largely unaware of all recent events and experiences in their lives
		They may retain some knowledge of their past lives but this is very sketchy
		They are generally unaware of their surroundings, the year, the season, and so on
		They may have difficulty in counting from 10, both backward and sometimes forward; they will require some assistance with activities of daily living (e.g., may become incontinent, will require travel assistance but occasionally will display ability to travel to familiar locations)

(continued)

TABLE 11.1. (continued)
Global Deterioration Scale

Stage	Clinical Phase	Clinical Characteristics
		Diurnal rhythms are frequently disturbed
		They almost always recall their own names
		They frequently continue to be able to distinguish familiar from unfamiliar persons in their own environment
		Personality and emotional changes occur; these are quite variable and include (a) delusional behavior (e.g., patients may accuse their spouses of being impostors, may talk to imaginary figures in the environment or to their own reflection in the mirror); (b) obsessive symptoms (e.g., person may continually repeat simple cleaning activities); (c) anxiety symptoms such as agitation may be present, and even previously nonexistent violent behavior may occur; and (d) cognitive abulia (e.g., loss of willpower because one cannot carry a thought long enough to determine a purposeful course of action)
7. Very severe cognitive decline	Late dementia	All verbal abilities are lost; frequently, there is no speech at all—only grunting
		They are incontinent of urine and require assistance in toileting and feeding
		They lose basic psychomotor skills (e.g., ability to walk); the brain appears to no longer be able to tell the body what to do
		Generalized cortical neurological signs and symptoms are frequently present

Source: Reisberg, Ferris, de Leon, and Crook (1982).

who has lost interest in initiating activities, engages in little meaningful activity, and deteriorates into a shell of a person can truly be experiencing any one of the three Ds. To further confuse matters, depressed older adults frequently complain about difficulties with attention, problem-solving competence, or memory that generate concern for family members as well as the patients themselves.

Contrary to popular belief, diagnosable depression is less common in older adults than in young adults. A very small percentage of community-dwelling older adults meet criteria for the most severe depression (Major Depressive Disorder) with only 1% experiencing the disorder during a 1-year period (Blazer, 1994; Wolfe, Morrow, & Fredrickson, 1996). Chronic, lower intensity depression (dysthymia) is found in 2% of older persons. Not surprisingly, prevalence rates are considerably higher in outpatient clinics, institutional settings, and hospitals (Blazer, 1994). Of considerable interest to clinicians and researchers, prevalence rates for minor, or subsyndromal depressions are quite high among older adults (20–30%). In other words, although older adults are less likely than younger adults to meet criteria for depressive disorders, there is a higher likelihood that older adults will experience a low level or subsyndromal depression that affects their pleasure in life but lacks the intensity required for formal diagnosis.

The causes of depression are multiple, and likely vary across individuals. Biological theories focus on genetic evidence and evidence of biochemical changes in the brains of depressed persons. Genetic evidence is drawn from family concordance studies that consistently report higher rates of depression in relatives of depressed persons than would be expected based on the base rate in the population. Similar data are now available for older adults, in which genetic factors account for approximately 30% of the variance in depression among aging twins (Gatz, Pedersen, Plomin, & Nesselroade, 1992). The second set of biological theories focuses on the biochemical changes in the brain that are believed to contribute to depression. In particular, the brains of persons who are depressed tend not to use neurotransmitters, such as catecholamines (e.g., norepinephrine) and indolamines (e.g., serotonin), effectively. With advanced age, structural and functional changes in the brain appear to compromise the very systems that manage the depression-related neurotransmitters leading some to believe that age predisposes persons to depression (Alexopoulos, 1993). However, the lower incidence of depression in older versus younger adults does not support that notion. Evidence for the biological factors as causal are limited to correlational studies of depression symptoms and brain changes, and evidence of the effectiveness of antidepressant medications. No biological markers of depression are yet available, nor is the evidence for the causal impact of biological changes in the brain as tight as is often believed.

The social factors that affect older adults' risk for depression have been organized by George (1994) into six categories. The first category includes demographic characteristics that demonstrate differential risk for depression. The second and third categories represent events and achievements that are distinguished from each other by their time referent (early or later in the life span). The fourth category contains potential risk factors that have been less commonly researched, but that are considered to hold considerable potential. The last two categories contain risk factors that have received the most research attention, with the distinction between the two categories primarily one of specificity (category six being the more specific). The specific variables that fall within these six categories have shown significant relationships to depression in many studies, although the effect is somewhat weaker in older adults than in younger. No single variable explains huge amounts of the variance in depression, but taken together, the variables represent a substantial set of causal factors.

Other causal factors include functional disabilities resulting from physical illness (Lichtenberg, 1994; Zeiss, Lewinsohn, Rohde, & Seeley, 1996), personality (Costa & McCrae, 1994), and institutionalization (Parmalee, Katz, & Lawton, 1989). Many physical illnesses create functional disabilities that restrict activity patterns and alter conceptions of self and self-worth. In addition, medications used to treat illnesses can produce depression as a byproduct of the biological changes characteristic of the illness or secondary to the medication used to treat the physical illness. For example, cardiovascular disease and a commonly described treatment for it, antihypertensive medications, both are known risk factors for depression (Cohen-Cole, 1989; Hurst, 1986). Personality is also a plausible contributor to depression. Based on evidence of long-term stability in trait characteristics, some argue that depressive traits are enduring personality characteristics that predispose individuals to clinical levels of depression (Costa & McCrae, 1994). Depression as a trait does not appear to increase in prevalence with age, nor does the prevalence of the clinical disorder. Personality data argue against conceptualizing depression as a discrete psychiatric disorder within a disease model. Instead, interindividual differences in personality are postulated to produce higher or lower intensity of depression symptoms. Institutionalization is another risk factor. Variations in the rate of depression across housing settings consistently show the highest rate of depression among older adults is in long term care (Ames, 1991). Institutional settings remove many elements of control that appear to be vital to mental well-being, thus resulting in induced dependency (Horgas, Wahl, & Baltes, 1996) that creates vulnerability to depression.

Depression can be assessed with self-report screening instruments or clinical interview. A clinical interview is necessary to establish a diagnosis, although self-report instruments are useful for screening purposes or to establish the intensity of distress. Many of the commonly used self-report instruments have been validated on older adults and norms are available for older adults living in a variety of contexts (e.g., nursing home, hospital, community-dwelling). For example, the Beck Depression Inventory (Beck, Ward, Mendelsohn, Mock, & Erbaugh, 1961) has been used extensively with older persons (Gallagher, 1986). A simpler self-report format is available in the Center for Epidemiological Studies Depression Scale (Radloff, 1977; Radloff & Teri, 1986) and the Geriatric Depression Scale (GDS) (Table 11.2; Yesavage, et al., 1983). The GDS is a popular instrument because it was designed for use with older adults and all items are appropriate for older adults. Although most clinicians conduct diagnostic interviews in an unstructured format, structured interviews such as the Structured Clinical Interview for DSM-IV (SCID; First, Spitzer, Gibbon, & Williams, 1995) provide a more rigorous evaluation of diagnostic classification.

Another purpose for assessment of depression is to generate information and a baseline for treatment planning and evaluation. Specific approaches to intervention require more specific assessment tools for these purposes. For example, the behavioral model of depression requires detailed assessment of daily mood and frequency of pleasant and unpleasant activities (Lewinsohn et al.,

TABLE 11.2.
Geriatric Depression Scale

Question	Yes	No
1. Are you basically satisfied with your life?	0	1
2. Have you dropped many of your activities and interests?	1	0
3. Do you feel your life is empty?	1	0
4. Do you get bored often?	1	0
5. Are you hopeful about the future?	0	1
6. Are you bothered by thoughts you can't get out of your head?	1	0
7. Are you in good spirits most of the time?	0	1
8. Are you afraid that something bad is going to happen to you?	1	0
9. Do you feel happy most of the time?	0	1
10. Do you often feel helpless?	1	0
11. Do you often get restless and fidgety?	1	0
12. Do you prefer to stay at home, rather than going out and doing new things?	1	0
13. Do you frequently worry about the future?	1	0
14. Do you feel you have more problems with memory than most?	1	0
15. Do you think it is wonderful to be alive now?	0	1
16. Do you often feel downhearted and blue?	1	0
17. Do you feel pretty worthless the way you are now?	1	0
18. Do you worry a lot about the past?	1	0
19. Do you find life very exciting?	0	1
20. Is it hard for you to get started on new projects?	1	0
21. Do you feel full of energy?	0	1
22. Do you feel that your situation is hopeless?	1	0
23. Do you think that most people are better off than you are now?	1	0
24. Do you frequently get upset about little things?	1	0
25. Do you frequently feel like crying?	1	0
26. Do you have trouble concentrating?	1	0
27. Do you enjoy getting up in the morning?	0	1
28. Do you prefer to avoid social gatherings?	1	0
29. Is it easy for you to make decisions?	0	1
30. Is your mind as clear as it used to be?	0	1

1984), whereas the cognitive approach to intervention requires detailed assessment of specific thoughts that are linked with depression (Thompson, 1996).

Clinical trials have established that treatment for depression is as effective for older adults as younger adults, with no one therapy being obviously superior to others. Across treatment modalities, approximately 50–70% of older adults with Major Depressive Disorder are treated successfully within 12–20 sessions (Rush et al., 1993). For psychosocial interventions, the effectiveness of psychological interventions for depression is quite high (0.79; Scogin & McElreath, 1994).

Depression is most commonly treated pharmacologically, because most treatment of depression is done by general physicians rather than mental health specialists. The range of available antidepressant medications has increased rapidly in recent decades. The tricyclic antidepressants (e.g., Imipramine) address primarily the norepinephrine and serontonin concentrations in the brain. Their side effects make them a drug to use cautiously with older persons because of the risks of sedation, undesirable cardiovascular effects, postural hypotension, and confusion. The Serotonin Selective Reuptake Inhibitors (SSRIs; e.g., Prozac, Paxil, and Zoloft) that target the serotonergic systems of the brain increase concentrations of that neurotransmitter while producing relatively few side effects. Currently, SSRIs are considered the first line medication choice for older adults (Newhouse, 1996). Monoamine oxidase inhibitors (MAO inhibitors) are effective with older adults, but require dietary restrictions that make them somewhat inconvenient. Their mechanism for treatment is unclear. Pharmacologic treatment effects are evident at about 12 weeks (Reynolds et al., 1992). Because depression is often a recurring problem, current research is establishing guidelines for maintenance therapies for persons to try to innoculate against future episodes (Reynolds, Frank, Perel, Mazumdar, & Kupfer, 1995).

Psychosocial interventions for treating depression show a similar or slightly better rate of effectiveness as the pharmacological treatments, but without the risk of side effects (Zeiss & Breckenridge, 1997). Empirically validated treatments for depression that also have been tested in clinical trials with older persons include behavior therapy, cognitive therapy, cognitive-behavioral therapy, interpersonal psychotherapy, and brief psychodynamic psychotherapy (Niederehe, 1994; Teri, Curtis, Gallagher-Thompson, & Thompson, 1994). Behavior therapy focuses on increasing the rate and pleasantness of pleasant events while decreasing the rate and unpleasantness of negative events and effective problem solving (Arean, Perri, Nezu, Schein, Christopher, & Joseph, 1993; Gallagher, Thompson, Baffa, Piatt, Ringering, & Stone, 1981; Lewinsohn et al., 1984; Thompson, Gallagher, & Breckenridge, 1987). Cognitive therapy attempts to eliminate depression-inducing cognitive models and automatic thoughts (Beck, Rush, Shaw, & Emery, 1979). Cognitive-behavioral therapy uses behavioral interventions and cognitive interventions to alter cognitions, behaviors, and emotions (Gallagher-Thompson & Thompson, 1996; Thompson, 1996). Interpersonal psychotherapy addresses four themes considered core to depression within the psychodynamic model: grief, interpersonal disputes, role transitions, and interpersonal deficit (Klerman et al., 1984; Sloane, Staples, & Schneider, 1985). The brief psychodynamic therapy that has been tested empirically with older adults is that of Horowitz and colleagues that focuses on responses to trauma (Horowitz & Kaltreider, 1979; Thompson, Gallagher, & Breckenridge, 1987). Other treatment modalities have also demonstrated promise, such as bibliotherapy (Scoggin, Jamison, & Davis, 1990) and reminiscence (Butler, 1974; Arean et al., 1993). Successful outcomes have also been demonstrated with medically ill outpatients and for inpatients (Zeiss & Breckenridge, 1997).

With the range of effective treatments available, how does one select a treatment to use? Guidelines now available from the Agency for Health Care Policy and Research (AHCPR) recommend medication as the first line of intervention because of the greater numbers of research studies demonstrating efficacy of medications, and attitudinal barriers to using psychotherapy among current older adults. The AHCPR guidelines suggest that medications should be chosen based on the following criteria: side effects, prior history of response to medication, history of first-degree relatives' response to medication, concurrent medications and illnesses that generate risk, likeliness of adherence to a medication regimen, interference with life style, cost, and preference (Rush et al., 1993). Psychological treatments may be selected based on the availability of a provider trained to treat older adults and trained to use a modality that is demonstrated to be effective, the client's preference, and the symptom profile.

The choice of medications versus psychosocial treatment has generated considerable controversy since the AHCPR guidelines were released, however. Zeiss and Breckenridge (1997) critique the recommendation to use medication as the first approach to treatment and present a well-reasoned argument for using psychosocial treatments instead. They demonstrate that the number of controlled outcome studies testing the efficacy of medications is actually the same as that for psychosocial treatment, with the same success rates. However, maintenance treatment is not shown to be necessary with psychosocial therapy (cognitive-behavioral therapy, in particular). Furthermore, surveys of the attitudes of older adults show that they prefer psychosocial treatment to medication (Rokke & Scoggin, 1995).

Other Mental Disorders and Concerns

Anxiety. Epidemiological data from community samples show that the prevalence of anxiety is much higher than previously believed, although still lower than is found in younger adults (Blazer, George, & Hughes, 1991; Himmelfarb & Murrell, 1984; Myers et al., 1984). The prevalence rates are somewhat controversial, ranging from 6 to 33%. Even at the lowest estimate, anxiety disorders are more prevalent than other disorders that are popularly believed to be more common (e.g., depression). The DSM-IV (American Psychiatric

Association, 1994) classification system for anxiety disorders includes 12 categories of disorders, including those listed here (in order of decreasing prevalence): phobias, generalized anxiety disorders, panic, obsessive-compulsive disorders, and posttraumatic stress disorder. As was the case for depression, older adults who do not meet criteria for the anxiety disorders still tend to report significant anxiety symptoms, generating concern that there may be either a subsyndromal anxiety condition or that older persons' tendency to underreport psychological symptoms leads to the lower prevalence of disorders (Blazer et al., 1991).

Anxiety disorders are particularly challenging to differentially diagnose because of the overlapping presentation of anxiety, depression, and physical illness. There are likely multiple directions in the causal relationships among these three kinds of disorders. That is, anxiety can exacerbate physical disorders (e.g., cardiac disease) or may be caused by physical disease or physiological responses to medications. Anxiety commonly cooccurs with depression, and the two classes of disorders share several symptoms in common. Indeed, the degree of overlap between depression and anxiety leads some to argue that they may reflect a single underlying disorder (Sheikh, 1992). Dementias often produce a restlessness or agitation that may be a unique type of anxiety, or may be simply a direct result of the disease's effect on the brain.

Anxiety has been conceptualized as being caused by biomedical, psychological, and social factors, similarly for younger and older adults. Theories of biological etiology of anxiety are far less well developed than the biological theories of depression. The evidence for variations in neurotransmitter concentrations in the brains of anxious older adults is quite inconsistent and thus inconclusive. Aging-related changes in brain function and structure also do not mimic the changes demonstrated in the brains of anxious younger or older adults. Thus, the biological models have yet to be developed into viable theories, and there is no reason at this point to believe that aging will play a unique role in any biological basis for anxiety.

Other hypothesized causes of anxiety in older adults include depression, medical illness, medication, environmental stressors, personality disorder, early onset dementing disorders, and other psychopathological disorders (e.g., paranoia, hypochondriasis) and substance abuse withdrawal (Shamoian, 1991). To date, the causes of anxiety disorders have received amazingly little research, especially within older adults, yielding little conclusive evidence for any particular etiology.

Assessment of anxiety disorders relies on clinical interviews, of which the structured forms such as the *Structured Clinical Interview for DSM IV Axis I Disorders—Version 2* (SCID-I/P; First et al., 1995) produce high reliability. Self-reporting ratings scales, such as the State-Trait Anxiety Inventory (Spielberger, Gorsuch, & Lushene, 1970) or the Beck Anxiety Inventory (Beck, Epstein, Brown, & Steer, 1988) are useful screening tools that are sensitive to the presence of clinical disorders although they do not result in a specific diagnosis. Unfortunately, norms for older adults are not available for most of these tests, and most fail to discriminate well between depression and anxiety (Sheikh, 1991).

Interventions for anxiety disorders in older adults are reported in the case study literature, but relatively few have been tested in rigorous clinical trials (Niederehe & Schneider, 1998). The benzodiazepines (e.g., Xanax or Valium), which are prescribed for over 50% of older adults experiencing anxiety, are the most frequently used intervention (Markovitz, 1993; Salzman, 1991). Other medications are also used (Buspirone, beta-blockers, antidepressants), with little data other than clinical reports to recommend them. These drugs should be used with great caution in older adults, because older adults metabolize medications idiosyncratically, leading to an increased risk of adverse drug reactions and to difficulties in conducting well-controlled clinical trials (Markovitz, 1993).

The database documenting the effectiveness of psychosocial interventions is also minimal. Treatment strategies for anxiety have been developed within the cognitive-behavioral model (Acierno, Hersen, & Van Hasselt, 1996), and the psychodynamic model (Verwoerdt, 1981), and from a more eclectic approach (Knight, 1992). Stanley, Beck, and Glassco (1997) report on the successful use of cognitive-behavioral therapy (CBT) and supportive psychotherapy for Generalized Anxiety Disorder in community-residing older adults. Using a small group format over a 14-week trial, the treatments produced significant decreases in worry, anxiety, and depression at posttreatment. The treatment gains were maintained at 6 month follow-up with additional gains in worry. This first controlled clinical trial of psychotherapeutic interventions with anxiety shows promise that needs to be extended in other rigorous clinical trials.

Substance Abuse.   Substance abuse with older adults is focused on a different set of substances than those abused by younger adults, with the exception of alcohol (Atkinson, Ganzini, & Bernstein, 1992). Older adults are less likely to abuse illegal drugs and more likely to misuse or abuse prescription medications and over-the-counter medications, as compared with younger adults. The impact of the substance abuse problem is no less serious, however, with alcohol and substance abuse ranking third among leading mental disorders in older Americans. Indeed, substance abuse accounts for 10–12% of those who receive services from mental health professionals (Segal, Van Hasselt, Hersen, & King, 1996).

Abuse of medications intended for therapeutic use is an equally serious area of concern. Older adults receive 30% of all prescribed medications and consume 40% of all over-the-counter (OTC) medications (HHS Inspector General, 1989). These high usage rates do not necessarily indicate abuse or misuse patterns, but certainly establish a vulnerability to substance-induced symptoms and disorders.

Cross-sectional comparisons of younger and older alcohol abusers inevitably confound patterns characteristic of a particular birth cohort with changes that may occur with age. Longitudinal data suggest that alcohol abuse patterns are relatively stable across the life span, although late onset alcohol abuse is also a serious problem. More recent birth cohorts use significantly more alcohol than earlier born cohorts. With expectations of stable use across the life span, alcohol abuse can be expected to be an even more prevalent problem among older adults in future decades.

The main barriers to identifying substance abuse in older adults result from denial of use and difficulty determining the exact amount of a substance that will result in intoxication. The tendency to deny use is consistent across adults of all ages, although the motivation for denial may vary. Denial can result from either a desire not to acknowledge the amount of a substance used or ignorance of the potential impact of substances on health (e.g., commonly used OTCs, such as laxatives or cold remedies, are often unrecognized as a potential source of misuse or abuse). The effects of chemical substances are particularly difficult to measure in older bodies because of the effects of aging on drug metabolism. The principles noted above with regard to antidepressants are pertinent to this discussion as well. Substances are metabolized idiosyncratically in older bodies, making appropriate dosages difficult to determine. Older adults who use prescribed and OTC medications report that they use them primarily to help cope with pain, insomnia, family problems, and other mental disorders (Finlayson, 1984). Professionals working with older adults need to be familiar with the impact of the most innocent of substances (e.g., aspirin) that can adversely affect mental and physical health (Smyer & Downs, 1995). Margaret's delirium symptoms that were described earlier are quite likely to be caused and exacerbated by the multiple medications she takes. Certainly, substance abuse and misuse and adverse drug reactions would be key foci of the assessment she needs.

Assessment of substance abuse is primarily done through clinical interviews. Unfortunately, the information usually has to be drawn out of the clients who do not want to report accurately their usage patterns. Self-report scales can be used to assess alcohol abuse [e.g., the Geriatric version of the Michigan Alcohol Screening Test (Blow et al., 1992) or the CAGE (Mayfield, McLeod, & Hall, 1974)], although self-report is particularly vulnerable to the effects of social desirability and denial. A structured behavioral assessment tool is also available (Gerontology Alcohol Project Drinking Profile; Dupree, Broskowski, & Schonfeld, 1984). Obviously, collateral reports are critical, because often it is the family member (as was the case with Margaret's son) who notices the change in behavior or the patterns of inappropriate usage. In addition, care must be taken to identify substance abuse and misuse patterns in older adults that may not fit well with the current DSM-IV classification criteria (Segal et al., 1996).

Treatment of substance abuse focuses on three goals: stabilizing and reducing substance consumption, treatment of coexisting problems, and arrangement of appropriate social interventions (Atkinson et al., 1992). With older adults, education is deemed a more useful tool than confrontation. Recent research on increasing medication compliance by altering the presentation of drug usage information (Park, Willis, Morrow, Diehl, & Gaines, 1994) may ultimately be useful in designing treatment programs for substance misuse due to misunderstanding of medications. Treatments designed to address coexisting problems draw on established methods of problem-solving therapies (e.g., Dupree & Schonfeld, 1996) and alcohol intervention studies (Janik & Dunham, 1983). Alcohol intervention research does show the benefit of using aging-specific groups rather than mixed-age groups to treat older alcohol abusers (e.g., Kashner, Rodell, Ogden, Guggenheim, & Karson, 1992).

Conclusion

The physiological, social, and psychological processes of aging require substantial adaptation in order to maintain optimum mental health and well-being. The case example of James and Claire illustrates the wide-ranging impact of physical illness, relocation, retirement, and functional impairments on mental well-being. Normative events, such as illness of one's spouse that Lonnie experienced, as well as nonnormative events, such as the untimely death of a loved one that Jeanette experienced, evoke specific stress-related responses that render a person more vulnerable to mental disorders. Of course, the vast majority of older adults cope with the challenges of aging and life's more distressing events successfully. As is clear by the fact that this chapter presents more materials on disorders than on mental well-being, much more research needs to be done to document the strategies of successful coping and adaptation and their outcomes that we call mental health and well-being.

One big surprise of the last couple of decades of research on mental disorders came from the epidemiological data that dispelled some myths about the inevitability of mental disorders in later life. Prevalence rates for disorders such as depression were much lower than anticipated, indeed were lower than for other age groups of adults. On the other hand, certain disorders appear more often than had been expected. For example, prevalence rates for anxiety were surprisingly higher than for depression, and the rates of cognitive impairment in nursing homes were extremely high. Finally, we are still struggling with some important questions about what is a disorder, as subclinical rates continue to appear with higher frequency than expected.

Assessment continues to be a challenge as the need to differentiate mental disorders from each other and from physical illnesses challenges researchers and clinicians alike. Differential diagnoses are often challenging because the essence of the entities being differentiated are not well-bounded constructs. In only a few areas are there assessment devices that are uniquely appropriate for older adults because they take into account special social, psychological, and biological conditions of either age or of this cohort. However, most tools that were developed for other adult populations appear to be valid with older persons as well. Again, much work remains to be done, but clinicians and researchers already have very useful assessment tools and strategies available to them.

Psychosocial and pharmacological treatments are currently available to assist older adults with most mental disorders. Each of the case examples presented in this chapter could benefit from a currently available treatment with demonstrated validity. There is certainly much work ahead—there are only one or two empirically tested approaches to treatment for many disorders. The field relies currently on adaptations of traditional treatment approaches to the needs and problems of older adults. As we come to know more about normal and optimal aging, new approaches to promoting well-being among older adults are also likely to emerge.

REVIEW QUESTIONS

1. What makes it challenging to differentiate dementia from delirium and depression?

2. Describe an assessment strategy that might differentiate dementia, delirium, and depression.

3. What cautions should be considered when using pharmacological interventions for mental disorders in older adults?

4. Describe common myths about mental well-being and mental disorders in older adults that have been demonstrated to be false in the empirical literature.

5. How does the aging process complicate efforts to define mental well-being in older adults?

References

Acierno, R., Hersen, M., & Van Hasselt, V. B. (1996). Anxiety-based disorders. In M. Hersen & V. B. Van Hasselt (Eds.), *Psychological treatment of older adults* (pp. 149–180). New York: Plenum.

Alexopoulos, G. S. (1993). Biological correlates of late-life depression. In L. S. Schneider, C. F. Reynolds, B. D. Lebowitz, & A. J. Friedhoff (Eds.), *Diagnosis and treatment of depression in late life* (pp. 101–116). Washington, DC: American Psychiatric Association.

American Psychiatric Association. (1994). *Diagnostic and statistical manual of mental disorders* (4th ed.). Washington, DC: American Psychiatric Association.

Ames, D. (1991). Epidemiological studies of depression among the elderly in residential homes and nursing homes. *International Journal of Geriatric Psychiatry, 6*, 347–354.

Aneshensel, C. S., Pearlin, L. I., Mullan, J. T., Zarit, S. H., & Whitlatch, C. J. (1995). *Profiles in caregiving*. San Diego, CA: Academic Press.

Arean, P. A., Perri, M. G., Nezu, A. M., Schein, R. L., Christopher, F., & Joseph, T. X. (1993). Comparative effectiveness of social problem-solving therapy and reminiscence therapy as treatments for depression in older adults. *Journal of Consulting and Clinical Psychology, 61,* 1003–1010.

Atkinson, R. M., Ganzini, L., & Bernstein, M. J. (1992). Alcohol and substance-use disorders in the elderly. In J. E. Birren, R. B. Sloane, & G. D. Cohen (Eds.), *Handbook of mental health and aging* (2nd ed., pp. 515–555). San Diego, CA: Academic Press.

Baltes, P. B., & Baltes, M. M. (1990). Psychological perspectives on successful aging: The model of selective optimization with compensation. In P. B. Baltes & M. M. Baltes (Eds.), *Successful aging: Perspectives from the behavioral sciences* (pp. 1–34). Cambridge, England: Cambridge University Press.

Beck, A. T., Epstein, N., Brown, G., & Steer, R. (1988). An inventory for measuring clinical anxiety: Psychometric properties. *Journal of Consulting and Clinical Psychology, 56,* 893–897.

Beck, A. T., Rush, J., Shaw, B., & Emery, G. (1979). *Cognitive therapy of depression.* New York: Guilford Press.

Beck, A. T., Ward, C. H., Mendelson, M., Mock, J., & Erbaugh, J. (1961). An inventory for measuring depression. *Archives of General Psychiatry, 4,* 561–571.

Birren, J. E., & Renner, V. J. (1980). Concepts and issues of mental health and aging. In J. E. Birren & R. B. Sloane (Eds.), *Handbook of mental health and aging* (pp. 3–33). Englewood Cliffs, NJ: Prentice-Hall.

Blazer, D. G. (1994). Epidemiology of late-life depression. In L. S. Schneider, C. F. Reynolds, B. D. Lebowitz, & A. J. Friedhoff (Eds.). *Diagnosis and treatment of depression in late life* (pp. 9–19). Washington, DC: American Psychiatric Association.

Blazer, D., George, L. K., & Hughes, D. (1991). The epidemiology of anxiety disorders: An age comparison. In C. Salzman & B. D. Lebowitz (Eds.), *Anxiety in the elderly: Treatment and research* (pp. 17–30). New York: Springer.

Blow, F. C., Brower, J. K., Sculenberg, J. E., Demo-Dananberg, L. M., Young, K. J., & Beresford, T. P. (1992). MAST-Geriatric Version (MAST-G): A new elderly specific screening instrument. *Alcoholism, 16,* 372.

Butler, R. (1974). Successful aging and the role of life review. *Journal of the American Geriatrics Society, 22,* 529–535.

Canadian Study of Health and Aging Working Group. (1994). Canadian Study of Health and Aging: Study methods and prevalence of dementia. *Canadian Medical Association Journal, 150,* 899–912.

Cohen-Cole, S. A. (1989). Depression in heart disease. In R. G. Robinson & P. V. Rabins (Eds.), *Depression in coexisting disease* (pp. 27–39). New York: Igaku-Shoin.

Costa, P. T., & McCrae, R. R. (1994). Depression as an enduring disposition. In L. S. Schneider, C. F. Reynolds, B. D. Lebowitz, & A. J. Friedhoff (Eds.), *Diagnosis and treatment of depression in late life* (pp. 155–167). Washington, DC: American Psychiatric Association.

Cummings, J. L., & Benson, D. F. (1992). *Dementia: A clinical approach* (2nd ed.). Boston: Butterworth-Heinemann.

Dupree, L. W., Broskowski, H., & Schonfeld, L. (1984). The Gerontology Alcohol Project: A behavioral treatment program for elderly alcohol abusers. *The Gerontologist, 24,* 510–516.

Dupree, L. W., & Schonfeld, L. (1996). Substance abuse. In M. Hersen & V. B. Van Hasselt (Eds.), *Psychological treatment of older adults* (pp. 281–297). New York: Plenum.

Erikson, E. H., Erikson, J. M., & Kivnik, H. Q. (1986). *Vital involvement in old age.* New York: Norton.

Finlayson, R. E. (1984). Prescription drug abuse in older persons. In R. M. Atkinson (Ed.), *Alcohol and drug abuse in old age* (pp. 61–70). Washington, DC: American Psychiatric Association.

First, M. B., Spitzer, R. L., Gibbon, M., & Williams, J. B. W. (1995). *The Structured Clinical Interview for Axis I DSM-IV Disorders—Patient Edition* (SCID-I/P, version 2.0). New York: New York State Psychiatric Institute, Biometrics Research Department.

Folstein, M. F., Bassett, S. S., Romanoski, A. J., & Nestadt, G. (1991). The epidemiology of delirium in the community: The Eastern Baltimore Mental Health Survey. *International Psychogeriatrics, 3,* 169–176.

Gallagher, D. (1986). Assessment of depression by interview methods and psychiatric rating scales. In L. W. Poon (ed.), *Handbook for clinical memory assessment of older adults* (pp. 202–212). Washington, DC: American Psychological Association.

Gallagher-Thompson, D., & Thompson, L. W. (1996). Applying cognitive-behavioral therapy to the psychological problems of later life. In S. H. Zarit & B. G. Knight (Eds.), *A guide to psychotherapy and aging* (pp. 61–82). Washington, DC: American Psychological Association.

Gallagher, D., Thompson, L. W., Baffa, G., Piatt, C., Ringering, L., & Stone, V. (1981). *Depression in the elderly: A behavioral treatment manual.* Los Angeles: University of Southern California Press.

Gatz, M., Kasl-Godley, J. E., & Karel, M. (1996). Aging and mental disorders. In J. E. Birren & K. W. Schaie (Eds.), *Handbook of the psychology of aging* (4th ed., pp. 365–382). San Diego, CA: Academic Press.

Gatz, M., Pederson, N. L., Plomin, R., & Nesselroade, J. R. (1992). Importance of shared genes and shared environments for symptoms of depression in older adults. *Journal of Abnormal Psychology, 101,* 701–708.

George, L. K. (1994). Social factors and depression in late life. In L. S. Schneider, C. F. Reynolds, B. D. Lebowitz, & A. J. Friedhoff (Eds.), *Diagnosis and treatment of depression in late life* (pp. 131–153). Washington, DC: American Psychiatric Association.

HHS Inspector General, U. S. Department of Health and Human Services. (1989). *Expenses incurred by medical beneficiaries of prescription drugs.* Washington, DC: U. S. Department of Health and Human Services.

Himmelfarb, S., & Murrell, S. A. (1984). Prevalence and correlates of anxiety symptoms in older adults. *Journal of Psychology, 116,* 159–167.

Horgas, A. L., Wahl, H., & Baltes, M. M. (1996). Dependency in late life. In L. L. Carstensen, B. A. Edelstein, & L. Dornbrand (Eds.), *The practical handbook of clinical gerontology* (pp. 54–76). Thousand Oaks, CA: Sage.

Horowitz, M., & Kaltreider, N. (1979). Brief therapy of the stress response syndrome. *Psychiatric Clinics of North America, 2,* 265–377.

Hurst, J. W. (1986). *The heart.* New York: McGraw-Hill.

Jahoda, M. (1958). *Current concepts of positive mental health.* New York: Basic Books.

Janik, S. W., & Durham, R. C. (1983). A nationwide examination of the need for specific alcoholism treatment programs for the elderly. *Journal of Studies on Alcohol, 4,* 307–317.

Jorm, A. F., Korten, A. E., & Henderson, A. S. (1987). The prevalence of dementia: A quantitative integration of the literature. *Acta Psychiatrica Scandinavica, 76,* 465–479.

Kashner, T. M., Rodell, D. E., Ogden, S. R., Guggenheim, F. G., & Karson, C. N. (1992). Outcomes and costs of two VA inpatient treatment programs for older alcoholic patients. *Hospital and Community Psychiatry, 43,* 958–989.

Klerman, G. L., Weissman, M. M., Rounsaville, B. J., & Chevron, E. (1984). *Interpersonal psychotherapy of depression.* New York: Basic Books.

Knight, B. G. (1992). *Older adults in psychotherapy: case histories.* Newberry Park, CA: Sage.

Lewinsoh, P., Antonuccio, D. O., Steinmetz, J. L., et al. (1984). *The coping with depression course.* Eugene, OR: Castalia.

Lichtenberg, P. A. (1994). *A guide to psychological practice in geriatric long-term care.* New York: Haworth Press.

Markovitz, P. J. (1993). Treatment of anxiety in the elderly. *Journal of Clinical Psychiatry, 54* (Suppl.), 64–68.

Marsiske, M., Lang, F. R., Baltes, P. B., & Baltes, M. M. (1995). Selective optimization with compensation: Life-span perspectives on successful human development. In R. A. Dixon & L. Backman (Eds.), *Compensating for psychological deficits and declines: Managing losses and promoting gains* (pp. 35–79). Mahwah, NJ: Erlbaum.

Mayfield, D., McLeod, G., & Hall, P. (1974). The CAGE questionnaire: Validation of a new alcoholism screening instrument. *American Journal of Psychiatry, 131,* 1121–1123.

Mittelman, M. S., Ferris, S. H., Steinberg, G., Shulman, E., Mackell, J. A., Ambinder, A., & Cohen, J. (1993). An intervention that delays institutionalization of Alzheimer's disease patients. *Gerontologist, 33,* 730–740.

Myers, J. K., Weissman, M. M., Tischler, G. L., Holzer, C. E., Lear, P. J., Orvaschel, H., Anthony, J. C., Boyd, J. H., Burke, J. D., Kramer, M., & Stolzman, R. (1984). Six month prevalence of psychiatric disorders in three communities: 1980–1982. *Archives of General Psychiatry, 41,* 959–967.

Newhouse, P. A. (1996). Use of serotonin selective reuptake inhibitors in geriatric depression. *Journal of Clinical Psychiatry, 57* (Suppl. 5), 12–22.

Niederehe, G. (1994). Psychosocial therapies with depressed older adults. In L. S. Schneider, C. F. Reynolds, B. D. Lebowitz, & A. J. Friedhoff (Eds.), *Diagnosis and treatment of depression in late life* (pp. 293–315). Washington, DC: American Psychiatric Association.

Niederehe, G. & Schneider, L. S. (1998). Treatment of depression and anxiety in the aged. In P. E. Nathan & J. M. Gorman (Eds.), *Treatments that work* (pp. 270–287). New York: Oxford University Press.

Park, D. C., Willis, S. L., Morrow, D., Diehl, M., & Gaines, C. L. (1994). Cognitive function and medication usage in older adults. *Journal of Applied Gerontology, 13,* 39–57.

Parmalee, P. A., Katz, I. R., & Lawton, M. P. (1989). Depression among institutionalized aged: Assessment and prevalence estimation. *Journal of Gerontology, 44,* M22–M29.

Pollock, B. G., Perel, J. M., Altieri, L. P., & Kirshner, M. (1992). Debrisoquine hydroxylation phenotyping in geriatric psychopharmacology. *Psychopharmacology Bulletin, 28,* 163–167.

Radloff, L. (1977). The CES-D Scale: A self-report depression scale for research in the general population. *Applied Psychological Measurement, 1,* 385–401.

Radloff, L., & Teri, L. (1986). Use of the Center for Epidemiological Studies—Depression scale with older adults. *Clinical Gerontologist, 5,* 119–135.

Reisberg, B., Ferris, S. H., De Leon, M. J., & Crook, T. (1982). The global deterioration scale for assessment of primary degenerative dementia. *American Journal of Psychiatry, 139,* 1136–1139.

Reynolds, C. F., Frank, E., Perel, J. M., Miller, M. D., Cornes, C., Rifai, A. H., Pollock, B. G., Mazum dar, S., George, C. J., Houck, P. R., & Kupfer, D. J. (1992). Combined pharmacotherapy and psychotherapy in the acute and continuation treatment of elderly patients with recurrent major depression: A preliminary report. *American Journal of Psychiatry, 149,* 1687–1692.

Reynolds, C. F., Frank, E., Perel, J. M., Mazumdar, S., & Kupfer, D. J. (1995). Maintenance therapies for late-life recurrent major depression: Research and review circa 1995. *International Psychogeriatrics, 7* (Suppl.), 27–39.

Rokke, P. D., & Scoggin, F. (1995). Depression treatment preferences in younger and older adults. *Journal of Clinical Geropsychology, 1,* 243–257.

Rush, A. J., Golden, W. E., Hall, G. W., Herrera, M., Houston, A., Kathol, R. G., Katon, W., Matchett, C. L., Petty, F., Schulberg, H. C., Smith, G. R., & Stuart, G. W. (1993). *Depression in primary care: Volume 2. Treatment of major depression. Clinical practice guideline, Number 5.* Rockville, MD: U. S. Department of Health and Human Services, Public Health Service, Agency for Health Care Policy and Research. AHCPR Publication No. 93-0551.

Salzman, C. (1991). Pharmacological treatment of the anxious elderly patient. In C. Salzman & B. D. Lebowitz (Eds.), *Anxiety in the elderly: Treatment and Research* (pp. 149–173). New York: Springer.

Salzman, C., & Nevis-Olesen, J. (1992). Psychopharamcologic treatment. In J. E. Birren, R. B. Sloane, & G. D. Cohen (Eds.), *Handbook of mental health and aging* (2nd ed., pp. 721–762). San Diego, CA: Academic Press.

Schulz, R., Visintainer, P., & Williamson, G. M. (1990). Psychiatric and physical morbidity effects of caregiving. *Journal of Gerontology: Psychological Sciences, 45,* P181–P191.

Scogin, F. R., & McElreath, L. (1994). Efficacy of psychosocial treatments for geriatric depression. *Journal of Consulting and Clinical Psychology, 62,* 69–74.

Scogin, F. R., Jamison, C., & Davis, N. (1990). Two-year followup of bibliotherapy for depression in older adults. *Journal of Consulting and Clinical Psychology, 58,* 665–667.

Segal, D. L., Van Hasselt, V. B., Hersen, M., & King, C. (1996). Treatment of substance abuse in older adults. In J. R. Cautela & W. Ishaq (Eds.), *Contemporary issues in behavior therapy: Improving the human condition* (pp. 69–85). New York: Plenum Press.

Shamoian, C. A. (1991). What is anxiety in the elderly? In C. Salzman & B. D. Lebowitz (Eds.), *Anxiety in the elderly: Treatment and research* (pp. 3–15). New York: Springer.

Sheikh, J. I. (1991). Anxiety rating scales for the elderly. In C. Salzman & B. D. Lebowitz (Eds.), *Anxiety in the elderly: Treatment and Research* (pp. 251–265). New York: Springer.

Sheikh, J. I. (1992). Anxiety and its disorders in old age. In J. E. Birren, R. B. Sloane, & G. D. Cohen (Eds.), *Handbook of mental health and aging* (2nd ed., pp. 409–432). New York: Academic Press.

Skoog, I., Nilsson, L., Palmertz, B., Andreasson, L., & Svanbor, A. (1993). A population-based study of dementia in 85-year-olds. *The New England Journal of Medicine, 328,* 153–158.

Sloane, R. B., Staples, F. R., & Schneider, L. S. (1985). Interpersonal therapy versus nortriptyline for depression in the elderly. In G. D. Burrows, T. R. Norman, & L. Dennerstein (Eds.), *Clinical and pharmacological studies in psychiatric disorders* (pp. 344–346). London: John Libbey.

Smyer, M. A., & Downs, M. G. (1995). Psychopharmacology: An essential element in educating clinical psychologists for working with older adults. In B. G. Knight, L. Teri, P. Wohlford, & J. Santos (Eds.), *Mental health services for older adults: Implica-*

tions for training and practice in geropsychology (pp. 73–83). Washington, DC: American Psychological Association.

Spielberger, C. D., Gorsuch, R. C., & Lushene, R. E. (1970). *Manual for the State-Trait Anxiety Inventory.* Palo Alto, CA: Consulting Psychologists Press.

Stanley, M. A., Beck, J. G., & Glassco, J. D. (1997). Generalized anxiety in older adults: Treatment with cognitive behavioral and supportive approaches. *Behavior Therapy, 27,* 565–581.

Teri, L., Curtis, J., Gallagher-Thompson, D., & Thompson, L. W. (1994). Cognitive-behavior therapy with depressed older adults. In L. S. Schneider, C. F. Reynolds, B. D. Lebowitz, & A. J. Friedhoff (Eds.), *Diagnosis and treatment of depression in late life* (pp. 279–291). Washington, DC: American Psychiatric Association.

Thompson, L. W. (1996). Cognitive-behavioral therapy and treatment for late-life depression. *Journal of Clinical Psychiatry, 57,* 29–37.

Thompson, L. W., Gallagher, D., & Breckenridge, J. S. (1987). Comparative effectiveness of psychotherapies for depressed elders. *Journal of Consulting and Clinical Psychology, 55,* 385–390.

Tune, L. E. (1991). Postoperative delirium. *International Psychogeriatrics, 3* 325–332.

Verwoerdt, A. (1981). *Clinical geropsychiatry* (2nd ed.). Baltimore, MD: Williams & Wilkins.

Wolfe, R., Morrow, J., & Fredrickson, B. L. (1996). Mood disorders in older adults. In L. L. Carstensen, B. A. Edelstein, & L. Dornbrand (Eds.), *The practical handbook of clinical gerontology* (pp. 274–303). Thousand Oaks, CA: Sage.

Yesavage, J. A., Brink, T. L., Rose, T. L., Lum, O., Huang, V., Adey, M., & Leirer, V. O. (1983). Development and validation of a geriatric depression screening scale: A preliminary report. *Journal of Psychiatric Research, 17,* 37–49.

Youngjohn, J. R., & Crook, T. H. (1996). Dementia. In L. L. Carstensen, B. A. Edelstein, & L. Dornbrand (Eds.), *The practical handbook of clinical gerontology* (pp. 239–254). Thousand Oaks, CA: Sage.

Zeiss, A. M., & Breckenridge, J. S. (1997). Treatment of late life depression: A response to the NIH Consensus Conference. *Behavior Therapy, 28,* 3–21.

Zeiss, A. M., Lewinsohn, P. M., Rohde, P., & Seeley, J. R. (1996). The relationship of physical disease and functional impairment to depression in the elderly. *Psychology and Aging, 11,* 572–581.

Additional Readings

Carstensen, L. L., Edelstein, B. A., & Dornbrand, L. (Eds.) (1996). *The practical handbook of clinical gerontology.* Thousand Oaks, CA: Sage.

Storandt, M., & VandenBos, G. R. (1994). *Neuropsychological assessment of dementia and depression in older adults: A clinician's guide.* Washington, DC: American Psychological Association.

Zarit, S. H. & Knight, B. G. (Eds.) (1996). *A guide to psychotherapy and aging.* Washington, DC: American Psychological Association.

12

Intergenerational Relationships in Later-Life Families: Adult Daughters and Sons as Caregivers to Aging Parents

Mary Ann Parris Stephens and Melissa M. Franks

The *Oxford English Dictionary* defines a family as a group of persons consisting of parents and their children, whether actually living together or not, or the unity formed by those who are connected by blood or affinity. A more psychosocial definition describes families as groups composed of individuals who have mutual obligations to provide a broad range of emotional and material support to one another (Dean, Lin, & Ensel, 1981). These two definitions most obviously characterize the nuclear family of parents rearing young children, in part because dependent children's need for support from their parents is highly salient.

These definitions of family, however, apply equally well to later life families. These families can be defined as those that include at least one member from the generation of older adults who are 65 years of age or older, and members from at least one younger generation. The bonds that exist between adult children and their aging parents and the support that parents receive from their adult children in times of illness are the principal themes around which this chapter is organized.

For the last two decades of the twentieth century, family gerontologists have paid considerable research attention to exchanges of support between parents and their adult children. This work has most often focused on exchanges of support that are transmitted in one direction (from adult children to their parents) under specific conditions (when parents need assistance because of illness). The primary purpose of this chapter is to review theory and research on adult daughters and sons as caregivers to their ill or dependent parents. To substantiate our view that parents and their children assist one another throughout their shared lives as adults, the first section provides an overview of several major changes occurring in American society during the twentieth century that have affected the nature of parent–adult child relationships.

329

The next two sections of this chapter examine the ways in which a parent's chronic illness or disabling health condition affects the patterns of support provided by their adult children. One of these sections focuses on adult daughters as caregivers, and reviews an extensive research literature on these middle generation women who often juggle demands from many roles in the domains of family and work while providing care to their ill parents. This section describes the many responsibilities of these women, as well as the repercussions of their involvement in parent care. The last section reviews the more limited body of research on adult sons who assume parent-care responsibilities. It focuses on research aimed at understanding why fewer adult sons than daughters are active support providers to their ill parents, as well as the consequences of providing such support for those sons who do assume an active role in parent care.

American Families in the Twentieth Century

Substantial societal changes have taken place during this century that have altered the nature of relationships among family members, in particular those between parents and their adult children. Perhaps the change that has had the most profound and pervasive impact on family life is increases in the number of years that people can expect to live. This change has occurred because medical advances have sharply reduced rates of mortality at both ends of the life span.

Increased life expectancy has created greater opportunities for family members to experience longer and more diverse relationships with one another. Although lower rates of death during the last century can, for the most part, be attributed to reduced infant mortality, many more adults also are surviving into older age. These shifts toward longer life expectancy have had both positive and negative consequences for interpersonal involvements among members of later-life families (Suitor, Pillemer, Keeton, & Robison, 1995).

On the positive side, a longer life span makes it possible for parents and children to develop and maintain adult relationships with one another over a greatly extended period of time. As an example, middle aged and older adults today are more likely to have living parents than at any time in history (Watkins, Menken, & Bongaarts, 1987). In addition to the possibility of having longer-term adult relationships with parents, increased life expectancy also affords greater opportunities for interactions across multiple generations. In American society today, having three living generations is far more common than in the nineteenth century. Moreover, demographic projections suggest that even early in the twenty-first century four-generation families will be normative (Kinsella, 1995).

Other societal changes that have altered the nature of the relationship between parents and adult children are the continuing trends toward urbanization and geographic mobility (Suitor et al., 1995). In the early years of the twentieth century, economic necessity was a key factor in continued involvement of parents and their adult children. It was common for the two generations to live in close proximity and to work together in occupations such as farmers and small business owners. Shared family employment, and the resulting economic interdependence of parents and adult children, is much less common in our contemporary urban society.

One corollary of this trend toward occupational and economic independence between generations is a dramatic increase in geographic mobility of the younger generation. Today, adult children often live and work at great distances from their aging parents. One important outgrowth of these economic and geographic changes for later-life families is that parent–child relationships have become far more voluntary and less obligatory (Suitor et al., 1995).

Such fundamental changes in the nature of later-life families have raised a variety of concerns about the quality of life for older adults. It has been reasoned that if adult children are not geographically proximate to their aging parents, and the norm of obligation is less widely held, older adults may ultimately be abandoned by their children and become social isolates. These concerns are often heightened in discussions concerning long-term care for those older adults who are ill or disabled.

Although American families have experienced substantial changes in the course of this century, the family remains an important interpersonal resource for many people. The closest and most intimate relationships continue to be those involving family members (Antonucci & Akiyama, 1993). A great deal of research conducted in recent years has also shown that concerns about families abandoning their older members is largely unwarranted.

Research and theory in gerontology and family studies has shown that many aging parents and their adult children value their relationship and expect to maintain this attachment throughout their lives. One indication of this enduring attachment is the frequency with which adult children and their parents are in contact with one another. Although most parents and their adult children prefer to reside in separate and independent households, they typically stay in frequent contact with one another. When adult children are not geographically proximate to their parents, research suggests that the form of contact is altered but the frequency of interactions remains constant (Peterson, 1989). When compared to adult children residing closer to parents, the contact of less proximal children consists of more phone calls and letters and of less frequent visits of longer duration. No evidence has been found to suggest that geographic distance alters the amount of affection felt between parents and their adult children.

Many of the negative consequences of longer life expectancy for parent–adult child relationships stem from the increasing likelihood that older family members will develop and suffer from chronic and disabling health conditions. It is estimated that 80% of adults over the age of 65 years suffer from at least one chronic illness (Jette, 1995). Many of these chronic health conditions ultimately reduce the functional independence of older parents. As a result, these individuals must rely on assistance from others to carry out even their most basic daily activities, such as personal care (e.g., dressing, bathing, toileting) and instrumental tasks (e.g., cooking, transportation, shopping). The assistance older adults receive from their families is a key factor in their ability to remain living in the community and to avoid institutional living (Shanas, 1979).

When the impairments resulting from such illness prevent older adults from continuing independent functioning, most turn to family for help (Cantor, 1983). Research on family caregiving clearly has demonstrated that the responsibility for the care of impaired older adults is most often assumed by one family member (Aneshensel, Pearlin, Mullan, Zarit, & Whitlatch, 1995; Gatz, Bengtson, & Blum, 1990), referred to as the primary caregiver. Other family members and friends, however, sometimes provide assistance to both the primary caregiver and to the impaired older adult, and are referred to as secondary caregivers.

Nearly two decades of research on family caregiving has identified an established hierarchy in determining who will become a *primary* caregiver to older family members. The responsibility for care typically falls first to the spouse of the impaired older adult. In situations in which a spouse assumes primary caregiving responsibilities, adult children often are involved as secondary caregivers. In this way, adult children may assist both of their parents (Bourgeois, Beach, Schulz, & Burgio, 1996). When a spouse is unavailable or unable to assume the role of primary caregiver, adult children are turned to next (Aneshensel et al., 1995; Gatz, et al., 1990).

Data from the Informal Caregivers Survey that used a nationally representative sample of caregivers to frail older adults reported that over one-third (37.4%) of all caregivers were adult children of the impaired person (Stone, Kafarata, & Sangl, 1987). Using data from this same survey, Figure 12.1 compares the proportions of sons and daughters who assume the parent-care role. Reading across the lower portion of the figure, among the daughters of these older adults, approximately one-fourth were involved in parent care. Of these daughter caregivers, nearly three-quarters assume the role of primary caregiver. Among adult children, daughters were three times as likely to assume the role of primary caregiver than sons. Moreover, among the most impaired parents, the disparity between daughters and sons increases such that daughters were four times as likely to assume the primary caregiver role (Stone & Kemper, 1989).

Because so many frail elderly are cared for by their daughters, it has been argued that parent care is becoming a "normative" experience in American families (Brody, 1985). This trend also has been widely publicized in the popular media (e.g., *New York Times*, 1989; Beck, 1990). Given that the vast majority of adult child caregivers are daughters, most research on intergenerational family caregiving has focused on adult daughters and their impaired parents. In the next section of this chapter, we focus on adult daughters who take on the parent-care role, and in the final section, we return to sons.

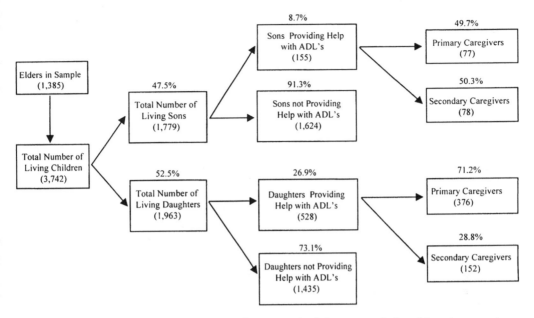

Figure 12.1. Comparison of the involvement of adult sons and daughters in parent care. From Coward, R. T., & Dwyer, J. W. (1990). The association of gender, sibling network composition, and patterns of parent care by adult children. *Research on Aging, 12,* 158–181. Copyright 1990 by Sage Publications, Inc. Reprinted with permission.

Adult Daughters Involved in Parent Care

As primary caregivers to an ill or disabled parent, daughters typically engage in a wide variety of support efforts. A large amount of caregiving research has emphasized the functional needs of older adults with dementia (i.e., those with cognitive and memory problems) who ultimately become totally dependent on others. However, those elders whose health conditions limit them only physically also have many needs for assistance with daily activities even though they remain cognitively intact. For example, stroke and arthritis often reduce a person's capacity for independence in mobility (e.g., walking and driving) and personal care (e.g., dressing and grooming).

The Informal Caregivers survey interviewed individuals who were providing assistance to older adults with dependencies caused by a diversity of health problems. Across all adult daughter caregivers, approximately 75% provided assistance to the impaired parent 7 days a week, and, on average, they did so for 4 hours per day (Stone et al., 1987). Approximately 69% of daughters helped their impaired parent with personal care activities and approximately 90% helped with instrumental activities, including household tasks, shopping, and transportation (Stone et al., 1987).

DATA OF DAUGHTER CAREGIVERS

In addition to providing assistance with activities of daily living, many family caregivers also provided help with supervision of the older relative (Stone et al., 1987). In some cases, supervision is needed because of the relative's cognitive impairment, often resulting in poor judgment or problematic and disruptive behavior (Aneshensel et al., 1995). In other cases, supervision is necessary to ensure the safety of the frail older adult, for example, to protect them against injury due to falls.

A smaller qualitative study of adult child primary caregivers (94% were daughters) also reported similar parent-care tasks. As in the national survey of informal caregivers, the adult children in this study spent an average of nearly 4 hours per day assisting their parent. When asked to identify the tasks they perform as part of their parent-care responsibilities, these caregivers most frequently mentioned helping the parent with bathing, dressing, cooking, administering medications, toileting, shopping, arranging doctor's visits, and getting the parent out of bed (Albert, 1991). Based on the compilation of caregivers' responses, three dimensions emerged as representative of the ways in which adult children characterize parent-care responsibilities: the type of impairment giving rise to the task (physical versus cognitive-emotional limitations), where the task is performed (within the household versus outside, involving others), and whether the task enhances parental autonomy or responds to a parent's incompetence.

The benefits to impaired older adults of receiving such support from their adult children are intuitively obvious, but the overall effects on the support providers appear to be less beneficial. A large research literature has accumulated to suggest that providing care to an impaired older adult can have deleterious effects on the psychological and physical well-being of primary caregivers (George & Gwyther, 1986; Schulz, Visintainer, & Williamson, 1990). The strongest evidence of negative effects, however, has been found for psychological well-being.

Two common approaches to determining the psychological consequences of providing care have been used. One approach compares the psychological adjustment of caregivers to that of population-based norms. The other approach compares the psychological adjustment of caregivers to that of age- and gender-matched individuals who are not caregivers. Many of these investigations have demonstrated greater psychiatric symptomatology for caregivers, in particular, elevated levels of depression (Schulz et al., 1990).

Although less consistent than the evidence for psychological adjustment, caregiving has been shown to have harmful consequences for caregivers' physical health. These negative health effects have been demonstrated by comparing caregivers to noncaregivers. In such comparisons, caregivers showed greater suppression of immune system functioning (Kiecolt-Glaser et al., 1987) and greater cardiovascular reactivity (King, Oka, & Young, 1994). Caregivers also tended to have more physician visits (Haley, Levine, Brown, Berry, & Hughes, 1987). Because most of the studies that were designed to assess the psychological and physical health consequences of caregiving used samples composed of many different family relationships (e.g., spouses and adult children), it has been difficult to determine the extent to which a particular type of caregiver is likely to suffer in this role.

Although little direct empirical evidence is available concerning the relative health consequences of caregiving for adult daughters versus other family members, these women are often assumed to be especially vulnerable to health effects from caregiving stress because they usually occupy many other social roles in addition to that of caregiver. Daughters who take on primary responsibility for parent care are often referred to as "women in the middle" (Brody, 1981). This label can refer to several dimensions (Brody, 1990). Sometimes it refers to the generational position of these women, in that they are between the older generation of their parents and the younger generation of children. It also can refer to their chronological age in that these women are usually in the middle years of the life span.

Another use of the term refers to the multiple roles of these women, in that they frequently occupy several major roles simultaneously, including caregiver, wife, mother, and employee. This label also indicates the conflicting societal values they often encounter between traditional values, which emphasize obligations to family, and newer values, which emphasize the importance of employment and other pursuits outside of the home. A woman can be considered to be "in the middle" for any or all of these reasons.

It was from this perspective that the "competing demands hypothesis" evolved to explain the negative impact that caregiving often has on adult daughters. This perspective argues that multiple role responsibilities create demands on these women that compete for their time and energy (Brody, 1981, 1990). Although this explanation has been widely accepted in the caregiving literature, it has not been subjected to extensive empirical testing.

Although not explicitly stated in the competing demands perspective, there usually is an implicit assumption that many women who are involved in parent care are also involved in many other roles at the same time. It is often reasoned that if there are many adult daughters providing care to their parents, and if these women have multiple family and employment roles that compete for their time and energy, the parent-care role can have widespread consequences at both the individual and societal levels. Thus, the validity of the assumption that women occupy many roles in addition to that of caregiver to an impaired parent has received a great deal of attention in gerontology (Rosenthal, Matthews, & Marshall, 1989; Spitze & Logan, 1990; Stone & Kemper, 1989).

In this section we examine evidence concerning women in the middle, in particular, their prevalence in the population of the United States, as well as the tenability of the competing demands hypothesis. Using census data and findings from community studies of middle-generation caregivers, we report estimates of the prevalence of American women who occupy multiple roles including that of caregiver. Second, we draw on both the literature concerning later-life caregiving and on research concerning women's multiple roles to determine how well the competing demands perspective describes the experiences of women involved in parent care.

Prevalence of Women in the Middle

Brody's (1981) definition of women in the middle does not explicitly include the parent-care role, but her use of this term always includes women who are giving care to a dependent older family member (most often a parent or parent-in-law). These women are conceptualized as having caregiving responsibilities in addition to other family and work roles. Brody's definition seems to imply at least two, sometimes overlapping, role constellations, caregiver and employee, and caregiver and mother (Boyd & Treas, 1989). In addition to these two constellations, the role of wife frequently is included in reference to women in the middle because many middle generation women who are caregivers, parents, and who participate in the work force, also are married.

National census data provide no information about the number of women who are caring for an impaired older parent or parent-in-law. They do, however, provide information on the numbers of women ages 25 to 64 who are married, or who have children living at home, or who are employed. It is also possible to obtain estimates of women who occupy various combinations of these three roles simultaneously. According to Census data, nearly 7 of 10 (69%) American women between the ages of 25 and 64 are married, have a child under age 18 living at home, and are in the labor force (U.S. Bureau of Labor, Women's Bureau, 1994).

For data on the number of women who might have an older relative needing care, one has to turn to different sources. Watkins et al. (1987) estimate that 89% of women between the ages of 40 and 55 have a living parent over the age of 65. Although their parents typically belong to the "young-old" cohort (ages 65–80), some research has indicated increased morbidity in this group of older adults (Crimmins, 1987), and 53% in this age range need help with one or more activities of daily living (Feller, 1983).

Surveys of caregivers to the frail elderly have shown that many middle generation women are likely to be involved in other roles in addition to that of caregiver. In a national survey, 75% of caregivers were women, the median age was 45, 66% were married, 39% had children residing in their homes, and 55% had a job outside of the home [American Association of Retired Persons (AARP), 1988]. Data from the informal caregivers survey revealed that of all adult daughter caregivers 24% had at least one child under the age of 18 living at home, 56% were married, and 44% were employed (Stone et al., 1987).

A community survey using a random probability sample estimated that 25% of women between the ages of 40 and 55 simultaneously occupy the roles of daughter, mother, wife, and employee (Spitze & Logan, 1990). Of those women who had at least one living parent (regardless of any other roles occupied), 14% provided at least 3 hours of assistance to the parent per week.

Because Spitze and Logan's estimates of daughters involved in caregiving did not consider other roles women occupied simultaneously, it could not be determined how many American women with these four roles were involved in parent care.

Life span research that has examined caregiving in the context of women's other roles across a 30-year period has shown that family caregiving is an increasingly likely role, both as women age and across birth cohorts (Moen, Robison, & Fields, 1994). In this study, caregiver referred to providing assistance to any ill, disabled or older family member, including a parent. Between the ages of 35 and 44, nearly one-fourth of women assumed the caregiver role, and between the ages of 55 and 64, over one-third took on this role. Slightly less than half (45%) of the women in the older cohort (born between 1905 and 1917) ever became caregivers, whereas nearly two-thirds (64%) of the youngest cohort (born between 1927 and 1934) did so. Thus, approximately 20% more of the younger women assumed caregiving responsibilities than their older counterparts. In addition, women were equally likely to become caregivers whether or not they were employed. These longitudinal findings illustrate some important changes that are taking place in American families as a result of longer life expectancy, and suggest that cross-sectional studies may have underestimated the prevalence of women who simultaneously are in the caregiver role and other important social roles.

There are other societal trends that suggest that the number of women with multiple role responsibilities is likely to increase. These trends include women delaying childbearing, adult children remaining at home for longer periods of time (U.S. Bureau of the Census, 1992), and increasing numbers of women in the labor force (U.S. Department of Labor, Women's Bureau, 1994). Thus, even though multiple role configurations that include the parent-care role may not be normative (in the sense of characterizing a majority of middle-aged women), there is an increasingly large number of women who are faced with these multiple role responsibilities. In addition, women who have these multiple role responsibilities may have special needs that deserve research attention (Boyd & Treas, 1989; Rosenthal et al., 1989; Stone & Kemper, 1990).

Theoretical Considerations on Multiple Roles

The competing demands hypothesis rests on assumptions similar to those of the scarcity hypothesis posited by some role theorists. The scarcity hypothesis assumes that individuals have limited personal resources, and that social organizations and role partners demand all of these resources (Goode, 1960). Thus, an individual's total role obligations are thought to be overly demanding, making role conflict normal.

The scarcity hypothesis has been challenged by the expansion hypothesis, which emphasizes the energy gains rather than the energy expenditures accrued by individuals with multiple roles (Marks, 1977; Sieber, 1974). This energy-expansion perspective predicts positive consequences due to the enhancement of personal resources such as mastery, self-esteem, identity, and social and material gains from various roles (Stoller & Pugliesi, 1989; Thoits, 1983). These energy-expansion perspectives also draw support from theories of interpersonal relationships that assume that individuals not only expend resources but also gain resources from any given role (Rook, 1990; Shinn, Lehmann, & Wong, 1984; Thibaut & Kelley, 1959). A growing literature on women's health has shown that occupying multiple roles (most often those of mother, wife, and employee) is associated with better overall well-being (Baruch, Barnett, & Rivers, 1983; Thoits, 1983; Verbrugge, 1983; Waldron & Jacobs, 1989).

Although the scarcity and expansion perspectives make different predictions about the effects of women's multiple roles, both are limited in that they focus on role occupancy alone or the number of roles occupied rather than on the quality of experiences that transpire within roles. Both perspectives, with their emphasis on quantity, predict a net gain or a net loss of resources, regardless of which roles a person occupies. In contrast, perspectives that emphasize the quality of role experiences would assert that two people could occupy similar roles yet experience different cost/benefit ratios within these roles. Such perspectives would, therefore, argue that in order to determine the quality of role experiences, the problems and rewards that occur within roles should be considered (Barnett & Baruch, 1985; Froburg, Gjerdingen, & Preston, 1986).

Quality refers to one's appraisals of the positive and negative aspects of experiences within a given role. There is an implicit assumption in the competing demands hypothesis that roles are inherently negative in quality and, thus, increase the stress women experience in fulfilling multiple roles. An alternative assumption is that any given role can have positive as well as negative qualities.

Gerontological theory and research in family caregiving generally have given little attention to the issue of role quality. The bulk of this research has tended to focus on the problems encountered in providing support to an impaired older adult, and has too often failed to recognize the more positive aspects of such support provision. Although some studies have reported that caregivers find certain aspects of their caregiving role to be satisfying (Boyd & Treas, 1989; Kinney & Stephens, 1989; Lawton, Kleban, Moss, Rovine, & Glicksman, 1989; Miller, 1989), how these positive experiences function in the stress process has not been well explained. On the basis of the role quality perspective, it could be argued that it is the amount of rewards that caregivers incur in their roles, in addition to the stress they encounter, that is important in determining the impact of role experiences on well-being.

The competing demands hypothesis assumes that roles outside of caregiving combine with the caregiver role to affect well-being negatively. Despite the popularity of this assertion, most research in caregiving has tended to examine the caregiver role in isolation from other roles. Moreover, when other roles have been considered, they often have not been given equal weight to that of the caregiver role (e.g., Lang & Brody, 1983; Stoller & Pugliesi, 1989). As such, little attention has been given to how these other roles influence well-being beyond the influence of the caregiver role.

Caregiving in the Context of Other Roles

Despite the widespread acceptance of the competing demands perspective, relatively few studies have examined ways in which caregivers' additional roles influence their well-being. One study examined the number of additional roles that adult child caregivers occupied, including marriage, parenthood, and employment (Skaff & Pearlin, 1992). Consistent with the energy-expansion hypothesis, the more roles adult children held outside of caregiving, the better their emotional health.

Most studies that have included caregivers other roles, however, examine the effects of one additional role at a time, usually the employee role. Investigations comparing employed and nonemployed caregivers have consistently shown that employment benefits caregivers' mental health. Adult child caregivers who are employed tend to experience less caregiver strain and better emotional health than those who are not employed (Brody, Kleban, Johnsen, Hoffman, & Schoonover, 1987; Miller, 1989; Skaff & Pearlin, 1992). Because these studies reveal that occupying this additional role can benefit caregivers' well-being, their findings are inconsistent with the predictions made by the competing demands hypothesis.

Studies that focus only on the occupancy of the employment role have indicated that employment per se is beneficial, but they do not offer insight into the characteristics of work experiences that might be responsible for these effects. To address this latter issue, some research has begun to examine the characteristics of work that are associated with caregivers' well-being (Scharlach & Fredriksen, 1994). Employed caregivers frequently report experiencing emotional, financial, and physical strain as they attempt to balance their caregiving and employment responsibilities. Caregivers who have highly demanding or stressful jobs (e.g., excessive work, insufficient time to get work done) have been shown to experience greater caregiver stress and general role strain. These results showed that adding one stressful role to another can reduce well-being and, as such, have lent some support to the competing demands hypothesis.

Little attention has focused on how caregivers' relationships with their spouse combines with parent care to influence caregivers' well-being. The evidence that does exist about these two roles, however, is not consistent with the competing demands perspective. One study compared adult daughter caregivers who were married with those who were not married (divorced, widowed, or never married) (Brody, Litvin, Hoffman, & Kleban, 1995). The results of this study showed that married women who are providing care to a parent have a mental health advantage over their counterparts who are not married.

Even less research attention has been given to the impact of holding the dual roles of caregiver and mother.

Over the past few years, we and our colleagues have focused considerable research attention on adult daughters who provide assistance to their chronically ill and disabled parents, and who simultaneously occupy other important social roles, such as mother, wife, and employee. We have been especially interested in two opposing questions: Do the roles that these women occupy in addition to the parent-care role have deleterious effects on their well-being (as the competing demands perspective assumes)? or Do these additional roles benefit their well-being (as the expansion perspective assumes)? To address these questions, we conducted a series of studies in which we conceptualize the parent-care role as an important family role that women often experience as a part of their larger family and work life.

Based on this conceptual framework, our work has been guided by three major assumptions about the nature of women's multiple roles. First, we have taken a role quality perspective and have assumed that experiences in any role can be both stressful and rewarding. Second, we have assumed that the effects of the parent-care role on well-being can best be understood when this role is considered in the context of other role experiences. Finally, we have assumed that experiences in any given role can affect well-being both independently and in combination with other roles. We first review our studies that have examined parent care and other roles as having independent effects on well-being, and then we discuss our studies that have examined the ways in which parent care and other roles influence one another to affect caregivers' well-being.

Most studies investigating the psychological impact of caregiving have assessed levels of depression in heterogeneous groups of family members and, thus, little information has been available about distress among adult daughter caregivers per se. We have used the Center for Epidemiologic Studies-Depression Scale (CES-D; Radloff, 1977) in several of our studies of women in the middle. A score of 16 on the CES-D is indicative of being at risk for clinical depression. The mean CES-D scores in our samples have ranged from 13 (Stephens & Townsend, 1997) to 17 (Stephens, Franks, & Atienza, 1997). Moreover, the percentages of women in our samples who have scored at or above the cut-off score of 16 have ranged from 32 (Stephens & Townsend, 1997) to 45 (Stephens et al., 1997). These values are similar to those reported in other caregiving research where specific family relationships were not the focus (e.g., Schulz et al., 1990), and suggest that many adult daughter caregivers are experiencing substantial emotional distress.

Role Quality.   To begin our exploration of women in the middle, it was first necessary to examine the quality of experiences associated with the role of principal interest, that of caregiver to an impaired older family member. The importance of our initial research was to demonstrate our most basic premise, that these women find their caregiving responsibilities to be stressful, but that they also find them to be rewarding. At the time we began this program of research, work on family caregiving had largely ignored the potential benefit derived from positive experiences in the parent-care role.

In our initial study of these issues, we examined 106 middle-aged women who served as caregivers to an impaired older family member (Franks & Stephens, 1992; Stephens, Franks, & Townsend, 1994). Most of these women (71%) were providing care to a parent, others (20%) were providing care to a parent-in-law, and the remainder (9%) were providing care to other family members, such as grandparents or aunts. We demonstrated that these women did indeed report experiencing both stressful and rewarding aspects of their caregiving role. The frequencies with which stressors and rewards were reported to have occurred in the parent-care role are shown in Tables 12.1 and 12.2.

Looking first at stressors reported in Table 12.1, all 12 were endorsed as having been at least slightly distressing by no fewer than half the respondents. Table 12.2 shows that rewards associated with the parent-care role were reported by a larger proportion of the women than were stressors. Of the 12 rewards, 8 were endorsed by three-quarters or more of the women.

TABLE 12.1.
Stressors Identified in the Parent-Care Role

Stressor	Percentage endorsing
Parent criticized or complained	71.6
Parent was unresponsive	67.4
Parent was uncooperative or demanding	67.4
Helped parent with personal care needs	67.3
Parent asked repetitive questions	67.3
Parent was agitated	66.4
Managed legal/financial affairs of parent	66.4
Parent's health declined	66.3
Supervised parent	63.1
Did not receive help with caregiving from friends or family	61.1
Had extra expenses due to caregiving	54.7
Parent was forgetful	53.6

From Stephens, M.A.P., Franks, M.M., & Townsend, A.L. (1994). Stress and rewards in women's multiple roles: The case of women in the middle. *Psychology and Aging, 9*, 45–52. Copyright 1994 by the American Psychological Association. Reprinted with permission of the publisher.

TABLE 12.2.
Rewards Identified in the Parent-Care Role

Reward	Percentage endorsing
Knew parent was well cared for	100.0
Fulfilled family obligation	93.7
Spent time in the company of parent	92.6
Gave care because wanted to not because had to	89.5
Saw parent enjoy small things	84.2
Parent showed affection or appreciation	81.1
Helped parent with personal care	81.0
Parent was cooperative or not demanding	77.8
Parent's good side came through despite the illness	73.7
Parent was calm or content	70.5
Relationship with parent became closer	64.2
Parent's health improved	47.3

From Stephens, M.A.P., Franks, M.M., & Townsend, A.L. (1994). Stress and rewards in women's multiple roles: The case of women in the middle. *Psychology of Aging, 9,* 45–52. Copyright 1994 by the American Psychological Association. Reprinted with permission of the publisher.

Most notable is the endorsement of helping the parent with personal care. More women endorsed this item as a reward (81%) than as a stressor (67.3%), and clearly some women endorsed this experience as both stressful and rewarding. Thus, the relative frequency with which these women experienced stressors and rewards in their caregiver role and the fact that some caregiving experiences were judged to have both positive and negative features emphasize the value of examining both the costs and benefits derived from providing parent care.

Because family caregiving research had focused almost exclusively on the stress that daughters encountered in the single role of caregiver, we were keenly interested in how stress in other family roles affected their well-being beyond experiences in the parent-care role. In our initial study, all women occupied not only the role of caregiver, but also simultaneously the roles of mother to children at home and wife. As with the parent-care role, these women reported experiencing stress in both of their additional roles. The stressors that were most often experienced in the mother role included heavy demands or responsibilities for the children, arguments with the children, and self-doubts about their own parenting skills. The stressors most frequently reported in the wife role included lack of companionship, conflict, and poor communication with the husband.

Our findings further demonstrated that these stressful aspects of women's roles as mother and wife detracted from their physical and psychological well-being even beyond the negative effects of stress in the caregiver role (Franks & Stephens, 1992). On the basis of these findings, we were able to support our contention that caregivers' additional roles should be considered in determining their well-being. It appeared, however, that the contributions of these other roles were largely negative, evidence that was in line with competing demands.

From the perspective of role quality, we had assumed that a more complete understanding of the impact of multiple role experiences would be possible when we considered the positive as well as the more problematic aspects of the women's additional roles. As with their parent-care role, the women in our initial study also reported experiencing many rewards in their roles as mother and wife. The rewards they reported most often in the role of mother were the meaning brought to their lives by being a mother and being loved and needed by their children. The rewards experienced most often in the role of wife included their husbands' contributions to family life as father and provider and support received from the husband. As with parent care, the rewarding aspects of these additional roles were reported more often by these women than were the stressful aspects.

Results from our study indicated that rewards in each of the three roles contributed to at least one aspect of well-being even after large portions of variance due to stress in all three roles had been accounted for. Although rewards derived from parent care were found to benefit well-being, the greatest benefit was associated with rewards stemming from the mother role (Stephens et al., 1994). These results thus provided evidence consistent with the expansion hypothesis, namely, that having multiple roles is not wholly detrimental to women's well-being.

From this initial study, we were able to demonstrate that a fuller appreciation of adult daughter caregivers' well-being could be achieved by examining their positive and negative experiences in multiple family roles, including parent care. However, we had considered only the independent contributions of experiences in each role, and did not examine the effects of combining multiple role experiences. Our next step was to focus on the ways in which caregivers' experiences in parent care together with experiences in other roles jointly relate to their well-being.

Role Combinations. Drawing from the assumptions made by the competing demands and expansion perspectives, we set out to explore the accumulation of stressful and rewarding roles. An "accumulation" of roles refers to the situation in which a woman has a large number of roles that are either primarily stressful or primarily rewarding. Based on the perspective of competing demands, we expected that stress in the mother and wife roles would further diminish well-being for those women experiencing higher levels of parent-care stress. Conversely, based on the perspective of energy expansion, we expected that rewards in the mother and wife roles would further enhance well-being among women experiencing higher levels of rewards in parent care.

Our results generally supported these expectations. Women experiencing higher levels of stress in only their parent-care role reported better well-being than did those women experiencing high stress in the parent-care role and one other role, or women with high stress in all three roles. An opposite pattern emerged for role rewards where women experiencing higher levels of rewards in only the parent-care role evidenced poorer well-being than did women with additional rewarding roles. Once again, our findings lent some support for both the competing demands and expansion perspectives.

In a subsequent study, we took another approach to examining the effects of combining women's additional roles with their parent-care responsibilities. This study focused on 296 women who simultaneously occupied the four roles of caregiver to an impaired parent (86% of women) or parent-in-law (14%), mother, wife, and employee (Stephens & Townsend, 1997). The aims of this study were to investigate whether the stress experienced in the additional roles of mother, wife, and employee might exacerbate (increase) the negative effects of parent-care stress on psychological well-being and whether the rewards experienced in these additional roles might buffer (decrease) the stress effects of parent care. Predictions about stress exacerbation and stress buffering were tested with a statistical interaction term (parent-care stress by stress in another role, or parent-care stress by rewards in another role).

We found clear evidence to support the stress exacerbation prediction in the mother role and to support the stress buffering prediction in the employee role. Women who experienced the combination of high parent-care stress and high stress in their mother role had poorer well-being, but no such effects were found for women with high parent-care stress and low mother-role stress. In contrast, women experiencing the combination of high parent-care stress and low rewards from employment had poorer well-being, but no such effects were found for women experiencing high parent-care stress and high levels of rewards from employment. Experiences in the wife role neither exacerbated nor buffered the effects of parent-care stress.

Our studies on combining parent care with women's additional roles suggest that experiences in these other roles can interact with experiences in parent care. Results from these studies suggest that if experiences in the additional roles are especially stressful, they can increase the harmful effects of parent-care stress on well-being. Conversely, if these additional roles involve especially rewarding experiences, however, they have the potential to ameliorate the harmful effects of parent-care stress. Our work on role combinations focused only on experiences occurring simultaneously in parent care and the other roles. As such, it cannot address the ways in which experiences in parent care alter (or are altered by) experiences associated with another role. Our studies on role spillover have dealt explicitly with these issues.

Role Spillover.   Some role theories have recognized the possibility that the stressful and rewarding experiences associated with any given role may not necessarily be confined to that role domain (e.g., Linville, 1987). Rather, because the boundaries between roles are sometimes ambiguous, it is possible for experiences in one role to "spill over" and color the experiences in another role (e.g., Bolger, DeLongis, Kessler, & Wethington, 1989; Linville, 1987; Repetti, 1987). This spillover is thought to be bidirectional in that experiences in one role have the potential to influence experiences in a second role, and vice versa. Furthermore, the influence of one role on another may be positive as well as negative.

From this theoretical perspective, we have considered spillover between women's parent-care role and two other roles, wife and employee. The competing demands and expansion hypotheses once again guided our conceptual framework. Consistent with competing demands, we conceptualized negative spillover as involving demands on time and energy in one role that influence the quality of experiences in the other role as well as psychological interference between the roles (e.g., Small & Riley, 1990). Conversely, consistent with the expansion perspective, we conceptualized positive spillover as involving feelings of attachment, mastery, and self-esteem in one role that influence the quality of experiences in the other role (Thoits, 1985; Verbrugge, 1983; Waldron & Jacobs, 1989).

We examined spillover between the parent-care and wife roles in 125 adult daughters, all of whom occupied both roles (Stephens & Franks, 1995). The type of negative spillover most frequently endorsed by these women was the limited time available for their husband because of caregiving responsibilities, followed by the interference in their marriage due to worries about caregiving. The spillover of self-esteem from the parent-care role to the wife role was the most frequently endorsed type of positive spillover, followed by the spillover of feelings of mastery gained through caregiving. Regarding negative and positive spillover in the other direction, very few women indicated that their marriage interfered with their parent-care responsibilities. In contrast, many women indicated that their marriage had helped to bolster their parent-care experiences.

In a subsequent study, we examined role spillover between parent care and employment among 105 employed daughter caregivers (Stephens et al., 1997). Exhaustion, difficulty concentrating, and work disruptions were the most frequently reported types of negative spillover from the parent-care role. In turn, the limited time and attention that could be provided to the parent because of employment were the most frequently reported types of negative spillover from the employment role. The most frequently endorsed type of positive spillover in both directions was being in a good mood in one role because of positive experiences in the other role.

In our two studies on role spillover, both negative and positive spillover were found to occur in both directions, from parent care to the other role and from the other role to parent care. Moreover, in both studies, women who experienced greater negative spillover (especially negative spillover from the parent-care role to the other role) tended to have poorer well-being, whereas women who experienced greater positive spillover (especially positive spillover from the parent-care role to the wife role or positive spillover from the employee role to the parent-care role) tended to have better well-being. Taken together, the results on role spillover suggest that a woman's parent-care role and her marriage or her employment have the potential not only to interfere with each other (as the competing demands hypothesis assumes), but also to enhance each other (as the role expansion hypothesis assumes).

Summary. Findings from our studies of role quality, role combinations, and role spillover have provided abundant evidence that the lives of these women cannot be easily captured by either the competing demands or expansion hypothesis alone. We find the strongest support for competing demands when we focus only on the problems and stressors encountered in the parent-care role and in other family and work roles. Likewise, we find the strongest support for energy expansion when we focus exclusively on the satisfying and rewarding aspects of role experiences.

A far more complex picture emerges when we consider problematic and rewarding role experiences simultaneously. Our studies have amply demonstrated that positive experiences in one role have the potential to offset the effects of negative experiences occurring in another role. This pattern of findings is not entirely consistent with either the competing demands or with the expansion perspectives.

Based on our accumulated findings, we have become convinced that the two questions that guided our original work in this area are more complementary to one another than opposing. Moreover, it is our contention that the processes governing the ways in which multiple roles affect well-being are more complicated than the ones proposed by either role theory. Thus, our research strongly suggests the need for a more comprehensive theoretical framework for understanding the lives of women who are in the middle of parent-care and other role responsibilities.

Adult Sons Involved in Parent Care

Although many more adult daughters than sons assume the role of caregiver to an impaired parent, some adult sons also take on the parent-care role. Because of the predominance of daughters in the role of caregiver, however, far less research attention has been given to explicating the caregiving activities of sons or to understanding how experiences in the parent-care role affect their psychological and physical well-being. A large portion of the research that has focused on adult son caregivers has been directed at explaining the gender differential in parent care. In this section, we review the research literature on parent care provided by adult sons, as well as research focusing on factors that may underlie the well-established gender difference in parent-care involvement of adult children.

Drawing on data from the Informal Caregivers Survey, it is evident that adult sons are less often involved in parent care than are adult daughters. As shown in the top portion of Figure 12.1, of all sons who are available to assist their parents, less than 10% are involved in parent care (compared with 27% of all daughters). Furthermore, of those sons who become caregivers, approximately half of them participate as primary caregivers. Considering the fact that three-quarters of daughter caregivers assume primary responsibility for their impaired parent, these data indicate that sons are more likely than daughters to serve as secondary caregivers.

Data from the Informal Caregivers Survey further indicate that when sons do become involved in parent care, their participation closely resembles that of daughters. Approximately 71% of adult son caregivers provide some assistance to their impaired parents 7 days a week, and, on average, they do so for 3.5 hours per day (Stone et al., 1987). About 54% of sons assist their parents with personal care, 74% assist with household tasks, and 94% assist with shopping and/or transportation.

Comparing the proportions of sons and daughters involved in these helping activities also reveals some divergence in the types of tasks each perform. Most notable are the differences in assistance with personal care, where daughters are much more likely to be helping. A smaller study (Horowitz, 1985) investigating parent care by sons and daughters also reported that sons were less likely to perform tasks that require intimate contact with the parent.

Further comparing the upper and lower portions of Figure 12.1 illustrates that, in part, the lower rate of participation of sons than daughters as primary caregiver stems from the fact that many fewer sons than daughters assume any responsibility for assisting their older parents. Two general approaches have been offered to explain this gender differential in parent care by adult children. One approach emphasizes the needs and preferences of the adult children and their ill or disabled parents. The other approach emphasizes the structure and composition of the family network.

From the perspective that focuses on the needs and preferences of family members, some theorists have assumed that adult daughters possess stronger feelings of attachment to their parents than do sons. Although when compared to sons, daughters often have been shown to have greater affection for their parents, there has been little evidence to suggest that these feelings of affection are linked to differences in support provided to aging parents (see review by Mancini & Blieszner, 1989; Silverstein, Parrott, & Bengtson, 1995). Thus, the attachment needs of adult children do not provide a wholly satisfactory explanation for the pervasiveness of daughters in parent care.

The extent to which adult children subscribe to societal norms of responsibility or obligation to aging parents also has been put forth to explain the gender differential in parent care. Some research based on this perspective has shown that sons and daughters do not differ in their beliefs about what adult children should do for their aging parents, including what should be done for parents in times of illness (Finley, Roberts, & Banahan, 1988). Although other research has shown adult daughters to have stronger feelings of filial responsibility than sons (Silverstein et al., 1995), this norm of responsibility was more strongly related to the support provided to parents by sons than by daughters.

Most of the research investigating filial obligation norms has emphasized the expectations about what adult children in general should do for aging parents. Therefore, it is possible that these generalized expectancies do not reflect an individual's personal feelings of obligation to help his or her own parents. However, research that has addressed adult children's beliefs about what they would do for their own parents if help were needed in the future also demonstrated no gender differences in personal expectations for providing parent care (Franks, Dwyer, Lamphere, & Mast, 1997). Thus, neither explanations relying on societal norms of obligation nor those relying on personal norms adequately account for differences in sons and daughters involvement in parent care.

Another potential explanation for differences in the proportions of son and daughter caregivers to parents is the presumed preference for gender consistency (Lee, Dwyer, & Coward, 1993). This argument derives from observations that more mothers than fathers receive care from adult children and that more daughters than sons are involved in parent-care. The reason that mothers are more often cared for by children stems from two demographic trends. Women tend to marry men older than themselves, and they have longer life expectancy than men. Thus, most spousal caregiving is done by wives. When older women need help, they frequently do not have a spouse available, and they most often turn to adult children for assistance.

Evidence was found to support the gender consistency hypothesis in a study examining relationships between the gender of the impaired parent and the gender of the adult child primary caregiver (Lee et al., 1993). This study reported that daughters more often than sons were primary caregivers to both parents but that they were even more likely to predominate in care to mothers than to fathers. Whereas 61% of all adult child primary caregivers to fathers were daughters, 77% of caregivers to mothers were daughters. It should be noted, however, that this study did not directly assess the preferences for gender consistency held by parents or their adult child caregivers. Therefore, the presumed preferences for gender consistency in caregiving remains a presumption.

Another approach to explicating the gender differential in sons and daughters involvement in parent care emphasizes the structure and gender composition of the sibling network (e.g., Coward & Dwyer, 1990; Lee et al., 1993). Rates of adult children involved in parent care were compared across single-child networks (families with only one child), single-gender networks (families with sons only or daughters only), and mixed-gender networks. It was expected that the gender difference in parent care would be attenuated in single-child and single-gender networks. Contrary to this prediction, research revealed that across all three types of networks, daughters remained more likely to assume the parent-care role than sons. In fact, the highest rate of sons participating in parent care was equal only to the lowest rate of participation by daughters. Thus, structure and gender composition of the sibling network does not explain the higher proportion of daughters than sons in parent care.

Structure and composition of the sibling network, however, were found to be related to the amount of caregiving stress and burden reported by son and daughter care providers. Overall, when compared to daughters, sons have been shown to experience less caregiving stress and burden (Coward & Dwyer, 1990) and fewer negative consequences from their parent-care role (Horowitz, 1985). When similar comparisons between sons and daughters were made separately by composition of their sibling network, gender differences in stress and burden emerged only in one type of network, those with mixed genders (Coward & Dwyer, 1990).

Because over half of all sibling networks consist of both sons and daughters, the particularly stressful nature of parent care for daughters from mixed-gender networks is compelling. One aspect of mixed-gender networks that may heighten caregiver distress is that sons and daughters have different approaches to participating in parent care (Matthews & Rosner, 1988). Whereas adult daughter primary caregivers described their sisters as providing more routine or predictable assistance with parent care, they described their brothers as less consistent participants in the parent-care system. Such differences in caregiving styles may result in conflict among brothers and sisters, thus increasing the stress of caregiving for adult daughter primary care providers from networks of mixed gender.

In sum, this review of research aimed at understanding why daughters more often take on parent-care responsibilities than sons reveals the complexity of the selection process. The preferences and needs of older adults and their adult children have provided the clearest insight into this differential selection process. Regardless of which factors best describe the lower likelihood that sons will become involved in parent care, when they do assume these responsibilities, their parent-care experiences tend to mirror those of caregiving daughters.

Summary

The extensive research literature on parent care by adult daughters and sons we have reviewed in this chapter suggests that despite changes in family relationships throughout this century, parents can and do rely on their adult children, especially in times of illness. Research on family caregiving clearly has established that involvement in parent care is not equally shared by daughters

and sons. Further, as revealed in this chapter, most research on parent care focuses only on the one adult child who assumes primary responsibility for the
impaired parent. If the contributions of and repercussions to all adult child
caregivers are to be more fully understood, research on the provision of care
to aging parents must extend beyond the primary caregiver. Broadening the
scope on parent-care activities and experiences beyond the parent and adult
child primary caregiver dyad will allow a more comprehensive view of intergenerational relations in later-life families.

REVIEW QUESTIONS

1. In the early part of the twenty-first century many children born after
   World War II (baby-boomers) will reach old age. How will this increase in
   the population of later-life families affect intergenerational relations?
   What other social and demographic trends may affect intergenerational
   relations in the next century?

2. Two theoretical perspectives, the competing demands and expansion hypotheses, have been used to describe the consequence for women with
   multiple role involvements. In the context of parent care, how well is each
   of these perspectives supported by empirical research findings?

3. Discuss how advances in medical care have influenced informal family
   caregiving.

4. Argue for or against the proposition that family caregiving is best conceptualized as a network of care providers rather than a dyadic relationship
   between a caregiver and an impaired older adult.

References

Albert, S. M. (1991). Cognition of caregiving tasks: Multidimensional scaling of the care-
   giver task domain. *The Gerontologist, 31*(6), 726–734.
American Association of Retired Persons. (1988). *National Survey of caregivers: Summary
   of findings*. Washington, DC: AARP.
Aneshensel, C. S., Pearlin, L. I., Mullan, J. T., Zarit, S. H., & Whitlatch, C. J. (1995). *Pro-
   files in caregiving: The unexpected career*. San Diego: Academic Press.
Antonucci, T. C., & Akiyama, H. (1993). Stress and coping in the elderly. *Applied and
   Preventive Psychology, 2*(4), 201–208.
Barnett, R., & Baruch, G. (1985). Women's involvement in multiple roles and psycho-
   logical distress. *Journal of Personality and Social Psychology, 49*, 135–145.
Baruch, G., Barnett, R., & Rivers, C. (1983). *Life prints: New patterns of love and work for
   today's woman*. New York: New American Library.
Beck, M. (1990). Aging: Trading places. *Newsweek*, July, pp. 48–54.

Bolger, N., DeLongis, A., Kessler, R.C., & Wethington, E. (1989). The contagion of stress across multiple roles. *Journal of Marriages and the Family, 51,* 175–183.

Bourgeois, M.S., Beach, S., Schulz, R., & Burgio, L.D. (1996). When primary and secondary caregivers disagree: Predictors and psychosocial consequences. *Psychology and Aging, 11*(3), 527–537.

Boyd, S. L., & Treas, J. (1989). Family care of the frail elderly: A new look at "women in the middle." *Women's Studies Quarterly, 1 & 2,* 66–74.

Brody, E.M. (1981). "Women in the Middle" and family help to older people. *The Gerontologist, 21,* 471–480.

Brody, E. M. (1985). Parent care as a normative family stress. *The Gerontologist, 25,* 19–29.

Brody, E. M. (1990). *Women in the middle: Their parent-care years.* New York: Springer.

Brody, E. M., Kleban, M. H., Johnsen, P. T., Hoffman, C., & Schoonover, C. B. (1987). Work status and parent care: A comparison of four groups of women. *The Gerontologist, 27,* 201–208.

Brody, E. M., Litvin, S. J., Hoffman, C., & Kleban, M. (1995). On having a "significant other" during the parent care years. *Journal of Applied Gerontology, 14*(2), 131–149.

Cantor, M. (1983). Strain among caregivers: A study of experience in the United States. *The Gerontologist, 23,* 597–604.

Coward, R. T., & Dwyer, J. W. (1990). The association of gender, sibling network composition, and patterns of parent care in adult children. *Research on Aging, 12*(2), 158–181.

Crimmins, E. M. (1987). Evidence on the compression of morbidity. *Gerontological Perspecta, 1,* 45–49.

Dean, A., Lin, N., & Ensel, W. M. (1981). The epidemiological significance of social support systems in depression. *Research in Community Mental Health, 2,* 77–109.

Feller, B. A. (1983). *Americans needing help to function at home* (#92). Washington, DC: Vital and Health Statistics of the National Center for Health Studies.

Finley, N. J., Roberts, M. D., & Banahan, B. F. (1988). Motivators and inhibitors of attitudes of filial obligation toward aging parents. *The Gerontologist, 28,* 72–78.

Franks, M. M., Dwyer, J. W., Lamphere, J. K., & Mast, B. (1997). *Expectations and provisions of parent care by daughters and sons.* Paper presented at the Annual Convention of the American Psychological Association, Chicago, IL.

Franks, M. M., & Stephens, M. A. P. (1992). Multiple roles of middle generation caregivers: Contextual effects and psychological mechanisms. *Journal of Gerontology: Social Sciences, 47,* S123–S129.

Froberg, D., Gjerdingen, D., & Preston, M. (1986). Multiple roles and women's mental and physical health: What have we learned? *Women and Health, 11,* 79–96.

Gatz, M., Bengtson, V. L., & Blum, M. J. (1990). Caregiving families. In J. Birren & K. Warren Schaie (Eds.), *The handbooks of aging* (pp. 404–426). San Diego, CA: Academic Press.

George, L. K., & Gwyther, L. P. (1986). Caregiver well-being: A multidimensional examination of family caregivers of demented adults. *The Gerontologist, 26*(3), 253–259.

Goode, W. J. (1960). A theory of role strain. *American Sociological Review, 25,* 483–496.

Haley, W. E., Levine, E. G., Brown, S. L., Berry, J. W., & Hughes, G. H. (1987). Psychological, social, and health consequences of caring for a relative with senile dementia. *Journal of the American Geriatric Society, 35,* 405–411.

Horowitz, A. (1985). Sons and daughters as caregivers to older parents: Differences in role performance and consequences.

The Gerontologist, 25, 612–617.

Jette, A. M. (1995). How does formal and informal care affect nursing home use? *Journal of Gerontology, 50B*(1), S4–S12.

Kiecolt-Glaser, J. K., Glaser, R., Shuttleworth, E. E., Dyer, C. S., Ogrocki, P., & Speicher, C. E. (1987). Chronic stress and immunity in family caregivers of Alzheimer's disease patients. *Psychosomatic Medicine, 49,* 523–535.

King, A. C., Oka, R. K., & Young, D. R. (1994). Ambulatory blood pressure and heart rate responses to stress of work and caregiving in older women. *Journal of Gerontology, 49*(6), 239–245.

Kinney, J. M., & Stephens, M. A. P. (1989). Hassles and uplifts of giving care to a family member with dementia. *Psychology and Aging, 4,* 402–408.

Kinsella, K. (1995). Aging and the family: Present and future demographic issues. In R. Blieszner & V. Hilkevitch Bedford (Eds.), *Handbook of aging and the family* (pp. 32–56). Westport, CT: Greenwood Press.

Lang, A. M., & Brody, E. M. (1983). Characteristics of middle-aged daughters and help to their elderly mothers. *Journal of Marriage and the Family, 45,* 193–201.

Lawton, M. P., Kleban, M. H., Moss, M., Rovine, M., & Glicksman, A. (1989). Measuring caregiving appraisal. *Journal of Gerontology: Psychological Sciences, 44,* 61–71.

Lee, G. R., Dwyer, J. W., and Coward, R. T. (1993). Gender differences in parent care: Demographic factors and same-gender preferences. *Journal of Gerontology: Social Sciences, 48*(1), 9–16.

Linville, P. W. (1987). Self-complexity as a cognitive buffer against stress-related illness and depression. *Journal of Personality and Social Psychology, 52*(4), 663–676.

Mancini, J. A., & Blieszner, R. (1989). Aging parents and adult children: Research themes in intergenerational relations. *Journal of Marriage and the Family, 51,* 275–290.

Marks, S. R. (1977). Multiple roles and role strain: Some notes on human energy, time and commitment. *American Sociological Review, 42,* 921–936.

Matthews, S. H., & Rosner, T. (1988). Shared filial responsibility: The family as the primary caregiver. *Journal of Marriage and the Family, 50,* 185–195.

Miller, B. (1989). Adult children's perceptions of caregiver stress and satisfaction. *Journal of Applied Gerontology, 8,* 275–293.

Moen, P., Robison, J., & Fields, V. (1994). Women's work and caregiving roles: A life course approach. *Journal of Gerontology, 49*(4), 176–186.

New York Times (1989). Juggling family, job and aged dependent, January, p. 18.

Peterson, E. T. (1989). Elderly parents and their offspring. In S. J. Bahr & E. T. Peterson (Eds.), *Aging and the family* (pp. 175–191). Lexington, MA: Lexington Books.

Radloff, L. S. (1977). The CES-D Scale: A self-report depression scale for research in the general population. *Applied Psychological Measurement, 1,* 385–401.

Repetti, R. L. (1987). Linkages between work and family roles. In S. Oskamp (Ed.), *Family processes and problems: Social psychological aspects* (Applied Social Psychology Annual, Vol. 7, pp. 98–127). Newbury Park, CA: Sage.

Rook, K. S. (1990). Stressful aspects of older adults' social relationships: Current theory and research. In M. A. P. Stephens, J. H. Crowther, S. E. Hobfoll, & D. L. Tennenbaum (Eds.), *Stress and coping in later-life families.* Washington, DC: Hemisphere.

Rosenthal, C. J., Matthews, S. H., & Marshall, V. W. (1989). Is parent care normative? The experiences of a sample of middle-aged women. *Research on Aging, 11,* 224–260.

Scharlach, A. E., & Fredriksen, K. I. (1994). Elder care versus adult care: Does care recipient age make a difference? *Research on Aging, 16,* 43–68.

Schulz, R., Visintainer, P., & Williamson, G. M. (1990). Psychiatric and physical morbidity effects of caregiving. *Journal of Gerontology: Psychological Sciences, 45*(5),
P181–P191.

Shanas, E. (1979). The family as a social support system in old age. *The Gerontologist, 19,*
169–174.

Shinn, M., Lehmann, S., & Wong, N. W. (1984). Social interaction and social support.
Journal of Social Issues, 40, 55–76.

Sieber, S. (1974). Toward a theory of role accumulation. *American Sociological Review, 39,*
567–578.

Silverstein, M., Parrott, T. M., & Bengtson, V. L. (1995). Factors that predispose middle-
aged sons and daughters to provide social support to older parents. *Journal of Marriage and the Family, 57,* 465–475.

Skaff, M. M., & Pearlin, L. I. (1992). Caregiving: Role engulfment and the loss of self.
The Gerontologist, 32, 656–664.

Small, S. A., & Riley, D. (1990). Toward a multidimensional assessment of work spillover
into family life. *Journal of Marriage and the Family, 52,* 51–61.

Spitze, G., & Logan, J. (1990). More evidence on women (and men) in the middle. *Research on Aging, 12,* 182–198.

Stephens, M. A. P., & Franks, M. M. (1995). Spillover between daughters' roles as caregiver and wife: Interference or enhancement? *Journal of Gerontology: Psychological
Sciences, 50B,* P9–P17.

Stephens, M. A. P., Franks, M. M., & Atienza, A. A. (1997). Where two roles intersect:
Spillover between parent care and employment. *Psychology and Aging, 12,* 30–37.

Stephens, M. A. P., Franks, M. M., & Townsend, A. L. (1994). Stress and rewards in
women's multiple roles: The case of women in the middle. *Psychology and Aging,
9,* 45–52.

Stephens, M. A. P., & Townsend, A. L. (1997). Stress of parent care: Positive and negative effects of women's other roles. *Psychology and Aging, 12*(2), 376–386.

Stoller, E. P., & Pugliesi, K. L. (1989). The transition to the caregiving role. *Research on
Aging, 11,* 312–330.

Stone, R., Cafferata, G. L., & Sangl, J. (1987). Caregivers of the frail elderly: A national
profile. *The Gerontologist, 27,* 616–626.

Stone, R. I., & Kemper, P. (1989). Spouses and children of disabled elders: How large a
constituency of long-term care reform? *The Milbank Quarterly, 67,* 485–506.

Suitor, J., Pillemer, K., Keeton, S., & Robison, J. (1995). Aged parents and aging children: Determinants of relationship quality. In R. Blieszner and V. Hilkevitch Bedford (Eds.), *Handbook of aging and the family.* Westport, CT: Greenwood Press.

Thibaut, J. W., & Kelly, H. H. (1959). *The social psychology of groups.* New York: Wiley.

Thoits, P. A. (1983). Multiple identities and psychological well-being: A reformulation
and test of the social isolation hypothesis. *American Sociological Review, 48,* 174–187.

Thoits, P. A. (1985). Social support and psychological well-being: Theoretical possibilities. In G. I. Sarason & B. R. Sarason (Eds.), *Social support: Theory, research, and applications* (pp. 51–72). Dordricht, The Netherlands: Martines Nijhoff.

U.S. Bureau of Labor: Women's Bureau. (1994). *1993 Handbook on women workers: Trends
and issues.* Washington, DC: U.S. Government Printing Office.

U.S. Bureau of the Census. (1992). *Classified index of industries and occupations.* Washington, DC: U.S. Government Printing Office.

Verbrugge, L. M. (1983). Multiple roles and physical health of women and men. *Journal of Health and Social Behavior, 24,* 16–30.

354 Stephens and Franks

Waldron, I., & Jacobs, J. A. (1989). Effects of multiple roles on women's health: Evidence from a national longitudinal study. *Women and Health, 15,* 3–19.

Watkins, S. C., Menken, J. A., & Bongaarts, J. (1987). Demographic foundations of family change. *American Sociological Review, 52,* 346–358.

Additional Readings

Abel, E. K. (1991). *Who cares for the elderly? Public policy and the experience of adult daughters.* Philadelphia: Temple University Press.

Beigel, D. E., Sales, E., & Schulz, R. (1990). *Family caregiving in chronic illness.* Newbury Park, CA: Sage.

Cook, J. A., Cohler, B. J., Pickett, S. A., & Buler, J. A. (1997). Life-course and severe mental illness: Implications for caregiving within the family of later-life. *Family Relations, 41,* 427–436.

Farkas, J. I., & Himes, C. L. (1997). The influence of caregiving and employment on the voluntary activities of midlife women and older women. *Journal of Gerontology: Social Sciences, 52B,* S180–S189.

Kaye, L. W., & Applegate, J. S. (1990). *Men as caregivers to the elderly: Understanding as aiding unrecognized family support.* Lexington, MA: Lexington Books/D.C. Heath.

Martire, L. M., Stephens, M. A. P., & Atienza, A. A. (1997). The interplay of work and caregiving: Relationships between role satisfaction, role involvement, and caregivers' well-being. *Journal of Gerontology: Social Sciences, 52B,* S279–S289.

Neal, M. B., Chapman, N. J., Ingersoll-Dayton, B., & Emlen, A. C. (1993). *Balancing work and caregiving for children, adults, and elders.* Newbury Park, CA: Sage.

Pavalko, E. K., & Artis, J. E. (1997). Women's caregiving and paid work: Causal relationships in late midlife. *Journal of Gerontology: Social Sciences, 52B,* S170–S179.

Pillemer, K., & Suitor, J. (1996). Family stress and social support among caregivers to persons with Alzheimer's disease. In G. R. Pierce, B. R. Sarason, & I. G. Sarason (Eds.), *Handbook of social support and the family* (pp. 467–494). New York: Plenum.

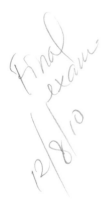

13

Work, Leisure, and Retirement

Harvey L. Sterns and Jennifer Hurd Gray

The life-span approach to work, leisure, and retirement emphasizes the possibility of behavioral changes at any point in the life span. Opportunities, choices, and decisions are not tied to any specific age. Individual differences in aging and development are also central to this perspective. The unique status of each individual results from age-graded, history-graded, and nonnormative life influences (Baltes & Graf, 1996). Organizations also age and undergo developmental changes in terms of life cycle, structure, and strategy. In particular, the latest period of downsizing and restructuring has created new relationships between organizations and employees. Despite the recent improvements in employment opportunities, these organizational changes have had enduring effects. It is apparent that workers of all ages need to be attentive to both their current work situations and personal plans for the future (Sterns & Miklos, 1995).

In response to changing social and organizational environments, self-management has emerged as a theme permeating the 1990s: self-management of career, leisure activities, and retirement. With workers changing occupations, employers, or jobs within their own company, greater individual responsibilities are required for maintaining and updating knowledge, skills, and abilities (Farr, Tesluk, & Klein, 1998; Sterns & Sterns, 1995). Hall and Mirvis (1995, 1996) capture this theme in their discussions of the protean career, which stresses continuous learning and self-direction of both one's life and career. One of the challenges to staying vital in one's work is finding the right balance between work, leisure, family, and other personal interests.

In terms of our nonwork lives, we are charged with greater responsibilities for managing our leisure pursuits, exercise regimens, and health promotion activities. In terms of leisure, the self-management theme is apparent in discussions of the "Ulyssean" adult. This view describes aging as a journey in which individuals seek out opportunities for growth and development (McGuire, Boyd, & Tedrick, 1996). Self-management of the nonwork domain of life also interacts with work-related activities. Through the emphasis on aging and growth, the Ulyssean perspective also encompasses both leisure and retirement. Decisions need to be made concerning what activities to carry over into retirement as well as what new opportunities to pursue.

The removal of mandatory retirement ages for most occupations has increased individual latitude and responsibility in choosing when and how to exit the workforce. More options than ever are available to individuals. The financial aspects of retirement planning in particular highlight self-management themes. Individuals may take more proactive stances due to increased opportunities for retirement savings (e.g., IRAs, ROTH IRAs, 401K plans). Consider also the self-management implications of the following illustrations: well-off retirees report their greatest regret as not having put more money into tax-deferred retirement savings while employed, although nearly 60% reported having invested the maximum allowed by law (Espinoza, 1997). A survey of 12,000 Americans (i.e., the Health and Retirement Study) indicated that in the 1990s, 40% of employed Americans aged 51 to 60 years would have no income other than Social Security were they to retire (Rich, 1993). Future changes in Social Security may also shift greater responsibilities to the individual. For example, one option discussed for restructuring the system is allowing individuals to set up private retirement accounts, thus giving greater freedom and responsibility for investment decisions to the individual (Schlesinger & Georges, 1998).

Self-management of career, leisure, and retirement entails a lot of responsibility. Some individuals may accept this responsibility and respond proactively with success. Others, however, may respond ineffectively or be unable to respond at all. These individuals may not have the needed skills or psychological resources, or may be constrained by their circumstances.

Our primary focus is to consider the interplay between the three life areas of work, leisure, and retirement in understanding the adult life span. We begin with a brief overview of industrial gerontology. Next, we discuss older worker stereotypes and how these perceptions may impact older workers. Illustrative comparisons are also drawn between older worker stereotypes and empirical research. Self-management issues in terms of changing organizational environments are also discussed. Work and leisure activities are considered to coexist and influence each other. The section on leisure addresses how early work/leisure relations carry over into later life.

Retirement is conceptualized as a process (see also Atchley, 1976; Ekerdt, DeViney, & Kosloski, 1996) that begins long before the actual act(s) and, therefore, also has reciprocal relations with work and leisure. Once retired, reciprocal relations are still seen between leisure, retirement, and any continued work activities. The discussion of retirement begins with a brief history of the concept, followed by illustrations of the changing nature of retirement. We then discuss a comprehensive model of retirement and related research with consideration of gender, decision making, adjustment, and satisfaction in postretirement life.

Origins of Industrial Gerontology

The field of industrial gerontology developed over 50 years ago in response to the need for research examining relations between aging, employment, and economic adaptation (Stagner, 1971; Sterns, 1986; Sterns & Alexander, 1987; Wellford, 1976). This field is an interdisciplinary approach to the study of aging and draws from industrial and organizational, developmental, and counseling psychology. Thus, many issues of aging and work such as selection, job performance and appraisal, training, career progression, work motivation, and retirement, have been embraced by this new area of psychology.

The knowledge and skills industrial gerontological professionals offer to this wide range of issues may be contrasted to an earlier view suggesting there is little need for such a specialized field (Stagner, 1971). That is, theories, models, and methods of personnel selection, training, and leadership were seen as applying to both younger and older workers and considering older workers as a distinct category was thought to be a less fruitful approach. Stagner (1971) recognized the major tasks for those interested in industrial gerontology were to dispel the widely held stereotypes of older workers and the acceptance of these stereotypes by older workers.

Work and Aging

"The effective, moving, vitalizing work of the world is done between the ages of twenty-five and forty—these fifteen golden years of plenty, the anabolic or constructive period, in which there is always a balance in the mental bank and the credit is still good" (Osler, cited in Graebner, 1980)

This passage from Osler's 1905 valedictory address at Johns Hopkins illustrates the starting point of a continuing debate regarding the changing capabilities of workers across the life span. We find in 1997 that approximately 3.8 million adults age 65 years and older were either working or actively seeking work (Administration on Aging/Profile of Older Americans: 1997 web page). This comparison between Osler's statements and older adult employment illustrates potential discrepancies between perceptions and actual characteristics of older workers. In particular, it raises the issue of older worker stereotypes and their applicability to the majority of older workers. In the following sections, we discuss older worker stereotypes and how these stereotypes may impact older workers, and compare these commonly held beliefs to the findings of empirical research. Career self-management, training, the changing nature of work, and future directions are also discussed.

Older Worker Stereotypes

The issue of stereotypes was recognized early as a main concern for the field of industrial gerontology (Stagner, 1971, 1985; Sterns, 1986). There still remains a continuing need for the careful evaluation of the way in which older worker stereotypes are researched and how these beliefs may change over time. In our discussions, we distinguish between older worker stereotypes, age bias, and age discrimination. Stereotypes are the traits and characteristics associated with older workers in general. Age bias may be considered the tendency to use age when forming impressions of others (Perry, Kulik, & Bourhis, 1996). Such tendencies are likely to result in systematic patterns between selection decisions and applicant age (Bass & Barrett, 1981). Age discrimination, as defined by the Age Discrimination in Employment Act (ADEA, 1967, amended 1976, 1978, 1986), is

> the failure or refusal to hire or to discharge any individual within the protected age bracket (i.e. 40+) or to otherwise discriminate against any such individual with respect to his compensation, terms, conditions or privileges of employment because of such individual's age; to limit, segregate, or classify employees in any way which would deprive any individual within the protected age bracket of employment opportunities, or otherwise adversely effect his status as an employee, because of such individual's age.

When discussing stereotypes in the context of work, it is important to recognize both older adult and older worker stereotypes. Although the content of these stereotypes undoubtedly overlaps, there are also differences. Older adult stereotypes seem to encompass older ages and include a wider range of contexts relative to older worker stereotypes. In comparison, older worker stereotypes encompass relatively younger ages and specifically relate to the work context. In discussions of work, older worker stereotypes take the forefront. Research examining the content of older worker stereotypes has revealed both negative and positive components. Older workers (i.e., 50s–60s) tend to be perceived as being deficient in terms of job performance (e.g., productivity, efficiency, motivation, ability, innovation, creativity, logic, accident avoidance), potential for development (e.g., ambition, eagerness, future oriented, capable of learning, adaptability, versatility), responsiveness to managerial influences, and certain job demands (e.g., innovative thinking, creativity, and risk taking) as compared to younger workers (i.e., 20s–30s) (Rosen & Jerdee, 1976a). On the positive side, older workers are also viewed as more reliable, dependable, trustworthy, honest, and less likely to quit or miss work due to personal reasons than younger workers (Rosen & Jerdee, 1976a).

Older worker stereotypes may negatively affect older workers in two ways. First, older workers may accept the stereotypes and integrate these characteristics into their self-concepts. Second, these stereotypes may impact the judgments and actions of organizational decision makers. That is, selection, job performance, or promotional decisions may be based on stereotypes of older workers rather than each worker's individual merits.

The acceptance of older worker stereotypes by older employees may potentially influence performance expectations and lead to self-fulfilling prophesies. For example, an individual's performance may be enhanced by altering self-expectations through explicit recognition of high performance potential (Eden, 1992). A self-fulfilling prophesy is seen in that the individual both expects more of himself or herself and demonstrates high performance. This superior performance level may be maintained over time through internalized higher self-expectations (Eden, 1992). Buying into the positive aspects of older worker stereotypes may increase self-efficacy and self-expectations and lead to enhanced performance in these areas. Individuals with higher self-efficacy also tend to set challenging goals, maintain strong goal commitment, and show heightened effort when confronted with setbacks or failures (Bandura, 1989).

In contrast, lowered self-expectations negatively affect performance. Over time, to the extent older workers buy into the negative aspects of the stereotype, self-efficacy and self-expectations regarding ability and job performance may be lowered. Individuals with lowered self-efficacy in a particular domain may avoid difficult tasks and have low aspirations, reduced motivation, and weak goal commitment (Bandura, 1989). Consequently, job performance may suffer.

Empirical evidence of age differences in the endorsement of older worker stereotypes suggests older workers may not be buying into these stereotypic beliefs. Older hourly employees have been found to hold more favorable attitudes about older workers than younger hourly employees (Bird & Fisher, 1986; Kirchner & Dunnette, 1954; Kirchner, Lindbom, & Patterson, 1952). In contrast, supervisor's age seems to be unrelated to attitude toward older workers (Bird & Fisher, 1986; Kirchner & Dunnette, 1954). Older respondents have also been found to perceive smaller age differences in performance capacity than younger respondents (Rosen & Jerdee, 1976b).

A second way stereotypes may affect older workers is through supervisors' acceptance of these beliefs. Stereotype endorsement by decision makers, however, does not necessarily translate into discriminatory decisions and actions. An individual may be aware of and/or believe these stereotypes but base employment decisions on an applicant's job-relevant qualifications rather than characteristics associated with age. Age bias may be one individual difference that influences the likelihood of using older worker stereotypes when forming impressions of others (Perry et al., 1996).

The behavioral implications of older worker stereotypes, the increasing numbers of older workers in the workforce, and the ADEA have been the impetus behind much of the research examining age-related bias in interview and performance appraisal settings. The more recent trends toward bridge employment, second, and third careers have also added to the importance of determining what influence, if any, older worker stereotypes and age biases may have on employment decisions.

In the arena of personnel selection, the impact of older worker stereotypes on employment decisions is not well understood. The research findings have been mixed, few well-developed theories are available for understanding age discrimination, and the mechanisms by which stereotypes may operate tend not to be clearly delineated (Finkelstein, Burke, & Raju, 1995; Perry et al., 1996).

To address these issues, Finkelstein and associates (1995) formulated several hypotheses on the basis of a cognitive model of social categorization (Fiske, Neuberg, Beattie, & Milberg, 1987) and examined these predictions through meta-analysis. An in-group bias hypothesis predicted raters would evaluate applicants who were of similar ages to themselves more favorably than those of dissimilar ages. In these analyses, older and younger raters ranged in age from 30 to 60 and 17 to 29 years, respectively. Older and younger applicants ranged in age from 48 to 65 years and 24 to 34, respectively.

The job information hypothesis predicted that job-relevant information about target applicants would impact the use of stereotypes. Specifically, older and younger applicants were expected to receive similar ratings in the presence of either positive or negative job information. When no job-relevant information was present, raters were predicted to rely on stereotypes and rate older applicants less favorably than younger applicants.

The salience hypothesis predicted that when applicant's ages were contrasted, raters would rely on stereotypes and rate older applicants less favorably than younger applicants. Lastly, the job stereotype hypothesis examined both age and job stereotypes. Older applicants were predicted to receive more favorable ratings than younger applicants when considered for older-typed jobs (i.e., jobs typically seen as being held by older workers; see Cleveland & Landy, 1983, 1987). Similarly, younger applicants were predicted to receive more favorable ratings when applying for younger-typed jobs.

In general, the findings provided some support for the in-group bias, job information, and salience hypotheses. Older applicants were rated less favorably than younger applicants in simulated employment decisions when raters were younger, no job-relevant information was present, and age was salient (i.e., raters evaluated both younger and older applicants). Older raters, however, did not rate older and younger applicants differently. The job stereotype hypothesis was not fully supported: evaluations of older and younger applicants were similar when applying for older-typed jobs. Although younger applicants were rated more favorably in younger-typed jobs, this finding was based on a very limited number of studies.

The correlations in these analyses ranged in size from zero to 0.81, with the average being around 0.26. The percentage of variance in ratings accounted for by applicant age was approximately 7%. This is similar to other work in which applicant age was determined to account for only 8% of the variance in interview ratings (Avolio & Barrett, 1987). Age may not be a major influence in selection evaluations (Avolio & Barrett, 1987).

To the extent these results generalize to organizational settings, the implications are that decision makers should be provided with job-relevant information regarding applicants and age-related information should be deemphasized (Finkelstein et al., 1995). Increasing numbers of older adults in applicants pools may also serve to reduce the salience of age (Cleveland, Festa, & Montgomery, 1988; Finkelstein et al., 1995); as the proportion of older adults in applicants pools increases, the salience of age may decrease.

Economic-based, as well as social-based, stereotypes may be working against older workers (Finkelstein et al., 1995). That is, older workers may be perceived as incurring greater organizational costs than younger worker in terms of higher salaries, health care, and other benefits. Recent research indicates that employers often view facilitating the retirement of older workers as cost effective due to perceptions that health care costs are higher (Hall & Mirvis, 1993). Several interesting issues arise when considering the potential operation of older workers stereotypes in employment settings. First, in organizational interview settings an applicant's age may be ambiguous. It might be necessary to infer age based on personal characteristics such as physical appearance or demeanor. Alternately, age may be estimated from information included in application forms, resumes, or vitas. This raises an interesting question: Are older workers stereotypes cued by age per se or by an applicant's physical appearance or other characteristics that are suggestive of age? Furthermore, consider the fact that people possess many characteristics. When is age more or less likely to serve as a cue instead of other characteristics? These multiple cues may also act together. For example, Kunda and Thagard (1996) propose that multiple stereotypes may influence each other's meanings and jointly affect impression formation. Similarly, stereotypes and individual specific information may be processed simultaneously and jointly influence both each other's meanings and impression formation (Kunda & Thagard, 1996).

Second, in comparison to the more straightforward categories of race and sex, age categories may be more complex. Although legal definitions and social norms suggest guidelines for defining older workers, individuals' conceptualizations may not adhere to these conventions (see Sterns & Doverspike, 1989 for a discussion of older worker definitions). For example, although ADEA designates 40 years as the legal demarcation of an older worker and the American Association of Retired People designates 50 years as eligibility for membership, individuals may use different age ranges to determine at what point they consider "workers" to become "older workers." The approximate age ranges included in one's conceptualization of younger, middle-aged, and older workers may vary with individual differences such as respondent age, age bias, and perceived retirement norms.

Stereotypes may be viewed as energy-saving devices that preserve cognitive resources for use in other processing tasks (Macrae, Milne, & Bodenhausen, 1994). Stereotypes and other heuristics are presumably learned and reinforced due to their general adequacy (Smith, 1994). This raises the question of the accuracy of older worker stereotypes. Even if stereotypes are accurate, however, it is imperative to evaluate each worker on his or her own merits rather than on the basis of social categories. In the following section, we examine the extent to which empirical research corroborates or disconfirms common older worker stereotypes. We focus specifically on stereotypes concerning job performance, training, withdrawal behaviors, and work attitudes.

Age and Job Performance.   One pervasive stereotype of older workers is the belief that this group demonstrates lower performance and productivity than younger workers (Rosen & Jerdee, 1976a). In a comprehensive literature review, Rhodes (1983) noted that research findings examining the relationship between age and job performance were inconsistent. Since this review, two different meta-analyses have summarized the primary studies examining this relation. Waldman and Avolio (1986) found age tended to be positively related to productivity ($r = 0.27$) and to peer ratings ($r = 0.10$) and negatively related to supervisor ratings ($r = -0.14$). Chronological age, however, accounted for only a small portion of the variance in job performance—regardless of the performance indicator. In a more comprehensive analysis, McEvoy and Cascio (1989) found a very weak, positive relation between age and performance ($r = 0.06$). In conjunction, these analyses suggest a small, positive, relation between age and job performance (see also Avolio, Waldman, & McDaniel, 1990)—at least for younger and middle-aged adults. Caution should be taken when generalizing this relation to the higher end of the age distribution. This tentativeness is due to the smaller and potentially nonrepresentative samples at this older age range (Sterns & McDaniel, 1994). At this point (i.e., 65+), there tends to be fewer workers represented in research samples. Additionally, the select group that remains employed may do so due to superior performance and/or health status. Selective dropout may also result in less stable correlations and the relation is more likely to be influenced by individuals with extreme scores.

To some extent, the relation between age and job performance across all age ranges may be largely a function of job knowledge gained through job experience (Sterns & McDaniel, 1994). For younger workers, small differences in job experience can translate into large differences in job performance. As workers age and gain experience, however, the additional experience contributes little to increasing overall job knowledge and performance. As a result, weaker relations between age and job performance would be evident for older workers.

The possibility of a nonlinear relation between age and job performance should also be considered (Warr, 1994). The results of Avolio et al. (1990) suggested that although the relation between age and job performance is adequately described by linear functions, the relation seems to be stronger for younger ages and weaker for older ages. Nevertheless, it is important to stress that the relation between these variables is near zero; a worker's age has little value for predicting job performance (Sterns & McDaniel, 1994).

Age and Training.   A second, common stereotype is the belief that older workers have lower potential for development, training, and learning than younger workers (Rosen & Jerdee, 1976a). Congruent with these beliefs, a recent meta-analysis revealed poorer job-related training performance for older than younger adults (Kubeck, Delp, Haslett, & McDaniel, 1996). Older adults tended to show less mastery of training material ($r = -0.26$; $d = -0.88$), completed final training tasks more slowly ($r = 0.28$; $d = 1.53$), and required more time to complete training programs ($r = 0.42$; $d = 0.139$) than younger adults. Interestingly, field studies tended to show smaller age effects than laboratory studies.

These findings were also translated into estimated mean training performance in order to illustrate the practical impact in organizational settings. In terms of training performance, 30, 40, 50, 60, and 70 year olds were estimated to be at 57th, 47th, 37th, 28th, and 20th percentiles, respectively. The authors also noted the likelihood of substantial individual differences and variance in training performance; some older adults will show similar or greater mastery than some middle-aged or younger adults.

Kubeck and associates (1996) suggested two potential explanations for the poorer mastery of training materials shown by older adults. First, older adults may begin training with a disadvantage by having less initial mastery of the material than younger adults. Consequently, even if older and younger adults gained similar amounts of knowledge through training, older adults would show less posttraining mastery due to initial knowledge differences. Second, differences may be due to less learning on the part of older adults. Potentially, older adults may need to unlearn previous information in order to acquire the new information (Sterns, 1986).

These explanations were investigated in a sample of 105 mid-level managers ranging in age from 27 to 58 years (Gray, Boyce, Hall, & McDaniel, 1996). Results indicated older workers had less pretraining knowledge of training materials than younger workers. Older workers also demonstrated less learning of the training materials than younger workers, even after controlling for pretraining knowledge. This suggests age differences in posttraining knowledge are partially due to pretraining knowledge differences. The unique contribution of age to explaining pretraining knowledge and posttraining mastery differences, however, was substantially decreased when education was controlled. This suggests the age differences noted in training may be due to a combination of factors, including well-documented age-associated cognitive changes as well as age differences in experience captured by proxy through the education variable.

Age and Work Withdrawal.　A positive older worker stereotype is the perception this group is less likely to quit or miss work due to personal reasons (Rosen & Jerdee, 1976a). A recent meta-analysis found a near zero relation ($r = -0.08$) between age and voluntary turnover (Healy, Lehman, & McDaniel, 1995). Age does not seem to be related to choosing to leave an organization.

Age, however, does seem to be related to certain types of absenteeism. Meta-analysis has found moderate, negative relations between age and two measures of voluntary absenteeism: attitudinal (i.e., the number of absences of 3 days or more, $r = -0.24$) and frequency (i.e., the number of absences, $r = -0.30$) (Hackett, 1990). Older employees tended to have fewer voluntary absences than younger employees. These relations changed very little when the effects of tenure were controlled. Furthermore, sex was found to moderate the

age/voluntary absenteeism relations. Older ages were related to fewer voluntary absences for men, whereas age and absenteeism was unrelated for women.
In contrast, age was unrelated to involuntary absence as measured by total time
lost from work.

Age and Work Attitudes. Older workers may also be viewed as being unin-
terested or uninvolved with their work and co-workers (Rosen & Jerdee, 1985).
This suggests older workers may hold less positive work-related attitudes than
younger workers. In particular we examine the relations between organizational commitment, job satisfaction, job involvement, occupational well-being,
and age.

Organizational commitment is a multidimensional construct with at least
two recognized components: attitudinal and continuance commitment. Attitudinal commitment is defined as an individual's "strong belief in and acceptance of the organization's goals and values, willingness to exert considerable
effort on behalf of the organization, and strong desire to maintain membership
in the organization" (Mowday, Steers, & Porter, 1979, p. 226). Older workers
may also demonstrate increased attitudinal commitment due to greater job satisfaction, having received more rewards from the organization, self-selection,
or having self-justified remaining with the organization by deciding they like
it (Meyer & Allen, 1984).

Continuance commitment reflects accumulated interests that would be lost
or diminished if the individual were to leave the organization (e.g., pensions,
seniority). This threat of loss is what binds the individual to the organization
(Becker, 1960). Continuance commitment has been hypothesized to increase
with age due to the accumulation of side bets over time (Ritzer & Trice, 1969).

Meta-analysis has found a moderate, positive relation between age and organizational commitment ($r = 0.20$) (Mathieu & Zajac, 1990). In general, organizational commitment seems to be stronger among older as compared to
younger workers. Commitment type was found to moderate this relation with
age being more strongly related to attitudinal than continuance commitment.
It is important to note that two scales often used to measure continuance commitment (i.e., Ritzer & Trice, 1969; Hrebiniak & Alutto, 1972) actually appear
to be measuring affective commitment (Meyer & Allen, 1984). Therefore, to the
extent these scales were present in the meta-analysis database, interpretation
of the relation between age and continuance commitment is less clear.

Correlations between age and job satisfaction typically range between 0.10
and 0.20 (Warr, 1994). The relations tend to be positive, but not particularly
strong. Examining facets of satisfaction may be more informative in understanding older adults' work experiences. Based on a review of the literature,
Warr (1994) concluded satisfaction with the work itself, intrinsic satisfaction,
and potentially pay satisfaction are greater for older as compared to younger
workers. Job involvement refers to an individual's psychological identification
with his or her job (Kanungo, 1982a, 1982b; Lawler & Hall, 1970; Lodahl &
Kejner, 1965; Saleh & Hosek, 1976), the degree to which job performance af-

fects an individual's self-esteem (Lodahl & Kejner, 1965; Saleh & Hosek, 1976) and active participation in the job (Saleh & Hosek, 1976). Similar to other work-related attitudes, job involvement is only weakly related to age. A recent meta-analytic study found only a small, positive correlation between these variables ($r = 0.16$) (Brown, 1996).

Warr (1992) examined potential curvilinear relations between age and two dimensions of occupational well-being: job anxiety–contentment and job depression–enthusiasm. The participants in this sample ranged from 18 to 64 years. U-shaped relations were found such that older workers tended to report the highest levels of contentment and enthusiasm, middle-aged workers reported the lowest levels, and the youngest workers reported higher levels than the middle-aged workers. This nonlinear component, however, become nonsignificant when job position (i.e., job tenure, job level), job characteristics, employment commitment, and education were taken into account. Warr (1992) also suggested the declines in job contentment and enthusiasm seen between the ages of 18 and 25 years may be partially accounted for by differences in perceived job characteristics.

Summary

In summary, only partial support is found for both the negative and positive aspects of the older worker stereotypes examined here. Empirical research does not support the perception that older workers perform more poorly on the job than younger workers. Age is weakly, albeit positively, related to job performance. Older workers do seem to be at a disadvantage relative to younger workers in training situations. This does not mean, however, that older workers are unable to learn training materials to the extent required to perform their jobs (Sterns, 1986; Sterns & Doverspike, 1989). In terms of the positive stereotypes, the research corroborates the belief that older workers are less likely to be voluntarily absent from work than younger workers. Worker age, however, was unrelated to voluntary turnover. Counter to common beliefs, older workers are neither more nor less likely to voluntarily leave their jobs than younger workers. Additionally, weak positive relations are found between age and work-related attitudes. Older workers seem to have only slightly more positive feelings toward their employing organizations and work.

The five stereotypic characteristics of older workers examined here do not overwhelmingly correspond to the empirical data. Stereotypes do not generalize to all older workers and may potentially impact workers in two ways. First, to the extent older workers include these perceptions in their self-concepts, they may unnecessarily limit themselves. In terms of career self-management, they may limit their avenues of exploration or not pursue certain opportunities. Alternately, they may not even engage in self-management activities. Second, to the extent organizational decision makers act on these perceptions, older workers' employment or career opportunities may be inappropriately limited. The most appropriate conclusion, however, is that each individual, regardless of age, should be evaluated (or self-evaluated) based on his or her own merits, skills, abilities, and motivation and not the stereotypic characteristics of a particular age group with which he or she happens to be associated.

Self-Management, Training, and Changing Organizations

Stereotypes are only one potential influence on older worker's employment experiences. Another influential factor is the work context itself. Workers do not exist in a static environment, and the changing nature of work and organizations is likely to impact older workers, their jobs, and careers.

As organizations transition from pyramid to flatter, more streamlined configurations through downswing and restructuring, employees may experience job loss, job plateauing, and skills obsolescence (Farr et al., 1998; Sterns & Miklos, 1995). Older workers may be singled out in downsizing efforts on the basis of stereotypic traits such as being unsuitable for retraining or fast-paced work environments (Mirvis & Hall, 1996a,b). Furthermore, depending on age of career entry, middle-aged and older workers may be more likely to occupy the mid-level managerial positions that are often the focus of downsizing and restructuring strategies. Additionally, slow company growth may lead to less opportunity for advancement (Farr et al., 1998). These changes suggest older workers may need to take increased involvement and responsibility in terms of career management.

Organizational changes are also altering the nature of the relationships between organizations and employees (Hall & Mirvis, 1996). Employers' commitment to employees may last only as long as there is a need for their skills and performance. Similarly, employees' commitment to the employer may last only as long as their expectations are being met. These changes place greater emphasis on employees' adaptability and abilities in learning to learn (Hall & Mirvis, 1996).

The idea of career self-management is well captured in the discussions of Hall and Mirvis (1996) of the protean career. A protean career is directed by the individual rather than the employing organization. Greater responsibility for learning, skill mastery, and reskilling is also placed on the individual (Hall & Mirvis, 1995). The individual is in charge, in control, and able to change the shape of his or her career at will—similar to a free agent in sports (Hall & Mirvis, 1996). This perspective and the goals of this type of career (e.g., psychological success, identity expansion, and learning) also recognize the artificiality of the distinction between work and nonwork life. Personal roles and career roles are highly interrelated and the boundaries between these roles tend to be fuzzy rather than clear cut (Hall & Mirvis, 1995). One disadvantage of protean careers is that an individual's identity is not likely to be tied to any one organization. Problems of self-definition may result in that one's personal identity is not connected to a formal organizational work role.

Mirvis and Hall (1996a) also suggest that taking on the responsibility of career self-management may hold special benefits for older workers. Greater tenure in a protean-type career may lead to increased value of older workers. It may be rather expensive to replace such knowledgeable, adaptable, and continuously learning employees with younger workers with less protean-type career experience. Protean careers may increase the organization's options for deploying older workers. Similarly, the options older workers may pursue in shaping their careers are also increased (Mirvis & Hall, 1996). Potential alternatives include moving to a new field (i.e., second or third careers), building new skills in their present field, changing organizations, phasing into retirement, or joining the contingent workforce.

Older workers, however, may also be at a disadvantage in terms of moving toward greater career self-management. Transitioning from a typical, organizational-driven career to a protean career may be a rather daunting task—particularly if an individual initially entered the workforce with a one career–one employer ideal. Additionally, stereotypic beliefs about older workers may lead to the underutilization of this group within the new relationships between organizations and employees (Mirvis & Hall, 1996a).

Organizational or technological changes can lead to changes in the knowledge, skills, and abilities required for a job. Sterns and Patchett (1984) discussed these issues, proposing that employees in fast-paced industries will have greater interest in career development because of an ongoing need to update skills. An individual's motivation may be an important factor in determining whether employees update skills. Shearer and Steger (1975) found that need for achievement and career expectations were both related to obsolescence. Lower levels of each were associated with greater obsolescence. Additionally, individuals with an external locus of control were move likely to be obsolete (Shearer & Steger, 1985).

McEnrue (1989) found that younger employees and those with a high level of organizational commitment expressed greater willingness to engage in self-development as a career management strategy than did other employees. The data suggested that organizational commitment may promote self-directed development among emloyees. Older employees saw less opportunity for advancement. This could account for older employees being less willing to engage in activities if they see no benefit from their efforts.

Dorsett (1994) found that age was a significant predictor of updating behavior. Contrary to stereotypes, older nurses (40 and over) were more apt to engage in updating behavior. However, the results suggested that motivation levels exerted the strongest positive effect on updating, followed by organizational climate and age. Her subjects were all nurses; there was no comparison across different jobs. However, her research was conducted before mandatory continuing education was implemented. Nurses are representative of professional roles but may not generalize to less skilled roles. Job characteristics that have been discussed as relevant to updating behavior are task diversity, complex and challenging work, and participation in decisions. Updating behavior is an area ripe for continued research to determine under what conditions younger and older workers are motivated to continue updating their skills.

This emphasis on updating and managing one's own career may be important in avoiding obsolescence and remaining employable for workers of all ages. Feldman (1989) suggests that managers and professionals today have a new set of career values. They no longer assume the organization has unilateral control over their careers, nor that organizations will take care of their employees in a parental fashion. This new careerism has led to employees being more critical in self-analysis, more assertive in seeking feedback, and more likely to refuse transfers or promotions that subvert career goals.

Although considerable research has examined aging within the context of work, at least one issue that deserves further attention is better understanding of the small age differences in job performance. For example, are older workers maintaining their performance through compensatory behaviors or are age-related cognitive and ability-related declines irrelevant to job performance (Sterns & McDaniel, 1994)? The conflicting findings regarding job performance versus training performance also deserve a closer look (Sterns & McDaniel, 1994). A paradox exists in that older adults seem to benefit less from training than younger adults, yet show equal, or slightly better, job performance.

Warr (1994) presented a framework that aids in understanding this paradox. Warr (see Table 13.1) suggested four categories of tasks differing on two dimensions: (1) workers' basic capacities are more exceeded with increasing

TABLE 13.1.
Warr (1994) Categories of Job Activity and Expected Relations of Performance with Age during Active Working Years

Task category	Basic capacities are exceeded to a greater degree with increasing age	Performance is enhanced by experience	Expected relationship with age job content	Illustrative
A	No	Yes	Positive	Knowledge-based judgments with no time pressure
B	No	No	Zero	Relatively undemanding activities
C	Yes	Yes	Zero	Skilled manual work
D	Yes	No	Negative	Continuous, processing

age and (2) performance is enhanced by experience. Positive relations between age and performance would be expected for tasks in which basic capacities are not exceeded with increasing age and performance is enhanced through experience. Negative or nonlinear relations would be expected for tasks in which basic capacities were exceeded and experience was not beneficial. No relation between age and job performance would be expected for the two remaining task categories. Physical changes can have a major affect on work performance. For a more extensive discussion, see Panek (1997) and Sterns, Sterns, and Hollis (1996).

This framework suggests training and everyday job demands may fall into different categories. That is, positive age–job performance relations may be found when job demands do not exceed older workers' capacities and experience is beneficial to performance. Negative age-training performance relations may be seen to the extent training demands exceed basic capacities or previous experience is not beneficial.

Summary

Organization and work changes set the stage for self-management of careers. Individuals may be motivated to engage in training and retraining as part of their updating. Organizations can support updating by providing an appropriate climate and providing training opportunities. Adult and older adult workers must continue to update to have the latest knowledge, skills, and abilities. Jobs can provide situations that stimulate the adult and older worker to grow and develop. Other job situations may place the worker at a disadvantage because growth opportunities do not exist at work. In the latter case, adult and older adult workers may need to seek new training on their own.

Work and Leisure

An emerging issue is the patterns of overcommitment to the work role. Each case must be looked at individually. People differ in the amount of energy they have available for work and nonwork tasks. A balanced life is often seen as a desired goal. In reality, ambitious, responsible people do not get ahead by leading so-called "balanced" lives. The line is fine between work behvior that is achievement and success oriented and work that is compulsive, driven, and cheerless (Lowman, 1993).

In life-span development and gerontology, the important role of leisure and activity in the well-being and life satisfaction of adults and older adults has been emphasized (Kaplan, 1979; Kelley, 1993, 1996; McGuire et al., 1996). Cutler and Hendrick (1990) believe technological changes and changing employment opportunities will lead to alterations between work and leisure over the next 20 years. They state that "to make sense of patterns of leisure and free time, they must be cast in a life-course perspective and interpreted in terms of an individual's movement across life and from one membership category to another. Furthermore, a strident work-leisure dicotomy is counterproductive, as it is the individual's perception that involves each with its most subjective meaningful quality" (Cutler & Hendrick, 1990, p. 169). Leisure provides an opportunity for important interaction with people who are significant others and can be crucial to one's self concept and sense of well-being. At midlife, there may be changes or shifts in how leisure is viewed.

Value orientation makes a difference in how an individual views leisure. This orientation is based on one's early social-cultural experience and has influence throughout life. What activities one chooses to engage in is based on one's past experience and one's perception as to what is socially appropriate. The opportunity to engage in leisure activities is being extended by new norms and increased free time.

Leisure participation, attitudes, and orientation depend on one's personal resources. Health is a major predictor determining activity level per se and preferences for involvement. Poor health may lead to more passive types of activity or to inactivity. Education level is also a predictor of future activity. Work provides an organizer around which leisure activities may be carried out. In retirement, many patterns of nonwork activities continue. Income is important because it offers choices in activities and locations.

Leisure as a form of consumption is a growing area of marketing research. The mature market, 50+, has been a growing area of study (Cole & Castellano, 1996; Sterns & Sterns, 1995). Leisure activities and related services have become important in our understanding of the life-styles of adults and older adults. Mature consumers display greater heterogeneity and diversity than any other age group. Following Neugarten's (1974) categories of young-old and old-old, the mature market is often divided into four major segments, based on age and life-cycle events.

The young-old are aged 55–64 and are generally active and healthy. Consisting of about 32.8 million consumers, these individuals are often preparing for retirement. They are "working to live—not living to work." Also called the "sandwich generation," the young-old are prime targets for products and services related to exercise equipment, health programs, and maintaining a youthful appearance. Consumers in this category are increasingly taking early retirement, changing careers (not all willingly), or working part-time.

The middle-old are 65–74 years old. Most of the 16.2 million consumers in this category are generally retired. They are prime targets for health and nutrition products/services, leisure products and activities (eating out, travel), and condos and retirement housing.

The old-old are 75–84 years old. Consisting of about 10.3 million consumers, this group is increasingly frail and displays greater health limitations with increasing age. Individuals in this category more often fit the "senior citizen" stereotype. Most are still healthy, although health may be increasingly problematic.

Age per se is a poor segmentation device (Morgan & Levy, 1993). A better way to segment older consumers is through health, use of time, money, and milestone events. Health segments mature Americans into three basic categories: healthy individuals who improve or maintain physical well-being with a wholly independent life-style, those who may need to make some life-style accommodations due to limitations posed by health status, and those with major limitations, requiring significant product and service purchases.

Time is another segmentation device, categorizing mature consumers into those who are still working full time and those who are working part-time or retired. Purchases of products and services often depend on the level of work or leisure. Money and attitudes toward money are still another means of segmenting the mature market. Only 13% of older adults fall below the poverty level; about 25% struggle financially.

Segmentation of the mature market as a means to predict purchase of services and leisure activities is perhaps more difficult than for younger age groups because of the heterogeneity and range of individual differences among older consumers. Mature market consumers are the most affluent group in the United States, and those aged 50–64 are the most affluent of all. Americans 50+ hold 77% of the nation's financial assets and 50% of all discretionary income. Per capita spending is about 2.5 times that of the population. Mature consumers tend to spend more money than do younger consumers on financial services, health, travel, and entertainment.

Retirement

Similar to work and leisure, retirement has also moved increasingly into the realm of self-management. The individual has become the focal point of the bulk of the responsibility in choosing when and how to retire (Avolio et al., 1990). Because retirement is a relatively new phenomenon, we begin by tracing the history of this institution and its transition from a rare to a normative event. We also discuss the changing nature of retirement, retirement definitions, and a comprehensive model of retirement with consideration of sex, decision making, adjustment, and satisfaction in postretirement life.

History of Retirement

A brief history of retirement in the United States illustrates the continual evolution of this institution. Through the 1700s and mid-1800s retirement was rather uncommon and about 70% of older men remained in the labor force. Many of these older workers held high status and prestigious positions (Atchley, 1982; Graebner, 1980). The aged were valued for their wisdom and experience and forced retirement was not supported by the social ideology of the time (Atchley, 1982).

The growth of retirement was influenced by at least two trends in the early industrial period: the emergence of labor unions and mandatory retirement (Atchley, 1982). Labor unions sought worker privileges based on seniority and, in response, management opposed these demands on the grounds that older workers were both less able and more expensive. Prevailing theories of older adults as worn out and useless reinforced beliefs that older adults were too incompetent to work (Richardson, 1993). Mandatory retirement emerged as a reflection of these beliefs and became a mechanism for removing older workers while simultaneously generating opportunities for younger workers.

In 1934, a union-sponsored railroad bill promoting compulsory retirement was unanimously passed by the U.S. Senate. One outcome of this bill was that many retirees were left in poverty due to the nonexistence of private pensions (Richardson, 1993). Workers who were mandatorily retired had little hope of finding another job and often had insufficient financial resources to support their retirement. In general, retirement was seen in an unfavorable light as it was associated with poverty and uselessness.

The Social Security Act of 1935 was passed in response to the growing number of older adults in poverty (Richardson, 1993). Both Social Security and employer pensions were seen as mechanisms to manage the labor market (i.e., facilitate the shedding of older workers and hiring of younger workers) and guarantee some basis of economic security in old age (Atchley, 1982; Quadagno & Hardy, 1996). A survey conducted in the early 1940s (Wentworth, 1945) revealed only 5% of the respondents reported retiring in good health because they wanted to do so. Over one-half reported retiring due to being laid-off and one-third retired due to poor health. Retirement in this time period continued to be viewed in a less than favorable light.

Retirement "came of age" between 1965 and 1980 (Atchley, 1982). In 1967 the ADEA was passed to protect workers aged 40 to 65 years and a 1978 amendment prohibited mandatory retirement before the age of 70 years. Policy changes in Social Security benefits and general increases in earnings also improved the financial status of retirees. The ADEA was again amended in 1986 to prohibit mandatory retirement ages in most occupations. Retirement was gradually viewed more favorably, as a right or privilege earned by working hard (Richardson, 1993).

Changing Nature of Retirement

Retirement is still evolving today as evidenced by changing transition patterns and ages of labor force exits. First, the transition from work to retirement is no longer clear cut. Retirement is not necessarily a complete withdrawal from the work force and work activities. An estimated one-third of retirees reenter the work force, although the likelihood of reentry decreases with age (Hayward, Hardy, & Liu, 1994). Postcareer bridge employment may involve changes in industry, occupation, hours, or salary (Ruhm, 1990). These multiple pathways from work to retirement highlight the importance of conceptualizing retirement as a process and studying the process over time. The retirement process may include an anticipatory period of the retirement decision (which may pre-date the decision and act by decades), the decision itself, the act(s) of retirement, and continual adjustment to retirement (see also Atchley, 1976; Ekerdt et al., 1996). Decisions pertaining to structuring and restructuring one's life and activities in retirement may continue for the rest of the life span.

In recognition of the multiple pathways of the retirement process, a recent study examined the frequency and antecedents of different exit patterns in a sample of 2226 white and black men aged 55 to 74 years (Mutchler, Burr, Pienta, & Massagli, 1997). Patterns of continuous work, continuous nonwork, crisp exits, and blurred exits were examined over a period of 28 months. A crisp transition is a single, unreversed, and clear-cut exit from the labor force. A blurred pattern is a gradual role transition marked by repeated reentries and exits and may encompass months or years. In this initial investigation, 10% of the sample was categorized as crisp transitioners and 15% as blurred transitioners. In comparison, approximately 34 and 41% of the sample reported continuous labor force participation and nonparticipation, respectively.

Crisp and blurred transitioners were also found to differ in terms of age, financial resources, and health status. Crisp transitioners tended to be younger than 65 years. Although not associated with any particular ages, blurred transitions tended to be uncommon past the age of 68 years. Limited financial resources (i.e., pension availability, nonwage income) were associated with blurred transitions as opposed to the crisp exit pattern. Inadequate income seemed to prompt individuals to maintain continued, although somewhat sporadic, labor force participation. Lastly, individuals with poor health were more likely to demonstrate blurred transitions as opposed to continuous labor force participation. Individuals with the poorest health, however, were more likely to demonstrate crisp exits or no labor force participation over the time course of the study. This research highlights the importance of examining exit patterns as opposed to single transitions in capturing the retirement process (Multcher et al., 1997). Considering retirement as a single transition no longer seems to adequately capture the complexity and the dynamic aspects of the process.

The continuously changing nature of retirement is also evidenced in retirement ages. The idea of a "normal" retirement age is an evolving concept and considering 65 years as a typical retirement age may no longer be appropriate as many individuals retire, initiate blurred transitions, or receive Social Security and pension income prior to this age (Cornman & Kingson, 1996; Multcher et al., 1997). Additionally, as the idea of a typical retirement age shifts to that of a range of ages (Cornman & Kingson, 1996), it becomes less clear how to distinguish "early" from "typical" from "late" retirement.

Retirement age trends show the "typical" retirement age for men and women has declined over the past 40 years. Between the late 1950s and the late 1980s, median retirement ages declined from about 66 to 63 years for both men and women (Gendall & Siegel, 1996). African-American men, Caucasian men, and Caucasian women all showed this 3-year decline. A larger drop (i.e., 4.6 years) was found for African-American women, although less confidence was placed on this estimate due to sampling issues. This decline seemed to level off in the 1980s for both Caucasian men and women, whereas an additional decrease of about 1 year was seen for both African-American men and women (Gendall & Siegel, 1996). A similar pattern was noted in the average age of initial receipt of Social Security retirement benefits. That is, an initial decline began in the late 1950s for all race and gender groups and leveled off no later than 1985 (Gendall & Siegel, 1996).

These illustrations demonstrate actual changes in retirement ages. Individuals, however, may or may not take these changes into account when assessing their own retirement timing. One's perceptions of typical ages may be very different from mathematically computed typical ages.

Trends in perceived retirement age norms also illustrate the changing nature of retirement. Based on data from the Health and Retirement Study, Ekerdt (1998) found almost 75% of workers aged 51 to 61 years recognized a typical or usual retirement age among their co-workers. These perceived ages tended to concentrate around both 62 and 65 years. Furthermore, 85% of workers indicated plans to retire at or before the perceived usual retirement age. Workers who planned partial retirements or job changes, as compared to complete exits, were also more likely to anticipate exiting their present jobs before the perceived typical retirement age. It seems that workers not only are retiring at actual younger ages, they are also planning to retire earlier than perceived norms.

Retirement Definitions

The previous illustrations hold implications for the conceptualization and definition of retirement. First, the way researchers define "retired" may be very different from how workers and retirees use the term. Second, relations between predictor and criterion variables may potentially differ depending on the definition and operation of retirement (Beehr, 1986; Howard, Marshall, Rechnitzer, Cunningham, & Donner, 1982; Palmore et al., 1982; Talaga & Beehr, 1995). Additionally, because not all researchers have made clear their working definition of retirement, it is difficult to understand this body of literature as a whole. The definition of retirement should be considered when comparing and integrating results across studies (Beehr, 1986; Palmore et al., 1982).

Talaga and Beehr (1995) outlined three retirement definitions typically found in the literature: self-attributions of work/retirement status, receipt of Social Security or pension income, and the number of hours worked per week for pay. The first two definitions are dichotomous measures. The third is a continuous measure indicating degree of retirement that explicitly recognizes the possibility of partial retirement. A partially retired category, however, may also

be included when measuring self-attributions. Although these definitions co-
vary with age in that older adults are more likely to consider themselves retired, receive Social Security or pension income, and work fewer hours (Talaga
& Beehr, 1995), they are not specifically tied to one particular age.

These three retirement indicators tend to be highly correlated (median r =
0.80) and demonstrate similar patterns of relations with demographic, health,
financial, work, family, and leisure variables (Talaga & Beehr, 1995). Degree of
retirement, however, tends to show somewhat smaller relations with these variables than self-attribution and Social Security/pension measures. Although the
results of this one study do not definitively support the empirical divergence
of the these retirement indicators, certain definitions may be more appropriate
for certain research questions. A theoretically appropriate measure may facilitate the interpretation of research results.

Retirement Processes

Retirement is best conceptualized as a decision-making process and behavioral
transition that occur over time and span both the work and leisure domains of
life. To fully understand these processes it is necessary to consider the antecedents and psychological processes leading up to the decision as well as the
consequences of the decision and actual retirement act(s). It is also important
to consider potential antecedents and consequences from a wide range of life
domains (e.g., work, family, friends, health, leisure). Only a limited view is
gained by examining a limited set of variables. For example, economists have
typically favored individual's preferences for leisure and consumption in predicting retirement, whereas sociologists have favored social opportunities and
behavioral constraints (Ekerdt, 1998). Considering variables from multiple life
domains facilitates a more comprehensive understanding of retirement
processes. Examining a wide range model also provides opportunities to examine the relative contributions of personal and environmental (i.e., work and
nonwork related) factors on retirement decisions and transitions.

Researching the process over time recognizes the possibilities that predictors of retirement may show changing relations over time. Some variables may
have greater or lesser influence on the decisions and transition processes as a
worker ages. Additionally, plans and decisions may change as workers explore
different options and situational contexts change (Ekerdt, 1998). Adjustment to
retirement may also be a dynamic process as retirees structure and restructure
their lives.

At least three comprehensive models of the retirement processes are found
in the literature (Atchley, 1979; Beehr, 1986; Feldman, 1994). An in-depth review of retirement models is outside the scope of this chapter, and therefore,
we focus on Beehr's (1986) model and associated research. Beehr (1986) presented a comprehensive model of the retirement decision and the subsequent
impact of this decision and exit type on the individual and the organization.

First, three continuums of retirement forms are recognized: voluntary versus involuntary, early versus on time, and partial versus complete. The voluntary/involuntary continuum may also be considered as degree of perceived volition (Talaga & Beehr, 1989). This continuum captures an individual's perceptions of his or her amount of choice concerning the exit decision. Perceptions of choice may be influenced by contextual factors such as a retirement incentive program, economic costs of not retiring (e.g., no pension advantage in working longer, window of opportunity to accept a retirement incentive package), work attitudes, perceived organizational and co-worker support, and not being able to find a job. Choice may also be influenced by friends, family, and health status. The early versus on-time dimension may also be considered as age of retirement (Talaga & Beehr, 1989). As mentioned earlier, the meaning of "early" and "on time" is becoming less clear due to the changing nature of retirement. This distinction, however, may be useful when considered in relation to an individual's perception of local retirement norms (e.g., Ekerdt, 1998). The third continuum, partial versus complete retirement, recognizes the different pathways to retirement (e.g., blurred versus crisp retirement transitions, Mutchler et al., 1997).

The Beehr (1986) retirement model highlights personal factors and two sets of environmental forces that influence preferences to retire, the retirement decision, and transition. Personal factors include personality, skill obsolescence, health status, and financial well-being. The environmental forces include both job factors (e.g., attainment of occupational goals, job characteristics) and non-job factors (e.g., marital/family life, leisure interests).

The model also recognizes the retirement transition as impacting both the individual and the organization. The three aspects of retirement (i.e., perceived volition, age, and degree of retirement) are proposed to have a direct impact on retirement adjustment (e.g., activities, psychological well-being). This impact may also depend on moderating factors such as retirement planning, retirement expectations, occupational status, health status, and financial well-being. For example, the relation between perceived volition and retirement satisfaction may be influenced by retirement planning. Individuals who feel they had little choice about retiring may be more satisfied in retirement if they have also planned adequately than those with no plans.

The three aspects of retirement were also proposed to influence organizational factors such as climate, employee motivation, and technical skills. That is, the exiting of experienced and knowledgeable workers, as well as incompetent and unmotivated workers, is likely to impact the organization's remaining human resource base. For example, if a large number of highly competent workers retire, the skills base of the organization may be disadvantaged. This situation may also have negative implications for employee motivation. If a large number of incompetent workers retire, the skills base may become a leveraging point through the hiring of competent workers. Although the inclusion of organizational consequences of retirement in this model is intriguing, little research has examined this aspect of retirement.

Research based on Beehr's model (and other comprehensive models) has facilitated a broader understanding of the retirement decision and process. For example, Taylor and Shore (1995) examined the impact of personal, psychological (i.e., nonjob factors), and organizational factors on planned retirement age in a sample of employees ranging in age from 19 to 71 years (mean age = 47). Of the personal variables examined, poorer health was related to an earlier planned exit age. Of the psychological variables, higher retirement self-efficacy was related to an earlier planned retirement age. Lastly, of the organizational variables, higher organizational commitment was related to later planned retirement ages. The psychological category demonstrated the strongest contribution to the prediction of planned retirement age, whereas the personal and organizational categories contributed to a lesser extent. Although not all factors within each category were significant predictors of planned retirement age, this study illustrates the importance of examining variables representing a wider scope of life domains.

Women, Men, and Retirement

The majority of retirement research has focused specifically on men's retirement decisions and adjustment. Less emphasis had been placed on women's retirement due to (1) the higher incidence of men's retirement, (2) assumptions that women's retirement was not problematic due to less significance of the work role, (3) beliefs that the retirement transition held greater significance to men than women (Gratton & Haug, 1983; Kasl, 1980; Seccombe & Lee, 1986; Szinovacz, 1987), and (4) assumptions that findings based on men's retirement would generalize to women (Sheppard, 1991).

The question has been raised if theoretical models of retirement are gender biased and if the "male model" of retirement aids in understanding of women's retirement (Calasanti, 1996). The male model assumes that not only do men and women have access to similar resources (e.g., occupational prestige, financial situation, education level, marital status), but they also use them in similar ways (Calasanti, 1996). Potential causes of gender differences in retirement decisions and adjustment may be due to women having later work force entries, more discontinuous work histories, less time in the work force, and the impact of these factors on financial resources (Belgrave, 1989; Gratton & Haug, 1983; Szinovacz, 1987; Talaga & Beehr, 1995).

Research examining potential gender differences in the retirement process have also benefited from the use of comprehensive retirement models (Calasanti, 1996; Talaga & Beehr, 1995). Talaga and Beehr (1995) examined personal (i.e., finances, health status), nonwork factors (i.e., number of dependents in the household, spouses health status, financial well-being, retirement status), and work-related factors (i.e., occupational status, work attachment), in predicting the retirement status of both men and women. Participants included employed and retired men and women ranging in ages from 50 to 70 years.

Retirement status was measured in terms of self-attributions, receipt of a pension, and degree of retirement.

Self-attributed retirement status was predicted by age, financial security, gender, spouse's perceived health, and the interaction between gender and spouse health. Older ages, greater financial security, being male, and higher perceived spousal health were related to considering oneself retired. Women whose husbands were in poor health were more likely to be retired than those whose husbands enjoyed better health. The opposite pattern, however, was found for men. The likelihood of husbands being retired increased as positive perceptions of their wives' health increased. Exploratory analyses suggested the relation between occupational level and self-attributed retirement may differ for men and women, and that these differences may be partially due to differences in financial security.

Pension retirement status was predicted by age, gender, and the interaction of gender and the number of dependents present in the household. Older individuals and men were more likely to be retired. The likelihood of being retired increased as the number of dependents increased for women, but slightly decreased for men.

The interplay between spouses' employment statuses was also examined. In terms of self-attributed and pension retirement status, having a retired spouse increased the likelihood of the other spouse also being retired. In contrast, gender differences were found when predicting degree of retirement. Men whose wives were retired reported working fewer hours per week than did women whose husbands were retired. When their spouses were employed, however, both men and women worked similar numbers of hours per week.

Calasanti (1996) also examined the appropriateness of assessing women's retirement adjustment through the "male model" of retirement. In addressing this issue, Calasanti (1996) suggested employment structures (i.e., years of training required for a particular occupation and the gender composition of a particular occupation) impact individual's labor market experiences and subsequent orientation carried into retirement. Labor market experiences were also thought to differ by gender. Primary labor markets were designated as requiring 4 or more years of training. Primary labor markets are also considered to be more stable, higher paid, and offer more opportunities for mobility than secondary labor markets (Calasanti, 1996). Occupations with 76% or more female incumbents were classified as female. Participants were categorized into four employment structures: primary, nonfemale; primary, female; secondary, nonfemale; and secondary, female. The average age of the participants was 69 years and retirement status was determined based on self-attributions.

In general, women tended to be more satisfied in retirement than men. Employment structure, however, did not account for these differences. Across the employment structures, some differences were found in the predictors of life satisfaction. Health was the only variable to predict satisfaction for all four categories. Being married predicted satisfaction for all categories except the secondary, female employment structure. Financial satisfaction predicted satisfaction only in the primary, nonfemale category and gender predicted satisfaction only for the secondary, nonfemale category.

Men and women within the same employment structure (i.e., primary, nonfemale) were also compared. Results indicated financial satisfaction, better health, being married, and higher educational attainment were beneficial to men's life satisfaction in retirement. In contrast, only financial satisfaction and better health were beneficial to women. Even within the same employment structure, gender differentiated the experiences of men and women and their subsequent life satisfaction in retirement (Calasanti, 1996). These results were interpreted as arguing against applying the same retirement adjustment models to both men and women.

Summary

Comprehensive retirement models provide a broader picture of the retirement process. The results of this research highlight the predictive contributions of variables representing different life domains as well as several gender differences. First, personal, work, and nonwork-related factors were found to influence planned retirement age (Taylor & Shore, 1995). Second, work, family (i.e., nonwork), and, more tentatively, personal factors were found to differ by gender in predicting planned retirement age and life satisfaction in retirement (Calasanti, 1996; Talaga & Beehr, 1995). The male model of retirement does not seem to be fully adequate for understanding women's retirement.

Planning, Decisions, and Adjustments

Predicting employees retirement decisions may be very useful in terms of organizational human resource planning and work force composition management. In particular, pension plans and retirement incentive plans may be viable labor force management mechanisms. For example, increases in the affordability of retirement have been found to be associated with increases in retirement. The trend of decreasing labor force participation in men under 62 years seems to be driven by employer pensions (Quadagno & Hardy, 1996). The purpose of these programs may be work force reduction, removal of ineffective or expensive employees, and expansion of opportunities for younger employees (Monahan & Greene, 1987).

Organizational influence as to which individuals retire, however, is limited. The Employee Retirement Income Security Act (ERISA) of 1974 prohibits employers from targeting specific employees for retirement. Benefits cannot be offered to one worker that are not offered to an entire class of workers. Uncertainty of who will retire may exist when early retirement or retirement incentive plans are offered to an entire class of workers. Plans introduced with the intention of reducing the work force or inducing ineffective workers to retire may backfire. Too many or too few workers may choose to retire or the most productive workers may retire and the least productive may remain. These types of uncertainties add to the importance of research examining what types of workers may be inclined to accept, as well as the response rates to, early retirement or retirement incentives (Davidson, Worrell, & Fox, 1996).

Organizations may also attempt to influence their work force through encouraging workers *not* to retire. Decreases in the numbers of skilled workers entering the work force may act to increase the importance of older workers as a resource for maintaining productivity (American Psychological Association, 1993). Knowing what factors influence workers' retirement decisions may help organizations in retaining skilled and effective older workers. Being able to predict what types of workers are and are not likely to retire and probable ages of retirement may also increase an organizations' flexibility in staffing, estimating pensions, and developing effective retirement planning programs (Taylor & Shore, 1995).

Examining predictors of retirement adjustment may help define important topics to include in retirement planning programs and key areas for intervention. This information would also facilitate identification of what types of older workers are most in need of planning and adjustment assistance (Mutran, Reitzes, & Fernandez, 1997). Additionally, predicting retirement adjustment may also add insight as to what types of employees may be more inclined to retire or accept retirement incentive packages.

Preparation for Retirement

People who plan for major life changes tend to be more successful in dealing with them. Since retirement is a major life change, it follows that those who are prepared for retirement will be better able to adapt to the retirement process. There are personal characteristics that indicate the degree to which an individual is prepared for retirement. For example, research has indicated that persons with higher income levels are better prepared and have a greater number of resources to utilize in retirement. Regardless of whether an individual has assets such as a high income, active planning for retirement can be undertaken to ease the transition. Some of the potential benefits of planning for retirement are more financial equity, the possibility of a healthier life-style, the opportunity to explore new leisure activities, and the possibility of exploring alternative housing (Atchley, 1996; Richardson, 1993; Sterns, Laier, & Dorsett, 1994).

One way to plan for retirement is to participate in a formal retirement preparation program, possibly one provided by an employer, a nonprofit organization, a consulting firm, or an independent retirement specialist. Unfortunately, surveys indicate that only a small percentage of workers participate in formal preretirement preparation programs, and the majority of organizations do not even offer such programs. Richardson (1993) found that only about 11% of employees attended a preretirement workshop.

Preretirement programs range in comprehensiveness from an individual session with an employee discussing benefits to several group sessions covering a broad array of topics (Feit & Tate, 1986). Studies have concluded that 59% of preretirement programs cover a broad range of topics (eight or more).

The most common topic covered in preretirement programs is financial planning (Rowen & Wilks, 1987). Other topics commonly covered in comprehensive programs include health issues, leisure, housing, interpersonal relationships, legal issues, the use of time, and adjustment to changing roles. These topics are important in planning a smooth retirement transation and should be included in retirement preparation programs (Richardson, 1993).

Although there has not been a great deal of research investigating the effectiveness of preretirement programs, there is some evidence that these programs do improve the retirement experience. Preretirement programs have been effective in improving participants' attitudes toward retirement, increasing the amount of planning behaviors, increasing participant's retirement knowledge, and raising satisfaction with retirement over time (Sterns et al., 1994).

Focusing on the effectiveness of formal preretirement programs neglects a very important form of retirement planning: informal planning. Individuals do not have to attend formal programs to prepare themselves for retirement. They can utilize informal means, such as consulting with advisors and getting support from retired friends and family members. This type of preparation is actually much more common than participating in formal programs.

A large amount of research has examined correlates of the retirement decision and subsequent adjustment. Reviews of the literature have consistently recognized health status as one of the principal influences of both men's and women's retirement decisions (Beehr, 1986; Davies, Matthews, & Wong, 1991; Feldman, 1994; Gratton & Haug, 1983; Hansson, DeKoekkoek, Neece, & Patterson, 1997; Howard et al., 1982; Kasl, 1980; Minkler, 1981; Quinn & Burkhauser, 1990; Ruhm, 1990; Sammartino, 1987; Talaga & Beehr, 1989) and adjustment (Davies et al., 1991; Howard et al., 1982; Talaga & Beehr, 1989). Individuals in poor health are more likely to retire and to be less satisfied in retirement than those with no health problems.

Previous reviews have also recognized financial variables as playing an important role in the decision to retire (Beehr, 1986; Davies et al., 1991; Feldman, 1994; Gratton & Haug, 1983; Hansson et al., 1997; Ruhm, 1990; Talaga & Beehr, 1989) and adjustment to retirement (Davies et al., 1991; Feldman, 1994; Howard et al., 1982; Talaga & Beehr, 1989). The conclusion has been that individuals with better financial resources or who are more satisfied with their financial resources tend to be retired as well as satisfied in retirement.

Some inconsistencies, however, are found in the relation between financial variables and the retirement decision. A recent study adds insight into possible reasons for these discrepant findings. Henretta, Chan, and O'Rand (1992) found that financial variables exert differential influences depending on the main reason for retirement. When wanting to retire or compulsory retirement were reported as the main reasons for leaving the work force, higher pension and social security values tended to increase the rate of retirement. In comparison, among those who retired mainly due to health limitations, greater pension and social security values were related to a decreased rate of retirement. When job loss was given as the main reason for retirement, pension and social security values were not related to retirement rate. Across all retirement reasons, higher wages were related to decreased retirement rates.

In general, attitudinal variables have received less attention than health and financial variables in research examining retirement decisions and adjustment. A more comprehensive picture of retirement may be gained through including such variables in terms of person characteristics, work, and nonwork-related factors. Work-related attitudes, however, seem to have received relatively more attention than other attitudinal variables.

Early retirement research hypothesized that the meaning individual's attached to their work would influence retirement attitudes (Simpson, Back, & McKinney, 1966; Friedmann & Havighurst, 1954). It was felt that positive work attitudes would be related to preferring work over retirement, later retirement ages, and dissatisfaction in retirement. Despite strong convictions of this relation, the research findings have been mixed and it has been suggested the relation between work attitudes and retirement attitudes has been overstated in the literature (Howard et al., 1982; Tornstam, 1992).

This suggestion was corroborated by a recent meta-analysis examining the relations between job satisfaction, job involvement, and retirement satisfaction (Gray & Citera, 1996). Job satisfaction and retirement satisfaction were essentially unrelated ($r = 0.01$) and a weak negative relationship was found between job involvement and retirement satisfaction ($r = -0.10$).

Among studies using longitudinal designs, job satisfaction ($r = 0.13$) and job involvement ($r = -0.01$) were only weakly related to retirement satisfaction. The majority of these longitudinal studies measured retirement status as participants' self-attributions. In general, these work-related attitudes do not have overwhelming implications for retirement satisfaction.

The previous sections discussed variables related to retirement adjustment, but tended to treat adjustment as a static condition. A recent longitudinal study examined men's retirement adjustment over a 6- to 7-year period (Gall, Evans, & Howard, 1997). At 1 year postretirement, retirees reported higher energy levels, financial satisfaction, interpersonal satisfaction, internal locus of control, and less distress as compared to their preretirement situations. This period was characterized as similar to Atchley's (1976) description of a "honeymoon" phase of retirement. In the period from 1 year postretirement to 6–7 years postretirement, interpersonal satisfaction, health satisfaction, and physiological health declined. Reported illnesses and internal locus of control increased, whereas financial satisfaction remained stable. The authors interpreted this period as a wearing off of the honeymoon effect or stabilization. Interestingly, life satisfaction remained stable over the entire time course of the study. This research illustrates the continual process of retirement adjustment and the importance of examining this processes well past the actual retirement act(s).

Summary

Work, leisure, and retirement influence each other through the adult life span. Individual characteristics, work-related, and nonwork-related factors impact work and leisure choices. These factors also influence anticipatory retirement planning and decision processes. The interplay between work, leisure, and retirement choices is likely to continue postretirement. Choosing to maintain connections with the labor force (e.g., second and third careers, part-time work, volunteer work), the types of leisure activities and life-style pursued, family, and health status are likely to influence retirement adjustment over time.

Conclusions

A life-span approach emphasizes opportunities, choices, and decisions regarding work, leisure, and retirement as not tied to any specific age. Self-management requires greater independent responsibility in these domains by workers of all ages. Stereotypes regarding older workers have been a continuing issue over the last five decades. These beliefs do not generalize to all older workers and may interfere with the accurate evaluation of adult and older adult workers. Each individual, regardless of age, should be evaluated based on his or her own knowledge, skills, and abilities.

The importance of career development and updating is emphasized as a lifelong endeavor. Organizational changes seem to be leading to continuing self-management on the part of employees. Older worker stereotypes may interfere with self-management activities. Individual motivation, organizational support, and job characteristics also hold implications for willingness to participate in, and actual engagement in updating behaviors as an integral part of career self-management.

A continuing issue is how one chooses to synthesize his or her work and leisure. Patterns of life satisfaction can begin earlier in life and carry into one's retirement years. New choices in later life can involve leisure activities, volunteerism, and part-time and full time work options. For example, individuals may have different balances between work and leisure, work and retirement, and leisure and retirement. The introduction of self-management of work, leisure, and retirement opens up new opportunities and freedoms, and places greater responsibilities on individuals.

Retirement is a process that is influenced by a complex array of factors. Health and financial well-being influence when and how individuals choose to retire or continue to work. Personal, organizational, and nonwork factors influence whether people have traditional careers or need to repeatedly enter the job market in later life. There are very different patterns evident. Some people choose to retire in their 50s while others feel a need to work longer. As is often said, there is no one way to grow old.

REVIEW QUESTIONS

1. Give examples of how older worker stereotypes may benefit older workers. Do you think the positive and negative aspects of these stereotypes may be differentially associated with different occupations (i.e., factory worker, museum curator, food server, CEO)?

2. When is a worker seen as older? What factors might influence this perception? What implications does this have for the worker?

3. You are working with an individual who is trying to decide whether or not to retire. What factors should the person consider?

4. An employer in a mid-sized company is interested in retaining his older workers for as long as possible. What options may be pursued in terms of training, employment policies, benefits, and scheduling of work?

5. How might career self-management benefit one's leisure and retirement process? How might career self-management hinder leisure and retirement?

References

Age Discrimination in Employment Act of 1967, 29 U.S.C. Sec. 621 et seq. (1976 & Supp V. 1978 & 1986).

American Psychological Association. (1993). *Vitality for life: Psychological research for productive aging.* Washington DC: American Psychological Association.

Atchley, R. C. (1976). *The sociology of retirement.* Cambridge, MA: Schenkman.

Atchley, R. C. (1979). Issues in retirement research. *The Gerontologist, 19,* 44–54.

Atchley, R. C. (1982). Retirement as a social institution. *American Review of Sociology, 8,* 263–287.

Atchley, R. C. (1996). Retirement. In J. E. Birren (Ed.), *Encyclopedia of gerontology: Age, aging, and the aged* (Vol. 2, pp. 437–449). San Diego, CA: Academic Press

Avolio, B. J., & Barrett, G. V. (1987). Effects of age stereotyping in a simulated interview. *Psychology and Aging, 2,* 56–63.

Avolio, B. J., Waldman, D. A., & McDaniel, M. A. (1990). Age and work performance in nonmanagerial jobs: The effects of experience and occupational type. *Academy of Management Journal, 33,* 407–422.

Baltes, P. B., & Graf, P. (1996). Psychology aspects of aging: Facts and frontiers. In D. Magnusson (Ed.), *The lifespan development of individuals: Behavioral, neurobiogocial and psychosocial perspectives* (pp. 427–460). Cambridge, UK: Cambridge University Press.

Bandura, A. (1989). Regulation of cognitive processes through perceived self-efficacy. *Developmental Psychology, 25,* 729–735.

Bass, B. M., & Barrett, G. V. (1981). *People, work, and organizations.* Boston: Allyn and Bacon.

Becker, B. S. (1960). Notes on the concept of commitment. *American Journal of Sociology, 66,* 32–42.

Beehr, T. A. (1986). The process of retirement: A review and recommendations for future investigation. *Personnel Psychology, 39,* 31–55.

Belgrave, L. L. (1989). Understanding women's retirement. *Generations, 13,* 49–52.

Bird, C. P., & Fisher, T. D. (1986). Thirty years later: Attitudes toward the employment of older workers. *Journal of Applied Psychology, 71,* 515–517.

Brown, S. P. (1996). A meta-analysis and review of organizational research on job involvement. *Psychological Bulletin, 120,* 235–255.

Calasanti, T. M. (1996). Gender and life satisfaction in retirement: An assessment of the male model. *Journal of Gerontology, 51B,* S18–S29.

Cleveland, J. N., Festa, R. M., & Montgomery, L. (1988). Applicant pool composition and job perceptions: Impact on decisions regarding an older applicant. *Journal of Vocational Behavior, 32,* 112–125.

Cleveland, J. N., & Landy, F. J. (1983). The effects of person and job stereotypes on two personnel decisions. *Journal of Applied Psychology, 68,* 609–619.

Cleveland, J. N., & Landy, F. J. (1987). Age perceptions of jobs: Convergence of two questionnaires. *Psychological Reports, 60,* 1075–1081.

Cole, & Castellano (1996). Consumer behavior. In J. E. Birren (Ed.) *Encyclopedia of gerontology: Age, aging, and the aged* (pp. 329–340). San Diego, CA: Academic Press.

Cornman, J. M., & Kingson, E. R. (1996). Trends, issues, perspectives, and values for the aging of the baby boom cohorts. *The Gerontologist, 36,* 15–26.

Cutler, S. J., & Hendricks, J. (1990). Leisure and time use across the life course. In R. H. Binstock & L. K. George (Eds.), *Handbook of aging and the social sciences* (3rd ed., pp. 169–185). San Diego, CA: Academic Press.

Davidson, W. N., Worrell, D. L., & Fox, J. B. (1996). Early retirement programs and firm performance, *Academy of Management Journal, 39,* 970–984.

Davies, D. R., Matthews, G., & Wong, C. S. K. (1991). Aging and work. In C. L. Cooper and I. T. Robertson (Eds.), *International Review of Industrial and Organizational Psychology* (Vol. 6, pp. 175–199). Chichester: John Wiley & Sons.

Dorsett, J. G. (1994). *Understanding the relationship between age and the updating process: The creation of a model.* Unpublished doctoral dissertation, The University of Akron, Akron, OH.

Eden, D. (1992). Leadership and expectations: Pygmalion effects and other self-fulfilling prophecies in organizations. *Leadership Quarterly, 3,* 271–305.

Ekerdt, D. J. (1998). Workplace norms for the timing of retirement. In K. W. Schaie & C. Schooler (Eds.), *Impact of work on older adults* (pp. 101–123). New York: Springer.

Ekerdt, D. J., DeViney, S., & Kosloski, K. (1996). Profiling plans for retirement. *Journal of Gerontology: Social Sciences, 51B,* S140–S149.

Espinoza, G. (1997). What to do now to retire rich. *Money, 26,* 82–89.

Farr, J. L., Tesluk, P. E., & Klein, S. R. (1998). Organizational structure of the workplace and the older worker. In K. W. Schaie & C. Schooler (Eds.), *Impact of work on older adults* (pp. 143–185). New York: Springer.

Feit, M. D., & Tate, N. P. (1986). NP: Health and mental health issues in preretirement programs. *Employee Assistance Quarterly, 1,* 49–56.

Feldman, D. C. (1989). Careers in organizations: Recent trends and future directions. *Journal of Management, 15,* 135–156.

Feldman, D. C. (1994). The decision to retire early: A review and conceptualization. *Academy of Management Review, 19,* 285–311.

Finkelstein, L. M., Burke, M. J., & Raju, N. S. (1995). Age discrimination in simulated employment contexts: An integrative analysis. *Journal of Applied Psychology, 80,* 652–663.

Fiske, S. T., Neuberg, S. L., Beattie, A. E., & Milberg, S. J. (1987). Category-based and attribute-based reactions to others: Some informational conditions of stereotyping and individuating processes. *Journal of Experimental Social Psychology, 23,* 399–427.

Friedmann, E. A., & Havighurst, R. J. (1954). *The meaning of work and retirement.* Chicago: University of Chicago Press.

Gall, T. L., Evans, D. R., & Howard, J. (1997). The retirement adjustment process: Changes in the well-being of male retirees across time. *Journal of Gerontology, 52B,* P110–P117

Gendell, M., & Siegel, J. S. (1996). Trends in retirement age in the United States, 1955–1993, by sex and race. *Journal of Gerontology, 51B,* S132–S139.

Graebner, W. (1980). *A history of retirement.* New Haven: Yale University Press.

Gratton, B., & Haug, M. (1983). Decision and adaptation: Research on female retirement. *Research on Aging, 5,* 59–76.

Gray, J. H., Boyce, C. A., Hall, R. J., & McDaniel, M. A. (1996). *Age differences in training: Less pre-training mastery or less learning?* Poster presented at the 11th annual conference of the Society for Industrial and Organizational Psychology, San Diego, CA.

Gray, J. H., & Citera, M. (1996). *A meta-analytical review of the relation between work attitudes and retirement attitudes.* Poster presented at the 10th annual meeting of the Society for Industrial and Organizational Psychology, San Diego, CA.

Hackett, R. D. (1990). Age, tenure, and employee absenteeism. *Human Relations, 43,* 601–619.

Hall, D., & Mirvis, P. (1993). How to overcome "barriers" to new older worker roles. *Perspective on Aging, Oct.–Dec.,* 15–19.

Hall, D. T., & Mirvis, P. H. (1995). The new career contract: Developing the whole person at midlife and beyond. *Journal of Vocational Behavior, 47,* 269–289.

Hall, D. T., & Mirvis, P H. (1996). The new protean career: Psychological success and the path with a heart. In D. T. Hall and associates (Eds.), *The career is dead—long live the career: A relational approach to careers.* (pp. 15–45). San Francisco: Jossey-Bass.

Hansson, R. O., DeKoekkoek, P. D., Neece, W. M., & Patterson, D. W. (1997). Successful aging at work: Annual review, 1992–1996: The older worker and transitions to retirement. *Journal of Vocational Behavior, 51,* 202–233.

Hayward, M. D., Hardy, M. A., & Liu, M. (1994). Work after retirement: The experiences of older men in the U.S. *Social Science Research, 23,* 82–107.

Healy, M. C., Lehman, M., & McDaniel, M. A. (1995). Age and voluntary turnover: A quantitative review. *Personnel Psychology, 48,* 335–345.

Henretta, J. C., Chan, C. G., & O'Rand, A. M. (1992). Retirement reason versus retirement process: Examining the reasons for retirement typology. *Journal of Gerontology, 47,* S1–S7.

Howard, J. H., Marshall, J., Rechnitzer, P. A., Cunningham, D. A., & Donner, A. (1982). Adapting to retirement. *Journal of the American Geriatrics Society, 30,* 488–500.

Hrebiniak, L. G., & Alutto, J. A. (1972). Personal and role-related factors in the development of organizational commitment. *Administrative Science Quarterly, 17,* 555–573.

Kanungo, R. N. (1982a). Measurement of job and work involvement. *Journal of Applied Psychology, 67,* 341–349.

Kanungo, R. N. (1982b). *Work alienation: An integrative approach.* New York: Praeger.

Kaplan, M. (1979). *Leisure: Lifestyle and lifespan,* Philadelphia: W. B. Saunders.

Kasl, S. V. (1980). The impact of retirement. In C. L. Cooper & R. Payne (Eds.), *Current concerns in occupational stress* (pp. 137–186). New York: John Wiley & Sons Ltd.

Kelly, J. R. (1993). *Activity and aging,* Newbury Park, CA: Sage.

Kelly, J. R. (1996). Activities. In J. E. Birren (Ed.), *Encyclopedia of gerontology: Age, aging, and the aged* (Vol. 1, pp. 37–49). San Diego, CA: Academic Press.

Kirchner, W. K., & Dunnette, M. D. (1954). Attitudes toward older workers. *Personnel Psychology, 7,* 257–265.

Kirchner, W. K., Lindbom, T., & Paterson, D. G. (1952). Attitudes toward the employment of older people. *Journal of Applied Psychology, 36,* 154–156.

Kubeck, J. E., Delp, N. D., Haslett, T. K., & McDaniel, M. A. (1996). Does job-related training performance decline with age? *Psychology and Aging, 11,* 92–107.

Kunda, Z., & Thagard, P. (1996). Forming impressions from stereotypes, traits, and behaviors: A parallel-constraint-satisfaction theory. *Psychological Review, 103,* 284–308.

Lawler, E. E., & Hall, D. T. (1970). Relationship of job characteristics to job involvement, satisfaction, and intrinsic motivation. *Journal of Applied Psychology, 54,* 305–312.

Lodahl, T. M., & Kejner, M. (1965). The definition and measurement of job involvement. *Journal of Applied Psychology, 49,* 24–33.

Lowman, R. L. (1993). *Counseling and psychotherapy of work dysfunctions.* Washington, DC: American Psychological Association.

Macrae, C. N., Milne, A. B., & Bodenhausen, G. V. (1994). Stereotypes as energy-saving devices: A peek inside the cognitive toolbox. *Journal of Personality and Social Psychology, 66,* 37–47.

Mathieu, J. E., & Zajac, D. M. (1990). A review and meta-analysis of the antecedents, correlates, and consequences of organizational commitment. *Psychological Bulletin, 108,* 171–194.

McEnrue, M. P. (1989). Self-development as a career management strategy. *Journal of Vocational Behavior, 34,* 57–68.

McEvoy, G. M., & Cascio, W. F. (1989). Cumulative evidence of the relationship between employee age and job performance. *Journal of Applied Psychology, 74,* 11–17.

McGuire, F. A., Boyd, R. K., & Tedrick, R. T. (1996). *Leisure and aging: Ulyssean living in later life.* Champaign, IL: Sagamore.

Meyer, J. P., & Allen, N. J. (1984). Testing the "side-bet theory" of organizational commitment: Some methodological considerations. *Journal of Applied Psychology, 69,* 372–378.

Minkler, M. (1981). Research on the health effects of retirement: An uncertain legacy. *Journal of Health and Social Behavior, 22,* 117–130.

Mirvis, P H., & Hall, D. T. (1996a). Career development for the older worker. In D. T. Hall and associates (Eds.), *The career is dead—long live the career: A relational approach to careers* (pp. 72–101). San Francisco: Jossey-Bass.

Mirvis, P. H., & Hall, D. T. (1996b). New organizational forms and the new career. In D. T. Hall and associates (Eds.), *The career is dead—long live the career: A relational approach to careers* (pp. 72–101). San Francisco: Jossey-Bass.

Monahan, D. J., & Greene, V. L. (1987). Predictors of early retirement among university faculty. *The Gerontologist, 27,* 46–52.

Morgan, C. M., & Levy, D. J. (1993). *Segmenting the mature market.* Chicago: Probus.

Mowday, R. T., Steers, R. M., & Porter, L. W. (1979). The measurement of organizational commitment. *Journal of Vocational Behavior, 14*, 224–247.

Mutchler, J. E., Burr, J. A., Pienta, A. M., & Massagli, M. P. (1997). Pathways to labor force exit: Work transitions and instability. *Journal of Gerontology, 52B*, S4–S12.

Mutran, E. J., Reitzes, D. C., & Fernandez, M. E. (1997). Factors that influence attitudes toward retirement. *Research on Aging, 19*, 251–273.

Neugarten, B. L. (1974). Age groups in American society and the rise of the young-old. *The Annals of the American Academy of Political and Social Science, 415*, 187–198.

Palmore, E., George, L., & Fillenbaum, G. (1982). Predictors of retirement. *Journal of Gerontology, 39*, 733–742.

Panek, P. E. (1997). The older worker. In A. D. Fisk & W. A. Rogers (Eds.), *Handbook of human factors and the older adult* (pp. 363–394). San Diego, CA: Academic Press.

Perry, E. L., Kulik, C. T., & Bourhis, A. C. (1996). Moderating effects of personal and contextual factors in age discrimination. *Journal of Applied Psychology, 81*, 628–647.

Quadagno, J., & Hardy, M. (1996). Work and retirement. In R.H. Binstock & L.K. George (Eds.), *Handbook of aging and the social sciences* (pp. 325–345). San Diego, CA: Academic Press.

Quinn, J. F., & Burkhauser, R. V. (1990). Work and retirement. In R. H. Binstock & L. K. George (Eds.), *Handbook of aging and the social sciences* (pp. 307–327). San Diego, CA: Academic Press.

Rhodes, S. R. (1983). Age-related differences in work attitudes and behavior: A review and conceptual analysis. *Psychological Bulletin, 93*, 328–367.

Rich, S. (1993). A grim outlook for retirement. *Akron Beacon Journal*, June 13, A12.

Richardson, V. E. (1993). *Retirement counseling*. New York: Springer.

Ritzer, G., & Trice, H. M. (1969). An empirical study of Howard Becker's side-bet theory. *Social Forces, 47*, 475–479.

Rosen, B., & Jerdee, T. H. (1976a). The nature of job-related age stereotypes. *Journal of Applied Psychology, 61*, 180–183.

Rosen, B., & Jerdee, T. H. (1976b). The influence of age stereotypes on managerial decisions. *Journal of Applied Psychology, 61*, 428–432.

Rosen, B., & Jerdee, T. H. (1985). *Older employees: New roles for valued resources*. Homewood, IL: Dow Jones-Irwin.

Rowen, R. B., & Wilks, C. S. (1987). Pre-retirement planning, a quality of life issue for retirement. *Employee Assistance Quarterly, 2*, 45–56.

Ruhm C. J. (1990). Career jobs, bridge employment, and retirement. In P.B. Doeringer (Ed.), *Bridges to employment* (pp. 95–107). Ithica, NY: IRL Press.

Saleh, S. D., & Hosek, J. (1976). Job involvement: Concepts and measurements. *Academy of Management Journal, 19*, 213–224.

Sammartino, F. J. (1987). The effect of health on retirement. *Social Security Bulletin, 50*, 31–47.

Schlesinger, J. M., & Georges, C. (1998). Use of surpluses to save social security gains fed chairman's support. *Wall Street Journal, 21*, A2–A5.

Seccombe, K., & Lee, G. R. (1986). Gender differences in retirement satisfaction and its antecedents. *Research on Aging, 8*, 426–440.

Shearer, R. L., & Steger, J. A. (1975). Manpower obsolescence: A new definition and empirical investigation of personal variables. *Academy of Management Journal, 18*(2), 263–275.

Sheppard, H. L. (1991) The United States: The privatization of exit. In J. Quadagno & D. Street (Eds.), *Aging for the twenty-first century: Readings in social gerontology* (pp. 351–377). New York: St. Martin's Press.

Simpson, I., Back., K., & McKinney, J. (1966). Orientations toward work and retirement, and self-evaluation in retirement. In I. Simpson & J. McKinney (Eds.), *Social aspects of aging*. Burham NC: Duke University Press.

Smith, E. R. (1994). Procedural knowledge and processing strategies in social cognition. *Human Behavior and Social Cognition*, 1, 99–151.

Stagner, R. (1971). An industrial psychologist looks at industrial psychology. *Aging and Human Development*, 2, 29–37.

Stagner, R. (1985). Aging in industry. In J. E. Birren & K. W. Schaie (Eds.), *Handbook of the psychology of aging* (pp. 789–817). New York: Van Nostrand Reinhold.

Sterns, A. A., Sterns, H. L., & Hollis, L. A. (1996). The productivity and functional limitations of older adult workers. In W. H. Crown (Ed.), *Handbook on employment and the elderly* (pp. 276–303). Westport, CT: Greenwood Press.

Sterns, H. L. (1986). Training and retraining adult and older adult workers. In J. E. Birren, P. K. Robinson, & J. E. Livingston (Eds.), *Age, health, and employment* (pp. 93–113). Engelwood Cliffs, NJ: Prentice-Hall.

Sterns, H. L., & Alexander, R. A. (1987). Industrial gerontology: The aging individual and work. In K. W. Schaie & C. Eisdorfer (Eds.), *Annual review of gerontology and geriatrics* (pp. 243–264). New York: Springer.

Sterns, H. L., & Doverspike, D. (1989). Age and the training and learning process. In I. L. Goldstein (Ed.), *Training and development in organizations* (pp. 299–332). San Francisco: Jossey-Bass.

Sterns, H. L., Laier, M. P., & Dorsett, J. G. (1994). Work and retirement. In B. R. Bonder & M. B. Wagner (Eds.), *Functional performance in older adults* (pp. 148–164). Philadelphia: F. A. Davis.

Sterns, H. L., & McDaniel, M. A. (1994). Job performance and the older worker. In S. E. Rix (Ed.), *Older workers: How do they measure up? An overview of age differences in employee costs and performances* (pp. 27–51). Washington, DC: Public Policy Institute. American Association of Retired Persons.

Sterns, H. L., & Miklos, S. M. (1995). The aging worker in a changing environment: Organizational and individual issues. *Journal of Vocational Behavior*, 47, 248–268.

Sterns, H. L., & Patchett, M. (1984). Technology and the aging adult: Career development and training. In P. R. Robinson & J. E. Birren (Eds.), *Aging and technology* (pp. 93–113). Englewood Cliffs, NJ: Prentice-Hall.

Sterns, R., & Sterns, H. (1995). Consumer issues: The mature market. In G. Maddox (Ed.), *The encyclopedia of aging* (2nd ed., pp. 222–224). New York: Springer.

Szinovacz, M. (1987). Preferred retirement timing and retirement satisfaction in women. *International Journal of Aging and Human Development*, 24, 301–317.

Talaga, J. A., & Beehr, T. A. (1989). Retirement: A psychological perspective. In C. L. Cooper & I. T. Robertson (Eds.), *International review of industrial and organizational psychology* (pp. 185–209). Chichester: John Wiley & Sons.

Talaga, J. A., & Beehr, T. A. (1995). Are there gender differences in predicting retirement decisions? *Journal of Applied Psychology*, 80, 16–28.

Taylor, M. A., & Shore, L. M. (1995). Predictors of planned retirement age: An application of Beehr's model. *Psychology and Aging*, 10, 76–83.

Tornstam, L. (1992). The quo vadis of gerontology: On the scientific paradigm of gerontology. *The Gerontologist*, 32, 318–326.

Waldman, D. A., & Avolio, B. J. (1986). A meta-analysis of age differences in job performance. *Journal of Applied Psychology*, 71, 33–38.

Warr, P. (1992). Age and occupational well-being. *Psychology and Aging*, 7, 37–45.

Warr, P. (1994). Age and employment. In H. C. Triandis, M. D. Dunnette, & L. M. Hough (Eds.), *Handbook of industrial and organizational psychology* (2nd ed., Vol. 4, pp. 485–550). Palo Alto, CA: Consulting Psychologists Press.

Wellford, A. T. (1976). Thirty years of psychological research on age and work. *Journal of Occupational Psychology, 49,* 129–138.

Wentworth, E. C. (1945). Why beneficiaries retire. *Social Security Bulletin, 8*(1), 16–20.

Additional Readings

Bass, S. A. (Ed.) (1995). *Older and active: How Americans over 55 are contributing to society.* New Haven, CT: Yale University Press.

Cleveland, J. N., & Shore, L. M. (1996). Work and employment. In J. E. Birren (Ed.), *Encylopedia of gerontology: Age, aging, and the aged* (pp. 627–639). San Diego, CA: Academic Press.

Crown, W. H.(Ed.) (1996). *Handbook on employment and the elderly.* Westport, CT: Greenwood Press.

Rix, S. E. (1990). *Older workers: Choices and challenges.* Santa Barbara, CA: ABC-CLIO.

Schaie, K. W., & Schooler, C. (Eds.) (1998). *Impact of work on older adults.* New York: Springer.

Sterns, H. L., Matheson, N. K., & Park, L. S. (1997). Work and retirement. In K. F. Ferraro (Ed.), *Gerontology: Perspectives and issues* (pp. 171–192). New York: Springer.

14

Older Adults' Decision-Making Capacity: Institutional Settings and Individual Choices

Michael A. Smyer and Rebecca Allen-Burge

Introduction

Several contexts influence psychological practice with older adults: the immediate clinical setting and its requirements for skill and care; the fiscal environment and its incentives and disincentives for particular therapeutic approaches; and the public policy environment, with often conflicting unintended consequences of policy initiatives. Long-term care settings, especially nursing homes, reflect the interaction of these contexts.

This chapter focuses on one area of clinical concern that illustrates the complexity of interacting contexts: Medical decision making in nursing homes. We begin with a brief description of decision-making capacity among older adults, highlighting the "legal fiction" that has developed in statutory language regarding older adults' ability to be involved in decision making. Next, we turn to the role that a number of long-term care settings play in our current care system. In doing so, we highlight nursing homes, since the combination of physical and mental disabilities among nursing home residents makes their decision-making capacity particularly problematic. In addition, nursing homes are highly regulated health care settings that must be responsive to the changing demands of federal and state legislation. In the third section, we review a recent public policy initiative that has underscored older adults' right to be involved in medical decision making: the Patient Self-Determination Act (PSDA) of 1990. Next, we focus on assessment approaches for gauging older adults' capacity to be involved in medical decision making, an area that represents the intersection of legal and clinical practice. Finally, we conclude with suggestions for integrating the older adult's own preferences and values into the decision-making process.

Older Adults' Decision-Making Capacity: A Changing "Legal Fiction"

In a recent review chapter, Sabatino (1996) suggested that legal approaches to older adults' decision-making capacity have been creating a "legal fiction" that is useful for both clinical and legal processes. Each state defines the capacity for being involved in medical decision making by outlining potential causes of *in*competency or *in*capacity.

There has been a progression of criteria for incapacity (Anderer, 1990; Sabatino, 1996). Once, most states equated advanced age with an inability to be involved in decision making; being old made one automatically at risk for decision-making incapacity. Over time, however, a more differentiated view of decision-making capacity emerged. A gradual change in statutory language replaced the simple reliance on advanced age as a basis for disability. Instead, various states listed specific disabilities (either mental or physical) that could serve as the basis for a judgment of decision-making incapacity (Anderer, 1990).

Eventually, some states moved beyond merely assessing the presence or absence of a disabling condition. Instead, the focus shifted to the functional impact of the disabling condition on the older adult's decision-making capacity.

Most recently, some jurisdictions have added an additional criterion for a finding of decisional incapacity: a clear necessity for action by the state. In short, some regulations require the state to limit its interventions to only those circumstances in which potential decisional incapacity represents a danger to himself or herself, or to others.

Sabatino (1996) pointed out that the District of Columbia Guardianship, Protective Proceedings, and Durable Power of Attorney Act of 1986 reflects these developments:

> The District of Columbia Guardianship, Protective Proceedings, and Durable Power of Attorney Act of 1986 incorporates necessity into an essential component of incapacity in the following way:

Cognitive test	"Incapacitated individual" means an adult whose ability to receive and evaluate information effectively or to communicate decisions is impaired
Behavioral test	to such an extent that he or she lacks capacity to manage all or some of his or her financial resources or to meet all or some essential requirements for his or her physical health, safety, habilitation, or therapeutic needs
Necessity test	without court assistance or the appointment of a guardian or conservator. (D.C. Code Ann. §21-2011(11))

> Sabatino (1996, pp. 18–19)

Long-Term Care Recipients: A Population at Risk

With these developments as the legal context, we now turn to the characteristics of long-term care recipients that make them a population potentially at risk for decision-making incapacity. In this section , we will review the changing role of a variety of settings in long-term care that are designed to accommodate the changing abilities of older adults. These settings reflect differing assumptions regarding appropriate levels of care and appropriate regulatory roles for state and federal governmental agencies.

We will outline the characteristics of recipients using four different care arrangements: home health agencies, assisted living settings, continuing care retirement communities, and nursing homes. The boundaries between and among these types of care arrangements are blurred. For example, one type of assisted living setting is a continuing care community. Similarly, all continuing care communities make provisions for nursing home care. In addition, the types of services provided by assisted living settings and home health care agencies may overlap significantly.

For our purposes, however, it will be useful to characterize the recipients of long-term care in a variety of settings. They have one element in common: They are facing the challenge of declining physical and functional abilities. For example, 85% of older adults have one or more chronic conditions, such as arthritis, hypertension, hearing impairment, or heart disease (Cassel, Rudberg, & Olshansky, 1992). At the same time, they often face functional impairment in their activities of daily living (ADLs) or instrumental activities of daily living (IADLs). ADLs and IADLs act as proxies for underlying cognitive and social abilities that allow the older person to continue to function independently in the community (Kemp & Mitchell, 1992). They also reflect key components of older adults' everyday decision-making capacity. Therefore, they are often used as eligibility criteria for services or to depict populations at risk (Wiener & Hanley, 1992).

Home Health Care

Home health care agencies provide care for almost 2 million older adults every year (Dey, 1996). Use of home health care is increasing rapidly, registering a 52% growth from 1992 to 1994. Drawing on data from the 1994 National Home and Hospice Care Survey, Dey reported that at any time in 1994 there were approximately 1.4 million elderly (age 65 or older) using home health care services. Fifty-seven percent of these elderly current patients were receiving help with at least one ADL. Sixty-one percent received help with at least one IADL, including 25% who reported assistance in taking medications.

These patterns are consistent with the serious nature of the health problems facing older adults using home health care. For men, among the most frequent diagnoses at admission were heart disease (32%), malignant neoplasms (10%), injury and poisonings (7%), and disease of the musculoskeletal system and connective tissues (5%). For women, among the most frequent primary diagnoses were diseases of the musculoskeletal system and connective tissue (17%), heart disease (13%), injury and poisonings (12%), and malignant neoplasms (6%) (Dey, 1996).

In short, these older adults have a variety of chronic diseases and functional limitations that may raise important health care decision-making issues for them. At the same time, their limited physical and functional abilities may cause us to question the "legal fiction" of decision-making capacity among home health care recipients. For example, 24% of men and 17% of women are discharged from home health care into either hospitals or nursing homes, settings that increasingly require attention to the patient's health care decision-making capacity.

Assisted Living Facilities

Assisted living facilities are care arrangements that fall somewhere between community-based care and nursing homes. These settings are designed to provide for or arrange for meals, personal and supportive services, health care, and 24-hour oversight of people living in a group setting. The focus is on residents who especially need help with ADLs (Gulyas, 1995).These settings come in different arrays: Some are stand-alone faciltities; others are part of continuing care communities, hospitals, or nursing homes.

Because of the broad range of settings and services that qualify as assisted living, it is difficult to arrive at precise estimates on the exact number of assisted living settings and care recipients. Recent estimates suggest, however, that there are currently between 30,000 and 40,000 such settings serving approximatley one million older adults in the United States (Assisted Living Facilities Association of America, 1993).

Older adults in assisted living settings are coping with physical and functional disabilities. However, they do not require the medical attention of a hospital or nursing home setting. The functional limitations in ADL and IADL areas suggest that assisted living residents may also be at risk for limitations in decision-making capacity.

Assisted living settings also differ from other long-term care arrangements in two other significant ways: their financing and their regulatory climate. Financially, older adults or their relatives pay for the majority of the costs of assisted living care (Gulyas, 1995). This is in contrast to the strong involvement of federal programs (Medicare and Medicaid) in other long-term care arrangements. Perhaps because of this lack of financial involvement, there are no federal regulations governing assisted living (Gulyas, 1995).

Continuing Care Retirement Communities

Continuing care retirement communities (CCRCs) or life care communities offer another option in long-term care. CCRCs are financed by a life care contract that includes both an entry fee (ranging from $35,000 to more than $120,000 depending on the size of the unit and the location) and a monthly service charge. For these fees, the life care community agrees to provide comprehensive health, housing, and support services to the older adult for life. The array of services typically includes nursing care, if needed, asistance with ADLs and IADLs, meal services, and, importantly, nursing home care. In essence, the CCRC is a self-insured community that pays for health care services through the fees it collects.

Life care communities are not for everyone. A little less than 10% of the elderly can afford the combination of entry fee and monthly fees (Cohen, Tell, Greenberg, & Wallack, 1987). Typically, CCRC residents trade home equity for long-term care equity: They sell their home and use the profit to pay the entry fee and to provide for the ongoing maintenance fees.

Many older adults seek a life care setting in anticipation of a shifting balance between capacity and incapacity. They seek a setting that will provide structure and support in the face of declining physical and mental abilities. Thus, in many ways they are seeking to prevent a crisis of incapacity, by putting themselves in a setting that will foster continued functioning as long as possible (Smyer, 1995). When that is no longer possible, the CCRC should be able to provide a continuity of care, consistent with the older adult's prior history and values.

Nursing Homes

Nursing homes play several roles in the health care system. They provide long-term, chronic care for older adults with a range of physical disabilities and impairments (Lair & Lefkowitz, 1990). For example, a national sample of nursing home residents found that more than half received help with ADLs and a large majority needed assistance with important IADLs (e.g., managing money and taking care of personal possessions) (Dey, 1997).

Nursing homes also play a major **mental** health treatment role. For example, estimates suggest that between 60 and 90% of nursing home residents have at least one mental disorder (Smyer, Shea, & Streit, 1994; Burns et al., 1993). Lair and Lefkowitz (1990) found that 29% of nursing home residents had dementia only, 14% had dementia in combination with one or more mental disorders, and 16% had a mental disorder without dementia. Similarly, Dey (1997) reported that 17% of nursing home residents had a **primary** diagnosis of mental illness at admission.The net result is that nursing home residents usually face a combination of mental and physical health problems.

Goodwin and her colleagues (1995) used the National Medical Expenditure Survey data to assess the link between nursing home residents' characteristics and the potential for decision-making incapacity. The Oklahoma statute served as a model with its definition of an "incapacitated person" based on a combination of a disability and a functional impairment. Goodwin et al. estimated that more than half of nursing home residents had a combination of physical or mental disability and functional impairment, placing them at risk for decision-making incapacity.

Nursing homes are also highly regulated health care settings. Because federal and state funds provide over half of the funds for nursing home care, Medicare and Medicaid regulations affect the care provided in nursing homes. In addition, other federal initiatives can have a large impact on nursing home care.

In the rest of this chapter, we will use nursing homes to illustrate the complexity of medical decision making in long-term care. Nursing homes represent the intersection of several aspects of care: residents who are at risk of impaired decision-making capacity because of a combination of mental and physical health problems; family members who bring their own expectations of care and decision-making roles; and public policy and regulations that place demands on the staff and residents of the setting. We turn to one of those policies next.

The Public Policy Context: The PSDA

The Patient Self-Determination Act (PSDA) went into effect on December 1, 1991. This legislation mandated that all facilities receiving Medicare and Medicaid funds (i.e., hospitals, nursing homes, home health care agencies, hospices, and health maintenance organizations) comply with five requirements regarding advance care planning. These included: (1) the provision of written information to individuals, at the time of their admission, about their right to make medical treatment decisions and to formulate advance directives; (2) the maintenance of written policies and procedures regarding advance directives; (3) the documentation of the execution of advance directives in the individual's medical chart; (4) compliance with state law regarding the implementation of advance directives; and (5) the provision of staff and community education regarding advance directives.

Proponents of legislation such as the PSDA believed that competent adults entering a facility such as a hospital or nursing home that received Medicare or Medicaid funds would be educated regarding end-of-life treatment issues and encouraged to complete advance directives (Emanuel, Weinberg, Gonin, Hummel, & Emanuel, 1993; Robinson, DeHaven, & Koch, 1993; Wolf et al., 1991; Zwahr, Allen-Burge, Willis, & Schaie, in preparation). Assessing the capacity of an individual to make medical treatment decisions remains one of the greatest challenges of medical ethics. These goals reflect the highest ethical standard of medical practice: the preservation of the autonomous wishes of the competent patient (American Geriatrics Society Ethics Committee, 1996; Brock, 1994). Theoretically, the use of advance directives ensures the preservation of individual autonomy by providing a mechanism for competent individuals to choose the types of medical treatment they would be willing to undergo in the future. By indicating treatment preference in advance of medical crisis, competent individuals may consider the consequences of their decisions in an unhurried manner.

When informed and competent autonomous decisions regarding medical care cannot be obtained, either the substituted judgment principle or the best interests principle is used to make medical decisions for the individual in question (Brock, 1994). The substituted judgment principle requires that the surrogate decision maker use available knowledge about the patient's values and wishes to decide as the person in need of treatment would have decided. If the surrogate decision maker does not know the person's values and wishes regarding medical care, the best interests principle is used (Brock, 1994). This directs the surrogate to choose the treatment alternative that best promotes the patient's interests as defined by the surrogate and/or by the state.

Descriptive studies have shown, however, that adults engage in informal advance care planning rather than formal execution of advance directives (Gamble, McDonald, & Lichstein, 1991; High, 1988, 1993; Sehgal, Galbraith, Chesney, Schoenfeld, Charles, & Lo, 1992). Individuals prefer family members to make treatment decisions for them if they become incapacitated (Gamble et al., 1991; High, 1993), and many want these surrogate family decision makers to be given leeway in the interpretation of advance directives even when such formal documents exist (Sehgal et al., 1992).

Simple educational interventions targeted at community-dwelling elderly with the purpose of increasing knowledge and execution of advance care documents have demonstrated little to no increase in formal advance directive use (Hare & Nelson, 1991; High, 1993; Sachs, Stocking, & Miles, 1992). Those community-dwelling individuals who execute formal advance care documents tend to be older (Emanuel, Barry, Stoeckle, Ettelson, & Emanuel, 1991; Emanuel et al., 1993; Fried, Rosenberg, & Lipsitz, 1995; Robinson et al., 1993; Sehgal et al., 1992; Schonwetter, Walker, Solomon, Indurkhya, & Robinson, 1996), sicker (Sachs, 1994), and more likely to engage in preventive health behaviors such as exercise (Zwahr et al., in preparation).

Thus, it is unlikely that at the time of nursing home placement, an individual will have executed a formal advance care document. At placement, family members (i.e., potential surrogate decision makers) may be approached by nursing home personnel and given information regarding advance directives. Since relocating to a nursing home is often an overwhelming series of transitions, the information given to individuals and their families at the time of admission (as mandated by the PSDA) is not likely to be fully processed. Although the provision of information regarding the use of advance directives was mandated by the PSDA, nursing home residents with cognitive impairments are not likely to benefit from such educational interventions. In fact, the very individuals whose civil rights the PSDA seeks to protect may not have the capacity to act in their own behalf in communicating end-of-life wishes either at the time of admission to a nursing home or when medical crises occur.

Assessing the "Fit" between Legislative Intent and Client Capacity

Although several promising means of assessing individual capacity to make medical treatment decisions or to complete advance directives have been identified, the problem of implementing these procedures in the nursing home remains. Problems in implementation are due primarily to the diversity of residents, potential surrogates, and nursing home facilities themselves. First, findings regarding the advance care planning activities of nursing home residents will be reviewed. Next, this section will specifically address the problem of assessing individual decision-making capacity, the lack of congruence between autonomous and surrogate medical decision making, and the lack of congruence between individual capacity and environmental demands. (For a broader discussion of geriatric assessment issues, see Edelstein and Kalish, Chapter 10, this volume.)

Many studies addressing capacity and legal/ethical issues of medical decision making have been conducted in nursing home settings (Batchelor, Winsemius, O'Connor, & Wetle, 1992; Cohen-Mansfield et al., 1991; Diamond, Jernigan, Moseley, Messina, & McKeown, 1989; Eleazer et al., 1996; Gerety, Chiodo, Kanten, Tuley, & Cornell, 1993; Kellogg, Crain, Corwin, & Brickner, 1992; Lurie, Pheley, Miles, & Bannick-Mohrland, 1992; Michelson, Mulvihill, Hsu, & Olson, 1991; Palker & Nettles-Carlson, 1995; Ouslander, Tymchuk, & Krynski, 1993; Terry & Zweig, 1994; Wetle, Levkoff, Cwikel, & Rosen, 1988). Unfortunately, most of the participants in these studies, while residing in long-term care institutions, were selected so that they did not demonstrate severe cognitive impairments. The selective omission of cognitively impaired residents is ironic because the prevalence of dementia exceeds 50% in most nursing homes (Ouslander, Osterweil, & Morley, 1997). Thus, results from these studies may not be generalizable to the entire range of nursing home residents.

Estimates of the prevalence of documented advance directives [e.g., Do Not Resuscitate (DNR) orders, living wills, durable power of attorney for health care] in the medical charts of nursing home residents range from 14.5% (Lurie et al., 1992) to 54% (Palker & Nettles-Carlson, 1995). The prevalence of DNR orders in nursing home settings may be slightly higher (36.3%) than more general advance directives (Terry & Zweig, 1994). Like older adults living in the community, nursing home residents report that a primary barrier to the completion of advance directives is the belief that family members, physicians, or others (e.g., God) will take care of their future health care needs (Palker & Nettles-Carlson, 1995).

Due to this tendency to prefer the involvement of others in planning their future medical treatment, Lurie and colleagues (Lurie et al., 1992) recommended that the process of advance planning for nursing home residents should respect individual differences in the desire for autonomous decision making. Wetle et al. (1988) investigated the perceptions of nursing home residents and their nurses regarding the adequacy of the amount of information given to residents regarding their medical condition. The cognitive status of participants was not formally assessed or reported; eligibility for participation was determined by resident nomination by nursing home staff. Results indicated that 40% of residents reported being told everything about their medical condition, but another 40% reported being told nothing. Sixty-six percent of residents, however, felt that the information they had been told regarding their condition was adequate. Of the 40% of residents who believed they were not involved in making decisions regarding their medical care, 80% considered that level of involvement appropriate.

Although some studies have failed to identify characteristics of residents who tend to informally or formally communicate advance care plans (Ouslander et al., 1993), several other investigations have identified characteristics of nursing home residents who discuss their advance care plans with others (i.e., informal plans) and/or who possess advance directives (i.e., formal plans). For example, Lurie et al. (1992) found that older residents were much less likely to have discussed their plans or treatment preferences with others. These older individuals were also much more likely to want their family members consulted in the event of medical crises necessitating a treatment decision (Lurie et al., 1992). Nursing home residents with formal advance directives are also older and have typically been admitted to their nursing facility after the enactment of the PSDA (Terry & Zweig, 1994). Individual characteristics associated with the documentation of DNR orders in the medical chart include increased age, the diagnosis of dementia, and the presence of advance directives (Terry & Zweig, 1994).

In a rare study including both cognitively intact and cognitively impaired residents, Diamond and colleagues (1989) reported that the mental status of nursing home residents was associated with life-sustaining treatment preference. Specifically, individuals having decisional capacity were more likely to choose to forego life-sustaining medical treatments, and those of questionable capacity were more likely to request aggressive treatment. Sixty-four percent of their sample were judged to have at least adequate mental competence scores, and 36% scored 24 or higher on the Mini-Mental State Examination (MMSE). Only 49% of participants, however, were judged to have decisional capacity based primarily on physician ratings.

Compounding the problem of resident diversity is the fact that individuals may not be competent to make medical decisions when they are in medical crisis (Dellasega, Smyer, Frank, & Brown, 1996; Frank, 1995; Uhlmann et al., 1987). For example, Dellasega and colleagues (1996) reported that medical inpatients demonstrated lower than normal specific cognitive abilities and decrements in everyday cognitive competence (Willis & Schaie, 1993; Marsiske & Willis, 1995). In fact, medical inpatients were able to understand specific medical treatment decisions only when information was presented in shorter segments and individuals obtained frequent feedback (Dellasega et al., 1996; Frank, 1995).

The Problem of Decision-Making Capacity

The literature on decisional capacity clearly states that capacity determinations are specific to each individual, each circumstance, and each medical decision. Pearlman (1996) cites the determination of decision-making capacity by physicians as the primary challenge facing physicians in the implementation of the American Geriatrics Society Ethics Committee guidelines. Pearlman also asserts the need for more effective intervention procedures to facilitate the completion of advance directives. He alludes to different legal and ethical standards for determining decisional incapacity.

Several investigators have identified levels of decisional capacity underlying treatment decisions in the context of informed consent (Drane, 1984; Grisso, 1994; Lidz, Appelbaum, & Meisel, 1988). Decisional capacity can be assessed at three levels according to these authors: (1) awareness and assent, (2) understanding of alternatives and choice, and (3) appreciation of consequences and rationality. Drane (1984) proposed that the level of decisional capacity required of an individual should be contingent on the level of medical risk involved in the treatment decision. Thus, he would advocate that the highest level of capacity (i.e., appreciation of consequences and rationality) should be demonstrated in cases of life-sustaining treatment decisions.

Rather than proposing a sliding scale of the assessment of capacity based on the medical decision to be made, Lidz et al. (1988) proposed a process model of medical decision making. Use of a process model recognizes that medical treatment decisions are not made at one discrete moment in time. Instead, these decisions are frequently made over time with input from multiple individuals (physicians, family members, clergy) and with the possibility of gleaning additional information (obtaining a second opinion, personal research). Lidz and colleagues (1988) caution that moving toward a process model of identifying capacity to consent to medical treatment would require (1) modification of the role expectations of both physicians and patients, (2) comparison and agreement among physicians and patients of internal representations of illness, and (3) the clarification of the values and quality of life expectations of both physicians and patients. This new dialogue between physicians and patients would necessarily occur across time at various phases of patient care, such as establishing mutual responsibility for outcome, defining the problem, setting treatment goals, selecting the appropriate treatment, and following through with the treatment plan.

This process model offers much if our primary goal remains the preservation of as much individual autonomy as possible in medical treatment decisions. The incorporation of autonomy, however, may need to become more lenient than fully informed consent. Perhaps some degree of personal autonomy can be preserved when personal preferences congruent with a more lenient legal standard of capacity are considered in medical treatment decisions.

Marson and colleagues have developed a method for assessing the capacity of older, community-dwelling adults for making medical treatment decisions at each of five different legal standards (Marson, Ingram, Cody, & Harrell, 1995a, 1995b; Marson, Chatterjee, Ingram, & Harrell, 1996). These standards, listed in order of the complexity of the cognitive processes required, include (1) providing a treatment choice, (2) making a reasonable treatment choice, (3) appreciating the consequences of one's choice, (4) providing rational reasons for the choice made, and (5) understanding the treatment situation and alternatives. These investigators have shown that individuals with mild to moderate Alzheimer's disease performed no differently than healthy, community-dwelling older adults on making a treatment choice, making a reasonable choice, and appreciating the consequences of their choice. Individuals with mild and moderate dementia, however, perform significantly worse on competency evaluations assessed at the level of providing rational reasons for choice and understanding treatment decisions. Marson et al. (1996) found that the simple ability to evidence a treatment choice was predicted by auditory comprehension. In contrast, frontal lobe functions may underlie the ability of individuals to provide a rational reason for their treatment choice (Marson et al., 1995b).

Few investigators have directly assessed the capacity of older adults living in long-term care settings to complete an advance directive. Molloy et al. (1996) compared five different measures of capacity to complete an advance directive among older adults living in congregate housing facilities and nursing homes. Their participants were English-speaking individuals assessed by their nurse caregivers as not so demented that they could not possibly participate in a medical treatment decision.

Molloy et al. (1996) compared capacity assessments made by a trained nurse specialist in collaboration with an interdisciplinary treatment team (Competency Clinic assessments), capacity assessments made by a geriatrician, measures of the ability to understand a generic or a specific advance directive document, and participants' scores on the Standardized Mini-Mental Status Examination (SMMSE). The determinations of capacity used in this study as the "gold standard" were the Competency Clinic assessments and the assessments made by the geriatrician. Results indicated that capacity assessments made by both the Competency Clinic and geriatricians compared favorably to assessments of decisional capacity based on the SMMSE. An SMMSE cut-off of 20, however, proved a more powerful method of differentiating individuals with the capacity to complete an advance directive from individuals with-out it.

Pruchno and her colleagues (1995) also assessed the decision-making capacity of nursing home residents, with a goal of identifying the most effective assessment battery. In a sample of 50 nursing home residents, they compared a clinician's assessment of the resident's competence for medical decision making with predictions developed from a composite of assessment approaches reflecting underlying abilities involved in decision making. The clinician's assessment was used as the "gold standard." Pruchno and her colleagues found that the best predictors of the clinician's assessment were the MMSE score and an information recognition score following procedures developed by Appelbaum and Grisso (1988). In addition, the Hopemont questionnaire (Edelstein, 1993) provided helpful information for residents who neither clearly lacked decision-making capacity nor clearly maintained this capacity. These three instruments (MMSE, recognition, and Hopemont) reflected the residents' abilities on key elements of decision making: comprehending a situation involving medical care, considering treatment options, and coming to a rational decision.

The Lack of Congruence between Autonomous and Surrogate Medical Decision Making

Another difficulty of implementing the PSDA in nursing home settings involves the diversity of surrogate involvement in advance planning activities and the inaccuracy of surrogate decisions in reflecting the wishes of the individual requiring treatment. Multiple studies across diverse settings have shown that the decisions made by a surrogate decision maker may not accurately reflect the decision that the individual in question would have made for him- or herself (Ditto et al., 1995; Eleazer et al., 1996; Karel & Gatz, 1996; McNabney, Beers, & Siebens, 1994; Seckler, Meier, Mulvihill, & Parris, 1991; Uhlmann, Pearlman, & Cain, 1988; Uhlmann & Pearlman, 1991; Zweibel & Cassel, 1989).

Among community-dwelling adults, Ditto and colleagues (1995) found that even with knowledge of prior written advance directives, the agreement between surrogate preferences and individual preferences for life-sustaining treatment is poor. In a multigenerational community survey regarding individual preferences and issues influencing life-sustaining treatment decisions, Karel and Gatz (1996) found that surrogates' views on treatment of an ill parent were more strongly related to the surrogates' treatment preferences for themselves than to the parents' autonomous wishes.

Among individuals in the primary care setting, Zweibel and Cassel (1989) investigated the concordance between treatment decisions made by older adults and their physician-designated surrogate decision makers. Particular strengths of this study include the appointment of surrogate decision makers by the attending physician (i.e., a likely real-world scenario), the inclusion of participants varying in ethnicity and cultural background, and the investigation of respondents' prior experience with life-sustaining treatment decisions. Many authors have found that variations in cultural background as reflected by ethnicity predict differences in medical treatment preferences in both community-dwelling older adults (Allen-Burge & Haley, 1997; Caralis, Davis, Wright, & Marcial, 1993; Garrett, Harris, Norburn, Patrick, & Davis, 1993; Schonwetter, Walker, Kramer, & Robinson, 1994) and older adults residing in long-term care settings (Eleazer et al., 1996). Interestingly, 85% of patients and 82% of surrogates in the Zweibel and Cassel (1989) study reported having at least one prior experience in making treatment decisions of this type. Results indicated that physician-appointed surrogates underestimated the older adult patient's desire for life-sustaining medical treatment. Zweibel and Cassel (1989) suggest that differences between patients and surrogates in the assessment of quality of life may underlie the differences in treatment preference ratings.

Seckler et al. (1991) also investigated the accuracy of substituted judgment in the context of a geriatric outpatient clinic. Inclusion criteria for participation were facility with the English language, MMSE score greater than 20, one visit to a health care provider in the previous year, and full comprehension of the concept of resuscitation. Thirty-nine percent of their respondents were Caucasian and 50% were African-American. These investigators found that a majority of older outpatients in this sample preferred the initiation of life-sustaining treatments, but neither family nor physician surrogate decision makers accurately reported the older individual's treatment preferences. Families tended to err on the side of providing unwanted treatment whereas physicians tended to withhold treatment that was desired. Only 16% of older outpatients had ever discussed their resuscitation preferences with family members, and only 7% of older individuals had such discussions with their physicians.

Among long-term care settings, Diamond et al. (1989) found that the concordance of patient-surrogate treatment preferences was poor. For example, 27% of surrogate-resident pairs in which the resident possessed decisional capacity reported discrepant treatment preferences. Seventy percent of surrogates in this study, however, reported that they were "very sure" of their substituted judgment. Only 45% of surrogates interviewed reported having had prior informal advance care planning discussions with the residents regarding the residents' treatment wishes.

Gerety et al. (1993) also investigated the concordance between life-sustaining treatment preferences of nursing home residents in comparison with surrogate decision makers in a sample drawn from a Veterans Affairs nursing facility (97% male). Treatment preferences were elicited for CPR, ventilation, and intensive care. Participants accepted treatment in 70% of all medical treatment scenarios. Participants' desire for the initiation of treatment declined with the health status scenario presented. Thirteen percent of respondents demonstrated inconsistent treatment preference decisions, represented by desiring treatment in a more fragile health state while declining treatment in more robust health. Treatment preferences were associated with depressive symptomatology such that individuals with more severe depressive symptoms were less likely to prefer the initiation of medical treatment. Concordance with surrogate decision makers was no greater than chance, but there appeared to be no systematic bias in surrogate treatment decisions in this study (i.e., surrogates were equally likely to opt for treatment when the resident would decline and to decline treatment when the resident would accept).

These studies clearly illustrate the lack of concordance between surrogate treatment preferences and the treatment preferences expressed by older adults themselves. They shed little light, however, on the issues underlying this lack of agreement between older adults and their potential surrogates. For example, although surrogate decision makers may rely on their assessments of the quality of life of patients in making treatment decisions (Uhlmann & Pearlman, 1991), patients may not rely on perceived quality of life when considering life-sustaining measures (Uhlmann & Pearlman, 1991; Pearlman et al., 1993). In a recent study regarding the issues influencing surrogate decision making, Allen-Burge and Haley (1997) found that characteristics of both the surrogate decision maker and the person for whom a decision was being made influenced surrogate treatment preference ratings for three different life-sustaining medical treatments (e.g., CPR, CPR and ventilation, or CPR and tube feeding). These authors asked individuals who were either currently caregivers for a community-dwelling individual with dementia or individuals who were not currently caregivers to make treatment preference ratings based on a vignette either describing an elderly man with healthy cognitive functioning or suffering symptoms of severe dementia. Only the cognitive status of the patient influenced treatment preference ratings for CPR (Allen-Burge & Haley, 1997). Decisions including the use of ventilation or tube feeding, however, were influenced not only by the cognitive status of the patient but also by the care giving status and race of the surrogate decision maker. Specifically, white caregivers were less likely than other groups to initiate either CPR and ventilation or CPR and tube feeding.

Although surrogate decision makers do not make treatment preference ratings that coincide with those made by older adults themselves, results from several studies indicate that one characteristic influencing surrogate treatment preference ratings is the cognitive status of the older adult for whom the decision is being made (Allen-Burge & Haley, 1997; Cohen-Mansfield, Droge, & Billig, 1992; Pearlman et al., 1993; Seckler et al., 1991; Uhlmann & Pearlman, 1991). This compounds the problem faced in nursing home settings, as new residents may not be able to communicate their own treatment wishes due to cognitive incapacity, and their cognitive incapacity may influence the treatment preferences of potential surrogate decision makers. These issues will be explored in the next section.

The Lack of Congruence between Capacity and Environmental Demands

Recent investigations have shown that the successful implementation of the PSDA varies greatly across hospital and nursing home sites (Park, Eaton, Larson, & Palmer, 1994; Zwahr, Park, Eaton, & Larson, 1996). Although the purpose of the PSDA was to increase the use of advance directives in acute and long-term care settings, few interventions have targeted health care staff and attempted to train these individuals to increase the prevalence of formal advance care plans among frail older adults. Kellogg and colleagues (1992) conducted a longitudinal intervention study designed to assess the impact of physician-initiated discussions on informed decision making and life-sustaining treatment preferences in 20 frail elderly home-bound adults. These investigators examined the relationship of physician-initiated discussion and psychological variables such as depression, life satisfaction, and control orientation. They found that formal advance care plans were extremely rare and that informal advance care plans were more frequent. They also found that after the initiation of a treatment preference discussion by a physician, older adults exhibited slightly lower depression scores. For those individuals with an internal control orientation, life satisfaction scores improved. The treatment decisions made by these individuals, however, were not stable and were likely to differ from their original preferences at 18 month follow-up (Kellogg et al., 1992).

Batchelor and colleagues (1992) conducted a longitudinal study of 424 nursing home residents after the initiation of a facility-wide policy on the documentation of advance directive status. Advance directive status was categorized as documentation in the chart of full code status, DNR status, or palliative care. Results indicated that restricted advance directive status (e.g., DNR or palliative care) was predicted by increased age and decreased functional and cognitive status of the resident, the presence of a surrogate decision maker, and having a nursing-home employed physician. Once again, the agreement between surrogate treatment preferences and resident preferences was low, with surrogates choosing restrictive directives 82% of the time and residents choosing restrictive directives only 62% of the time.

Willis (1996) postulated a model of everyday competence that incorporates and theoretically links the functional abilities of the individual whose capacity is questioned and the demands and resources of the environment in which the individual lives. Dellasega et al. (1996) extended the application of Willis' model to medical decision-making capacity assessments among older hospitalized adults. These authors noted that the demands of a hospital environment are great and the resources of acutely ill elders are low, making life-sustaining medical treatment decisions more complex in this setting. Likewise, nursing home residents vary widely in possession of the resources necessary to maintain everyday competence and nursing home settings vary in the ability to provide the environmental structures necessary to optimize resident functioning. Since these two components of capacity may be incongruent in the nursing home setting, a rethinking of the imperative of full individual patient autonomy as the most important ethical standard may be in order. Policy-makers and legislators interested in medical treatment decisions among older nursing home residents must resolve how to incorporate the reserve capacities, values, and preferences of incapacitated older nursing home residents in their medical treatment plans (Smyer, 1996).

Attempts by professional groups to resolve this conflict in capacity and environmental demands have already begun. For example, the Position Statement published by the AGS Ethics Committee states that an attempt should always be made to ascertain the cognitively incapacitated older adult's ability to participate in the medical decision-making process (American Geriatrics Society Ethics Committee, 1996). Along with others, Michelson et al. (1991) demonstrated that alert, nondemented nursing home residents are able to respond to medical treatment decisions presented in a case-study format and to make a treatment choice among the alternatives proposed to them. Marson and his colleagues have shown that even moderately demented older adults with preserved auditory comprehension are able to state a treatment preference, but more complex cognitive abilities involving executive functions are necessary to appreciate the consequences of such a decision and to understand treatment alternatives (Marson et al., 1995, 1996).

Problems arise in nursing home settings when health care staff must integrate the incapacitated older adults' stated treatment preferences and input (or lack of input) from surrogate decision makers. The American Geriatrics Society Ethics Committee (1996) states that in cases in which no appropriate surrogate decision maker can be identified, a multidisciplinary team of health care professionals should undertake the task of medical decision making using the "best interests" ethics standard. These guidelines call for institutions to develop policies and procedures for making medical decisions and for greater uniformity across jurisdictions in the approach to surrogate medical decision making. Special consideration should be given to the individual's prior history and cultural milieu. One primary goal of the Position Statement is to protect the individual's ability to die naturally and comfortably.

Resolving the Dilemma: How Do We "Gauge Success"?

In summary, the problems in implementing the PSDA in nursing home settings reflect the challenges of medical decision making in all long-term care settings. These include the capacity and willingness of residents to execute advance directives or participate in treatment decisions, the variability and inaccuracy of surrogate involvement in the treatment planning and daily activities of nursing home residents, and the variability in the execution of advance care planning on the part of staff (Batchelor et al., 1992; Kellogg et al., 1992). Given the complexities and incongruities between the reality of medical decision making in long-term care settings and the goals of current legislative mandates, how do we gauge the success of our efforts to resolve the inconsistencies?

Consistent with the AGS guidelines, the resolution of this medical-ethical dilemma will involve the integration of information from a variety of sources and the consolidation of information on a variety of levels. Health care professionals must know and communicate with patients well enough to know the individual's treatment goals. Optimally, the health care team will develop effective ethics committees with a standardized approach to ethical dilemmas (Pearlman, 1996).

The reserve capacity of the individual also must be considered. Thus, the treatment preference of the incapacitated older adult should always be elicited and should help to focus the medical decision making of a surrogate decision-making body. Additional individual characteristics factoring into such decisions will include an assessment of prior experience with such decisions, personal values and spirituality, culture, and perceived quality of life. Environmental circumstances influencing such decisions should include an assessment of the resources available in a given setting to maximize the approximation of individual autonomy.

Lawton (1996) offers a multidimensional model of quality of life that could be usefully incorporated in medical treatment decisions for incapacitated older nursing home residents. Means of assessing individual and environmental indicators of quality of life suggested by Lawton (1996) include the Affect Rating Scale (Lawton, Van Haitsma, & Klapper, 1996), the Pleasant Events Schedule—AD (Logsdon & Teri, 1997), and observational ratings of an individual's mood and surrounding environment (Scilley, Burgio, Stevens, Hardin, & Hsu, 1996). Future research should explore the usefulness of such quality of life assessments for models of autonomous and surrogate medical decision making in nursing homes.

Long-term care contexts need an infrastructure for responding to medical and ethical crises as they arise among residents. The idea proposed here revolves around an interdisciplinary team that can plan the institution's response prior to medical or ethical crises among incapacitated residents. Such an ethics team could use information regarding the residents' previous and current values and stated treatment preferences as well as objective criteria indexing the residents' quality of life in considering judgments regarding aggressive treatment versus palliative care. In doing so, nursing home residents, relatives, and staff would acknowledge Cohen's (1993) dictum: biography is as important as biology in responding effectively to impaired older adults.

REVIEW QUESTIONS

1. What cognitive functions underlie older adults' decision-making capacity?

2. What are the most effective means of assessing the core components of older adults' decision-making capacity?

3. What is the impact of disease and disability on older adults' ability to be engaged in medical decision making?

4. What is the "legal fiction" of a competent older person and how has it changed in the last three decades?

5. What is the most effective and appropriate way to engage older adults' family members in decision making in long-term care settings?

6. Compare and contrast two styles of assessing older adults' decision-making capacity: an all-or-nothing model that assumes the older person must be totally competent to be involved and a modified approach that assumes that the older person must be involved within the limits of his or her ability. What are the advantages and disadvantages of each?

7. What are the ethical principles followed in medical decision making? Who makes decisions under each ethical principle and how are these principles different?

8. How well do surrogate treatment preferences match older adults' autonomous wishes regarding life-sustaining medical treatment? Across care settings (i.e., community, primary care, nursing homes), what issues have been shown to be related to surrogate treatment preferences?

9. Explain the potential incongruity of resident capacity and environmental demands for medical decision making in nursing home settings.

References

Allen-Burge, R., & Haley, W. E. (1997). Individual differences and surrogate medical decisions: Differing preferences for life-sustaining treatments. *Aging and Mental Health, 1*(2), 121–131.

American Geriatrics Society Ethics Committee. (1996). Making treatment decisions for incapacitated older adults without advance directives. *Journal of the American Geriatrics Society, 44*, 986–987.

Anderer, S. J. (1990). *Determining competency in guardianship proceedings*. Washington, DC: American Bar Association.

Appelbaum, P. S., & Grisso, T. (1988). Assessing patients' capacities to consent to treatment. *New England Journal of Medicine, 319*, 1635–1638.

Assisted Living Facilities Association of America. (1993). *An overview of the assisted living industry*. Fairfax, VA: Assisted Living Facilities Association of America.

Batchelor, A. J., Winsemius, D., O'Connor, P. J., & Wetle, T. (1992). Predictors of advance directive restrictiveness and compliance with institutional policy in a long-term-care facility. *Journal of the American Geriatrics Society, 40*, 679–684.

Brock, D. W. (1994). Good decisionmaking for incompetent patients. *Hastings Center Report: Special Supplement*, S8–S11.

Burns, B. J., Wagner, H. R., Taube, J. E., Magaziner, J., Permutt, T., & Landerman, L. R. (1993). Mental health service use by the elderly in nursing homes. *American Journal of Public Health, 83*(3), 331–337.

Caralis, P. V., Davis, B., Wright, K., & Marcial, E. (1993). The influence of ethnicity and race on attitudes toward advance directives, life-prolonging treatments, and euthanasia. *The Journal of Clinical Ethics, 4*(2), 155–165.

Cassel, C.K., Rudberg, M. A., & Olshansky, S.J. (1992). The prices of success: Health care in an aging society. *Health Affairs, 11*(2), 87–99.

Cohen, E. S. (1993). Comprehensive assessment: Capturing strengths, not just weaknesses. *Generations, XVII*(1), 47–50.

Cohen, M.A., Tell, E.J., Greenberg, J.N., & Wallack, S.S. (1987). The financial capacity of the elderly to insure for long-term care. *The Gerontologist, 27,* 494–501.

Cohen-Mansfield, J., Droge, J. A., & Billig, N. (1992). Factors influencing hospital patients' preferences in the utilization of life-sustaining treatments. *The Gerontologist, 32,* 89–95.

Cohen-Mansfield, J., Rabinovich, B. A., Lipson, S., Fein, A., Gerber B., Weisman, S., & Pawlson, L. G. (1991). The decision to execute a durable power of attorney for health care and preferences regarding the utilization of the life-sustaining treatments in nursing home residents. *Archives of Internal Medicine, 151,* 289–294.

Dellasega, C., Smyer, M., Frank, L., & Brown, R. (1996). Commentary: Decision-making capacity in the acutely ill elderly. In M. A. Smyer, K. W. Schaie & M. B. Kapp (Eds.), *Older adults' decision-making and the law.* (pp. 142–161). New York: Springer Publishing Co. Inc.

Dey, A.N. (1996). Characteristics of elderly home health care users: Data from the 1994 National Home and Hospice care survey. *Advance data from vital and health statistics; no. 279.* Hyattsville, MD: National Center for Health Statistics.

Dey, A.N. (1997). Characteristics of elderly nursing home residents: Data from the 1995 National Nursing Home Survey. *Advance data from vital and health statistics; no. 289.* Hyattsville, MD: National Center for Health Statistics.

Diamond, E. L., Jernigan, J. A., Moseley, R. A., Messina, V., & McKeown, R. A. (1989). Decision-making ability and advance directive preferences in nursing home patients and proxies. *The Gerontologist, 29,* 622–626.

Ditto, P. H., Coppola, K. M., Klepac, L. M., Danks, J. H., Moore, K. A., & Smucker, W. D. (1995). *Do advance directives improve the accuracy of substituted judgment?* Paper presented at the meeting of the Gerontological Society of America, Los Angeles, CA.

Drane, J. F. (1984). Competency to give an informed consent: A model for making clinical assessments. *Journal of the American Medical Association, 252,* 925–927.

Edelstein, B. (1993). *Hopemont Capacity Assessment Inventory.* Unpublished manuscript.

Eleazer, G. P., Hornung, C. A., Egbert, C. B., Egbert, J. R., Eng, C., Hedgepeth, J., McCann, R., Strothers, H., Sapir, M., Wei, M., & Wilson, M. (1996). The relationship between ethnicity and advance directives in a frail older population. *Journal of the American Geriatric Society, 44,* 938–943.

Emanuel, E. J., Weinberg, D. S., Gonin, R., Hummel, L. R., & Emanuel, L. L. (1993). How well is the Patient Self-Determination Act working?: An early assessment. *The American Journal of Medicine, 95,* 619–628.

Emanuel, L. L., Barry, M. J., Stoeckle, J. D., Ettelson, L. M., & Emanuel, E. J. (1991). Advance directives for medical care—A case for greater use. *New England Journal of Medicine, 324,* 889–895.

Frank, L. B. (1995). *Psychological and legal considerations in the assessment of decision-making capacity of older adults.* Unpublished doctoral dissertation, The Pennsylvania State University, University Park.

Fried, T. R., Rosenberg, R. R., & Lipsitz, L. A. (1995). Older community-dwelling adults' attitudes toward and practices of health promotion and advance planning activities. *Journal of the American Geriatrics Society, 43,* 645–649.

Gamble, E. R., McDonald, P. J., & Lichstein, P. R. (1991). Knowledge, attitudes, and behavior of elderly persons regarding living wills. *Archives of Internal Medicine, 151,* 277–281.

Garrett, J. M., Harris, R. P., Norburn, J. K., Patrick, D. L., & Danis, M. (1993). Life-sustaining treatments during terminal illness: Who wants what? *Journal of General Internal Medicine, 8,* 361–368.

Gerety, M. B., Chiodo, L. K., Kanten, D. N., Tuley, M. R., & Cornell, J. E. (1993). Medical treatment preferences of nursing home residents: Relationship to function and concordance with surrogate decision-makers. *Journal of the American Geriatrics Society, 41,* 953–960.

Goodwin, P. E., Smyer, M. A., & Lair, T. I. (1995). Decision-making incapacity among nursing home residents: Results from the 1987 NMES Survey. *Behavioral Sciences and the Law, 13,* 405–414.

Grisso, T. (1994). Clinical assessments for legal competence of older adults. In M. Storandt & G. R. VandenBos (Eds.), *Neuropsychological assessment of dementia and depression in older adults: a clinician's guide* (pp. 119–140). Washington, DC: American Psychological Association.

Gulyas, R.A. (1995). *AAHSA's position on assisted living.* Washington, DC: American Association of Homes and Services for the Aging.

Hare, J., & Nelson, C. (1991). Will outpatients complete living wills? A comparison of two interventions. *Journal of General Internal Medicine, 6,* 41–46.

High, D. M. (1988). All in the family: Extended autonomy and expectations in surrogate health care decision-making. *The Gerontologist, 28,* 46–51.

High, D. M. (1993). Advance directives and the elderly: A study of intervention strategies to increase use. *The Gerontologist, 33,* 342–349.

Karel, M. J., & Gatz, M. (1996). Factors influencing life-sustaining treatment decisions in a community sample of families. *Psychology and Aging, 11,* 226–234.

Kellogg, F. R., Crain, M., Corwin, J., & Brickner, P. W. (1992). Life-sustaining interventions in frail elderly persons: Talking about choices. *Archives of Internal Medicine, 152,* 2317–2320.

Kemp, B.J., & Mitchell, J.M. (1992). Functional impairment in geriatric mental health. In J.E. Birren, R.B. Sloane, & G.D. Cohen (Eds.), *Handbook of mental health and aging* (pp. 671–697). San Diego, CA: Academic Press.

Lair, T., & Lefkowitz, D. (1990). Mental health and functional status of residents of nursing and personal care homes. DHHS Pub. No. PHS90–3470. Rockville, MD: Department of Helath and Human Services, Agency for Health Care Policy and Reserch.

Lawton, M. P. (1996). *Assessing quality of life.* Unpublished manuscript.

Lawton, M. P., Van Haitsma, K., & Klapper, J. (1996). Observed affect in nursing home residents with Alzheimer's disease. *Journal of Gerontology: Psychological Sciences, 51B,* P3–14.

Lidz, C. W., Appelbaum, P. S., & Meisel, A. (1988). Two models of implementing informed consent. *Archives of Internal Medicine, 148,* 1385–1389.

Logsdon, R. G., & Teri, L. (1997). The Pleasant Events Schedule—AD: Psychometric properties and relationship to depression and cognition in Alzheimer's disease patients. *The Gerontologist, 37,* 40–45.

Lurie, N., Pheley, A. M., Miles, S. H., & Bannick-Mohrland, S. (1992). Attitudes toward discussing life-sustaining treatments in extended care facility patients. *Journal of the American Geriatrics Society, 40,* 1205–1208.

Marsiske, M., & Willis, S. L. (1995). Dimensionality of everyday problem solving in older adults. *Psychology and Aging, 10,* 269–283.

Marson, D. C., Chatterjee, A., Ingram, K. K., & Harrell, L. E. (1996). Towards a neurologic model of competency: Cognitive predictors of capacity to consent in Alzheimer's disease using three different legal standards. *Neurology, 46*(3), 666–672.

Marson, D. C., Ingram, K. K., Cody, H. A., & Harrell, L. E. (1995a). Assessing the competency of patients with Alzheimer's disease under different legal standards: A prototype instrument. *Archives of Neurology, 52*, 949–954.

Marson, D. C., Ingram, K. K., Cody, H. A., & Harrell, L. E. (1995b). Neuropsychologic predictors of competency in Alzheimer's disease using a rational reasons legal standard. *Archives of Neurology, 52*, 955–959.

McNabney, M. K., Beers, M. H., & Siebens, H. (1994). Surrogate decision makers' satisfaction with the placement of feeding tubes in elderly patients. *Journal of the American Geriatrics Society, 42*(2), 161–168.

Michelson, C., Mulvihill, M., Hsu, M. A., & Olson, E. (1991). Eliciting medical care preferences from nursing home residents. *The Gerontologist, 31*, 358–363.

Molloy, D. W., Silberfeld, M., Darzins, P., Guyatt, G. H., Singer, P. A., Rush, B., Bedard, M., & Strang, D. (1996). Measuring capacity to complete an advance directive. *Journal of the American Geriatrics Society, 44*, 660–664.

Omnibus Budget Reconciliation Act of 1990, P.L. 101–508, 4206, and 4751, codified at 42 U.S.C. 1395cc (a) (1) (q), 1395 mm (c) (8), 1395cc (f), 1396a (57), (58), 1396a (w).

Ouslander, J. G., Osterweil, D., & Morley, J. (1997). *Medical care in the nursing home* (2nd ed.). New York: McGraw-Hill.

Ouslander, J. G., Tymchuk, A. J., & Krynski, M. D. (1993). Decisions about enteral tube feeding among the elderly. *Journal of the American Geriatrics Society, 41*, 70–77.

Palker, N. B., & Nettles-Carlson, B. (1995). The prevalence of advance directives: Lessons from a nursing home. *Nurse Practitioner, 20*(2), 7–19.

Park, D. C., Eaton, T. A., Larson, E. A., & Palmer, H. T. (1994). Implementation and impact of the Patient Self-Determination Act. *Southern Medical Journal, 87*, 971–977.

Pearlman, R. A. (1996). Challenges facing physicians and healthcare institutions caring for patients with mental incapacity. *Journal of the American Geriatrics Society, 44*, 994–996.

Pearlman, R. A., Cain, K. C., Patrick, D. L., Appelbaum-Maizel, M., Starks, H. E., Jecker, N. S., & Uhlmann, R. F. (1993). Insights pertaining to patient assessments of states worse than death. *Journal of Clinical Ethics, 4*(1), 33–41.

Pruchno, R. A., Smyer, M. A., Rose, M. S., Hartman-Stein, P. E., Henderson-Laribee, D. L. (1995). Competence of long-term care residents to participate in decisions about their medical care: A brief, objective assessment. *The Gerontologist, 35*(5), 622–629.

Robinson, M. K., DeHaven, M. J., & Koch, K. A. (1993). Effects of the Patient Self-Determination Act on patient knowledge and behavior. *The Journal of Family Practice, 37*, 363–368.

Sabatino, C. (1996). Competency: Redefining our legal fictions. In M. Smyer, K. W. Schaie, & M. Kapp (Eds.), *Older adults' decision-making and the law* (pp. 1–28). New York: Springer.

Sachs, G. A. (1994). Increasing the prevalence of advance care planning. *The Hastings Center Report, Special Supplement,* S13–S16.

Sachs, G. A., Stocking, C. B., & Miles, S. H. (1992). Empowerment of the older patient? A randomized, controlled trial to increase discussion and use of advance directives. *Journal of the American Geriatrics Society, 40*, 269–273.

Schonwetter, R. S., Walker, R. M., Kramer, D. R., & Robinson, B. E. (1994). Socioeconomic status and resuscitation preferences in the elderly. *Journal of Applied Gerontology, 13*(2), 157–171.

Schonwetter, R. S., Walker, R. M., Solomon, M., Indurkhya, A., & Robinson, B. E. (1996). Life values, resuscitation preferences, and the applicability of living wills in an older population. *Journal of the American Geriatrics Society, 44,* 954–958.

Scilley, K., Burgio, L. D., Stevens, A., Hardin, J. M., & Hsu, C. (1996). Observed affect as a measure of quality of life for elderly nursing home residents. In R. G. Logsdon (Chair), *Quality of life in Alzheimer's disease: Implications for research.* Symposium conducted at the meeting of the Gerontological Society of America, Washington, DC.

Seckler, A. B., Meier, D. E., Mulvihill, M., & Paris, B. E. C. (1991). Substituted judgment: How accurate are proxy predictions? *Annals of Internal Medicine, 115,* 92–98.

Sehgal, A., Galbraith, A., Chesney, M., Schoenfeld, P., Charles, G., & Lo, B. (1992). How strictly do dialysis patients want their advance directives followed? *Journal of the American Medical Association, 267,* 59–63.

Smyer, M.A. (1995). Formal support in later life: Lessons for prevention. In L.A. Bond, S.J. Cutler, & A. Grams (Eds.), *Promoting successful and productive aging* (pp. 186–202). Thousand Oaks, CA: Sage.

Smyer, M. A. (1996). Afterword: Decision-making capacity among older adults: Person, process, and context. In M. A. Smyer, K. W. Schaie, & M. Kapp (Eds.), *The impact of the law on older adults' decision-making capacity* (pp. 283–287). New York: Springer.

Smyer, M. A., Schaie, K. W., & Kapp, M. (Eds.) (1996). *Older adults' decision making and the law.* New York: Springer.

Smyer, M. A., Shea, D., & Streit, A. (1994). The provision and use of mental health services in nursing homes: Results from the National Medical Expenditure Survey. *American Journal of Public Health, 84*(2), 284–287.

Terry, M., & Zweig, S. (1994). Prevalence of advance directives and do-not-resuscitate orders in community nursing facilities. *Archives of Family Medicine, 3,* 141–145.

Uhlmann, R. F., Clark, H., Pearlman, R. A., Downs, J. C. M., Addison, J. H., & Haining, R. G. (1987). Medical management decisions in nursing home patients. *Annals of Internal Medicine, 106,* 879–885.

Uhlmann, R. F., & Pearlman, R. A. (1991). Perceived quality of life and preferences for life-sustaining treatment in older adults. *Archives of Internal Medicine, 151,* 495–497.

Uhlmann, R. F., Pearlman, R. A., & Cain, K. C. (1988). Physicians' and spouses' predictions of elderly patients' resuscitation preferences. *Journal of Gerontology: Medical Sciences, 43,* M115–121.

Wetle, T., Levkoff, S., Cwikel, J., & Rosen, A. (1988). Nursing home resident participation in medical decisions: Perceptions and preferences. *The Gerontologist, 28,* 32–38.

Wiener, J.M., & Hanley, R.J. (1992). Caring for the disabled elderly: There's no place like home. In S.M. Shortell & U.E. Reinhardt (Eds.), *Improving health policy and management: Nine critical research issues for the 1990s* (pp. 75–110). Ann Arbor, MI: Health Administration Press.

Willis, S. L. (1996). Assessing everyday competence in the cognitively challenged elderly. In M. Kapp, K. W. Schaie, & M. A. Smyer (Eds.), *Older adults' decision-making and the law* (pp. 87–127). New York: Springer Publishing Co.

Willis, S. L., & Schaie, K. W. (1993). Everyday cognition: Taxonomic and methodological considerations. In J. M. Puckett & H. W. Reese (Eds.), *Lifespan developmental psychology: Mechanisms of everyday cognition* (pp. 33–53). Hillsdale, NJ: Erlbaum.

Wolf, S. M., Boyle, P., Callahan, D., Fins, J. J., Jennings, B., Nelson, J. L., Barondess, J. A., Brock, D. W., Dresser, R., Emanuel, L., Johnson, S., Lantos, J., Mason, D., Mezey, M., Orentlicher, D., & Rouse, F. (1991). Sources of concern about the Patient Self-Determination Act. *New England Journal of Medicine, 325,* 1666–1671.

Zwahr, M. D., Allen-Burge, R., Willis, S. L., & Schaie, K. W. (In preparation). Individual differences in possession of living wills: Relationships with preventive health behaviors.

Zwahr, M. D., Park, D. C., Eaton, T. A., & Larson, E. J. (1996). Knowledge about advance directives: What is known and what is learned from hospital information. *The Gerontologist, 36* (Special Issue), 282.

Zweibel, N. R., & Cassel, C. K. (1989). Treatment choices at the end of life: A comparison of decisions by older patients and their physician-selected proxies. *The Gerontologist, 5*, 615–621.

Additional Readings

American Geriatrics Society Ethics Committee. (1996). Making treatment decisions for incapacitated older adults without advance directives. *Journal of the American Geriatrics Society, 44*, 986–987.

Batchelor, A. J., Winsemius, D., O'Connor, P. J., & Wetle, T. (1992). Predictors of advance directive restrictiveness and compliance with institutional policy in a long-term-care facility. *Journal of the American Geriatrics Society, 40*, 679–684.

Brock, D. W. (1994). Good decisionmaking for incompetent patients. *Hastings Center Report: Special Supplement*, S8–S11.

Grisso, T. (1994). Clinical assessments for legal competence of older adults. In M. Storandt & G. R. VandenBos (Eds.), *Neuropsychological assessment of dementia and depression in older adults: a clinician's guide* (pp. 119–140). Washington, DC: American Psychological Association.

High, D. M. (1993). Advance directives and the elderly: A study of intervention strategies to increase use. *The Gerontologist, 33*, 342–349.

Kellogg, F. R., Crain, M., Corwin, J., & Brickner, P. W. (1992). Life-sustaining interventions in frail elderly persons: Talking about choices. *Archives of Internal Medicine, 152*, 2317–2320.

Marson, D. C., Chatterjee, A., Ingram, K. K., & Harrell, L. E. (1996). Towards a neurologic model of competency: Cognitive predictors of capacity to consent in Alzheimer's disease using three different legal standards. *Neurology, 46*(3), 666–672.

Pruchno, R. A., Smyer, M. A., Rose, M. S., Hartman-Stein, P. E., & Henderson-Laribee, D. L. (1995). Competence of long-term care residents to participate in decisions about their medical care: A brief, objective assessment. *The Gerontologist, 35*(5), 622–629.

Smyer, M. A., Schaie, K. W., & Kapp, M. (Eds.) (1996). *Older adults' decision making and the law*. New York: Springer.

15

~

Public Policy Issues

Robert H. Binstock

Introduction

From the New Deal to the present public policies have substantially improved the well-being of older Americans. But as the twentieth century comes to a close, policies on aging are approaching an important set of crossroads. Many older persons are highly dependent on government programs as safety nets for income, health care, long-term care, and various other needs. Others still need further help to meet their basic needs of daily survival. Yet our political system may not maintain all the help that is currently provided, and may not respond to additional needs.

After many decades of creation and expansion of an "Old Age Welfare State"[1] the present climate of American politics and public discourse is such that the future of governmental programs benefiting older persons is problematic. Today, public resources are perceived as scarce. The importance of "balancing the budget" of the federal government is a mainstay of contemporary domestic politics.

The benefits provided to elderly persons through federal programs and the continuing growth of the older population are commonly viewed as major obstacles to balancing the budget in the twenty-first century. Benefits to older Americans already account for approximately two-fifths of federal expenditures in 1997[2] and would be a greater proportion in the future if present policies remain as they are.

The total of older Americans eligible for benefits from programs on aging will increase tremendously when the Baby Boom —a cohort of 75 million persons born between 1946 and 1964—reaches the ranks of old age in 2010 and beyond. By the year 2030, the number of persons aged 65 and older will have more than doubled from 31 million in 1990 to about 70 million, and will comprise 20% of the population (Hobbs, 1996).

Accordingly, there is much anxiety about costs of governmental benefits to the aging, now and in the future. Contemporary apostles of "apocalyptic demography"[3] (e.g., Callahan, 1987; Schneider & Guralnik, 1990; Wattenberg, 1987) generate foreboding economic implications of populating aging. For example, distinguished economist Lester Thurow, using extrapolation from present policies as a mode of prediction, has stated that as soon as 2013 benefits to the elderly and interest payments on the national debt will take up 100% of the federal budget (Thurow, 1996). As exemplified by this statement, extrapolation from the present is a poor mode of prediction (see Bell, 1964). Especially so with respect to public policies, which, in fact, change very frequently. Nonetheless, a great many contemporary discussions of domestic policy issues portray an artificially homogenized constituency of "the aged" as in conflict with other groupings of Americans, and as a growing and unsustainable burden that will undermine our national well-being.

Moreover, many contemporary journalists, as well as scholars who are experts in subjects other than politics, fear that older people will constitute a sufficiently powerful political force in an aging society to ensure, selfishly, that their needs will be met through the auspices of government at the expense of other societal needs (e.g., Thurow, 1996). Consequently, in the view of these commentators, it will be impossible to substantially refashion Social Security, Medicare, Medicaid, and other policies benefiting the elderly because of the political power of older people.

This chapter examines the future of policies on aging and the politics that affects them. It starts with an account of how the political context of policies on aging has changed over the years. Then it examines, in turn, the challenges posed by the aging of the Baby Boom for the future of Social Security, Medicare, and the financing of long-term care through Medicaid and other means, and various reform options for meeting these challenges. Finally, it considers whether the political behavior of older persons and the organizations that purport to represent them will make it impossible or very difficult to undertake such reforms.

The Changing Political Contexts of Policies on Aging

An official boundary between adulthood and old age in the United States was first established by the New Deal's Social Security Act of 1935, enacted some quarter of a century after similar public pension programs had been enacted in most of the industrial world (Hudson & Binstock, 1976). Even as early twentieth century laws regulating child labor and the age of sexual consent marked boundaries between childhood and adulthood, Social Security—by designating age 65 as an eligibility requirement for retirement benefits—publicly institutionalized an age norm for retirement, and set a major precedent for the notion that older Americans need help from government.

During the more than half a century since then American policies toward older persons have been adopted and amended in a number of different social, economic, and political contexts. The reasons why each policy was originally enacted and subsequently altered have been subject to widely variant interpretations (see Binstock & Day, 1996). But one feature common to most of them is that they have used old age as sweeping, convenient markers for designating a category of American citizens as in need of governmental assistance.

1935 To 1978: The "Old Age Welfare State"

From the New Deal until about 20 years ago, public policy issues concerning older Americans were framed by an underlying *ageism* (see Palmore, 1990)— the attribution of the same characteristics, status, and just deserts to a heterogeneous group that has been artificially homogenized, packaged, labeled, and marketed as "the aged."

The stereotypes of ageism—unlike those of racism and sexism—have not been wholly prejudicial to the well-being of their objects, the aged. Indeed, ageism has been expressed through a number of policies—such as Medicare health insurance and "senior citizen" discounts—that treat all older persons the same by providing them with benefits and protection simply on the basis of old age (see Kutza, 1981).

Prior to the late 1970s the predominant stereotypes of older Americans were compassionate. Elderly persons tended to be seen as poor, frail, socially dependent, objects of discrimination, and above all "deserving" (see Kalish, 1979). For more than 40 years—dating from the Social Security Act of 1935— American society accepted the oversimplified notion that all older persons are essentially the same and all are worthy of governmental assistance. The lowest levels of economic status, health, and functional capacities that could be found among older persons became familiar as common denominators (Neugarten, 1970).

The American polity implemented this compassionate construct by adopting and financing major age-categorical benefit programs, and tax and price subsidies for which eligibility is not determined by need. Through the New Deal's Social Security, the Great Society's Medicare and Older Americans Act (an omnibus social service program), special tax exemptions and credits for being aged 65 or older, and a variety of other measures enacted during President Nixon's New Federalism, the elderly were exempted from the screenings that are applied to welfare applicants to determine whether they are worthy of public help.

During the 1960s and 1970s just about every issue or problem affecting just some older persons that could be identified by advocates for the elderly became a governmental responsibility: nutritional, legal, supportive, and leisure services; housing; home repair; energy assistance; transportation; help in getting jobs; protection against being fired from jobs; public insurance for private pensions; special mental health programs; a separate National Institute on Aging; and on, and on, and on. By the late 1970s, if not earlier, American society had learned the catechism of compassionate ageism very well and had expressed it through a great many policies; a committee of the U.S. House of Representatives, using loose criteria, was able to identify 134 programs benefiting the aging, overseen by 49 committees and subcommittees of Congress (U.S. House of Representatives, 1997).

Emergence of the Aged as Scapegoat

Starting in 1978, however, the long-standing compassionate stereotypes of older persons began to undergo an extraordinary reversal. Older people came to be portrayed as one of the more flourishing and powerful groups in American society and, yet, attacked as a burdensome responsibility. The immediate precipitating factor was a serious cash flow problem in the Social Security system that emerged within the larger context of a depressed economy during President Carter's administration (see Estes, 1983; Light, 1985).

Two additional elements contributed importantly to this reversal of stereotypes. One element was tremendous growth in the amount and proportion of federal dollars expended on benefits to aging citizens, which at that time had come to be more than one quarter of our annual budget and comparable in size, to expenditures on national defense. Journalists (e.g., Samuelson, 1978) and academicians (Hudson, 1978) began to notice and publicize this phenomenon in the late 1970s.

A second element in the reversal of the stereotypes of old age was dramatic improvements in the aggregate status of older Americans, in large measure due to the impact of federal benefit programs. Social Security, for example, has helped to reduce the proportion of elderly persons in poverty from about 35% four decades ago (Clark, 1990) to 10.5% today (Baugher & Lamison-White, 1996). The success of such programs had improved the economic status of aged persons to the point where journalists and social commentators could—with superficial accuracy (see Quinn, 1987)—describe older people, on average, as more prosperous than the general population.

Throughout the 1980s and into the 1990s the new stereotypes, readily observed in popular culture, depicted older persons as prosperous, hedonistic, politically powerful, and selfish. For example, "Grays on the Go," a 1988 cover story in *Time*, was filled with pictures of senior surfers, senior swingers, and senior softball players. Older persons were portrayed as America's new elite—healthy, wealthy, powerful, and "staging history's biggest retirement party" (Gibbs, 1980).

A dominant theme in such accounts of older people was that their selfishness was ruining the nation. The *New Republic* highlighted this motif with a drawing on the cover caricaturing older persons with the caption "greedy geezers." The table of contents "teaser" for the story that followed announced that "The real me generation isn't the yuppies, it's America's growing ranks of prosperous elderly" (Fairlie, 1988). This theme has been echoed widely in recent years, and the epithet "greedy geezers" has become a familiar adjective in journalistic accounts of federal budget politics (e.g., Salholz, 1990). In the early 1990s *Fortune* declaimed that "The Tyranny of America's Old" is "one of the most crucial issues facing U.S. society" (Smith, 1992).

In this unsympathetic climate of opinion the aged emerged as a scapegoat for an impressive list of American problems. Demographers and advocates for children blamed the political power of elderly Americans for the plight of youngsters who have inadequate nutrition, health care, education, and insufficiently supportive family environments (see, e.g., Preston, 1984). One children's advocate even proposed that parents receive an "extra vote" for each of their children, in order to combat older voters (Carballo, 1981). Former Secretary of Commerce Peter Peterson (1987) suggested that a prerequisite for the United States to regain its stature as a first-class power in the world economy was a sharp reduction in programs benefiting older Americans.

Widespread concerns about spiralling U.S. health care costs were redirected, in part, from health care providers, suppliers, administrators, and insurers—the parties that were responsible for setting the prices of care—to elderly persons for whom health care is provided. A number of academicians and public figures—including politicians—have expressed concern that health care expenditures on older persons will absorb an unlimited amount of our national resources and crowd out health care for others as well as various worthy social causes. Some of them even proposed that old-age-based health care rationing is necessary, desirable, and just (see Binstock & Post, 1991).

Equity as an "Intergenerational" Construct

The various problems for which elderly people had become a scapegoat were thematically unified as issues of so-called "intergenerational equity" through the efforts of Americans for Generational Equity (AGE). Formed as an interest group in 1985, with backing from the corporate sector as well as a handful of Congressmen who led it, AGE recruited some of the prominent "scapegoaters" to its board and as spokespersons. According to its annual reports, most of AGE's funding came from insurance companies, health care corporations, banks, and other private sector businesses and organizations that are in financial competition with Medicare and Social Security (Quadagno, 1989).

Central to AGE's credo was the proposition that today's older people are (and tomorrow's will be) locked in an intergenerational conflict with younger age cohorts regarding the distribution of public resources. AGE's basic view was that the large aggregate of public transfers of income and other benefits to today's cohorts of older persons, financed through unfairly burdensome taxes on the contemporary labor force, are unlikely to be available in the future as old age benefits (e.g., Social Security and Medicare) when Baby Boomers become elderly retirees (Longman, 1987). The organization disseminated this viewpoint from its Washington office through press releases, media interviews, a quarterly publication, and periodic conferences on subjects such as Children at Risk: Who Will Support an Aging Society? and Medicare and the Baby Boom Generation. Although AGE faded from the scene at the end of the decade, its message was taken up shortly thereafter by the Concord Coalition (1993), a new organization founded by former Senators Paul Tsongas and Warren Rudman.

As the 1980s came to a close, the themes of intergenerational equity and conflict were adopted by the media and academics as routine perspectives for describing many social policy issues (Cook, Marshall, Marshall, & Kaufman, 1994). The intergenerational themes also gained currency in elite sectors of American society and on Capitol Hill. The President of the prestigious American Association of Universities, for instance, asserted: "[T]he shape of the domestic federal budget inescapably pits programs for the retired against every other social purpose dependent on federal funds, in the present and the future" (Rosenzweig, 1990).

Within this political climate of the 1980s and early 1990s the age-categorical principle for distributing benefits and burdens among older people that had created an Old-Age Welfare State began to erode. Starting in 1983, Congress made a number of incremental changes in Social Security, Medicare, the Older Americans Act, and other programs and policies reflecting the diverse economic situations of older people (Binstock, 1994). Some of these reduced benefits to comparatively wealthy older people; others targeted benefits toward relatively poor older people.

The Contemporary Political Context: Balancing the Budget

With the advent of a Republican-dominated 104th Congress in 1995 a new era in the politics of aging began to emerge. Issues concerning programs on aging have now become framed by a much larger political agenda than concerns with the status of older people or issues of generational equity.

Congress and the President began acting on the principle that the annual budget of the federal government should be brought into balance. In turn, this interest in balancing the budget brought a great deal of attention to issues of reforming programs that benefit older Americans, both in the short term and the long term, because these programs loom very large in terms of projected federal expenditures.

Congress looked to long-term budgetary concerns by establishing a Bipartisan Commission on Entitlement and Tax Reform (1995), which issued a report examining the fiscal implications of the Baby Boom cohort becoming eligible for Social Security and Medicare in the early decades of the twenty-first century. Short-term concerns were addressed throughout 1995 and 1996 in Congressional bills designed to achieve large reductions in projected Medicare and Medicaid expenditures and to make significant structural changes in the programs. But President Clinton vetoed the legislation, purportedly because of his disapproval of proposed structural changes.

In 1997 the President and Congress enacted the Balanced Budget Act of 1997 (Public Law No. 105-33, 1997), designed to bring the federal budget into balance by 2002. It included measures to trim the growth of Medicare spending by $115 billion over 5 years, the largest savings package ever imposed on Medicare. This alleviated a short-term "crisis" in Medicare's Part A, Hospital Insurance (HI) program. The Federal Insurance Contributions Act (FICA) payroll taxes that finance Part A and the HI trust fund reserves had been projected to be inadequate to pay the program's obligations by 2001. With the new legislation, Medicare Part A is projected to be solvent until 2007. [Part B of Medicare, Supplementary Medical Insurance (SMI), is financed by a combination of premiums from program participants—about 25% of the total—and general revenues of the United States.]

Nonetheless, the matter of substantially reforming old age programs will remain on the public agenda in the years immediately ahead. The aging of the Baby Boom has major fiscal implications if Social Security, Medicare, and Medicaid policies remain largely as they are today. In fiscal year 1996, federal spending on these programs was $630 billion, amounting to 8.4% of the nation's gross domestic product (GDP). By 2030, when most of the Baby Boom will have reached old age, these three programs are projected to consume 16% of GDP, nearly twice the present proportion (Congressional Budget Office, 1997a, p. xiii). Proposals abound for reforming these policies to reduce projected outlays, and they generate many complex issues.

The Future of Social Security

At present Social Security's Old-Age and Survivors Insurance (OASI) program is very sound financially. In 1996 it paid benefits to 37.7 million Americans—26.9 retired workers, 8.5 million other adults, and 2.3 million children (National Academy on Aging, 1997). The total federal expenditure for these benefits was $303 billion. The average retired worker received $745 per month. Social Security's retired-worker payments to lower-income older persons are their major source of funds and enable the majority of them to remain above the poverty line (Crystal, 1996)—although 10.5% of the population aged 65 and older has incomes that are below the poverty line (Baugher & Lamison-White, 1996).

Most of OASI's financing, 89%, comes from the FICA payroll tax on employers and employees. Taxes on the OASI benefits received by upper-income beneficiaries yields another 2%. And the balance comes from interest paid by the federal government on loans from the OASI Trust Fund, which houses the surplus in the program's income that is not needed to pay current benefits. In 1966 the total income for OASI was $363 billion, and the surplus added to the Trust Fund for the year was $60 billion. The accumulated total surplus in OASI was projected to be $628 billion for fiscal 1997 (Congressional Budget Office, 1997b, p. 40).

The long-term picture for OASI is not so rosy. Between 2010 and 2030 the percentage of GDP spent on Social Security will increase by one-third, from 4.8% to 6.4% (Congressional Budget Office, 1997a, p. 29). According to the Trustees of the OASI Trust Fund, the cost of paying benefits is projected to exceed payroll tax receipts in 2012. Interest on Trust Fund reserves will need to be drawn on in 2012, and the reserves themselves will need to be drawn on starting in 2019; the reserves are projected to be fully depleted in 2029. Thereafter, under current law, payroll taxes would be able to fund OASI benefits at only about 77% of their current levels (Board of Trustees of the Old Age and Survivors Insurance and Disability Insurance Trust Funds, 1997).

A number of options have been identified to date for dealing with this situation (see, e.g., Kingson & Schulz, 1996; Steurle & Bakija, 1997). Some would reduce future OASI benefits. Others involve raising revenues for OASI. And still others involve compensating for reduced benefits by partially "privatizing" Social Security. Most of them are likely to be politically difficult to implement in the current political climate.

Raising the Retirement Age

One option for reducing OASI benefit obligations is to raise Social Security's retirement age, which would effectively reduce benefits by delaying their inception. At present a worker becomes eligible for full retirement benefits at age 65. Under current law, this "normal retirement age" (NRA) is scheduled to increase gradually in 2003 and reach age 67 in 2027. Members of Congress and others have recommended that the implementation of this change to age 67 could be accelerated and/or the NRA could be raised to age 70 by 2002. The Congressional Budget Office (1997a, p. 34) calculates that such approaches would reduce OASI outlays from 3% to 8% in 2030. Proponents of this type of reform argue that in terms of life expectancy and health status, age 70 today is an equivalent retirement age to the 65 year old NRA established by Social Security during the New Deal (see, e.g., Chen, 1994).

Reducing the Size of Benefits

OASI benefits could also be lowered by changing the formula through which they are calculated. In 1996, for example, workers who had average earnings throughout their career were eligible for an annual retired-worker benefit of about $10,700, which replaced 43.2% of their previous annual earnings. Under current law, which includes inflation adjustment for benefits, the average worker who retires at age 65 (receiving what will then be reduced "early retirement benefits") in 2030 will receive about $12,000 dollars (in 1996 dollars), a replacement rate of 36.4%; an average worker who retires at the then NRA of age 67 would have a replacement rate of 42.8%, which is not much below the current average (Board of Trustees of the Federal Old-Age and Survivors Insurance and Disability Insurance Trust Funds, 1996). A reform that would reduce retired-worker benefits by 1% a year starting in 1998 would provide beneficiaries who became eligible for benefits in 2032 and thereafter with about 70% of their benefits under current law, or about $2,000 (in 1996 dollars) below what present NRA average retirees receive today. This would achieve an estimated 19% reduction in OASI outlays in 2030 (Congressional Budget Office, 1997a, p. 32).

Reducing Inflation Adjustments

Another way to cut program outlays is to reduce the rate at which OASI beneficiaries receive cost-of-living adjustments (COLAs) in their benefits. Each year benefits are automatically adjusted to reflect increases in the consumer price index (CPI). For example, the COLA that became effective in December 1996 was 2.9% based on the CPI increase of that magnitude over a 12-month period (Congressional Budget Office, 1997b, p. 34).

But a recent Advisory Commission to Study the Consumer Price Index, established by Congress, estimated that the measures used to determine the CPI result in an upward bias of 1.2 percentage points a year (Advisory Commission to Study the Consumer Price Index, 1996). If so, OASI beneficiaries have been receiving COLAs that are higher than necessary to keep up with inflation. For instance, if CPI measures were adjusted to reflect the Commission's estimate, the December 1996 C0LA would have been 1.7% rather than 2.9%.

Reducing the COLA would result in substantial savings in OASI benefit obligations, either by adopting new measures to determine the CPI or by legislating that the COLA should be less than the CPI. The Advisory Commission estimated that a 1.2 percentage point COLA reduction starting in 1998 would save $60 billion in benefits by 2002. Such reductions, however, would also have a big impact on the OASI income of retired workers. The Congressional Budget Office estimates that with a 1 point reduction persons who retired at age 65 today who reached the age of 74 would effectively experience 11% less in benefits, and 19% less by the time they reached age 84 (Congressional Budget Office, 1997a, p. 35).

Expanding Taxation of Benefits

Additional income for paying benefits could be raised by expanding the current taxation of OASI benefits. This approach, of course, would also effectively reduce the after-tax income available to OASI beneficiaries.

Under current law OASI benefits are subject to taxation if a taxpayer's adjusted gross income (AGI) exceeds certain thresholds. Up to 50% of benefits are subject to taxation when an individual's AGI exceeds $25,000 and a couples' exceeds $32,000; up to 85% of benefits are taxable when an individual's income is over $34,000 and a couple's is over $44,000.

Various options for expanding taxation of benefits are under discussion, and some of them would raise substantial income for the Social Security system. One option, for example, would be to eliminate the income thresholds altogether, making 85% of benefits for all OASI recipients taxable; this would raise $116 billion between 1998 and 2002 (Congressional Budget Office, 1997c, p. 355). Another option would be to eliminate the lower thresholds and require all beneficiaries below the present upper thresholds ($34,000 and $44,000) to pay taxes on 50% of benefits; this would raise $58 billion in the same period (Congressional Budget Office, 1997c, p. 356).

Increasing Payroll Taxes

More income could also be obtained, of course, by raising the OASI payroll tax. At present, workers are taxed at the rate of 5.35% of salary or wages up to $65,400 in such earnings per year. Employers are also taxed at 5.35%, so the total rate is 10.7%. Raising the tax rate by a percentage point or two could yield significant returns. In 1996, a two percentage point increase (one percentage point for both employer and employee) would have yielded an additional $60 billion.

The government could also obtain additional FICA revenue by eliminating the ceiling on the amount of annual earnings that are taxed (as is already the case with the portion of the payroll tax that funds the Medicare HI Trust Fund). But the amount of money raised through this measure would be small because about 87% of wages and salaries subject to FICA already fall below the ceiling (Steurle & Bakija, 1997, p. 55).

Using General Revenues to Pay Benefits

Additional funds could be found by using general revenues of the United States, as well as the payroll tax, to pay OASI benefits. Traditional supporters of the U.S. Social Security system feel that this would undermine political support for the entire program. They argue that the payroll contribution feature of the system ensures political solidarity for it by reinforcing the notion that it is a universal "social insurance" program rather than a welfare program. In effect, virtually everyone contributes premiums and virtually everyone benefits. Supporters of exclusive use of payroll-financing fear that the use of general revenues would stigmatize the program, thus eroding its wide base of popular support. Yet this argument is not very compelling. Most industrialized nations throughout the world already use general revenues to fund their Social Security systems. Moreover, in this country, part of Medicare's Part B has been funded by general revenues (currently at the rate of 75%) for over three decades without any indication that political support for it has eroded to date.

Funding the Reserves in the Trust Fund

Most of the options discussed above would be difficult to implement politically, and would have a substantial deleterious impact on the incomes of those persons who will be primarily dependent on OASI for their income in old age. Yet, various combinations of these options would do much to meet the challenge of maintaining the financial viability for OASI in the twenty-first century as the dimensions of the problem have been depicted by the Social Security Trustees in their annual reports.

But the challenge is much graver than portrayed by the Trustees. Although official projections are that OASI income and Trust Fund reserves will sustain benefits through the year 2029, the broader financial picture is actually much worse.

The reserves that will need to be drawn on to sustain benefits through 2029 consist of loans that the trust fund has made to the federal government to fund other activities. These loans, in the form of government bonds, are presently earning interest for the Trust Fund. But when the reserves need to be drawn on after 2019, additional revenue will have to be raised to pay off the bonds so that reserve funds will be liquid. To be sure, the full faith and credit of the United States stands behind these bonds, but the revenue to make them good will have to come from somewhere.

The amount of money that will need to be raised for paying off the bonds will be significant. For example, the CBO projects that the size of the federal debt owed to the OASI trust fund as early as 2007 will be $1.7 trillion (Congressional Budget Office, 1997b, p. 44). In that same year, the total federal budget is projected to be $2.6 trillion. So, if the bonds in the trust fund had to be paid off in that year, a sum equal to an additional 65% of the budget would have to be raised (Congressional Budget Office, 1997b, p. 29). (CBO budget projections do not extend beyond 2007.)

When the redemption of the bonds begins in 2019 and thereafter, some form of federal taxes will have to be raised, or spending on programs other than Social Security will need to be drastically curtailed, or the U.S. Treasury will have to sell other bonds. Selling other bonds would increase the national debt considerably, as well as interest payments on that debt. OASI payroll taxes have been a major factor in keeping the federal budget close to balanced in recent years and will continue to be so until the reserves are drawn on. The excess funds raised from the payroll tax, which become trust fund reserves, are counted as income in the annual federal balance sheet. In 1997 the annual excess is expected to be $78 billion; by 2007 it is projected to be $132 billion (Congressional Budget Office, 1997b, p. 46). If the present political consensus on the importance of a balanced federal budget persists over the next two decades, it may shatter when the challenge of paying off the bonds in the Trust Fund is at hand.

"Privatizing" Social Security

Some analysts and commentators have suggested during the past few decades that Social Security should be "privatized," fully or in part, by replacing the OASI program with some forms of private insurance or investment. Among the various arguments offered in favor of such proposals are that privatization would increase the rate of economic growth, increase the nation's competitiveness in the global economy, protect Social Security reserves from being spent to finance general government consumption, increase the rate of return to retired workers on FICA contributions made when they were workers, protect future workers against sharp rises in the FICA tax rate when the Baby Boom retires, and protect Baby Boomers against sharp reductions in their OASI benefits. Strong arguments can be made against each of these propositions (see Williamson, 1997).

Until recently, privatization has been advocated by few, relatively isolated voices, primarily libertarians and organizations that express their viewpoint such as the Cato Institute (Ferrara, 1985). In 1997, however, it became much more of a mainstream view when a special Advisory Council on Social Security appointed by the U.S. Secretary of Health and Human Services issued its report (1994–1996 Advisory Council on Social Security, 1997).

The Advisory Council's charge was to develop recommendations for improving the long-range financial status of OASI. Unable to reach a consensus, the Council presented three separate plans: a "Maintenance of Benefits" plan, an "Individual Accounts" plan, and a "Personal Security Accounts" plan.

The privatization element in the Maintenance of Benefits plan calls for investing up to 40% of the OASI reserves in equities rather than U.S. bonds. The federal government would invest the funds in a broad index (or indices) of market performance rather than in specific equities. The theory behind this is that the rate of return on investment would be higher and shore up the trust fund for paying benefits to the Baby Boom. Other elements in this plan are a slight reduction in OASI benefits, higher payroll taxes beginning about the year 2045; and redirecting the portion of the payroll tax that now goes to the HI (Medicare Part A) Trust Fund to OASI. (This latter measure, of course, would exacerbate the problems faced by the HI trust fund.)

The privatizing component in the Individual Accounts plan would involve an additional 1.6% payroll tax on workers only (up to the OASI ceiling for the year). This new revenue would be placed into an individual mandatory account for each worker, which would be held by the government for investment in equity index funds, or other approved options, and then annuitized on retirement. In short, these accounts would be similar to existing employer-sponsored defined contribution pension plans, with the government as investment manager for each worker. Again, the Advisory Council recommendation assumes that these accounts will yield workers a higher rate of return than government bonds. Another major element in the Individual Accounts Plan is a cut in OASI benefit payments which would reduce them by a projected 16% in 2030 (as compared with current law). Proponents of this measure assume that the decreases in benefits will be offset by annuities from the new Individual Accounts.

The Personal Security Accounts (PSA) plan offers the most radical proposal for privatization (see Schieber, 1997). It would require that 5 percentage points of the worker's payroll tax (about 47% of the present combined worker/employer total OASI tax) be redirected to individual accounts and invested in the various financial instruments that are widely available in financial markets. The accounts would be held for retirement purposes, outside the government, and individuals would decide how the money in their accounts would be invested. This feature would mean that individuals who invest the same amount of money are likely to end up with widely different results; the distribution of retirement benefits would be drastically different from that in the current Social Security system. The PSA plan also calls for phasing out the current OASI benefit formula and replacing it with a smaller, flat benefit (indexed to keep pace with average wage growth) for future retirees who are now under age 55. The returns from the PSAs are expected to at least compensate for these reductions.

Although public discussion about these privatization proposals has been limited to date, they are sure to be hotly debated when the challenge of dealing with the long-term problems of Social Security are seriously addressed by public officials in the years immediately ahead. Social Security traditionalists will argue that privatization will not only be risky for worker/retirees, but will also undermine the "social insurance" principle that has maintained solid public support for the system over many decades. On the other side of the argument will be the vested interests in the world of finance, pleased at the thought of tens to hundreds of billion additional dollars being invested each year in the private sector.

The Future of Medicare

The future fiscal outlook for Medicare—the national health insurance program for persons aged 65 and older (as well as for persons who receive federal disability benefits and those who have end-stage renal disease)—is far worse than for Social Security. Between 2010 and 2030 federal spending for Medicare, as a percentage of GDP, is projected to increase by 73% as compared to a one-third increase in the percentage of GDP projected for OASI spending in the same period.

To be sure, the number of Baby Boomers who will become eligible for Medicare is roughly comparable to those who will be eligible for Social Security. But, whereas OASI costs per beneficiary are determined by law, the majority of Medicare's costs under its current program structure—much of which is on a fee-for-service basis—are largely determined by the amounts and kinds of health care that beneficiaries receive and the expenses involved in providing it. In 1996, spending on Medicare was 2.4% of GDP; by 2030 it is projected to approximately triple, to 7.1% (Congressional Budget Office, 1997a, p.38).

Demography Is Not Destiny

Based on such projections, a national commission established by Congress has depicted health care costs of the elderly in the twenty-first century as an unsustainable economic burden for our nation (Bipartisan Commission on Entitlement and Tax Reform, 1994). Biomedical ethicist Daniel Callahan has expressed this view in rather apocalyptic terms, depicting the elderly population as "a new social threat" and a "demographic, economic, and medical avalanche...one that could ultimately (and perhaps already) do [sic] great harm" (Callahan, 1997, p. 20). Accordingly, he has proposed old-age-based health care rationing—specifically that Medicare reimbursement for life-saving care be categorically denied to anyone aged 80 and older (cf. Binstock & Post, 1991).

The few studies that have focused on population aging as a factor in U.S. health care costs have found that the impact of aging and other demographic changes on expenditures in recent decades has been dwarfed by the combined effects of other factors, such as increases in the intensity and utilization rates of health services, health-sector-specific price inflation, and general inflation (Arnett, McKusick, Sonnefeld, & Cowell, 1986; Getzen, 1992; Mendelsohn & Schwartz, 1993; Pfaff, 1990; Sonnefeld, Waldo, Lemieux, & McKusick, 1991). These empirical studies, however, have been retrospective and contemporary.

One cross-national study attempted to anticipate the potential impact of the aging of the Baby Boom on U.S. health care expenditures (Binstock, 1993). It looked at the experience of 12 industrialized nations including some, such as Sweden, in which, compared to the United States, a much higher percent-

age of the population is aged 65 and older. Others, like Japan, have a much
higher rate of population aging. It found no relationship between population
aging and the amount of national wealth spent on health care. Rather, it concluded that the structural features of health care systems—and behavioral responses to them by citizens and health care providers—are probably far more
important determinants of a nation's health care expenditures.

In short, demography is not destiny with respect to health care expenditures. The amount of expenses that is "caused" by population aging can be
controlled by policy reforms that change the structural features of a health care
system. But the options for reforming Medicare to meet the long-term problems of financing adequate health care for aged Baby Boomers are not as clear
or as plentiful as they are for dealing with Social Security.

Contemporary Structural Changes in Medicare

A number of recent policy changes have been made to contain Medicare costs.
Although they may have some impact in holding down costs, they also pose
distinct risks for older persons in terms of access to and quality of health care.

The general approach in these reforms is an attempt to transition from the
program's traditional open-ended fee-for-service approach to paying for health
care to a situation in which as much as possible of Medicare operates with fixed
budgets that cap program costs. The primary strategy now in place for carrying out this approach is to encourage both the proliferation of and enrollment
in Medicare managed care organizations (MCOs) that receive a flat per capita
fee for providing health care for each beneficiary enrolled in the plan. The
amount of the per capita fee is based on the average fee-for-service reimbursement for Medicare patients in a geographic area in the previous year
(termed the "adjusted average per capita cost"). This strategy places managed
care organizations and health care providers at financial risk and reduces the
government's exposure to open-ended costs.

About 13% of Medicare participants are already enrolled in MCOs and the
number is expected to grow in the years immediately ahead as the federal government encourages the proliferation of Medicare managed-care contractors
(Pear, 1997a). The financial incentives of managed care organizations, however,
foster undertreatment of patients (see Kane & Kane, 1994; Mechanic, 1994).
Studies have already indicated that outcomes for older people who are poor
and have chronic diseases and disabilities are worse in HMOs than when provided through fee-for-service payments (Nelson, Brown, Gold, Ciemnecki, &
Docteur, 1997; Shaugnessy, Schlenker, & Hittle, 1994; Ware, Bayliss, Rogers,
Kosinski, & Tarlov, 1996). Even relatively healthy older persons in HMOs seem
to have been underserved in certain respects (Wiener & Skaggs, 1995).

The Balanced Budget Act of 1997 (BBA97) expanded this cost-containment
strategy and introduced others by creating a Medicare Part C "Medicare +

Choice" program (Public Law No. 135-33, 1997). Part C offers a panoply of new options for Medicare participants.

Some of these choices continue the MCO strategy. One of them, designed to encourage more program participants to enroll in MCOs, offers a "point-of-service" option that enables patients to see doctors who are not part of the MCO in which they have enrolled. Two other MCO selections—provider-sponsored coordinated care and preferred provider organizations—are designed to eliminate costs that are presently paid to "middlemen" by Medicare under current MCO arrangements. At present, Medicare's per capita fee payment goes to a so-called Third Party Administrator (TPA) with which it has contracted, typically an insurance company. The TPA subsequently makes contracts with health care provider organizations to provide care for a fixed sum to each Medicare participant the TPA enrolls. In the process, the TPA takes a sum off the top of each per capita payment when making its financial arrangements with provider organizations. BBA97, by authorizing Medicare to contract directly with health care providers, makes possible the elimination of the costs of financing TPA middlemen. No doubt, as providers contract directly with Medicare, the per capita fee will subsequently be reduced to reflect the elimination of the funds that are being retained by TPAs.

Although Medicare + Choice retains traditional fee-for-service as an option, it also seeks to reduce program costs through another strategy that encourages program enrollees to choose "private fee-for-service." One such option is simply to allow persons to opt out of Medicare reimbursement completely and make their own contracts with providers. Another includes such private contracts, but also retains a limited amount of Medicare reimbursement.

Finally, Medicare + Choice lays the groundwork for another mechanism that would place program enrollees on fixed budgets. It includes a 5-year demonstration program (limited to 390,000 enrollees) that establishes Medicare Medical Savings Accounts (MSAs) plans. MSA plans include high-deductible (as high as $6,000) health insurance policies; Medicare will pay an annual per capita fee into the plan on a "defined contribution" basis after the insurance premium is paid. But expenditure of these Medicare funds for health care can take place only after the enrollee incurs "countable" expenses equal to the annual insurance deductible. Countable expenses include those payable customarily under Part A and Part B, as well as deductibles and copayments that would have been paid under traditional fee-for-service. At the plan's option, other expenses that are not reimburseable by Medicare (such as prescription drugs) may also be counted.

Most policy analysts expect that relatively healthy and wealthy individuals will choose this option. Unused balances in such plans can be retained by Medicare participants as ongoing investments, spent, and even passed on through inheritance. Medicare's contributions into MSAs will be exempt from taxes, and so will earnings from the account. Withdrawals will not be taxed either if they are used to pay for medical expenses that are ordinarily deductible under Internal Revenue Code. MSA funds used in other ways must be included in an individual's gross income for tax purposes. Such nonmedical expenditures will be subject to an additional 50% penalty if they exceed a threshold based on the amount of the MSA balance and the MSA plan insurance deductible for the year of withdrawal.

It is also a distinct possibility, however, that poorer older people would select the MSA option, too. The sum paid into MSAs by Medicare—say, $5,000 in some urban areas—may be perceived as a substantial cash windfall by older people who are either below the poverty line, which is $9,220 for an elderly couple (Baugher & Lamison-White, 1996), or only a few thousand dollars above it. Those poorer people who elect the MSA may well forego needed medical care in order to preserve the windfall, even though poorer old people tend to be relatively unhealthy (Robert & House, 1994).

One certain cumulative effect of the various Medicare + Choice plans established by BBA97 is that Medicare enrollees face a bewildering array of choices as they make their annual enrollment decisions. The theory is that beneficiaries will compare the various options on the basis of quality, service, and price. To this end, the Secretary of Health and Human Services was required by the legislation to prepare and disseminate information to program participants regarding each option, including items and services covered, cost-sharing, and comparative plan information (including premiums, quality, disenrollment procedures, and consumer satisfaction). Whether consumers are able to use these data for truly informed choices is problematic.

Other Options for Reforming Medicare

These contemporary changes in Medicare may contain the growth of federal expenditures on the program somewhat in the years immediately ahead. And they may do so without severely affecting access to and quality of care for older persons. Yet, whatever savings these measures achieve will be far from sufficient to deal with projected expenditures for the decades when the Baby Boom reaches old age. Even if a very high percentage of Medicare participants choose Medicare + Choice options that predetermine costs to the program (even as OASI benefit costs are predetermined), the fact remains that by 2030 the number of older persons eligible for the program will have doubled. The challenge of paying for their health care is enormous.

One logical strategy for further containment of Medicare expenditures, of course, is to cut back on reimbursements to health care providers. However, a great deal has already been done in this vein. In 1984 Medicare initiated a prospective fixed-payment system for reimbursing hospitals on the basis of a patient's diagnosis, which eliminated the capacity of providers to set the charges for hospital stays. The Omnibus Budget Reconciliation Act of 1993 trimmed an estimated $55 billion in payments to hospitals, physicians, and other health care providers over the period 1994–1998 (Congressional Budget Office, 1993). BBA97 cut another $115 billion in estimated provider reimbursement from 1998 through 2002. As these cutbacks are combined with the growth of per capita payments to providers, further cutbacks in provider reimbursements might seriously compromise quality of care.

Another option, considered in an early version of BBA97, was to raise the age of eligibility for Medicare to 67. To do this in a fashion that implements the reform rather immediately, say in one or several years, would probably be unfeasible politically. But it could be done gradually, as is the case with the normal retirement age for OASI benefits, which is already scheduled to be gradually increased to age 67 over a 25-year period. This option for Medicare, which is likely to surface again, is estimated to reduce Medicare spending by about 5% by 2025 (Congressional Budget Office, 1997a, p. 41). Some members of Congress have even suggested that the age might be raised to 70; this would reduce Medicare spending about 13% by 2030 (Congressional Budget Office, 1997a, p. 47). The use of age 67 is more likely, however, because it has the appeal of matching the scheduled age change in OASI. The downside of such a change is that many workers retire from firms that do not provide retiree health insurance, and those employers that do provide it are seeking to eliminate it as a fringe benefit.

Another approach would be to increase the Part B premiums paid by Medicare enrollees so that the portion of Part B financed in this fashion would grow substantially, thereby reducing the portion financed by general revenues. The Congressional Budget Office has looked at this option in terms of increasing the premium-financed portion from its current level of 25% to 50% by 2010, thus reducing the general revenues-financed portion by 50% every year thereafter. With this approach, however, the income status of many enrollees would be sharply affected. The premiums paid by enrollees currently are 3% of their average income. Under the CBO plan, premiums would be 30% of average income by 2030 (Congressional Budget Office, 1997a, p. 47). An alternative would be to replace the current flat premium approach with sliding-scale premiums based on the financial status of enrollees.

Still another reform would be to increase taxes to pay for Medicare. This could be done by using general revenues, or by increasing the rate of the FICA payroll tax that finances Part A.

If each of the reform options described above were implemented in some form, they could have a cumulative impact sufficient to solve the long-term challenge of public financing for Medicare. Any one of them, however, may be politically difficult to adopt. It is not surprising that BBA97 called for the establishment of a bipartisan commission to explore long-term policy options for restructuring Medicare. The commission, appointed in December 1997, will be sorely tasked. The organization and financing of American health care are changing very rapidly, and it is difficult to envision with any confidence just what the nation's health care system will look like a decade or two hence.

The Future of Long-Term Care

Comparable to the projections for Medicare spending when the Baby Boom reaches old age are estimates of spending on long-term care in nursing homes and in home and other community-based settings. The Congressional Budget Office, using 1990 as a baseline year, has estimated that total national costs of long-term care will almost double by 2010 and more than triple by 2030 (Congressional Budget Office, 1991).

In addition to the sheer size of the Baby Boom, the need for long-term care will increase in the twenty-first century because the older population is aging within itself. The population aged 75 and older will have grown from 13 million in 1990 to 32 million in 2030, and those aged 85 and older will have tripled from 3 million to 9 million (Hobbs, 1996). Prevalence rates of morbidity and disability increase markedly in advanced old age. For example, whereas 22.6% of the population aged 65 to 74 experiences difficulties with functional activities of daily living (ADLs), the rate is 44.5% among those aged 85 and older. Similarly, the rate of Alzheimer's disease increases markedly in the older age ranges. According to recent estimates, 6% of people between the ages of 65 and 74 have Alzheimer's disease; among those age 85 and over, as many as 50% show signs of it (National Academy on Aging, 1994).

A reflection of such prevalence rates in advanced old age can be found in the present rates of nursing home use in different old-age categories. About 1% of Americans aged 65 to 74 years are in nursing homes; this compares with 6.1% of persons 75 to 84 and 24% of persons aged 85 and older. Similarly, disability rates increase in older old-age categories among persons who are not in nursing homes, from nearly 23% of those aged 65 to 74 who experience difficulties with ADLs to 45% of those aged 85 and older.

Whether rates of disability in various old-age categories will increase or decline in the future is a matter on which experts disagree. Assuming no changes in age-specific risks of disability, Cassel, Rudberg, and Olshansky (1992) calculate a 31% increase between 1990 and 2010 in the number of persons aged 65 and older experiencing difficulties with ADLs. Using the same assumption, the Congressional Budget Office projects that the nursing home population will increase 50% between 1990 and 2010, double by 2030, and triple by 2050 (Congressional Budget Office, 1991). However, even those researchers who report a recent decline in the prevalence of disability at older ages emphasize that there will be large increases in the absolute number of older Americans needing long-term care in the decades ahead (see, e.g., Manton, Corder, & Stallard, 1993, 1997).

Out-of-Pocket Financing

The challenges of financing long-term care seem formidable, now and in the future. Out-of-pocket payments by functionally dependent elders and their families already account for one-third of long-term care expenditures. The average annual cost of a year's care in a nursing home averaged more than $46,000 in 1995 (Levit et al., 1996), a sharp increase from the $37,000 average cost in 1993 (Wiener & Illston, 1996). Although the use of a limited number of services in a home or other community-based setting is less expensive, noninstitutional care for patients who would otherwise be appropriately placed in a nursing home is not cheaper and is often more expensive (Weissert, 1990).

For a high percentage of older people the prices of long-term care are simply unaffordable. Among person aged 65 and older, 40% have a pretax income of less than 200% of the poverty threshold—under $14,618 for an individual and $18,440 for a married couple in which the man is aged 65 or older (Baugher & Lamison-White, 1996). Under one-tenth of older persons in nursing homes can finance a year of care from their income (Hanley, Wiener, & Harris, 1994).

The Role of the Family

A number of research efforts have estimated that about 80–85% of the long-term care provided to older persons outside of nursing homes is provided on an in-kind basis by family members —spouses, siblings, adult children, and broader kin networks (see Hanley, Alecxih, Wiener, & Kennel, 1990). About 74% of dependent community-based older persons receive all their care from family members or other unpaid sources: about 21% receive both formal and informal services; and only about 5% use just formal services (Liu, Manton, & Liu, 1985). The vast majority of family caregivers are women (see Brody, 1990; Stone, Cafferata, & Sangl, 1987). The family also plays an important role in obtaining and managing services from paid service providers. Caregiving by families does not tend to decline significantly even when they are able to supplement their caregiving with formal, paid services (Edelman & Hughes, 1990; Tennstedt, Crawford, & McKinlay, 1993).

The capacities and willingness of family members to care for disabled older persons, however, may decline when the Baby Boom cohort reaches old age because of a broad social trend. The family, as a fundamental unit of social organization, has been undergoing profound transformations that will become more fully manifest over the next few decades as Baby Boomers reach old age. The striking growth of single-parent households, the growing participation of women in the labor force, and the high incidence of divorce and remarriage (differentially higher for men) all entail complicated changes in the structure of household and kinship roles and relationships. There will be an increasing number of "blended families," reflecting multiple lines of descent through multiple marriages and the birth of children outside of wedlock through other partners. This growth in the incidence of step- and half-relatives will make for a dramatic new turn in family structure in the coming decades. Already, such blended families constitute about half of all households with children (National Academy on Aging, 1994).

One possible implication of these changes is that kinship networks in the near future will become more complex, attenuated, and diffuse (Bengtson, Rosenthal, & Burton, 1990), perhaps with a weakened sense of filial obligation. If changes in the intensity of kinship relations significantly erode the capacity and sense of obligation to care for older family members when the Baby Boom cohort is in the ranks of old age and disability, demands for governmental support to pay long-term care may increase accordingly.

The Role of Private Insurance

Private insurance policies that cover long-term care—a relatively new product—are very expensive for the majority of older persons. A typical good-quality policy will provide benefits of $100 a day for nursing home care and $50 a day for home health care or adult day health care (at a program outside the home). The benefits are limited, however, with respect to when they first become available and how long they will be paid. From the time that eligibility for benefits is determined there is usually a 90-day "waiting period" before benefits are paid; in effect, this is a deductible amounting to $9,000 for nursing home care and $4,500 for home and adult day health care. There is also the problem of price inflation. Policies do offer inflation protection for an additional premium, but this additional coverage may not be enough to cover the full rate of inflation in long-term care costs over time.

Only about 4–5% of older persons have any private long-term care insurance, and only about 1% of nursing home costs are paid by private insurance (Wiener, Illston, & Hanley, 1994). A number of analyses have suggested that even when the product becomes more refined, no more than 20% of older Americans will be able to afford it (Crown, Capitman, & Leutz, 1992; Friedland, 1990; Rivlin & Wiener, 1988; Wiener, Illston, & Hanley, 1994).

The Role of Government

About 57% of long-term care expenditures is financed by federal, state, and local government, and the bulk of this portion is paid for by Medicaid, the federal-state program for the poor. Nationwide, the federal government finances about half of Medicaid and state governments finance the rest. Medicaid paid $22.5 billion for nursing home and home care services in 1995, which was 37.9% of all expenditures for long-term care (Levit et al., 1996). Medicaid finances the care—at least in part—of about three-fifths of nursing home patients and 28% of home and community-based services (American Association of Retired Person, 1994). Eligibility for Medicaid subsidy is determined by income and asset tests administered by state governments. Although many patients are poor enough to qualify for Medicaid when they enter a nursing home, a substantial number become poor after they are institutionalized (Adams, Meiners, & Burwell, 1993). Persons in this latter group deplete their assets in order to meet their long-term care bills, eventually "spending down" and becoming sufficiently poor to qualify for Medicaid.

Medicare also pays for some nursing home and home care. The services covered are for postacute or "subacute" care and not a broader range of nonmedical long-term care services that is often needed by a functionally disabled older person. Following a hospitalization of a few days or longer, Medicare pays for up to 100 days of care in a skilled nursing facility as long as the care includes skilled nursing and/or rehabilitation on a daily basis. After the first 20 days, however, the patient is required to pay up to $95 a day. In 1995 Medicare paid $7.3 billion for nursing home care, which was 10% of all payments to nursing homes (Levit et al., 1996). In addition, Medicare reimburses fully for part-time or intermittent home care therapy or skilled health care if a physician continues to authorize the need for such care. In the early 1990s the interpretation of "part-time" and "intermittent" became more lenient than previously, and the program's expenditures for home care grew substantially. Consequently, the program's outlays for home care increased by 176% from 1991 to 1995, from $4.2 billion to $11.6 billion. Medicare reimbursements in 1995 accounted for 44% of all home care payments (Levit et al., 1996).

Contemporary increases in public long-term care spending have already engendered efforts to contain costs. In 1995 Congress initially proposed to cap the rate of growth in Medicaid expenditures in order to achieve projected savings of $182 billion by 2002, and then put forward versions that involved a smaller amount of savings. These proposals were vetoed by President Clinton. They resurfaced in 1996 with proposed reductions of $72 billion, but no legislation was enacted that year. After his reelection in 1996, however, President Clinton proposed containing the growth of federal Medicaid expenditures at an annual level equivalent to the nation's increase in per capita economic output for each year (Pear, 1997b). This approach remains on the policy agenda, although governors oppose it because of the pressure it would place on state Medicaid budgets.

If federal expenditures on Medicaid are capped, many states are unlikely to use their own funds to make up any gaps between the federal funds they would have received and the amounts they actually get. According to one analysis (Kassner, 1995), the 1995 Congressional proposals for limiting Medicaid's growth would have trimmed long-term care funding by as much as 11.4% by 2000, which meant that 1.74 million Medicaid beneficiaries would have lost or been unable to secure coverage. In addition, this analysis assumed that states would make their initial reductions in home and community-based care services (because nursing home residents have nowhere else to go), and concluded that such services would be substantially reduced from their current levels. Five states were projected to completely eliminate home and community-based services by the end of the century and another 19 to cut services by more than half. Whether such specific predictions might come true if Medicaid is capped, ongoing federal and state efforts to control Medicaid costs are highly likely to have adverse consequences for the quality of Medicaid-financed care and access to it (see, Cohen & Spector, 1996; Holahan et al., 1995; Liebig, 1997; Wiener, 1996).

Federal measures to limit Medicare funding of home care have already been undertaken. The Balanced Budget Act of 1997 required that prospective payment reimbursement for the program's home health care be implemented by 1998 with rates set on the basis of the case-mix service requirements for individual service recipients. An additional reform likely to be adopted in the near future is to change the current policy, under which Medicare home health care is fully reimbursed, by establishing co-payments and deductibles. This would not only reduce the amount of reimbursement per payment, but might also discourage patients from using the program's home health care benefits as much as they do now.

Overall Outlook

In summary, the challenges of financing long-term care in the next century appear to be severe. Out-of-pocket payments for care are becoming larger and increasingly unaffordable for many. Neither the projected income and asset status of members of the Baby Boom cohort nor the dynamics of the market (at this time) indicate that these trends will abate. Broad societal trends suggest that informal, unpaid care by family members may become less feasible in the future than it is today. Only a minority of older persons may be able to afford premiums for private long-term care insurance. It is possible that low-tech and high-tech innovations in the provision of care could reduce costs while maintaining or enhancing the quality of care (see Binstock & Spector, 1997; Cluff, 1996), but little effort has been invested to date in the development of such innovations.

When members of the Baby Boom reach the ranks of old age in the decades ahead many of them and their families may look to government to subsidize their long-term care. Yet, even the safety net that government programs now provide by financing long-term care for the poor is seriously threatened by contemporary federal and state budgetary politics. The political context is such that public resources for long-term care are likely to be even less available—in relation to the need for care—than they have been to date.

Perhaps the entrance of the Baby Boom into the ranks of old age may precipitate a grassroots movement that will revitalize political awareness of the problems of long-term care financing as a major issue in American society. Such a movement might well be joined by millions of younger disabled persons and their advocates, although the constituencies of the elderly and the disabled have a checkered history of working effectively as allies because of differing philosophical and political concerns (Binstock, 1992a).

The prospects of success for such a grassroots movement will probably depend on effective promulgation of the notion that long-term care is an essential part of *health care* (a notion that traditionally has been anathema to the younger disabled constituency). This would make it possible for long-term care to receive adequate attention in more general policy debates about the future of American health care.

Policy Reforms and the Politics of Aging

Assuming that adequate economic resources will be available, will the politics of the early twenty-first century be such as to enable resources to be transferred substantially to older people at a level consistent with today's policies?

For several decades it has been an axiom among many journalists and political commentators that older people are an exceptionally strong force in American politics and, therefore are able to promote and defend their self-interests successfully. Accordingly they believe that it will virtually impossible to implement major reforms in Social Security, Medicare, and other policies on aging in accordance with some of the options outlined above. Economist Lester Thurow expressed what is perhaps the strongest statement of this view, to date:

> No one knows how the growth of entitlements for the elderly can be held in check in democratic societies. . . . Will democratic governments be able to cut benefits when the elderly are approaching a voting majority? Universal suffrage . . . is going to meet the ultimate test in the elderly. If democratic governments cannot cut benefits that go to a majority of their voters, then they have no long-term future. . . . In the years ahead, class warfare is apt to be redefined as the young against the old, rather than the poor against the rich. (Thurow, 1996, p. 47)

Central to this viewpoint is a so-called "senior power" model of politics, which assumes that the political behavior of older people is dominated by their self-interests, and that they all perceive their interests to be the same. Applying this model, one expects older people to be homogeneous in political attitudes and voting behavior, and, through sheer numbers, to be a powerful, perhaps dominating force.

The "senior power" model, however, is neither empirically valid nor conceptually sound. Consider Sweden, for example, which presently has the highest proportion of people aged 65 and older, about 18%. During the past two decades there have been substantial cutbacks in Sweden's benefits to the aging as part of a general retrenchment of that nation's welfare state (Sundstrom, 1995).

Political Attitudes and Voting Behavior

Numerous studies, involving many different birth cohorts, have established that the attribute of old age has little impact on political attitudes and behavior (Binstock & Day, 1996). Attitudinal differences *between* age groups are far less impressive than those *within* age groups. Numerous polls have shown that older people are nearly indistinguishable from younger adults [both the middle-aged and younger categories] on most issues—including aging policy issues. In fact, socioeconomic characteristics and partisan attachments are the best predictors of political attitudes among adults of all ages.

Although older persons vote at much higher rates than younger age groups, they do not vote as a monolithic bloc, any more than middle-aged persons or younger persons do. The aged are not a single-issue voting constituency. Older people distribute their votes among candidates in about the same proportions as do younger age groupings of citizens (see Binstock, 1992b, 1997a).

That the attitudes and votes of older persons distribute in the same fashion as those of younger persons should not be surprising. There is no sound theoretical reason to expect that a cohort—constituted of all religions, ethnic groups, economic and social statuses, political attitudes, and every other characteristic in society—would suddenly become homogenized in its political behavior when it reaches the "old age" category. Moreover, as Nobel Laureate Herbert Simon (1985) has pointed out, the very assumption that mass groupings of citizens, such as elderly people, vote primarily on the basis of self-interested responses to a single issue or cluster of issues is, in itself, problematic. Even to the extent that policy issues might have an impact within *heterogeneous* groups such as older persons, self-interested responses to any single issue are likely to vary substantially.

Old-Age-Based Interest Groups

The "senior power" model also assumes that old-age-based political organizations, interest groups, and splinter political parties that purport to represent the interests of all older people are powerful in affecting old-age policy, and will become more so in the future. Here again, the evidence suggests otherwise.

The major old-age programs in the United States have been enacted over the years through the initiatives of political elites, not interest groups (Binstock & Day, 1996). And important retrenchments and reforms in old-age policies have been accomplished despite the opposition of old-age groups. To be sure, policymakers prefer to have the assent of these organizations when such changes are under way. But the old-age interests have not proved to be a formidable obstacle when they oppose such reforms.

We have experienced more than a decade of policy reforms in old-age programs that many of the several dozen old-age interest groups have viewed with disfavor (Binstock, 1994). Most notable of these groups is the American Association of Retired Persons (AARP). It has 33 million members, an annual budget approaching $500 million, 1,700 employees, 4,000 local chapters, and extensive contacts with the White House and Congress (Binstock, 1997b). The press describes AARP as the 800-pound guerrilla of American politics that can get anything it wants.

Yet AARP has rarely tried to cohere the votes of its members and has failed to do so when it has tried. It has experienced strong protests and even resignations from within its heterogeneous membership whenever it has taken a reasonably specific position on policy issues, and it is very moderate in its political tactics: no massive rallies or protests and no significant mass media campaigns. In fact, AARP maintains its 33 million membership and large revenues through the material and associational incentives that it provides to its members, rather than through political incentives. The political activities of AARP are essentially marketing strategies, and do not include controversial and militant tactics that threaten to jeopardize the stability of the organization's membership size and financial resources (see Binstock, 1997b; Binstock & Day, 1996; Day, 1995).

The Future of Old Age Political Cohesion?

In summary, regarding the politics of aging, there is no evidence to date that "senior power" will, as Thurow and others suggest, imperil the future of democracy. Yet, things could change.

Some social scientists (e.g., Cutler, 1977) have argued for several decades that by the twenty-first century an age-group consciousness would develop among older people, to the extent that they would behave in a cohesive political fashion to dominate our political systems and establish gerontocracies. Perhaps this could happen. Perhaps the class warfare among young and old that Thurow envisions could emerge.

Suppose, for example, that propositions for official old-age-based health care rationing become more prominent and reach the policy agenda as the Baby Boom approaches old age. If so, age-group consciousness might very well develop among older people, and they may act in a cohesive political fashion in attempts to counter such proposals. Other radical propositions regarding Social Security and Medicaid could have the same effect.

Age-group consciousness and political cohesiveness, and age-group conflict, could well emerge in the twenty-first century. If our economy is not productive in the aging society, we may find ourselves contemplating the destruction of the fragile moral and ethical principles regarding the sanctity and dignity of human life, which our cultures have developed laboriously over many centuries. Consider what might happen, for instance, if Callahan's proposal that denying life-saving care categorically on the basis of an old-age threshold became a public policy. We could experience the ascendence of a *new* morality, in which older people are set aside (categorically) as unworthy of the humanistic protection and support that we have tried to make available to all of our citizens. And this, in turn, could lead us down the clichéd "slippery slope" in which various other categories of citizens— grouped, perhaps, by race, ethnicity, religion, and disabling conditions and diseases—are also deemed unworthy of life-saving care.

The preeminent challenge for our nation regarding public policies on aging in the twenty-first century will be to maintain, actively, a range of moral perspectives with which we can frame our public policy issues and discussions. *This would not mean* being overly preoccupied by issues framed in terms of intergenerational equity—conflict between heterogeneous cohorts of young versus old, to the exclusion of other important frameworks. *It would mean* the maintenance of frameworks of equity that generate, for example, issues of rich versus poor, or the conditions of some racial and ethnic groups versus others, among people of all ages.

Acknowledgment

Portions of this chapter have been adapted from R. H. Binstock (1998). Public policies on aging in the 21st century. *Stanford Law and Policy Review*, 9(2), 311–28.

Notes

1. The term "Old Age Welfare State" was coined by J.F. Myles. (1983). Conflict, crisis, and the future of old age security. *Milbank Memorial Fund Quarterly/Health and Society, 61,* 462–472.
2. This percentage is calculated by the author on the basis of federal outlays, by category, estimated for fiscal year 1997 [Congressional Budget Office. (1997). *The economic and budget outlook: An update.* Washington, DC: U.S. Government Printing Office] as modified by more detailed information from *Health Care Financing Review, Medicare and Medicaid Statistical Supplement, 1996,* and U.S. Social Security Administration, *Social Security Bulletin, Annual Statistical Supplement, 1996.*
3. The term "apocalyptic demography" was coined by A. Robertson. (1991). The politics of Alzheimer's disease: A case study in apocalyptic demography. In M. Minkler & C.L. Estes (Eds.), *Critical perspectives on aging; The political and moral economy of growing old* (pp. 135–150). Amityville, NY: Baywood Publishing Co.

REVIEW QUESTIONS

1. How has the political context of policies on aging changed over the years?

2. What are the problems projected for Social Security's Old Age and Survivors Insurance (OASI) program and its beneficiaries when the Baby

Boom birth cohort reaches old age? What policy reforms might help maintain the OASI program? What impact might they have on program participants?

3. What are the contemporary public policy strategies for containing government expenditures for the Medicare program?

4. What are the problems projected for the Medicare program when the Baby Boom birth cohort reaches old age? What policy reforms might help reduce these problems?

5. How is long-term care presently financed? What problems are associated with the various financing mechanisms?

6. What are longer-term problems of financing long-term care?

7. What are the key elements of what is known about the political behavior of older people and old age-based interest groups? How might these elements affect efforts to reform policies on aging? What circumstances might change these elements of political behavior in the future?

References

1994–1996 Advisory Council on Social Security (1997). *Report of the 1994–1996 Advisory Council on Social Security, Volume I: Findings and recommendations.* Washington, DC: U.S. Government Printing Office.

Adams, E. K., Meiners, M. R., & Burwell, B. O. (1993). Asset spend-down in nursing homes: Methods and insights. *Medical Care, 31,* 1–23.

Advisory Commission to Study the Consumer Price Index. (1996). *Toward a more accurate measure of the cost of living.* Final report to the Senate Finance Committee. Washington, DC: U.S. Government Printing Office.

American Association of Retired Persons, Public Policy Institute (1994). *The costs of long-term care.* Washington, DC: American Association of Retired Persons.

Arnett, R. H., III, McKusick, D. R., Sonnefeld, S. T., & Cowell, C. S. (1986). Projections of health care spending to 1990. *Health Care Financing Review, 7*(3), 1–36.

Baugher, E., & Lamison-White, L. (1996). *Poverty in the United States: 1995.* U.S. Bureau of the Census, Current Population Reports, Consumer Income, P60–194. Washington, DC: U.S. Government Printing Office.

Bell, D. (1964). Twelve Modes of prediction—a preliminary sorting of approaches in the social sciences. *Daedalus, 93,* 845–880.

Bengtson, V. L., Rosenthal, C., & Burton, L. (1990). Families and aging: Diversity and heterogeneity. In R. H. Binstock & L. K. George (Eds.), *Handbook of aging and the social sciences* (3rd ed., pp. 263–287). San Diego, CA: Academic Press.

Binstock, R. H. (1992a). Aging, disability, and long-term care: The politics of common ground. *Generations, 16*(2), 83–88.

Binstock, R. H. (1992b). Older voters and the 1992 presidential election. *Gerontologist, 32,* 601–606.

Binstock, R. H. (1993). Health care costs around the world: Is aging a fiscal "black hole"? *Generations, 18*(4), 37–42.

Binstock, R. H. (1994). Changing criteria in old-age programs: The introduction of economic status and need for services. *Gerontologist, 34,* 726–730.

Binstock, R. H. (1997a). The 1996 election: Older voters and implications for policies on aging. *Gerontologist, 37,* 15–19.

Binstock, R. H. (1997b). The old-age-lobby in a new political era. In R. B. Hudson (Ed.), *The future of age-based policy* (pp. 57–74). Baltimore, MD: Johns Hopkins University Press.

Binstock, R. H., & Day, C. L. (1996). Aging and politics. In R. H. Binstock & L. K. George (Eds.), *Handbook of aging and the social sciences* (4th ed., pp. 362–387). San Diego, CA: Academic Press.

Binstock, R. H., & Post, S. G. (Eds). (1991). *Too old for health care?: Controversies in medicine, law, economics, and ethics.* Baltimore, MD: Johns Hopkins University Press.

Binstock, R. H., & Spector, W. D. (1997). Five priority areas for research on long-term care. *Health Services Research, 33,* 715–730.

Bipartisan Commission on Entitlement and Tax Reform. (1994). *Commission findings.* Washington, DC: U.S. Government Printing Office.

Bipartisan Commission on Entitlement and Tax Reform. (1995). *Final report.* Washington, DC: U.S. Government Printing Office.

Board of Trustees of the Federal Old-Age and Survivors Insurance and Disability Insurance Trust Funds. (1996). *1996 annual report.* Washington, DC: U.S. Government Printing Office.

Board of Trustees of the Federal Old-Age and Survivors Insurance and Disability Insurance Trust Funds. (1997). *1997 annual report.* Washington, DC: U.S. Government Printing Office.

Brody, E. M. (1990) *Women in the middle: Their parent care years.* New York: Springer.

Callahan, D. (1987). *Setting limits: Medical goals in an aging society.* New York: Simon & Schuster.

Carballo, M. (1981). Extra votes for parents?, *Boston Globe,* December 17, 35.

Cassel, C. K., Rudberg, M. A., & Olshansky, S. J. (1992). The price of success: Health care in an aging society. *Health Affairs, 11*(2), 87–99.

Chen, Y.-P. (1994). "Equivalent retirement ages" and their implications for Social Security and Medicare financing. *Gerontologist, 34,* 731–735.

Clark, R. L. (1990). Income maintenance policies in the United States. In R. H. Binstock & L. K. George (Eds.), *Handbook of aging and the social sciences* (3rd ed., pp. 382–397). San Diego, CA: Academic Press.

Cluff, L. E. (1996). The role of technology in long-term care. In R. H. Binstock, L.E. Cluff, & O. von Mering (Eds.), *The future of long-term care: Social and policy issues* (pp. 96–118). Baltimore, MD: Johns Hopkins University Press.

Cohen, J. W., & Spector, W. D. (1996). The effect of Medicaid reimbursement on quality of care in nursing homes. *Journal of Health Economics, 15,* 32–48.

Concord Coalition. (1993). *The zero deficit plan: A plan for eliminating the federal budget deficit by the year 2000.* Washington, DC: The Concord Coalition.

Congressional Budget Office. (1991). *Policy choices for long-term care.* Washington, DC: U.S. Government Printing Office.

Congressional Budget Office. (1993). *The economic and budget outlook: An update.* Washington, DC: U.S. Government Printing Office.

Congressional Budget Office. (1997a). *Long-term budgetary pressures and policy options.* Washington, DC: U.S. Government Printing Office.

Congressional Budget Office. (1997b). *The economic and budget outlook: Fiscal years 1998–2007.* Washington, DC: U.S. Government Printing Office.

Congressional Budget Office. (1997c). *Reducing the deficit: Spending and revenue options.* Washington, DC: U.S. Government Printing Office.

Cook, F. L., Marshall, V. M., Marshall, J. E., & Kaufman, J. E. (1994). The salience of intergenerational equity in Canada and the United States. In T. R. Marmor, T. M. Smeeding, & V. L. Greene (Eds.), *Economic security and intergenerational justice: A Look at North America.* (pp. 91–129). Washington, DC: Urban Institute Press.

Crown, W. H., Capitman, J., & Leutz, W. N. (1992). Economic rationality, the affordability of private long-term care insurance, and the role for public policy. *Gerontologist, 32,* 478–485.

Crystal, S. (1996). Economic status of the elderly. In R. H. Binstock & L. K. George (Eds.), *Handbook of aging and the social sciences* (4th ed., pp. 388–409). San Diego, CA: Academic Press.

Cutler, N. E. (1977). Demographic, social-psychological, and political factors in the politics of aging: A foundation for research in "political gerontology." *American Political Science Review, 71,* 1011–1025.

Day, C. L., (1995). *Old-age interest groups in the 1990s: Coalition, competition, and strategy.* Paper presented at the annual meeting of the American Political Science Association, Chicago, IL, September 2.

Edelman, P., & Hughes, S. (1990). The impact of community care on provision of informal care to homebound elderly persons. *Journal of Gerontology: Social Sciences, 45,* S874–S884.

Estes, C. L. (1983). Social Security: The social construction of a crisis. *Milbank Memorial Fund Quarterly/Health and Society, 61,* 445–461.

Fairlie, H. (1988). Talkin' 'bout my generation. *New Republic, 198,* 19–22.

Ferrara, P. J. (1985). Social Security and the super IRA: A populist proposal. In P. Ferrara (Ed.), *Social Security: Prospects for real reform* (pp. 193–220). Washington, DC: Cato Institute.

Friedland, R. (1990). *Facing the costs of long-term care: An EBRI-ERF policy study.* Washington, DC: Employee Benefits Research Institute.

Getzen, T. (1992). Population aging and the growth of health expenditures. *Journal of Gerontology, 4,* S98–S104.

Gibbs, N. R. (1980). Grays on the go. *Time, 131*(8), 66–75.

Hanley, R. J., Alecxih, L. M. B., Wiener, J. M., & Kennel, D. L. (1990). Predicting elderly nursing home admissions: Results from the 1982 National Long-Term Care Survey. *Research on Aging, 12,* 199–228.

Hanley, R. J., Wiener, J. M., & Harris, K. M. (1994). *The economic status of nursing home users.* Washington, DC: The Brookings Institution.

Hobbs, F. B. (1996). *65+ in the United States.* U.S. Bureau of the Census, Current Population Reports, Special Studies, P23–190. Washington, DC: U.S. Government Printing Office.

Holahan, J., Coughlin, T., Liu, K., Ku, L., Kuntz, C., Wade, M., & Wall, S. (1995). *Cutting Medicaid spending in response to budget caps.* Washington, DC: Kaiser Commission on the Future of Medicaid.

Hudson, R. B. (1978). The "graying" of the federal budget and its consequences for old age policy. *Gerontologist, 18,* 428–440.

Hudson, R. B., and Binstock, R. H. (1976). Political systems and aging, in R. H. Binstock and E. Shanas, eds., *Handbook of aging and the social sciences,* 369–400. New York: Van Nostrand Reinhold.

Kalish, R. A. (1979). The new ageism and the failure models: A polemic. *Gerontologist, 19,* 398–407.

Kane, R. L., & Kane, R. A. (1994). Effects of the Clinton health reform on older persons and their families: A health care systems perspective. *Gerontologist, 34,* 598–605.

Kassner, E. (1995). *Long-term care: Measuring the impact of a Medicaid cap.* Washington, DC: American Association of Retired Persons.

Kingson, E. R., & Schulz, J. H. (Eds). (1996). *Social Security in the 21st century.* New York: Oxford University Press.

Kutza, E. (1981). *The benefits of old age.* Chicago: University of Chicago Press.

Levit, K. R., Lazenby, H. C., Braden, B. R., Cowan, C. A., McDonnell, P. A., Sivarajan, L., Stiller, J. M., Won, D. K., Donham, C. S., Long, A. M., & Stewart, M. W. (1996). National health expenditures, 1995. *Health Care Financing Review, 18*(1), 175–214.

Liebig, P. S. (1997). Policy and political contexts of financing long-term care. In K. H. Wilber, E. L. Schneider, & D. Polisar (Eds.), *A secure old age: Approaches to long-term care financing* (pp. 147–177). New York: Springer.

Light, P. C. (1985). *Artful work: The politics of Social Security reform.* New York: Random House.

Liu, K., Manton, K. M., & Liu, B. M. (1985). Home care expenses for the disabled elderly. *Health Care Financing Review, 7*(2), 51–58.

Longman, P. (1987). *Born to pay: The new politics of aging in America.* Boston, MA: Houghton Mifflin.

Manton, K. G., Corder, L. S., & Stallard, E. (1993). Estimates of change in chronic disability and institutional incidence and prevalence rates in the U.S. elderly population from the 1982–1984, and 1989 National Long-Term Care Survey. *Journal of Gerontology: Social Sciences, 48,* S153–S166.

Manton, K. G., Corder, L. S., & Stallard, E. (1997). Chronic disability in elderly United States populations: 1982–1994, *Proceedings of the National Academy of Sciences USA, 94,* 2593–2598.

Mechanic, D. (1994). Managed care: Rhetoric and realities. *Inquiry, 31,* 124–128.

Mendelsohn, D. B., & Schwartz, W. B. (1993). The effects of aging and population growth on health care costs. *Health Affairs, 12*(1), 119–125.

National Academy on Aging. (1994). *Old age in the 21st century.* Washington, DC: Syracuse University.

National Academy on Aging. (1997). Social Security: The Old Age and Survivors Trust Fund, 1997. *Gerontology News,* June, unpaginated insert.

Nelson, L., Brown, R., Gold, M., Ciemnecki, A., & Docteur, E. (1997). Access to care in Medicare HMOs, 1996. *Health Affairs, 16*(2), 148–156.

Neugarten, B. L. (1970). The old and the young in modern societies. *American Behavioral Scientist, 14,* 13–24.

Palmore, E. B. (1990). *Ageism: Negative and positive.* New York: Springer.

Pear, R. (1997a). House panel votes changes to try to keep Medicare solvent. *New York Times,* June 10, A19.

Pear, R. (1997b). Medicare cuts would trim at-home care for patients. *New York Times*, February 9, 16.

Peterson, P. (1987). The morning after. *Atlantic, 260*(4), 43–49.

Pfaff, M. (1990). Differences in health care spending across countries: Statistical evidence. *Journal of Health Politics, Policy, and Law, 15*, 1–67.

Preston, S. H. (1984). Children and the elderly in the U.S. *Scientific American, 251*(6), 44–49.

Public Law No. 105-33. (1997). The Balanced Budget Act of 1997.

Quadagno, J. (1989). Generational equity and the politics of the welfare state. *Politics and Society, 17*, 353–376.

Quinn, J. (1987). The economic status of the elderly: Beware the mean. *Review of Income and Wealth, 33*(1), 63–82.

Rivlin, A. M., & Wiener, J. M. (1988). *Caring for the disabled elderly: Who will pay?* Washington, DC: The Brookings Institution.

Robert, S. A., & House, J. S. (1994). Socioeconomic status and health over the life course. In R. A. Abeles, H. C. Gift, & M. G. Ory (Eds.), *Aging and the quality of life* (pp. 253–274). New York: Springer.

Rosenzweig, R. M. (1990). *Address to the president's opening session.* 43rd Annual Meeting of the Gerontological Society of America, Boston, MA, November 16.

Salholz, E. (1990). Blaming the voters: Hapless budgeteers single out "greedy geezers." *Newsweek*, October 29, 36.

Samuelson, R. J. (1978). Aging America: Who will shoulder the growing burden? *National Journal, 10*, 1712–1717.

Schieber, S. J. (1997). A new vision for Social Security: Personal security accounts as an element of Social Security reform. In R. B. Hudson (Ed.), *The future of age-based public policy* (pp. 134–143). Baltimore, MD: Johns Hopkins University Press.

Schneider, E. L., & Guralnik, J. M. (1990). The aging of America: Impact on health care costs. *Journal of the American Medical Association, 263*, 2335–2340.

Shaugnessy, P. W., Schlenker, R. E., & Hittle, D. F. (1994). Home health care outcomes under capitated and fee-for-service payment. *Health Care Financing Review, 16*(1), 187–222.

Simon, H. A. (1985). Human nature in politics: The dialogue of psychology with political science. *American Political Science Review, 79*, 293–304.

Smith, L. (1992). The tyranny of America's old. *Fortune, 125*(1), 68–72.

Sonnefeld, S. T., Waldo, D. R., Lemieux, J. A., & McKusick, D. R. (1991). Projections of national health expenditures through the year 2000. *Health Care Financing Review, 13*(1), 1–27.

Steurle, C. E., & Bakija, J. M. (1997). Retooling Social Security for the 21st century. *Social Security Bulletin, 60*, 37–60.

Stone, R., Cafferata, G. L., & Sangl, J. (1987). Caregivers of the frail elderly: A national profile. *Gerontologist, 27*, 616–626.

Sundstrom, G. (1995). Ageing is riskier than it looks. *Age and Ageing, 24*, 373–374.

Tennstedt, S. L., Crawford, S. L., & McKinlay, J. B. (1993). Is family care on the decline?: A longitudinal investigation of the substitution of formal long-term care services for informal care. *Milbank Quarterly, 71*, 601–624.

Thurow, L. C. (1996). The birth of a revolutionary class. *New York Times Magazine*, May 19, 46–47.

U.S. House of Representatives, Select Committee on Aging. (1977). *Federal responsibility to the elderly: Executive programs and legislative jurisdiction.* Washington, DC: U.S. Government Printing Office.

Ware, J. E., Bayliss, M. S., Rogers, W. H., Kosinski, M., & Tarlov, A. (1996). Differences in 4-year health outcomes for elderly and poor, chronically-ill patients treated in HMO and fee-for-service systems: Results from the medical outcomes study. *Journal of the American Medical Association, 276,* 1039–1047.

Wattenberg, B. J. (1987). *The birth dearth.* New York: Pharos Books.

Weissert, W. G. (1990). Strategies for reducing home care expenditures. *Generations, 14*(2), 42–44.

Wiener, J. M. (1996). Can Medicaid long-term care expenditures for the elderly be reduced? *Gerontologist, 36,* 800–818.

Wiener, J. M., & Illston, L. H. (1996). Health care financing and organization for the elderly. In R. H. Binstock & L. K. George (Eds.), *Handbook of aging and the social sciences* (4th ed., pp. 427–445). San Diego, CA: Academic Press.

Wiener, J. M., Illston, L. H., & Hanley, R. J. (1994). *Sharing the burden: Strategies for public and private long-term care insurance.* Washington, DC: The Brookings Institution.

Wiener, J. M., & Skaggs, S. (1995). *Current approaches to integrating acute and long-term care financing and services.* Washington, DC: Public Policy Institute, American Association of Retired Persons.

Williamson, J. B. (1997). A critique of the case for privatizing Social Security. *Gerontologist, 37,* 561–571.

Additional Readings

Binstock, R. H., Cluff, L. E., & von Mering, O. (1996). *The future of long-term care: Social and policy issues.* Baltimore, MD: Johns Hopkins University Press.

Binstock, R. H., & George, L. K. (Eds.). (1996). *Handbook of aging and the social sciences* (4th ed.). San Diego, CA: Academic Press.

Hickey, T., Speers, M. A., & Prohaska, T. R. (1997). *Public health and aging.* Baltimore, MD: Johns Hopkins University Press.

Hudson, R. B. (Ed.). (1997). *The future of age-based policy.* Baltimore, MD: Johns Hopkins University Press.

Marmor, T. R., Smeeding, T. M., & Greene, V. L. (Eds.). (1994). *Economic security and intergenerational justice: A look at North America.* Washington, DC: The Urban Institute Press.

McManus, S. A. (1996). *Young v. old: Generational combat in the 21st century.* Boulder, CO: Westview Press.

Moon, M. (1996). *Medicare now and in the future.* Washington, DC: The Urban Institute Press.

Peterson, P. G. (1993). *Facing up: How to rescue the economy from crushing debt and restore the American dream.* New York: Simon & Schuster.

Pratt, H. J. (1993). *Gray agendas: Interest groups and public pensions in Canada, Britain, and the United States.* Ann Arbor, MI: University of Michigan Press.

Schulz, J. H. (1995). *The economics of aging* (6th ed.). Westport, CT: Auburn House.

Schulz, J.H., Borowski, A., & Crown, W.H. (1991). *Economics of population aging: The "graying" of Australia, Japan, and the United States.* New York: Auburn House.

Torres-Gil, F. M. (1992). *The new aging: Politics and change in America.* New York: Auburn House.

Wiener, J. M., Illston, L. H., & Hanley, R. J. (1994). *Sharing the burden: Strategies for public and private long-term care insurance.* Washington, DC: The Brookings Institution.

Index

AARP. *See* American Association of Retired Persons
Abercrombie, J., 216
absolute fit indexes, 54
accidents, 158; and alcohol use, 159–60
acetylcholine, and Alzheimer's disease, 309–10
Achenbaum, W. A., 224
activities of daily living (ADLs), 146, 278, 289, 393–95, 432
activity theory of aging, 23
acute physical symptomatology, and death anxiety, 168
AD. *See* Alzheimer's disease
Adams, C., 254
adaptive functioning, assessment of, 278–79
ADEA. *See* Age Discrimination in Employment Act
ADLs. *See* activities of daily living
Administration on Aging, 357
adulthood, 243, 248, 252; as cultural category, 70; Piaget's view of, 250
advance directive option for medical care, 174–77
Advisory Commission to Study the Consumer Price Index, 422
Advisory Council on Social Security, 425–26
aerobic capacity, and aging, 98–99
Affect Rating Scale, 407
AGE. *See* Americans for Generational Equity
age, 4–6; bias, 358–59; deficits, and cognitive aging, 188–91, 195, 199; discrimination, 358–59; and job performance, 362–69; norms, 20, 24; as variable in research, 38, 41–44

Age and Achievement (Lehman), 228
Age Discrimination in Employment Act (ADEA), 358–59, 361, 372
age-fair intelligence tests, 217
Age Game, 72
ageism, 280–81, 416
Agency for Health Care Policy and Research (AHCPR), 318
aging, 4–6; and culture, 65–86; and life expectancy, 75–76; and modernization, 83–84; and public policies, 415–20; as a skill, 186–87; theories of, 1–26; and value systems, 78–79; variable factors in, 38; and work, 357–69
Agitation Behavior Mapping Instrument, 288
agnosia, as characteristic of dementia, 309
Agreeableness (A), as general personality factor, 256–57
AGS. *See* American Geriatrics Society
AIDS, 3, 171
alcohol, 147; abuse of, 159–60, 320–21; and bone loss, 96; consumption of, and ethnicity, 70; and pseudodementia, 129; and suicide, 178; and undernutrition, 136
Allen, M. J., 271
Allen-Burge, R., 404
allergies, and antibodies, 125
Alzheimer's Association, 21
Alzheimer's disease, 4, 9, 25, 47, 129, 401; and central nervous system changes, 104; and cognitive decline, 214; and depression, 291; estrogen replacement therapy for, 130, 133; as prevalent dementia, 309, 432; and strokes, 134; and WAIS, 219

Hollis, L. A., 369
Holmes, Eleanor R., 81, 83
Holmes, Lowell D., 81, 83
holocultural research, 77–78
home health care, 164, 393–94
Hopemont Capacity Assessment
 Interview, 278
Hopemont questionnaire, 402
hormonal: changes, and benign prostatic
 hyperplasia, 139; deficiencies, and
 cognitive impairment, 147; diseases,
 and hypertension, 133
hormone replacement therapies (HRT),
 132–33, 147
Horn, John, 220
Horowitz, M., 318
hospice care, 170–74
Hospital Insurance (HI) program, 420,
 426
hostility, and trait theorists, 255
Hoyer, W., 198–99
human leukocyte-associated (HLA)
 proteins, 125
humoral immune response, 10, 125
Huntington's disease, 11
hypersecretion, 138
hypersomnia, as symptom of depression,
 310
hypertension, 133–34, 140, 145, 283, 393
hyperthermia, 106
hyperthyroidism, 123, 131, 291
hypochondriasis, as cause of anxiety, 319
hypokalemia, 140
hyponatremia, 140
hypothalmus, 7, 131
hypothyroidism, 123, 131, 274

IADLs. *See* instrumental activities of
 daily living
identification: as consideration in SEM,
 54; Freud's notion of, 244
identity: development, 16–17, 240; as
 psychosocial quality, 44; sense of, and
 aging, 91–93
identity theory of aging, 22
Ikels, C., 70, 79
Imipramine, and depression, 317
immigrant families, and change, 239–40
immune function, 7, 127–28

immunity and disease processes, and
 optimal aging, 123–47
immunoglobulins, 125
immunosenescence, 126–27
immunosuppression, 128
impotence, 104, 140
"incapacitated person," definition of, 396
incapacity, criteria for, 392
incontinence. See fecal incontinence;
 urinary incontinence
incremental fit indexes, 54
independence: and development, 240; as
 goal in aging, 78–79
independent variable, 35, 46
indirect effect, in SEM, 53–54
Individual Accounts plan, for improving
 OASI, 425–26
individualism, vs. relatedness, 240–41
individual psychology, and
 modernization theory, 83
individuals, and culture, 70–75
individuation, 243, 246
indolamines, and depression, 314
industrial gerontology, 357
industrialization, and aging, 20
infant mortality rates, and life
 expectancy, 76
infections, and cognitive impairment, 146
inflation adjustments, reduction in,
 422–23
influenza, 138, 158
Informal Caregivers Survey, 332–33, 347
information-loss model, 14
information-processing model of
 cognition, 13
informed consent, 60–61, 400
Ingeneri, D. G., 80
in-group bias hypothesis, 360
inhibition deficit hypothesis, 192
insomnia, 283, 310
Institutional Review Boards, 60–61
institutional settings, and choices of
 older adults, 391–407
instrumental activities of daily living
 (IADLs), 146, 278, 393, 394–95
Instrumental Activities of Daily Living
 (IADL) Scale, 282
insulin, 131–32
integumentary system, diseases of, 143–44

LaVergne, TN USA
16 August 2010
193387LV00001B/2/A